Seminars in General Adult Psychiatry

Volume 1

College Seminars Series

Series Editors

Professor Hugh Freeman, Honorary Professor, University of Salford, and Honorary Consultant Psychiatrist, Salford Health Authority

Dr Ian Pullen, Consultant Psychiatrist, Dingleton Hospital, Melrose, Roxburghshire

Dr George Stein, Consultant Psychiatrist, Farnborough Hospital, and King's College Hospital

Professor Greg Wilkinson, Editor, *British Journal of Psychiatry*, and Professor of Liaison Psychiatry, University of Liverpool

Other books in the series

Seminars in Alcohol and Drug Misuse. Edited by Jonathan Chick & Roch Cantwell

Seminars in Basic Neurosciences. Edited by Gethin Morgan & Stuart Butler

Seminars in Child and Adolescent Psychiatry. Edited by Dora Black & David Cottrell

Seminars in Clinical Psychopharmacology. Edited by David King

Seminars in Liaison Psychiatry. Edited by Elspeth Guthrie & Francis Creed

Seminars in Practical Forensic Psychiatry. Edited by Derek Chiswick & Rosemarie Cope

Seminars in Psychiatric Genetics. By Peter McGuffin, Michael J. Owen, Michael C. O'Donovan, Anita Thapar & Irving Gottesman

Seminars in the Psychiatry of Learning Disabilities. Edited by Oliver Russell

Seminars in Psychology and the Social Sciences. Edited by Digby Tantam & Max Birchwood

Forthcoming titles

Seminars in Psychiatry for the Elderly. Edited by Brice Pitt & Mohsen Naguib

Seminars in Psychotherapy. Edited by Sandra Grant & Jane Naismith

Seminars in General Adult Psychiatry

Edited by
George Stein & Greg Wilkinson

with the assistance of
Rosalind Ramsay

Volume 1

GASKELL

British Library Cataloguing-in-Publication Data
A catalogue record for this book is available from the British Library.
ISBN 0 902241 91 5 (Boxed set of 2 volumes)
ISBN 1 901242 11 0 (Vol. 1)

Distributed in North America
by American Psychiatric Press, Inc.
ISBN 0 88048 577 9

Gaskell is an imprint of the Royal College of Psychiatrists,
17 Belgrave Square, London SW1X 8PG
The Royal College of Psychiatrists is a registered charity, number 228636

The views presented in this book do not necessarily reflect those of the Royal College of Psychiatrists, and the publishers are not responsible for any error of omission or fact. College Seminars are produced by the Publications Department of the College; they should in no way be construed as providing a syllabus or other material for any College examination.

Printed by Bell & Bain Ltd., Thornliebank, Glasgow

Contents

Contributors

Dr Morris Bernadt, Department of Psychological Medicine, Kings College Hospital, Denmark Hill, London SE5 9RS

Dr Jonathan Bird, Burden Neurological Hospital, Stoke Lane, Stapleton, Bristol, Avon BS16

Sharon Borrows, Sleep Centre, Papworth Hospital, Papworth Everard, Cambridge CB3 8RE

Dr Tom Brown, St John's Hospital at Howden, Howden Road West, Livingston, West Lothian EH54 6PP

Professor Patricia Casey, Department of Psychiatry, Mater Hospital, 62–63 Eccles Street, Dublin 7, Republic of Ireland

Dr John Cookson, The Royal London Hospital, 2A Bow Road, London E3 4LL

Dr Lynne M. Drummond, Department of Psychiatry, St George's Hospital Medical School, Cranmer Terrace, Tooting, London SW17 0RE

Dr Tom Fahy, The Maudsley Hospital, Denmark Hill, London SE5 8AZ

Professor Nicol Ferrier, Department of Psychiatry, School of Neurosciences, The Royal Victoria Infirmary, Queen Victoria Road, Newcastle upon Tyne, Tyne and Wear NE1 3LP

Dr Alistair G. Hay, Craig Dunain Hospital, Inverness IV3 6JU

Dr Frank Holloway, Maudsley Hospital, Denmark Hill, London SE5 8AZ

Dr Roger Howells, Maudsley Hospital, Denmark Hill, London SE5 8AZ

Dr Robin Jacobson, Department of Psychiatry, Jenner Wing, St George's Hospital Medical School, London SW17 0RE

Dr Michael Kopelman, Academic Unit of Psychiatry, United Medical and Dental Schools, St Thomas's Hospital, Lambeth Palace Road, London SE1 7EH

Dr Alan Lee, Department of Psychiatry, University Hospital, Queen's Medical Centre, Nottingham NG7 2UH

Dr Peter F. Liddle, Department of Psychiatry, University of British Colombia, 2255 Westbrook Mall, Vancouver, British Colombia V6T 2A1, Canada

Professor Clive Mellor, PO Box 399, Chilliwack, British Colombia V2P 6J7, Canada

Professor Harold Merskey, London Psychiatric Hospital, 850 Highbury Avenue, PO Box 2532, London, Ontario N6A 4H1, Canada

Dr Stirling Moorey, Hackney Hospital, Homerton High Street, London E9 6BE

Professor Gethin Morgan, Department of Mental Health, University of Bristol, 41 St Michael's Hill, Bristol, Avon BS2 8DZ

Dr John Owen, Cossham Hospital, Lodge Hill, Kingswood, Bristol, Avon BS15 1LF viii

Dr David Cunningham Owens, Royal Edinburgh Hospital, Kennedy Tower, Morningside Park, Edingurgh, Lothian EH10 5HF

Dr Jeremy Pfeffer, Department of Psychiatry, London Hospital, Whitechapel, London E1 1BB

Dr Rosalind Ramsay, St Thomas's Hospital, Lambeth Palace Road, London SE1 7EH

Dr Mary Robertson, Academic Department of Psychiatry, Wolfson Building, The Middlesex Hospital, London W1N 8AA

Professor Jan Scott, Department of Psychiatry, School of Neurosciences, The Royal Victoria Infirmary, Queen Victoria Road, Newcastle upon Tyne, Tyne and Wear NE1 3LP

Dr Philip Sedgwick, St George's Hospital Medical School, Cranmer Terrace, London SW17 0RE

Dr George Stein, Kings College Hospital, Farnborough Hospital, Farnborough Common, Orpington, Kent BR6 8ND

Dr Richard Stern, Springfield Hospital, 61 Glenburnie Road, London SW17 7DJ

Professor Michael Stone, Suite 114, 225 Central Park West, New York City, NY 10024, USA

Dr George Szmukler, The Maudsley Hospital, Denmark Hill, London SE5 8AZ

Dr Mark Tattersall, Huntercombe Manor Hospital, Huntercombe Lane South, Taplow, Berkshire SL6 0PQ

Dr Janet Treasure, Institute of Psychiatry, Denmark Hill, London SE5 8AF

Dr Christopher Vassilas, Department of Old Age Psychiatry, Wedgwood Unit, West Suffolk Hospital, Bury St Edmunds, Suffolk IP33 2QZ

Professor Greg Wilkinson, Academic Department of Psychiatry, Royal Liverpool University Hospital, Liverpool L69 3BX

Dr Peter Woodruff, Institute of Psychiatry, De Crespigny Park, London SE5 8AF

Foreword

Series Editors

The publication of *College Seminars*, a series of textbooks covering the breadth of psychiatry, is very much in line with the Royal College of Psychiatrists' established role in education and in setting professional standards.

College Seminars are intended to help junior doctors during their training years. We hope that trainees will find these books useful, on the ward as well as in preparation for the MRCPsych examination. Separate volumes will cover clinical psychiatry, each of its subspecialities, and also the relevant non-clinical academic disciplines of psychology and sociology.

College Seminars will make a contribution to the continuing professional development of established clinicians.

Psychiatry is concerned primarily with people, and to a lesser extent with disease processes and pathology. The core of the subject is rich in ideas and schools of thought, and no single approach or solution can embrace the variety of problems a psychiatrist meets. For this reason, we have endeavoured to adopt an eclectic approach to practical management throughout the series.

The College can draw on the collective wisdom of many individuals in clinical and academic psychiatry. More than a hundred people have contributed to this series; this reflects how diverse and complex psychiatry has become.

Frequent new editions of books appearing in the series are envisaged, which should allow *College Seminars* to be responsive to readers' suggestions and needs.

Hugh Freeman
Ian Pullen
George Stein
Greg Wilkinson

Preface

Psychiatry, according to Johann Christian Reil (1759–1813) the German anatomist who first coined the term, consists of the meeting of two minds, the mind of the patient with the mind of the doctor. As patients tell their story, it is the task of the doctor to recognise the tale, and to do so with some compassion. Pattern recognition lies at the heart of the diagnostic process; common trends in the rich tapestry of the patient's experiences are summarised in the many clinical syndromes and disorders of psychiatry. This book, intended for doctors in training beginning their career in psychiatry, places its greatest emphasis on detailed descriptions of the common psychiatric disorders. We hope such a clinical descriptive approach will help the doctor recognise patterns and so make a sound psychiatric diagnosis. Our intention is that this book will serve as a useful basis for trainees preparing for their Membership examinations, but in addition it should engage those who have passed that hurdle.

Diagnostic acumen separated from therapeutic skill is of little use to patients or their families. When Reil first introduced the word psychiatry, he meant it in a therapeutic sense, in that the psyche of the doctor would act as a healing agent on the mind of the patient. While the initial meetings between doctor and patient usually have a diagnostic purpose, later contacts involve treatment. Throughout the book we have tried to provide guidelines on the management of common disorders. Our approach to treatment has been eclectic, but at the same time we have tried to describe each of the many treatments now available in some depth. The more specialised psychotherapies, once shrouded in a mystique requiring years of specialised training, are now gradually being replaced by briefer, less intensive treatment more readily grasped by trainees. We have described these newer treatments in some detail (for example, with behaviour therapy for the treatment of phobias, or cognitive therapy for depression). Physical treatments are accorded equal weight and separate chapters describe the physical treatments of both depression and schizophrenia.

Our hopes for better understanding and new treatments lie in scientific research. Sometimes, the scientific advances of the previous decades have been spectacular, such as the introduction of new drugs to treat depression or schizophrenia; in other cases developments have been less dramatic but as important, such as the gradual realisation that much of the depression found in the community is socially determined. At one time, a medical advance was deemed to have occurred if a charismatic professor at an ancient university announced a new classification; if another professor, perhaps from a different school of psychiatry, disagreed, it was hailed as a medical controversy. Today, this is no longer possible and rigorous scientific evidence is required before any new information can be incorporated into the fabric of existing knowledge. This applies to both the biological and psychosocial dimensions of the spectrum of knowledge.

We have tried to balance the essential clinical descriptive information and its supporting scientific evidence, with some of the more interesting but still speculative recent findings, hopefully without overwhelming the reader with too many studies. In this lies a dilemma, because the needs of the beginner and those with experience can be at variance. The novice must assimilate the body of existing knowledge while the established clinician is more interested in the advancing front of knowledge, even if many of the new findings eventually prove ephemeral.

Our guiding principle in editing the book has been to remain close to clinical issues and to answer the two questions "What disorder is it?" and "How can we help?" The third and often the most tantalising question "Why is it" remains unanswered, at least for most conditions, and so we have tended to focus less on aetiological considerations.

An era is now passing when doctors bear sole responsibility for the treatment of patients under their care. Modern psychiatric treatment is a team effort and this change is to be welcomed, not least because it helps to ease the burden on the doctor. Medical authority no longer rests on a position in the hierarchy, but rather on greater knowledge and wider clinical experience. Increasingly patients, relatives, carers, managers and other members of the psychiatric team question the doctor's decisions and treatment, and as a consequence of these wider changes this book is rooted in an evidence base and comprehensively and extensively referenced.

The *College Seminars* series has separate volumes for each of the sub-specialities of psychiatry, and this structure has given the editors and contributors considerable freedom, permitting us to concentrate solely on general psychiatry. General psychiatry is now too vast a subject for a single person to be an expert in all its aspects and this inevitably means a comprehensive text must be multi-authored. We believe that many of the chapters are works of great scholarship by leading experts in their fields, and their length and detail bear witness to long hours of toil. For this the editors express their deepest gratitude. In other chapters the clinical acumen, diagnostic nuances and imaginative therapeutic strategies have an immediacy which brings the whole book to life, while offering the clinician new ways to help patients and their families. We hope our readers will derive both pleasure and wisdom from this book.

We would like to thank the American Psychiatric Association and the World Health Organization for permission to publish tables from DSM–IV and ICD–10. The editors are particularly grateful for the assistance of Dr Rosalind Ramsay throughout the preparation of this book, first for keeping the editors in touch with the needs of the readership, and second for critically scrutinising the text. Much of this book was edited in the library of the Maudsley Hospital, which houses a unique collection of psychiatric journals and books; we would like to thank the librarian, Mr Martin Guha, and his staff for their unfailing support. Numerous junior doctors from Farnborough Hospital, the London Hospital and the University of Liverpool have read earlier drafts of the chapters in this book and their comments have helped us greatly to sharpen the focus of the text. Special thanks are due to Penny Nicholson at Farnborough Hospital who typed and re-typed many of the manuscripts as well as coordinating the whole project, ably assisted in this task by Christine Scotcher. The technical and publishing expertise of Lesley Bennun, Dinah Alam and Andrew Morris at the College is also acknowledged with much gratitude.

George Stein
Greg Wilkinson

1 Clinical features of depressive disorders

Alan Lee

---

*Classic phenomenology ● Clinical features of depressive disorders ●
Diagnostic criteria ● Classification ● Measurement ● Course and
outcome ● Bereavement*

Classic phenomenology

Robert Burton published *The Anatomy of Melancholy* in 1621, and immediately it enjoyed great popularity. Samuel Johnson declared it to be the only book that ever raised him from his bed two hours sooner than he wished to rise. The writings of Milton, Byron and Lamb were all strongly influenced by it.

In his account of melancholy, Burton undertook to describe a state of mind that had been familiar to many before him, and must have found its resonances in the experiences of a large number of his readers. Here was a systematic account of the mental phenomena that had centuries before led the psalmist David to declare:

> "I am a worm and no man, a reproach of men and despised of the people...I am poured out like water and all my bones are out of joint: my heart is like wax; it is melted in the midst of my bowels. My strength is dried up...Thou has brought me into the dust of death" (Psalm 22, v6–15).

Similarly, Job had described:

> "wearisome nights are appointed to me...I am full of tossings to and fro unto the dawning of the day...When I say my bed shall comfort me, my couch shall ease my complaint; then thou scarest me with dreams and terrifiest me through visions...I have sinned...I am a burden to myself...thou shalt seek me in the morning but I shall not be" (Job, ch7, v3–21).

Melancholy, literally the 'Black Humour', had been one of Hippocrates' four categories of madness, and it had been established as such throughout medieval teaching. In the 13th century Bartholomeus Angelicus wrote:

> "The patients are faint and fearful in heart without cause, and oft sorry...feeling like earthen vessels they dread to be touched lest they should break...they feel they have the world upon their heads and shoulders for it is about to fall"(cit Hunter & Macalpine, 1963, p1)

1

For many of Burton's predecessors, melancholy had been regarded with ambivalence. While few welcomed its ravages, many believed it to be a sign of great sensibility, and some even believed that the melancholic "are accounted as the most fit to attempt matters of weighti charge and high attempt" (Du Laurens, 1599, cit Hunter & Macalpine, 1963).

In keeping with this, Burton gave to melancholy a bitter-sweet character. In his rhyming prologue, alternate verses had the refrain "Naught so sweet as melancholy", but he left his readers in no doubt as to the terrifying quality of its most severe forms. He wrote: "If there is a hell on earth, it is to be found in a melancholy man's heart".

After Burton, more than 300 years elapse before there is an account of the phenomenology of melancholy which matches his in both scope and quality. Emil Kraepelin's *Manic Depressive Insanity and Paranoia*, published in English in 1921, is filled with vivid descriptions which confirm for the reader the appropriateness of Burton's use of the words "Hell on Earth". His text is still widely quoted. A decade after Kraepelin, *The Journal of Mental Science* published Aubrey Lewis's "Melancholia, a clinical survey of depressive states". In about 100 pages, this paper combines meticulous phenomenological analysis with an empirical study of 61 carefully documented patients seen in his practice at the Maudsley Hospital. Taken together, these works of Burton, Kraepelin and Lewis render an account of the clinical features of the depressive disorders that is unlikely ever to be equalled.

Nineteenth and early 20th century psychiatry saw a shift in terminology from Burton's Melancholy to the current usage of the word depression. The nature and context of this change has been well described by Berrios (1992). The term depression was favoured by physicians who heard in it echoes of a more physiological disorder. Kraepelin legitimised its use by giving it adjectival status in "depressive insanity". Adolf Meyer was an enthusiastic proponent of the more modern usage. The word depression, however, still has its passionate detractors. In *Darkness Visible* (1991), William Styron wrote:

> "Melancholia would still appear to be a far more apt and evocative word for the blacker forms of the disorder, but it was usurped by a noun with a bland tonality and lacking any magisterial presence, used indifferently to describe an economic decline or a rut in the ground, a true wimp of a word for such a major illness....for over 75 years the word (depression) has slithered innocuously through the language like a slug, leaving little trace of its intrinsic malevolence and preventing by its very insipidity, a general awareness of the horrible intensity of the disease when out of control."

Clinical features of depressive disorders

"The Tower of Babel never yielded such confusion of tongues, as
this chaos of melancholy doth variety of symptoms" (Burton, 1621,
p. 240).

Many phenomena can be identified as features of depressive disorders.
These vary both in the patterns in which they occur and in their intensities.
In severe forms symptoms may be pervasive and unchanging. In milder
forms they may shift constantly in ways which reflect the dynamic
relationships between them.

Some phenomena are exaggerations of normal experience, for example
feelings of sadness or guilt. These become significant as symptoms either
because of their intensity, or their frequency, or their inappropriateness.
Other phenomena involve impairments of normal capacities, for example
loss of the ability to feel pleasure. A third group of phenomena emerge
as developments from other symptoms, as is seen when marked feelings
of guilt evolve into delusions.

There have been many attempts to classify symptoms but none has
been widely accepted. This account follows the traditional order of
presentation within the mental state, except that appearance and
behavioural features are considered separately at the end, along with an
account of histrionic features and depressive stupor. Impaired
concentration and memory are discussed alongside other impairments
of feeling, energy and thinking, these together with vegetative (bodily)
changes are often referred to as the associated features of depression.

Painful affects

Depressed mood

"Sorrow sticks by them still continuously, gnawing as the vulture
did..." (Burton, 1621).

Depressed mood is the commonest symptom to be found in depressive
disorders. It has an obvious claim to be the central feature of the disorder,
but it is not essential for diagnosis and it is not easy to delineate. Most
definitions refer to sadness, misery or dejection. The mood is painful and
oppressive, and is frequently without apparent cause. It can be
distinguished from the normal feelings of sadness or unhappiness which
accompany loss or failure by its greater intensity, duration and
pervasiveness. A special quality is often described, as if a black cloud were
descending. Sufferers feel heavy-hearted and weighed down with their
miseries. Tears come unexpectedly and at times for no reason. The severely
depressed may be beyond tears, in a state of frozen misery.

This extremely unpleasant state is usually coloured by depressive thinking, and is experienced as gloom, hopelessness, despair, insufficiency, loneliness or unwantedness. One sufferer wrote: "The grey drizzle of horror induced by depression takes on the quality of physical pain...I feel the horror like some poisonous fogbank, rolling in on my mind, and forcing me to bed" (Styron, 1991).

Some patients successfully conceal their mood change, and very few offer their depressed mood as a presenting complaint. It is extremely rare for a first time sufferer to use the words "I feel depressed". Sometimes the symptom of depressed mood is absent. In other cases it may be masked, due to irritability, problems with introspection, or a cultural tendency to show depression in forms other than mood disturbance.

Anxiety

> "A kind of panic and anxiety overtook me, accompanied by a visceral queasiness...A flight of birds caused me to stop, riveted with fear...I have felt the wind of the wings of madness." (Styron, 1991)

Anxiety is also one of the commonest symptoms in depressive disorders, although sufferers rarely complain of it by name. Often it is experienced as an apprehensive foreboding, as if something terrible is going to happen. Sufferers usually do complain of the autonomic accompaniments which include a dry mouth, palpitations, tremulousness, sweating, blushing, butterflies or a knot in the stomach, choking, difficulty getting breath, dizziness, and giddiness. The pattern of autonomic symptoms varies widely. They may be misinterpreted as evidence of a physical illness, and this may lead to escalating anxiety. Panic attacks and phobic avoidance may develop. Many wake early with anxious ruminations and autonomic symptoms, feeling unable to face the day. This is a very useful diagnostic pointer to the presence of a depressive illness.

The feeling of anxiety can be coloured by cognitive features, in particular pessimistic thinking, low self-esteem, and a preoccupation with death. Danger is imminent, as is loss and disgrace. Every man encountered is a potential thief or is out to pick a quarrel. Friends or relatives will die. The world is upon the sufferers' shoulders and it is about to fall. There is a fear of collapse, of madness, of death or eternal damnation.

Agitation

Agitation is marked anxiety combined with excessive motor activity. Sufferers feel anxious and restless and complain that they cannot keep still. They may continually wring their hands, or fidget with a convenient object. They may constantly shift positions. In more severe forms they cannot remain seated, and pace up and down, or pick feverishly at their clothes. They often appear scared or startled with wide eyes and a half open mouth.

Agitation is often accompanied by worrying. The sufferer cannot escape from a round of painful thoughts ridden with anxiety. Subjectively, agitated patients report feeling frantic, always wanting to be somewhere else but not knowing where to go to. One man described feeling dreadful, badgered and worried. Another woman felt she was getting into a terrible state of feverish nervous excitement: "I know that something has to be done. I don't know what to do."

Agitation must be distinguished from akathisia (motor restlessness occurring as an extrapyramidal side-effect of neuroleptic medication), from states of gross excitement, and from stereotypies. In akathisia, anxiety is usually less prominent and often absent. Gross excitement usually has an aggressive or explosive quality. Motor stereotypies involve the exact repetition of patterns of movement and tend to be comforting, leading to a reduction of anxiety.

Agitated and retarded depressions are usually distinguished but the two phenomena can occur together.

Irritability

Alongside sadness and fear, those who are depressed may complain of increased irritability. This may be experienced as a lowered threshold for annoyance and anger in the face of frustration. Sufferers may keep it to themselves, or may show it in the form of increased argumentativeness, uncharacteristic shouting and quarrelling, outbursts of temper, throwing or breaking things, or in extreme cases, violence to others.

Changes in mood

Fluctuations in mood are common, and may be both abrupt and extreme. About 50% of sufferers show a regular pattern. Most of these feel worse in the mornings, but some show regular mid-afternoon or evening exacerbations. Diurnal variation with the mood lowest in the morning is often considered typical of the melancholic sub-type of depression, as is loss of reactivity to the environment. Changes in mood are often seen also in association with the menses.

Reactivity to the environment is often harder to assess in hospital, but reactive patients often show an improvement immediately following admission, and further marked changes following visits from relatives, visits home, changes in other patients, and attempts at therapy. Reactivity does not imply a less serious depression, for it is not unknown for patients to be cheerful one moment, misleading those around them as to the need for vigilance, and then unexpectedly to hang themselves.

Impairments of feeling, energy and thinking

Anhedonia: loss of capacity for enjoyment

> "They are utterly unable to rejoice in anything. They cannot apprehend, believe or think of anything that is comfortable to them."
> (Richard Baxter, 17th century clergyman, cit Hunter & Macalpine, 1963, p241)

This is the second most common symptom in depressive disorders. Whereas painful sadness is the psychological opposite of pleasure, anhedonia refers to its negation – the absence of pleasure. Anhedonia is part of a wider phenomenon as Jaspers (1963) describes: "the feeling of having lost feelings", associated with a "terrible emptiness – a subjectively felt void". It is closely linked to feelings of dulled perception, depersonalisation and derealisation, and also to feelings of insufficiency and lack of vitality.

Those with anhedonia do not experience pleasure even if something good happens. They are not cheered by fine weather, receiving a compliment, winning a game, or by a surprise windfall. They cannot enjoy the company of friends, and are not happy spending time at their previous hobbies and interests. Kraepelin captures the phenomenon well:

> "(he is)...indifferent to relatives and to what he formerly liked best. Every comfort and every gleam of light is shut out. Everything is disagreeable to him; everything wearies him; company, music, travel, his professional work. Life appears to be aimless and meaningless. All the joy (of nature) cannot pump a drop of bliss from his heart up to his brain".

Lewis (1934) comments on the "especial distress" experienced by his patients from rural districts when they were unable to enjoy the sight of the fields, the sky, the trees and the flowers.

Anergia: loss of energy

Kraepelin's description of "total lack of energy" in a depressed man has never been bettered:

> "He drags himself with difficulty from one day until the next. He lacks spirit and willpower. He cannot rouse himself, cannot work any longer, has to force himself to everything. The smallest bit of work costs unheard of effort, even the most everyday arrangements, getting up, washing, dressing, are accomplished with the greatest difficulty and in the end are left undone. Work, visits, important letters, business affairs are like a mountain in front of the patient, and are just left because he does not find the power to overcome the opposing inhibitions. Finally he gives up all activities and sits

doing nothing with his hands in his lap, brooding to himself in utter dullness. Sometimes a veritable passion for lying in bed occurs."

Kraepelin did not view loss of energy as tiredness or fatigue, but rather as one manifestation of 'psychic inhibition', the sufferer being unable to overcome opposing inhibitions to action, which themselves may have resulted from excessive fear and pessimism. Janet (cit Lewis, 1934) held a similar view: "The feeling of inadequacy is essentially a fear of action, a flight from action, a checking regulation which stops one action, seeks to replace it with its opposite, and in doing so causes a failure of the action."

Today these concepts would be regarded by many as closer to the phenomenon of obsessional slowness. Loss of energy is now usually framed in terms of unpleasant inappropriate tiredness, listlessness, and exhaustion, which cannot be overcome voluntarily. Others, for example the authors of the Present State Examination (Wing *et al*, 1974), view anergia as a mild form of retardation. There may also be an important overlap with feelings of loss of energy and hypochondriasis.

Although these observations suggest that anergia may not refer to a unitary phenomenon, the description "fatigue or loss of energy, nearly every day" remains as one item of the DSM–IV operational definition for major depression. Equally "decreased energy or increased fatiguability" is a central feature of the ICD–10 criteria. A useful probe is : "Have you been getting exhausted or tired-out during the day or evening, even when you have not been working very hard." It is important to distinguish this symptom from anergia due to a physical disorder, and it may also be useful, though extremely difficult, to try and separate subjective and objective elements.

Sufferers complain of sluggishness, of feeling sapped and drained, or of lacking strength. Their limbs feel like lead, they have lost their vitality, or they feel insufficient in some way. They may describe themselves as worn out, exhausted, or even too weak to move. They may feel slowed down almost to the point of paralysis. Styron (1991) wrote that it was as if psychic energy was throttled back to zero. Informants report neglect of children, meals, housework, personal cleanliness and tidiness. Depressed people are often sent home from work because of inefficiency. The combination of exhaustion with inability to sleep may be particularly hard to bear.

Retardation

About half of depressed patients feel that their movements are slowed down. This phenomenon is retardation. Those affected may also appear slow. They may, for example, walk very slowly or sit perfectly still throughout an interview. Speech may also be slowed, hesitant and laboured, with few sentences longer than ten words, and seldom more than one sentence. There may be long pauses before replying (response latency) and also between each word.

Loss of energy, inefficient thinking and retardation have often been viewed as being unified by the concept of psychic inhibition. Many textbooks follow this line and refer to a generalised slowing of thought and action as psychomotor retardation. This practice has been criticised as leading to an overemphasis on objective signs, at the expense of the core phenomenon of the subjective experience of slowness. Lewis argued that observed slowness in speech and task performance was usually not due to slowness in thought, but rather to inattention, preoccupation or difficulty in thinking. None of his patients said that their thoughts were slower or fewer. Many of those whose talk appeared slowed described their thoughts as racing. Also many complaints of slowed movement were not born out by objective testing. These observations lead one to consider restricting the use of retardation to describing the subjective feeling of slowed movement, but there is as yet no consensus on this, and it is observable slowness that forms part of the DSM–IV and ICD–10 criteria.

Inefficient thinking/impaired concentration

> "They are inconstant...persuaded to and fro on every small occasion...Wavering, irresolute, unable to deliberate through fear...As a man that is bitten by fleas, their restless minds are tossed and vary" (Robert Burton, 1621).

There are several components to the difficulty in thinking found in depression. Indecisiveness, a tendency to ruminate, and an inability to sustain attention, are all important factors. There is often a difficulty in ordering and calling up thoughts and memories, and occasionally slowness. Most of Lewis's patients described a constant press of thoughts, their thoughts running on, their brain never stopping. Kraepelin similarly described his patients as feeling that too much was in their head, fresh thoughts were always coming, leading to confusion. As a result their thinking was unclear, muddled and lacking in focus. In many patients when thinking is seen to be laborious and slow it is found to be due to disorganisation of thoughts rather than any slowness of the thoughts themselves.

Other patients will describe their lack of concentration by saying that their thoughts just drift off. In severe cases those affected cannot read more than a few lines, follow a television programme for more than a few minutes, or follow a conversation. Depressed persons feel that they cannot take things in, cannot collect or pull together their thoughts, their heads feel heavy, their minds stupid and confused. They often feel they have no memory and that they have lost their command of previous knowledge. They may have problems remembering where they lay things. This difficulty may interact with an increased sensitivity to losses, so that "each momentary displacement fills the person with a frenzy of dismay" (Styron, 1991). Indecision may show itself as inconstancy or appear as paralysis, with sufferers considering at length the simplest matters.

Loss of interest

> "the enthusiast gradually gives up his hobby, the gardener leaves the weeds alone, the golfer lets his clubs rust." (Max Hamilton, 1982)

In both major diagnostic systems (ICD–10 and DSM–IV), this symptom is combined in a single criterion together with loss of pleasure. Most definitions also refer to a marked reduction in the range and intensity of interests and hobbies, including work and domestic activities, leisure pursuits, keeping well informed and maintaining an interest in clothes, food and personal appearance.

By these definitions the symptom is a composite phenomenon, related to both feeling and activity. It has three components:

1) inability to enjoy interests (anhedonia)
2) loss of anticipatory pleasure and concern (apathy)
3) reduction of activities.

The distinction between the first two of these, anhedonia and apathy, may reflect disorder of different neurophysiological mechanisms. Apathy also has an element of helpless futility. The third component, reduction of activities, follows from anhedonia and apathy, but also may result from inefficient thinking, inability to sustain concentration, phobic avoidance, fatigue and loss of energy, and motor retardation. Despite the fact that it is not a unitary phenomenon, it is loss of interests as defined by behavioural change that is most easily identified and rated, and therefore this is likely to remain in clinical use.

Bodily symptoms

Disturbance of appetite/weight loss

As a rule there is little appetite for food or drink, and food lacks any flavour. Occasionally, there may be increased appetite or episodes of ravenous hunger and bingeing. Attitudes to eating and drinking may change quickly and will usually range from a mild disinclination due to lack of appetite, to outright refusal. Carers may need to use much persuasion and cajolery. Reluctance to eat or drink may result directly from a delusional belief that the food is poisoned. Refusal to accept fluids can quickly become life-threatening.

Kraepelin described marked fluctuations in body weight, suggesting changes in fluid balance. Today the most common clinical picture before treatment is of weight loss due to poor appetite, and not due to dieting or physical illness. Symptom criteria usually specify losses of more than 5% of the body weight in a month or two pounds a month for several months. Typically, a depressed person's weight stabilises after a loss of about one stone, unlike the continuing decline seen in anorexia nervosa and occult malignancy. Sometimes weight is lost without any apparent reduction in food intake. In about 10% of depressive episodes there is a similar degree of weight gain, and this is often associated with hypersomnia.

Constipation is a common complaint, which may be due to reduced intestinal motility, to reduced food intake, or to the side-effects of antidepressant drugs. The complaint may also reflect hypochondriacal cognitive distortions in the mental state.

Disturbance of sleep

Hippocrates described his melancholic patients as having little or no sleep. Several had not slept for over two years. Kraepelin's patients typically lay sleepless for hours in bed, tormented by painful ideas, confused and anxious dreams, waking dazed, worn out and weary. They would get up late and might lie in bed for days or even weeks.

Three patterns are traditionally described. Initial insomnia or delayed sleep is present when there is more than a one hour delay in sleeping after settling down. A delay of two hours or more marks a severe disturbance. Middle insomnia is also common, with either frequent wakening, or a prolonged period of being unable to return to sleep. It is not unusual to find a depressed person falling asleep shortly before they are due to arise. The third pattern, which is traditionally associated with the melancholic sub-type, is early morning wakening. This is present when waking occurs at least one hour earlier than normal. Waking two or more hours earlier than usual marks a severe disturbance, and this is required to satisfy the symptom criterion in DSM–IV Melancholia. Sufferers are often at their lowest in mood after waking early and this is a time when the risk of suicidal behaviour may be high.

Occasionally there is an increased duration of sleep (hypersomnia) or an inverted sleep pattern with long periods of sleep during the day. There may be discrepancies between observed and reported sleep, which may reflect confusion, histrionic exaggeration, or hypochondriacal and nihilistic features of the mental state. Today the clinical picture is often distorted by hypnotic medication. A fuller account of the disorders of sleep in depression will be found on page 1214.

Loss of libido

This symptom is rarely complained of directly although it is frequently present. A tactful approach is often needed to elicit it, and combining enquiries with routine questions about sleep and appetite is often helpful. There is usually a lack of interest in sexual activity compared with normal, and this will probably be reflected in a diminished frequency of sexual intercourse. Men may suffer from erectile impotence, and women may report loss of sexual pleasure. Very occasionally libido is increased. Amenorrhoea may also accompany severe depressive states.

Disorders of thought content: depressive cognition

Alongside feelings of sadness and anxiety, and together with impaired enjoyment, energy, thinking, and bodily symptoms, there are usually changes in thought content. These include morbid preoccupations and disturbances of judgement. In severe depression distorted thinking can result in overvalued ideas and delusions, which may have a melodramatic or even fantastic quality.

Cognitive distortions may relate to the past, present or future, and to the self or the outside world. Thinking about the past is often dominated by self-reproach and guilt. In the present the self is often viewed as worthless, and helpless. Hypochondriacal ideas may be prominent. The outside world is seen as useless, meaningless, and occasionally persecutory. The future is viewed with apprehension, pessimism, hopelessness and even nihilism. Thoughts of death are common. Suicidal ideas may follow, particularly in the setting of acute hopelessness and despair, but sometimes they arise independently and unexpectedly.

Thoughts and feelings of guilt

> "Their phantasy most erreth in aggravating their sins. They are continual self accusers apprehending themselves forsaken of God." (Richard Baxter, 1716, cit Hunter & Macalpine, 1963)

Guilt is one of the most striking features of depressive disorders. Seventy-five per cent of sufferers feel it to some degree. Three phenomena can be distinguished.

Pathological guilt: those affected blame themselves for some action which others would not take very seriously. They often recognise that this is out of proportion but they cannot help feeling self-blame and dwelling upon it. They may blame themselves for neglecting their children, bills having not been paid, duties having been ignored. Friends have been let down, unwise decisions are regretted intensely. Sweets were stolen as a child. They have been ungrateful to their parents. Characteristically, sufferers also feel blame for bringing an illness upon themselves. Ideas of worthlessness and self-deprecation are closely associated.

Guilty ideas of reference: those affected feel that others are blaming them, and in more severe forms they feel accused. Insight is preserved and the feeling is recognised as their own. Intense forms shade into persecutory delusions.

Delusions of guilt: as depressive states deepen, ideas of guilt become less realistic, and insight into their pathological nature is lost. Patients magnify their own role in events and may give an entirely false account of a serious misdemeanour (delusional memory). Delusional guilt sometimes has the quality of glorifying self-aggrandisement. One patient claimed "I am the chief sinner, there never was anyone in the world as wicked as me". Patients may believe that they have committed adultery or incest, that they have killed their families, that they have caused a train crash or air disaster, or that they have become possessed by the Devil. Patients may give themselves up repeatedly to the police. Delusional guilt may also involve feelings of responsibility for others. One patient was convinced that she was making other patients ill. Another believed that whenever he ate, someone was executed.

Great care should be taken to distinguish between delusional memories and accurate recall of painful events for which feelings of guilt are appropriate. Guilt over past incest may be delusional, or it may be a highly significant disclosure.

Thoughts of worthlessness and self-depreciation

"I am a worm and no man." (Psalm 22, v 6)

In depressive states any premorbid tendency to feelings of inferiority and low self-worth is amplified. Raised standards are applied to the self without a corresponding change with regard to others. Compensatory merits are discounted. Severely depressed people often regard themselves as worthless and as total failures. Delusions of poverty, such as the belief that one is bankrupt, are less common.

Sufferers describe themselves as unwanted, unloved, and not worthy of having friends. They feel discontented with themselves. They lack confidence. They have failed at everything, they will lose their jobs, they face ruin. Requests for lists of personal strengths and weaknesses often result in catalogues of faults with no redeeming features. In severe states, feelings border on self-loathing and self-hatred.

It can be hard to distinguish depressive self-deprecation from insight and from longstanding attitudes to the self. For example, there may have been failures at work as a result of impaired concentration, indecisiveness and lack of energy. There may always have been a lack of confidence and low self-esteem. Depressive colouring is identified by its fluctuation with mood, by its intensity, and by the fact that it is a change from the normal.

Hypochondriasis

> "Some are afraid that they shall have every fearful disease they see others have, hear of or read." (Robert Burton, 1621)

Depressed people have many good reasons to feel that they are physically ill. They may have experienced low mood, loss of appetite and fatigue during a previous physical illness. Depressed mood or muscular tension may be felt as a physical pain in the chest or head. The autonomic symptoms of anxiety all suggest physical disorder, and in panic the sufferer often fears that he will die.

These experiences may lead a person to suspect a physical illness, but this does not amount to hypochondriasis. However, when there is also anxious foreboding and a worried, pessimistic mood, hypochondriacal phenomena are likely to emerge. Together with a loss of interest in the external world, there may be a heightened awareness of bodily sensations, and an abnormally intense and painful preoccupation with the possibility of a fearful disease. There may also be a growing conviction of an unhealthy, rotten, or diseased body. In extreme forms there may be beliefs that the sufferer has one or more physical illnesses in the face of evidence to the contrary. Such hypochondriacal delusions can take on a fantastic and even nihilistic quality. The illness may be viewed as a deserved punishment.

Kraepelin described patients believing that they were incurably ill and expecting slow and painful deaths. Some claimed they had lung disease or cancer, others had tapeworms, others could not swallow. Lewis's patients were particularly concerned with their bowels: "they have all gone wrong......the food just wedges in". One patient had a sudden blank feeling across his forehead and was sure it was a stroke. More fantastic ideas have involved organs being withered, burnt or rotten, brains melting, skulls full of filth, bones out of joint, insects breeding inside. Patients have reported excruciating pains, disfiguring eruptions on the face, testicles being crushed, food falling down between intestines into the scrotum. Nihilistic hypochondriacal delusions have included beliefs that the body is hollow, that stomach and bowels are no longer there, that no urine is passed, and that genitals have disappeared.

Hopelessness – tedium vitae – suicidal thoughts/plans/acts

> "My days are swifter than a weavers shuttle and are spent without
> hope...so that my soul chooseth strangling, and death rather than
> my life." (Job, ch 7, vs 6 & 15)

The future can appear bleak and without comfort. Life may seem pointless
and not worth living (tedium vitae), there being little or no hope of
recovery, so that more pain and anguish will follow. Fleeting thoughts of
suicide are common, and often plans are made. When hope is lost, suicide
may begin to appear as a logical solution, as a relief from intolerable pain,
and even as an atonement for real or delusional guilt. Thoughts of joining
loved ones who have already died are particularly ominous, as is the writing
of a suicide note, settling one's affairs, and taking precautions against
being found. Threats to take the lives of children or a partner to save them
from the effects of the suicide should also be taken very seriously. While
suicidal acts usually arise out of a sense of extreme despair, they may
emerge suddenly and without warning in states of milder depression, often
in association with impaired impulse control, and with the sufferer unable
to account for his own motives.

Many risk factors for suicide have been identified, but these can be
difficult to apply in practice. Three useful clinical predictors are
hopelessness, suicidal plans and previous attempts. Kraepelin regarded
psychic inhibition as protective against suicide, and warned against the
increasing risk when retarded patients recovered their volition whilst
remaining hopeless. Many clinicians have experienced the unexpected
suicide of a patient who appeared to be recovering. The decision to take
one's life is often accompanied by a sense of calmness, and suicidal
plans may be concealed behind apparently cheerful behaviour. A detailed
account of suicide is given in chapter 12.

Suicidal thoughts and acts are not the only results of depressive thinking
about the future. If recovery is felt to be unlikely, or impossible, then
compliance with treatment may be poor. Pessimism may interact with
perceptions of the world as cruel and desolate, and with an extremely
apprehensive mood. The resulting thought-content can range from regret
that society's values are decaying to a conviction of imminent global
catastrophe.

The self may be perceived as potentially dangerous. One patient,
reported by Du Laurens (1597, cit Hunter & Macalpine, 1963), believed
that if he were to pass water then his whole town would be drowned by
the volume of his urine. He was reported as being treated by his attendants
convincing him that the town was engulfed in a raging fire which needed
his intervention. Today patients are more likely to be convinced of
impending nuclear holocaust or financial ruin, and some would claim
that altruism can no longer be relied upon for a cure. Delusions of
catastrophe often have a nihilistic quality. Everything will be destroyed.

Nothing can be done. In extreme forms, as Jaspers describes, the future vanishes.

Delusions

As has already been shown, these will sometimes occur as an end point of severe cognitive distortion. Five main types can be identified:

(1) delusions of guilt
(2) delusions of poverty
(3) hypochondriacal delusions
(4) delusions of catastrophe
(5) nihilistic delusions.

All of these are regarded as mood congruent. Persecutory delusions, delusional jealousy, and delusions of bodily change are also sometimes found in depressive illnesses.

Examples of delusions of guilt, poverty, hypochondriasis, and catastrophe have already been given.

Cotard (1882) described a syndrome of *nihilistic delusions* often associated with hypochondriasis. The central feature was the delusion of negation, so that for example a patient went beyond the belief that his bowels were not working to the point where he declared that his bowels did not exist. As already illustrated, such nihilistic delusions can refer to parts of the body, the self, the world, or even the future.

Persecutory delusions commonly take the form of beliefs that the patient is under surveillance, that there is a plot, an organisation such as the CIA is pursuing, other patients are detectives or secret agents, food is poisoned. The persecution is usually felt to be justified, as a development from guilty ideas of reference, but some patients show resentment at its unjust nature, and some may even loudly proclaim their innocence.

Disorders of experience

Depersonalisation

Depersonalisation is not a common symptom of depression, but when present it is striking. Sufferers feel unreal, as if they were acting a part, or as if they were a robot. Insight into the abnormality of this phenomenon is retained. The feeling is highly unpleasant, but difficult to describe. Metaphor is often used. One patient said " I've got this dreadful feeling as if I'm unreal, a sort of dead feeling, wooden inside, I've changed, I do things mechanically".

Jaspers analysed depersonalisation as resulting from a loss of sense of awareness; of the self as an active agent; of temporal continuity of the self and of the distinction between the self and the outside world. Depersonalisation is also closely linked to the phenomena of anhedonia, increased self-consciousness, and hypochondriacal and nihilistic thinking. It should be distinguished from:

(1) a perception of parts of the body as unfamiliar
(2) dysmorphophobia (the perception of one's appearance as changed)
(3) delusions of bodily change
(4) nihilistic delusions of non-existence.

One should always ask for a subject's own explanation of feelings of depersonalisation and derealisation (see below). Sometimes this enquiry will reveal previously hidden delusions.

Depersonalisation is by no means a diagnostic sign of depression. It sometimes occurs in healthy persons under stress, in association with intense anxiety, or following sensory deprivation. It may occur in many other psychiatric conditions including organic disorders (especially temporal lobe seizures), schizophrenia, and both generalised and phobic anxiety disorders. Very occasionally it occurs as a primary phenomena alongside derealisation. It is categorised as such in ICD–10 as the depersonalisation–derealisation syndrome, and in DSM–IV as depersonalisation disorder, a subclass of the dissociative disorders. Theories of the mechanisms underlying depersonalisation have been well reviewed by Sedman (1970).

Derealisation

This is another uncommon but often striking feature. In mild forms of derealisation, the person's surroundings lack colour and life and other people may seem to be pretending their emotions. In more severe forms everything seems artificial or unreal, like a stage set populated with actors. One patient described: "People seem changed, like machines, things look mysterious. It's as if I were in a dream, watching a film." Lewis analysed the phenomenon as a combination of various changes, including:

(1) altered perceptions of the environment, for example appearances of unreality, mystery, acting and soullessness
(2) changes in consciousness, for example, bewilderment, muddle, impressions of mystery and confusion
(3) loss of the ability to recall images with vividness
(4) changes in the experience of time.

Derealisation should be distinguished from nihilistic delusion. Derealisation is an experience, not a belief, and insight into its abnormal nature is retained.

Obsessive–compulsive phenomena

Obsessive–compulsive symptoms occur in 20–35% of depressive episodes, often as an exaggeration of premorbid tendencies. A few of those who gain obsessions during a depressive episode fail to lose them on recovery. Several groups can be distinguished:

(1) obsessional checking and repeating
(2) obsessional orderliness
(3) obsessional thoughts of harm or accident to self or others
(4) obsessional cleanliness
(5) obsessional ideas, ruminations and feelings of incompleteness.

Central to all of these is the experience of intrusive thoughts or impulses which are recognised as one's own, and which are entertained or carried out against conscious resistance. The sufferer recognises them as senseless and tries to stop but cannot. In time the experience of conscious resistance may fade.

Checking once or twice may be normal. Many depressed persons cannot remember whether they have locked doors or not, they may therefore return and check. This is not an obsession unless they can remember locking the door, but still need to check one more time to satisfy some lingering doubt.

Obsessional orderliness and cleanliness may be exaggerations of normal traits, and the threshold for identifying symptoms is usually when they become overly time consuming or interfere with other activities. Bathing twice a day or more is likely to be an obsessional symptom, but if so, the person should feel that it is in reality unnecessary to bathe again and should try to stop doing so. Ordering and cleaning rituals often act to neutralise some obsessional fear, for example of harming someone or of contracting a serious disease. Severely affected patients may wash their hands until they are raw.

Obsessional thoughts in depressive disorders usually have aggressive or obscene themes. Knives may be avoided for fear of harming the self or others. There may be a strong impulse to shout obscenities whilst in a church service. There may be recurrent and apparently senseless thoughts of killing one's family. The obsessional nature of these thoughts is usually protective against harmful actions, but any switch from an obsessional to a delusional quality in thoughts with suicidal or homicidal themes is extremely ominous.

Many clinicians have hypothesised a link between obsessional phenomena and the development of psychosis. Obsessional symptoms may have a dual role in depression, acting both as markers of a propensity for psychosis, and also as defences against disintegration of the psyche (Stengel, 1945).

Hallucinations

In states of normal grief, seeing and hearing the deceased is not uncommon, but hallucinations are rare in depressive illnesses. When they occur they are usually auditory, second person and consistent with depressive themes of guilt, death, personal inadequacy, disease, nihilism or deserved punishment. They are often isolated phenomena and are seldom in the foreground of the clinical picture. Often there is little more than an indistinct muttering. Kraepelin reported his patients as hallucinating the crackling of hell, or the hammering of a gallows being erected. When a voice is recognised it is often that of a relative or partner, only a few words are recognised. A typical example is the voice of a parent saying in a condemnatory tone: "You have let everybody down" or "you are a nasty lazy man" or "you deserve to die". On closer examination, many of these phenomena prove not to be true hallucinations, but rather illusions, auditory misinterpretations, or pseudohallucinations which are heard within the mind and not located in physical space. Kraepelin describes vividly how the vascular murmur of the ear becomes a reproach: " Whore, whore, whore..." which is then attributed to the Devil. When true hallucinations do occur they are often more frequent at night and are often described as emanating from the sufferer's body, for example as a voice speaking from inside the stomach.

Command hallucinations also occur, most often instructing the patient to harm his or herself, or others. These should be examined carefully for evidence of passivity phenomena in which the patient feels impelled to act under the controlling influence of an outside force. The association of command hallucinations with passivity phenomena is an extremely dangerous development.

Visual distortions are sometimes seen, for example faces can take on an ominous or spectral quality. A shadow may be seen at the window. Worms may swarm in the patient's food. True visual hallucinations are rare, but they may appear as an invitation or enticement to suicide. One patient saw a clear vision of a noose and believed this was a signal that she should hang herself. Hallucinations in other modalities are even rarer. One example is the perception of a strong smell of putrefaction emanating from a house or from the person's own body. Very occasionally hallucinations occur simultaneously in more than one sensory sphere.

Mood incongruent psychotic features

One encounters patients whose illnesses appear to be typically depressive, but who show somatic hallucinations, or passivity experiences, or describe thought insertion, or express bizarre nonsensical or absurd delusions, or delusions of external influence, or persecutory delusions unrelated to deserved punishment. Both Kraepelin and Lewis reported such features in their classic descriptions of melancholy, and they were especially prominent in Kraepelin's categories of paranoid and fantastic melancholy. Along with third person auditory hallucinations, many of these phenomena constitute first rank symptoms of schizophrenia, and their occurrences in illnesses which appear otherwise to be typically depressive, pose diagnostic problems. A helpful development has been to group together such cases under the broad heading of mood incongruent psychotic depressive illness. There is now increasing evidence (Kendler, 1991) that this grouping may best be considered as a distinct sub-type of depressive illness rather than as a variant of schizophrenia.

Histrionic features

Kraepelin wrote that hysterical disorders were observed "extraordinarily often" in melancholia. Aubrey Lewis devoted many paragraphs to 'neurotic features' which comprised a mixture of psychosomatic and conversion symptoms and histrionic behaviours. Although such features are familiar to most clinicians they now receive scant recognition in many textbooks.

Kraepelin's account included noises in the ears, shivering in the back, and special sensitivity to the influence of the weather. He also described fainting fits, giddiness, hysterical convulsions, choreiform clonic convulsions, and psychogenic tremor. Lewis portrayed many conversion type symptoms such as vomiting or headaches under stress or in unwelcome situations. His account of histrionic behaviour included exaggerated and melodramatic talk, attitudes of extreme dependence, threatening a hunger strike, clutching arms with a very appealing manner, seeking endless sympathy, and pedantic formality. He described over-intimacy, letters like novelettes, and strong affective relations which quickly changed from strong attachment to active dislike. Some of his patients were "always seeking attention, calling out, asking for interviews, self-pitying, and copying symptoms from others." Others were "laughing and crying alternately with neither giving the impression of much depth." One patient was always stealing another patient's pillows, another's eyes kept revolving. Many were worried about their eyes, their ears, and multiple pains which cleared up quickly.

Such features can be regarded as pathoplastic effects of a histrionic premorbid personality, or as a re-emergence of childhood and infantile behavioural patterns with acute fears of abandonment, fierce attachments and possessiveness. One should be cautious about assuming the former, for it is striking how apparently histrionic 'personality' features often disappear completely when a patient recovers fully from a depressive illness.

Depressive stupor

Kraepelin described stupor as a syndrome rather than a symptom. His patients usually lay mute and motionless in bed, at most withdrawing timidly from approaches, sometimes demonstrating catalepsy, sometimes merely aimless resistance. They sat helpless before food, but often allowed themselves to be spoon-fed. They held fast what was pressed into their hand, turning it slowly about without knowing how to get rid of it. Unable to care for their bodily needs they frequently became dirty. Now and then periods of excitement were interpolated. Kraepelin described how, after the return of consciousness, memory was "very much clouded and often quite extinguished".

Depressive stupor is usually conceptualised either as an end point of severe retardation, or as an extreme form of psychic inhibition. Very severe forms, with a complete failure to respond to the surroundings, are now very rarely seen. More commonly patients present in a pre-stuporous phase, having stopped eating and drinking, still speaking a few words, but spending most of their time staring into space. When patients recover they usually give a clear account of their experiences, describing the state as an extremely painful one. The fact that Kraepelin's stuporous patients had only patchy recall on recovery has led to suggestions that some were showing clouding of consciousness, perhaps due to dehydration or nutritional factors. Stupor is also discussed on page 1000.

Appearance, behaviour and talk

The appearance of depression is usually easier to recognise than it is to describe. It is often identified directly rather than inferred from any combination of elements. Systematic description is important in clinical practice as part of the mental state. The following features are common, but few may be present, and the subject may even be smiling and apparently jocular.

Most of those suffering from depressive disorders appear sad, dejected, downcast, miserable, or guilty, much of the time. The term "depressive facies" is sometimes used. Their posture is often stooped or drooping, and they may sit head in hands, looking at the floor. They may look stony faced, frightened or apprehensive. Worry may be evidenced by a furrowed brow, and the corners of the mouth may be turned down. They may be close to tears, crying, weeping or even sobbing. Their general manner may signal an attitude of dependency, hostility, or even indifference.

Evidence of self-neglect is common. Those affected may be untidy and unkempt, dirty, and smelling, with unwashed hair. Clothes may be unusually drab, or dirty and stained. Nightclothes may be worn in the middle of the day. There may be signs of weight loss or dehydration, or evidence of self-harm, with scars or bruises. Agitation or retardation may be apparent, as described previously. There may be a poverty of movement, gesture, and speech. Talk is likely to be soft or monotonous, and may die away, often leaving sentences incomplete. There may be hesitancy, monosyllabic replies or even muteness.

Changes in social behaviour

Depressive illnesses can provoke many changes in social behaviour, and these are often the most prominent features of the clinical presentation.

Inefficiency at work may lead to threats of redundancy or to unemployment. Unpaid bills and failure in budgeting may cause financial crises. Irritability, loss of feeling and social withdrawal can lead to a breakdown of relationships with friends or family. Marital discord is a common presenting problem. It may be hard to distinguish between cause and effect in a chronically depressed person who complains of an unhappy marriage.

Alcohol and other drugs are often used to provide relief from depressive symptoms, especially low mood, anxiety and insomnia. A presentation with alcohol or drug abuse may mask an underlying depressive illness. Equally, a hidden alcohol problem commonly underlies treatment resistant depression. Antisocial behaviours are sometimes released by depressive illnesses. Shoplifting, promiscuity, sexual aberrations, violence, and physical and sexual abuse can all be ways in which a depressive illness can present itself.

Hypochondriacal features may lead to repeated medical consultations, especially when somatic symptoms closely mimic a physical illness. This is a fairly common mode of presentation of depressive disorders, particularly in those who have difficulty in describing their feelings.

Most importantly of all, depressive illnesses can result in increased risk taking, self-harm, suicide, and even homicide. An episode of deliberate self-harm is one of the commonest ways in which a depressive illness may draw attention to itself.

Of course, phenomena such as unemployment, marital discord, anti-social behaviour and deliberate self-harm can have many other causes. They are sometimes associated with depressive illnesses, and when they occur, one possibility among many is that the individual is suffering from a primary depressive illness.

Diagnostic criteria

None of the features outlined above is either necessary or sufficient for the diagnosis of a depressive episode. For each feature, one can find episodes where the phenomenon is absent and yet most would agree that the diagnosis is still one of depression. Conversely each of these features can occur as a symptom of another disorder. Depressive disorders therefore show a pattern of family resemblances, and diagnoses are best made using polythetic criteria, with multiple elements. Both ICD–10 (World Health Organization, 1992) and DSM–IV (American Psychiatric Association, 1994) employ this approach.

There have been many attempts to isolate core features. The most obvious candidate is depressed mood, which is identified in many accounts ranging from *The Anatomy of Melancholy* to most current textbooks. Burton, however, was very aware that depressed mood was not essential. He wrote: "Some indeed are sad and not fearful, some fearful and not sad; some neither fearful nor sad".

Kraepelin does not appear to have viewed depressed mood as a central feature at all. He believed that the underlying process was a depression of function: "simple psychic inhibition". Bleuler and Janet held similar views, Janet stressing the importance of a feeling of inadequacy. Jaspers (1963) argued for two independent central features: "an unmotivated profound sadness" and "a retardation of psychic events".

Recently two more features, low self-esteem and anhedonia have found support as candidates for core features of the disorder. Anhedonia has been particularly identified as a potential marker for the melancholic sub-type of depression (Snaith, 1987).

DSM–IV and ICD–10 criteria include both depressed mood and anhedonia as core features. DSM–IV requires that at least one of these must be present for a diagnosis of a depressive syndrome. ICD–10 is closer to the Jasperian tradition, including increased fatiguability as a third core feature and requiring two out of three features as necessary. Thus in both current systems there can be patients diagnosed as depressed who are 'neither fearful nor sad'. Robert Burton would have approved.

Classification

The bewildering range of depressive disorders has led to a search for organising principles. Variation can be accounted for by differences in severity and by the shaping (pathoplastic) effects of personality and circumstances. However, many psychiatrists believe that there must also be a heterogeneous group of disorders behind the variability, and there have been many attempts to find a useful and valid division into subtypes. Few areas in psychiatry have generated more heated debate and yet remained for so long in a state of confusion. There have been two main themes running through the literature.

From endogenous depression to DSM–IV melancholia and beyond

Firstly, is it possible to make a single division of depressive illnesses into two main types on the combined basis of aetiology, clinical features and response to treatment?

Timothy Bright (1586) noted "how diverslie the word melancholy is taken". He identified cases where melancholy was "not moved by any adversity present or imminent", in which "the melancholy humour...abuseth the mind" and for which physical treatment was needed. He also described a second type of melancholy where "the perill is not of body" but "proceedeth from the mind's apprehension" requiring "cure of the minde", that is psychotherapy. Over four centuries, Bright's distinction between endogenous and exogenous forms has reappeared in various guises, in particular as the distinction between endogenous and reactive depressions, and as the distinction embodied in the International Classification of Diseases (up to and including ICD–9), between 'psychotic' and 'neurotic' depression.

With hindsight we can see how this apparently sensible and simple distinction has led to confusion. Three main elements characterise Bright's endogenous category:

(1) the absence of an external cause
(2) a biological clinical picture
(3) response to physical treatment.

Problems arise when cases meet one of these criteria but not the others. For example, Paykel *et al* (1984) have shown that the clinical picture of depressive illnesses is mostly independent of the presence or absence of an external cause. It follows that the aetiological division between endogenous and reactive depression may bear little relation to the biological clinical picture or to response to particular forms of treatment.

Further problems have arisen from the use of the terms 'psychotic' and 'neurotic' to attempt to identify the distinction that Bright made. Kendell (1968) has described how the patients encountered in asylum practice by Kraepelin, and identified as suffering from manic depressive psychosis, differed from those seen in the consulting rooms of early psychoanalysts who described their patients as suffering from depressive neuroses. This selective experience by different groups of clinicians with very different aetiological models may have led to an artificial polarisation between two forms of what may nevertheless have been the same illness.

In addition, both 'psychotic' and 'neurotic' have several meanings. A diagnosis of 'manic-depressive psychosis' or 'psychotic depression' according to Kraepelin and the tradition of the International Classification of Diseases (before ICD–10), does not require the presence of hallucinations or delusions. However for many psychiatrists the term psychotic is used to convey precisely the fact that hallucinations or delusions are present. Further confusion surrounds the use of the term 'neurotic'. This can be used to refer to milder depressive episodes, to episodes showing 'neurotic' clinical features, to 'reactive' episodes, to chronic fluctuating depressive disorders, to depressive disorders which respond to psychotherapeutic interventions, or to depressive episodes arising on the background of a neurotic personality. It is no surprise to find that the diagnosis of 'neurotic' depression lacks both reliability and validity.

One escape route from this confusion would be to adopt the position argued by Lewis (1938), namely that all the variability in depressive illness is due to the effects of severity and pathoplastic factors, together with a variation between episodic and chronic forms. However, others remained strongly wedded to the notion of two distinct illnesses. The Newcastle Scale was developed in the 1960s to distinguish between endogenous and reactive (non-endogenous, neurotic) depression. Based on previous history and phenomenology, it gave rise to a bimodal distribution of scores and was shown to predict response to ECT (Carney *et al*, 1965). The Newcastle group thus argued strongly for a categorical approach to diagnosing endogenous and reactive depression, claiming that there were definitely two different types of disorder. Meanwhile Kendell (1968), following Lewis's tradition, and studying consecutive admissions to the Maudsley Hospital, derived an index which placed illnesses on a unimodal continuum from 'neurotic to 'psychotic' depression and which also predicted response to physical treatments. This set the scene for a vigorous debate between the lumpers (all forms of a single illness) and the splitters (definitely two types of illness) which was finally resolved only when both camps were able to prove the correctness of their own views.

One of the very useful things that did emerge from this controversy was a growing precision in the definition of a biomedical sub-type. Discriminant function and factor analytic studies, such as those conducted by Kendell and the Newcastle Group, produced a surprisingly consistent picture of features which were to be found in the type of depression that responded best to physical treatments. The discovery that the presence or absence of an external cause was of little relevance to the phenomenology of depression or to its response to treatment, led to attempts to restrict these defining characteristics to clinical features alone.

The advent of the Research Diagnostic Criteria (RDC) in America marked a further development (Spitzer *et al*, 1978). Neurotic depression was discarded as an amorphous category, and depressions were divided into major and minor on the basis of severity. "Psychotic" major depression was restricted to cases showing delusions or hallucinations. A separate category of endogenous depression (RDC) or melancholia (in the subsequent DSM criteria) was established and operational criteria for these included pervasive anhedonia, loss of reactivity, early morning wakening and weight loss. DSM–III–R (APA, 1987) further introduced a classification of depressions into three levels of severity; mild, moderate and severe, and this has remained in DSM–IV.

A similar approach was followed in ICD–10, with three levels of severity, and 'psychotic' being restricted to hallucinations, delusions, or depressive stupor. 'Melancholic' features were designated as "somatic". Biological features had been considered as an alternative to somatic symptoms and this would reflect the usage of many psychiatrists, but somatic symptoms remained in the final version.

Following criticisms that melancholic subtyping had limited predictive value in DSM–III (APA, 1980), the operational criteria for melancholia were extended in DSM–III–R. These went beyond phenomenological items such as pervasive anhedonia and early morning wakening, to encompass previously 'normal' personality, previous episodes with complete recovery, and previous response to physical treatments. Critics observed that the new criteria introduced an element of circularity into validation research, and confounded illness and personality. ICD–10 has continued to be restricted to phenomenological items in its definitions of the 'somatic symptoms' sub-type, and DSM–IV has reverted to this approach. The authors of ICD–10 acknowledge that the status and future of the biomedical pole of Timothy Bright's distinction is still uncertain, but they observe that there remains widespread clinical interest in its survival.

Unipolar and bipolar disorders

The second major theme running through the history of the classification of the affective disorders involves the relationship between mania and depression. Circular forms of alternating manic and depressive states were described in 1854 by the French psychiatrists Baillarger (la folie a double form) and Falret (la folie circulaire). The question arose as to whether the depressive episodes seen in such patients reflected the same disorder as that to be found in others who showed only depressive episodes. Kraepelin believed that mania and depression were definitely "manifestations of a single morbid process", and he argued strongly for their unification in a single disorder, manic-depressive insanity. This term was to be used even where no manic attacks ever occurred. Many believe that this synthesis was as significant as the separation of manic-depressive insanity from dementia praecox, but it has always had its critics, most notably Adolf Meyer. Nevertheless diagnoses in ICD–9 (WHO, 1978) followed Kraepelin, so that a single episode of severe depression was described as manic-depressive psychosis: depressed type. This often misled the lay public who wrongly interpreted the diagnosis as implying that manic attacks were to be expected.

Leonhard (published in English in 1979) has been credited with rediscovering the distinction between unipolar and bipolar affective disorders. Most of the more recent research has emphasised the differences between those patients who show unipolar depressive histories and those who show bipolar histories of both depression and mania. Two independent empirical studies embodying this distinction appeared almost simultaneously (Angst, 1966; Perris 1966) and their remarkably consistent findings have had a major impact on the psychiatric literature.

Almost all studies find that bipolar disorders show an earlier age of onset, and more frequent but shorter episodes. Whereas unipolar depression is twice as common in women as men, the incidence of bipolar illness is almost equal between the sexes. Combined rates of unipolar and bipolar disorders found in first degree relatives of bipolar probands (e.g. Angst 21%, Perris 20%) are significantly greater than those found in first degree relatives of unipolars (Angst 11.7%, Perris 14.6%). Bipolar probands also show increased risks of bipolar disorders alone in first degree relatives whereas unipolar probands do not. The twin study of Bertelsen *et al*, (1977) found a greater monozygotic to dizygotic concordance ratio for bipolar disorder (4.9) compared with unipolar disorder (2.3).

Despite these findings, as yet there has been no clear difference shown in clinical features or pathophysiology between unipolar and bipolar depressive episodes. Most of the evidence remains consistent with the hypothesis that bipolar illness represents no more than an increased genetic loading for a unitary affective disorder. Kraepelin may therefore yet be proved to have had an equally penetrating insight, but the unipolar/bipolar distinction is now widely regarded as the most robust sub-classification of the affective disorders. It was no surprise to find that ICD–10 followed the DSM approach in distinguishing between unipolar and bipolar disorders.

Further subdivisions of bipolar disorders have been suggested. Perris did not include those who showed short-term euphoria associated with treatment in his bipolar group, but these patients together with those who have shown depressive episodes and short hypomanic episodes not requiring hospital treatment have been identified in the American literature as bipolar II (Dunner *et al*, 1976). This subdivision has been incorporated in DSM–IV.

The two main classificatory systems

DSM–IV (American Psychiatric Association, 1994)

One of the advantages of the DSM–III–R classification of mood disorders was the clear and explicit distinction made between symptoms, syndromes, episodes and disorders. Symptoms comprise the clinical features described earlier in this chapter, differing from the normal by virtue of their intensity, pervasiveness, and inappropriateness. These are combined as elements of operational criteria to define mood syndromes. Mood syndromes can occur as part of any disorder, but when they occur on the basis of a mood disorder the result is a mood episode. Episodes occurring singly or in combination define a mood disorder. These distinctions are less explicit in DSM–IV, but the structure remains.

DSM–IV criteria for a *depressive syndrome* are shown in Box 1.1. These insist on the presence of either depressed mood or loss of interest or pleasure, and require that at least five of a list of clinical features are present for at least two weeks and represent a change from normal functioning. Symptoms 'clearly' due to a physical disorder or mood incongruent psychosis are to be excluded.

DSM–IV criteria for a *depressive episode* require a depressive syndrome sufficient to cause clinically significant distress or impairment in functioning. They exclude cases where the syndrome is induced by a substance (e.g. a drug of abuse or a medication) or by an organic factor, or is part of normal bereavement.

DSM–IV also gives further criteria which enable descriptions of severity (mild, moderate or severe), of the presence or absence of psychotic features, of the character of any psychotic features (mood congruent or mood incongruent), of the degree of any remission, and of chronicity. These are shown in Box 1.2 (page 29).

DSM–IV allows for the specification of melancholic features, and the criteria for this are shown in Box 1.3 (page 30).

Box 1.1 An outline of DSM–IV criteria for a major depressive syndrome

At least five of the following symptoms during the same two week period. One should be either depressed mood, or loss of interest or pleasure.

(1) Depressed mood most of the day, nearly every day
(2) markedly diminished interest or pleasure in all, or almost all, activities most of the day, nearly every day
(3) significant weight loss or weight gain when not dieting (e.g. more than 5% of body weight in a month), or decrease or increase in appetite nearly every day
(4) insomnia or hypersomnia nearly every day
(5) psychomotor agitation or retardation nearly every day (observable by others)
(6) fatigue or loss of energy nearly every day
(7) feelings of worthlessness or excessive and inappropriate guilt nearly every day
(8) diminished ability to think or concentrate, or indecisiveness, nearly every day
(9) recurrent thoughts of death (not just fear of dying), recurrent suicidal ideation, or a suicide attempt or specific plan.

Adapted with permission from DSM–IV. Copyright 1994 American Psychiatric Association.

In DSM–IV, the move from depressive episodes to bipolar and depressive disorders appears complicated but follows simple rules. If a manic episode has occurred then a current episode of depression is classified as bipolar disorder, most recent episode depressed. If no manic episodes have occurred, then it is classified under the depressive disorders, which are further divided into single episode and recurrent forms. Other criteria specify seasonal pattern (see Box 1.6), atypical features, catatonic features, rapid cycling, and postpartum onset (within four weeks of childbirth).

ICD–10 (World Health Organization, 1992)

The ICD–10 classification follows broadly the same lines as the DSM approach. It is thus a radical departure from ICD–9, finally abandoning the distinction between manic-depressive psychosis and depressive neurosis. Strict operational definitions are confined to a separate set of research criteria, but the descriptive elements are mostly identical to DSM–IV, and the classificatory headings are similar, differing in terminology and organisation rather than in substance. The main points of difference are:

(1) There is a lower threshold for 'mild' depressive episodes in ICD–10 (four symptoms rather than five).
(2) Diagnosis of a depressive episode requires two out of three essential features (sadness, anhedonia, anergia), compared with the one out of two (sadness, anhedonia) required in DSM–IV.
(3) Melancholic features are termed somatic symptoms, and there are several differences in the criteria (see Box 1.3).
(4) Psychotic symptoms include depressive stupor alongside delusions and hallucinations.

Other classifications

Recurrent and nonrecurrent depression

The majority who suffer a single depressive episode will experience further episodes (Angst, 1988). But there may be a distinct sub-group for whom the risk of recurrence is much less. Conversely, those who have had previous episodes show higher risks of further recurrences. Such findings raise the possibility that there may be two distinct subtypes, namely single episode and recurrent depressive disorders. This is reflected in both DSM–IV and ICD–10. If nonrecurrent and recurrent depressive disorders could be identified at first presentation, this would be of great clinical value.

Box 1.2 An outline of DSM–IV criteria for severity of depressive episode

(1) Mild: five or six symptoms and only minor impairment in occupational functioning or in usual social activities or relationships with others.
(2) Moderate: symptoms or functional impairment between 'mild' and 'severe'.
(3) Severe: without psychotic features: several symptoms in excess of those required to make the diagnosis, and marked impairment of functioning.
(4) With psychotic features: delusions or hallucinations.
   Mood-congruent psychotic features: delusions or hallucinations whose content is entirely consistent with the typical depressive themes of personal inadequacy, guilt, disease, death, nihilism, or deserved punishment.
   Mood-incongruent psychotic features: delusions or hallucinations whose content does not involve typical depressive themes of personal inadequacy, guilt, disease, death, nihilism, or deserved punishment. Included are persecutory delusions (not directly related to depressive themes), thought insertion, thought broadcasting, and delusions of control.
(5) In partial remission: intermediate between "in full remission" and "mild", and no previous dysthymia.
(6) In full remission: no significant signs or symptoms during the past two months.

Specify chronic if the full criteria for a major depressive episode have been met continuously for at least the past two years.

Adapted with permission from DSM–IV. Copyright 1994 American Psychiatric Association.

Persistent disorders: cyclothymia/dysthymia

In Chapter seven of *Manic-Depressive Insanity*, Kraepelin identified four fundamental states which he regarded as "permanently slighter" forms of the disorder. These were expressed in the forms of depressive, manic, irritable, and cyclothymic 'temperaments'. He believed that these occurred in about one third of his manic-depressive patients, and that they provided evidence of the illness even during the 'free' intervals between attacks. He also maintained that such states occurred in others who had never displayed an attack.

Box 1.3 A comparison of DSM–IV criteria for specifying melancholic features with ICD–10 criteria for somatic symptoms

DSM–IV
During the most severe period of the current episode, either
(1) loss of interest or pleasure in almost all activities
or:
(2) lack of reactivity to usually pleasurable stimuli
and at least three of the following:
(3) early morning awakening (at least two hours before usual)
(4) depression regularly worse in the morning
(5) marked objective psychomotor retardation or agitation
(6) significant anorexia or weight loss
(7) distinct quality of depressed mood
(8) excessive or inappropriate guilt.

ICD–10
At least four of the following:
(1) marked loss of interest or pleasure
(2) loss of emotional reactions
(3) waking in the morning two hours or more before usual time
(4) depression worse in the morning
(5) objective evidence of marked psychomotor retardation or agitation
(6) marked loss of appetite
(7) weight loss (5% or more of body weight in the past month)
(8) loss of libido.

Adapted with permission from DSM–IV. Copyright 1994 American Psychiatric Association.

Two of these fundamental states are to be found in modern classifications, depressive 'temperament' appearing as dysthymia, with cyclothymia appearing unchanged. DSM–IV criteria are given in Boxes 1.4 and 1.5. There is no uniformity now as how to regard these disorders, though they probably include a mixture of sub-clinical mood disorders, chronic reactions to adverse circumstances, partial remissions of mood episodes, and disorders of personality structure (Akiskal, 1983). The term "double depression" has been coined to describe a depressive episode occurring against the background of dysthymia (Keller & Shapiro, 1983).

Dysthymia is common, with an onset typically in adolescence or early adult life, and can give rise to considerable subjective distress and disability. There is evidence of familial aggregation with other depressive disorders, and women are more commonly affected than men.

Box 1.4 An outline of DSM–IV criteria for dysthymia

(1) Depressed mood for most of the day, more days than not, as indicated either by subjective account or observation, for at least two years.
(2) Presence, while depressed, of at least two of the following:
    (a) poor appetite or overeating
    (b) insomnia or hypersomnia
    (c) low energy or fatigue
    (d) low self-esteem
    (e) poor concentration or difficulty making decisions
    (f) feelings of hopelessness.
(3) During a two-year period of the disturbance, never without the symptoms in (1) and (2) for more than two months at a time.
(4) No major depressive episode during the first two years of the disturbance.
(5) Has never had a manic or hypomanic episode, or met criteria for cyclothymia.
(6) Not exclusively during the course of a chronic psychotic disorder, such as schizophrenia or delusional disorder.
(7) The symptoms are not due to direct physiological effects of a substance or general medical condition.
(8) The symptoms cause clinically significant distress or impaired functioning.

Early onset: before age 21.
Late onset: at age 21 or later.

Adapted with permission from DSM–IV. Copyright 1994 American Psychiatric Association.

Cyclothymia typically begins early and shows a chronic course. Its lifetime prevalence has been estimated as between 0.4% and 3.5%, with men and women equally affected. There is a familial aggregation with both unipolar and bipolar disorders, and some of those with cyclothymia go on to develop frank bipolar illnesses. Mood swings are typically unrelated to life events, and cyclothymia may be difficult to diagnose without prolonged assessment or an exceptionally good account of previous behaviour. Psychoactive substance abuse is a frequent concomitant.

Recurrent brief depressive disorder

Not all episodes of depression last for two weeks or more, some remit after just a few days. Thus, while some brief episodes can meet criteria for mild,

---

Box 1.5 An outline of DSM–IV criteria for cyclothymia

(1) For at least two years: numerous hypomanic episodes, and numerous periods with depressive symptoms that did not meet criteria for a major depressive episode.

(2) During the same two-year period, never without hypomanic or depressive symptoms for more than two months at a time.

(3) No major depressive, mixed or manic episode during the first two years of the disturbance.

(4) The symptoms in (1) are not better accounted for by schizo-affective disorder and are not superimposed on a chronic psychotic disorder, such as schizophrenia or delusional disorder.

(5) The symptoms are not due to direct physiological effects of a substance or general medical condition.

(6) The symptoms cause clinically significant distress or impaired functioning.

Adapted with permission from DSM–IV. Copyright 1994 American Psychiatric Association.

---

moderate or even severe depressive syndromes, they may fail to be classified as major depressive episodes because of their short duration. When such brief depressions recur frequently the cumulative morbidity may be very significant. There has been a growing recognition of the extent of this morbidity, and recurrent brief depressive disorder has been found to be common (Angst *et al*, 1990). As a result, criteria for its definition are included in ICD–10. These require brief depressive episodes to occur at least once a month over the previous year, and not solely in relation to the menstrual cycle. In contrast to dysthymia, patients with recurrent brief depressive disorder are not depressed most of the time. Taken together, dysthymia and recurrent brief depressive disorder encompass most of those disorders previously categorised as depressive neurosis or minor depression. The earlier terms, 'neurosis' and 'minor' have been abandoned now because of their unreliable application in both clinical practice and research.

Seasonality: seasonal affective disorder

For over 2000 years there has been speculation about seasonal influences on the incidence of mania and melancholia, and in particular about the possible connection between the winter months and depression. Broadly based epidemiological studies have shown at best only mild seasonal peaks which explain very little of the variance in incidence rates (Angst, 1988). However most clinicians are aware of individual patients whose bipolar illnesses or recurrent depressive illnesses show a remarkably consistent seasonal pattern, and it is possible that such patients constitute a significant sub-type of the mood disorders. During the decade 1980–90 this idea received a major impetus from the finding that patients with winter depression may respond to a specific treatment, phototherapy. As a result criteria for seasonal pattern were incorporated into DSM–III–R, and these have been modified in DSM–IV (see Box 1.6).

Summer and winter depressions have been recognised, but it is winter depression that has been most studied, and popularised as seasonal affective disorder (SAD) (Wehr & Rosenthal, 1989). Patients with SAD typically describe lowered levels of energy and activity, anxiety, dysphoria and irritability, impaired concentration, social withdrawal and decreased libido. Most also report a distinctive constellation of symptoms which include hypersomnia, increased appetite and over-eating, and carbohydrate craving. Most are mild to moderate in severity but a significant number (11% in one series) require in-patient treatment. In Washington DC, at latitude 38.9, the illness has been reported as beginning in November when the hours of daylight fall below ten. Untreated episodes usually resolve by springtime and some sufferers report mild euphoria and increased levels of energy, activity and libido, with decreased need for sleep in the summer months. Most meet the criteria only for unipolar disorders, some meet bipolar II criteria and very occasionally bipolar I disorders are found. Over 50% of sufferers report a history of an affective disorder in at least one first degree relative.

About one half of patients studied have shown a clinically significant response to a week of treatment with bright light. Response has been

---

Box 1.6 An outline of DSM–IV criteria for seasonal pattern

(1) There has been a regular temporal relationship between the onset of an episode and a particular time of the year, and this is not obviously due to seasonal-related psychosocial stresses.
(2) Full remissions (or a change from depression to mania or hypomania) also occur at a particular time of the year.
(3) In the last two years, two episodes have occurred as in (1) and (2), and no non-seasonal episodes have occurred.
(4) Seasonal major depressive episodes, as described above, outnumber all non-seasonal episodes.

shown to depend both on the intensity of light and its duration. 2500 lux for two hours daily is recommended, but briefer, and proportionately more intense light may be equally effective. Morning treatment may be better. It has been found that exposure of the patient's eyes to the bright light is important, absorption by the skin alone is much less effective. Patients who respond are usually advised to continue light treatment until the springtime, and prophylactic treatment beginning in the autumn has been advocated. Conventional antidepressant treatments have also been reported to be effective in SAD. There were early hopes that the seasonal pattern and response to phototherapy could be explained in terms of changes in melatonin secretion, but attempts to explore such hypotheses have been disappointing.

Agitated and retarded depression

There has been a traditional distinction between cases with prominent agitation and those with prominent retardation. This has encouraged polarisation: "Is this agitated or retarded depression?", and has led to neglect of the fact that these two phenomena can co-exist. RDC subtypes of agitated and retarded major depression have failed to meet validating criteria, and the distinction has been dropped from later classifications. However it is still used clinically in cases where phenomena are very striking. Both agitation and retardation are important components of the criteria for melancholic features and somatic symptoms. There has recently been renewed interest in the phenomenon of retardation as a possible predictor of response to ECT and subsequent bipolarity.

Involutional melancholia

This term was used by Kraepelin to describe the clinical picture of depression occurring in late middle-age with agitated and often hypochondriacal features on the background of a personality with obsessional features. It has been shown repeatedly not to meet validating criteria and is now obsolete. Interestingly, Kraepelin abandoned it in later editions of his textbook.

Primary and secondary depression

This distinction is widely accepted in the United States, but has been received with less enthusiasm in the UK. The rationale for its introduction was to enable the definition of more homogeneous groups of depressive disorders for research purposes. Primary depressions are those not preceded by any other psychiatric disorder (or some physical disorders in early versions of the primary/secondary criteria). The division has been made less relevant by the clear distinctions between syndrome, episode and disorder in the DSM approach. Validating evidence for the distinction is weak, and it appears to many clinicians to be of limited use.

Classification on the basis of family history

One of the best ways of resolving the problem of classifying depressive disorders would be to demonstrate genetic heterogeneity. There have been tantalising glimpses of this possibility. Winokur and colleagues (1971) distinguished two groups on the basis of age of onset. The first, with age of onset before 40, comprised predominantly of females. This group showed a higher incidence of alcoholism and sociopathy in male relatives, and a higher incidence of depression in female relatives. The second group showed a predominance of males with a family history of depressive disorders alone. On this basis, he and co-workers proposed a division into those with a family history of depression alone (pure depressive disease), those with a history of alcoholism or sociopathy in first degree relatives (depressive spectrum disease), and 'non-genetic' cases (sporadic depressive disease). This subdivision has received some support with findings of neuroendocrine and treatment correlates, but attempts at replication have been inconsistent, so that Winokur's classification has not yet been widely adopted. Recent developments in molecular genetics have opened up new horizons for similar strategies, but as yet no practical classification has emerged.

A unitary psychosis?

In the late 19th century Kraepelin distinguished manic depressive insanity from dementia praecox on the basis of long-term course, and argued that here were two separate disorders with distinct pathophysiologies. This has been very widely accepted as an advance on previous views such as that of Griesinger (1861) who saw all psychiatric disorders as successive symptom clusters reflecting the oscillations of a vital principle. Nevertheless there remain those who argue that all psychoses do have a common basis. In the late 20th century Crowe (1991), amongst others, has assembled genetic evidence inviting us to revisit this controversy.

Measurement

The severity of a depressive syndrome depends on the number of symptoms, their intensity, their frequency, their duration and their pervasiveness. Subjective distress and impairments in functioning are also relevant. Not all of these factors co-vary and some may be negatively correlated. Despite this, experienced clinicians and their patients are able to make global assessments of severity which correlate surprisingly well.

An example of guidelines for global assessment is given in the DSM–IV criteria for distinguishing mild, moderate and severe depressive episodes (see Box 1.2).

Most scientific approaches to the measurement of depression involve rating instruments. These are of two types. Observer ratings involve an examination of the subject, and ratings are completed by the interviewer. Self-ratings are made directly by the subject. While self-rating scales are more economical and are therefore useful for large scale surveys, they have disadvantages, with milder depressives tending to overrate their symptoms and psychotic depressives under-rating themselves. Good scales show test–retest and inter-rater reliability and have face validity, predictive validity and internal consistency (see chapter 26). Data should be available for normative populations and to enable comparison with other instruments. Effective scales are short, clear and easy to administer, but if they are too short then reliability is sacrificed.

Hamilton Depression Rating Scale (Hamilton, 1960)

After over 30 years of use, this is still the most popular observer rating scale for measuring the severity of depression. It meets most of the above criteria, except that some have criticised it for being too long. Seventeen items are rated on scales of either 0–4 or 0–2, using a clinical interview and all available information. The assessment refers to the previous one to two weeks, and this limits its usefulness as a repeated measure of progress. Some argue that it is biased towards biological features of depression; over half of the 17 items relate to either anxiety, somatic features, or insomnia. Nevertheless it remains for many the instrument of choice for rating severity in those diagnosed as suffering from a depressive episode. The accuracy of other scales is often tested by the strength of their correlation with the Hamilton Scale.

Montgomery–Åsberg Depression Rating Scale (MADRS; Montgomery & Åsberg, 1979)

This shorter observer rating scale was derived from the Scandinavian comprehensive psychiatric rating scale. Ten items were selected as the most sensitive to change in depressed patients responding to treatment. It satisfies most of the above criteria and although it also requires a clinical interview, it is in theory easier to administer than the Hamilton, and can be completed in under 20 minutes. It is widely used to measure change in depressed patients.

Beck Depression Inventory (Beck *et al,* 1961)

The BDI is probably the best known self-rating scale for depression, and it too has retained its popularity for over 30 years. It was designed to be read to the subject who chose from set responses. In this way it overcame the main objection to self-rating scales, namely the uncertainty that the subject is following the instructions correctly. Now it is usually given in a self-report form. It satisfies most criteria mentioned above, but lacks discriminatory power amongst very severely ill depressives. In contrast to the Hamilton scale, all but six of the 21 items relate to psychological phenomena. It can be repeated after short intervals and can be seen as complementary to the Hamilton and MADRS.

Zung Self-rating Depression Scale (Zung, 1965)

This 20 item self-rating scale avoided the imbalance towards psychological phenomena found in the BDI, and also took steps to avoid response bias. Its widespread use has declined following reports of poor correlations with observer ratings and insensitivity to change during treatment response.

Wakefield Self-assessment Inventory and Leeds Scale (Snaith *et al,* 1971 & 1976)

The Wakefield Inventory was developed as an improvement on the Zung Scale. It comprises 12 self-rating items carefully constructed to avoid response bias. Whilst it has proved useful to screen for depressive symptoms it was limited in its ability to discriminate between different degrees of severity. It has been superceded by the Leeds Scale, which was derived from it but also includes an anxiety scale. The depressive sub-scale of the Leeds scale is reported to have overcome the problems of its predecessor.

Visual Analogue Scale (Zealley & Aitken, 1969)

This is one of the easiest ways of estimating global severity or the severity of individual symptoms. The rating can be made by either the clinician or subject. A 10 cm line is drawn and the end points are identified as the extremes of the phenomena to be measured. When rating sadness the end points might be 'not sad at all' and 'as sad as I can imagine'. The rater makes a mark at the point on the line that best represents the present state. Despite its simplicity, this technique can produce useful information that correlates well with more sophisticated instruments. It is very useful for making repeated measures of a rapidly changing phenomenon such as diurnal variation in mood. One drawback is that ratings suffer from contrast effects, rapid changes being rated higher than slower ones.

Course and outcome

In *The Anatomy of Melancholy*, Burton devoted most of his chapter on 'prognostics' to suicide. Suicide does remain "the greatest, most grievous calamity" which is "a frequent thing and familiar" amongst depressives, and is "the doom of all physicians" (Burton, 1621). It is considered in chapter 12 in this volume.

Regarding course and outcome, Burton quoted Montanus:

> "This malady doth commonly accompany them to the grave: Physicians may ease it, and it may lay hid for a while, but they cannot quite cure it, but it will return again more violent and sharp than at first."

Three hundred years later, a more optimistic perspective was provided by Kraepelin who separated manic depressive insanity from dementia praecox on the grounds that it was a 'remitting' disorder.

Throughout most of the 20th century an optimistic view held sway, despite follow up studies in the first three decades which catalogued an impressive array of long-term morbidity and mortality (e.g. Poort, 1945). The advent of modern 'effective' treatments, and the promising results of short-term therapeutic trials reinforced the optimism and it was widely assumed that the prognosis of depressive illnesses had improved. However, few of the therapeutic trials lasted longer than two years, so that if later recurrence and long-term chronicity were a feature of the natural history of depressive disorders, it would rarely have been recorded. Recent long-term follow up studies of depressed in-patients (Kiloh *et al*, 1988; Lee & Murray, 1988) have revealed a picture similar to that found in the pre-treatment era. These studies, taken together with prospective studies showing cumulatively high rates of relapse and failure to recover (Keller *et al*, 1986), have led to a less sanguine, but perhaps more realistic appraisal of the serious long-term import of a severe depressive illness.

Clinical prognosis studies

Knowledge of the course and outcome of psychiatric disorders is gained by combining clinical experience with the findings of clinical prognosis studies. Ideally, the follow up of a typical cohort of sufferers will allow useful estimation of the rates at which patients recover, of the likelihood of recurrence, of the chances of chronicity and other complications, and of the risks of increased mortality from suicide and other causes.

While shorter-term follow up studies (one to seven years) give a fairly accurate picture of recovery and early relapse, they underestimate recovery amongst apparently chronic patients. More importantly, they also underplay the long term risks of recurrence. Longer follow up studies give a clearer picture of the life-time impact of a disorder, by showing the risks of poor outcome due to repeated recurrences, cumulative chronicity, accumulating secondary handicaps, and the evolution of secondary disorders. While such long-term studies will almost certainly be naturalistic, that is subjects will be followed with no attempt to control for treatments, this may have the advantage of giving a clearer picture of the likely ranges of outcomes under normal clinical conditions.

A well designed follow up study will prospectively ascertain a representative cohort, make diagnoses according to well established criteria, and will follow this series closely and comprehensively. Outcomes will be established according to clearly defined criteria, and analyses will use actuarial techniques in order to allow for deaths and patients lost to follow up. There should be sufficient numbers to allow for generalisable findings, but not so many that intensive follow up becomes impossible. Where predictors of outcome are sought, then the follow up examinations should be conducted blind to initial assessments. These are the requirements for a perfect clinical prognostic study, and not surprisingly there are very few, if any, long-term investigations that can fulfil them all.

In an 18 year follow up of a consecutive series of 89 Maudsley in-patients prospectively ascertained and diagnosed with primary depressive illnesses by R E Kendell in 1965–66, we were fortunate to be able to trace all except one of the series in 1983–84, to personally interview 94% of the survivors with standardised research instruments and to establish corroborated outcome data for 98% of the series (Lee & Murray, 1988). We found that less than one fifth of the survivors had remained well and over one third had suffered unnatural death or chronic severe distress and handicap. The vital importance of comprehensive follow up was emphasised by the finding that over half of the severely ill survivors were out of contact with mental health services and that many of these were amongst the most difficult to trace. Some of our doubts as to the representativeness of the Maudsley series were allayed by the simultaneous publication of an 18 year follow up of a consecutive series of depressed in-patients from Sydney, Australia which reported very similar, although perhaps slightly less gloomy, findings (Kiloh *et al*, 1988).

Outcome of depressive disorders: recovery

Kraepelin (1921) described depressive episodes which ranged in length from days to more than a decade. Illnesses lasting several years were very common. Since 1945 the median length of depressive episodes has fallen to six months. Recovery rates are often thought to depend on severity of illness, but there has been no convincing demonstration that out-patients recover at different rates to in-patients (Angst, 1988).

In the early months of an episode the cumulative likelihood of recovery rises quickly, so that by six months about half of episodes have remitted. By two years about three-quarters have remitted, and the remainder are classified as chronic. Chronic depressive episodes continue to remit slowly, so that by five years a further 15% of the initial cohort will have recovered, making 90% in all. The remaining 10% may show very prolonged episodes but the chances of eventual remission never disappear entirely. In our Maudsley series of 89 patients, ten showed unremitting depressive episodes at 15 years, but one of these recovered dramatically in the 16th year.

Recovery has been shown to be faster in bipolar patients and in melancholic episodes. Secondary depressive episodes tend to be slower to remit, although successful treatment of underlying disorders can lead to rapid recovery. The presence of hallucinations or delusions predicts a slower recovery as do neurotic personality traits, as shown by high neuroticism scores on testing with the Eysenck Personality Inventory during or after the episode. Mood incongruent features and hypochondriacal symptoms have also been shown to predict slower recovery. Whilst the pattern of previous episodes is a useful guide to future course, this can be misleading as a recurrent disorder with short episodes can unexpectedly become chronic.

The bodily symptoms of depression may remit more rapidly than the cognitive ones such as pessimism and low self-esteem. Cognitive distortions can be persistent and troublesome, as may continuing phobic avoidance, obsessional features, and impairments of concentration. Many symptoms remit in a gradual and fluctuating way which can be very disheartening to sufferers who fear that they are never going to make a full recovery. Social impairments may also persist with loss of confidence, social withdrawal, and difficulties both at work and in personal relationships. These social changes are sometimes found even where there is complete symptomatic remission. Most experts agree that about a quarter of all apparently recovered depressives show significant and enduring residual problems of one kind or another.

Recurrence

Many of those who recover from a depressive episode experience a recurrence. Recurrence rates are best described using survival analysis, a technique borrowed from the life table approach used by insurance companies. There are two phases to the cumulative risk of recurrence, the first occurring within a few months and understandable as a re-emergence of the original episode. It has been proposed that the term 'relapse' be kept for this, whilst 'recurrence' be used for those cases where a new episode of illness occurs after a longer period of full remission. As many as one third of depressive episodes may show the phenomenon of relapse.

Estimates of recurrence rates vary depending on the samples studied, and the length of follow-up. Most community studies show life time risks of around 50%, but Angst (1988) has argued that this may be an underestimate, and that if followed long enough and closely enough virtually all moderate and severe depressive episodes will lead to recurrence. Risk is increased in those with previous recurrences, an earlier age of onset, in bipolar patients, and in the melancholic sub-type. Our own study of depressed Maudsley in-patients found 95% had shown at least one recurrence after 18 years, whilst 60% had required re-admission. Those with recurrent melancholia had an 85% likelihood of re-admission by 18 years, and a 50% risk of re-admission within two years. Kiloh *et al* (1988) in Sydney also found 50% of those with recurrent melancholia re-admitted within two years. Figures such as these suggest that for some depressed people little may have changed since Burton's quotation from Montanus.

Very poor global outcome

Very poor long-term outcome can result from a failure to recover, or from an interaction between residual symptoms and secondary handicaps such as unemployment, divorce and social isolation. Alcoholism may be a complicating factor. A very small number of sufferers also develop chronic schizophrenic illnesses, or chronic paranoid states, and very occasionally a chronic defect state occurs without other schizophrenic symptomatology. In our Maudsley series a quarter of the survivors showed one or other of these various forms of very poor outcome after 18 years. Those with very poor outcome fell into two groups, the divorced and single who had multiple hospital admissions, and those with very unhappy marriages, few admissions and a relative isolation from mental health services. We found that an index diagnosis of melancholia was strongly predictive of very poor outcome in the long term, despite the fact that it had predicted good outcome in the shorter term. This finding has not yet been replicated.

There is an increasing consensus for the DSM–IV definition of chronicity, that is an episode lasting longer than two years. The cumulative risk of such chronicity may be as high as one in three (Keller *et al*, 1986). Factors predicting chronicity are outlined above as being associated with slower recovery. A positive family history, previous episodes, accumulating life events, and thyroid disorder in women have also been implicated (Scott, 1988).

Mortality

The risk of mortality for depressive in-patients is doubled (Tsuang & Woolson, 1977), due both to suicide and to an increased risk of physical disorders especially arteriosclerotic and other vascular disorders (Angst, 1988). Several studies have linked depressive episodes to the later development of auto-immune and neoplastic disease, but findings have as yet been inconclusive. Fifteen per cent of in-patient depressives eventually end their lives by suicide (Guze & Robins, 1970), and whilst most of these suicides occur outside hospital, the risk is at its highest in the two years following discharge. The increased risk of suicide in less severely ill out-patients may be confined to those who show comorbid alcoholism or disorders of personality (Martin *et al*, 1985) but this finding has not yet been replicated.

Switches from unipolar to bipolar disorder

One in ten of those who begin with a depressive episode go on to develop an episode of mania. The likelihood of such a switch drops markedly after the third episode of depression, by which time more than two-thirds of those who will show a bipolar disorder have already done so. Research criteria for unipolar disorder were initially set on this basis to require three episodes of depression, but these are now often relaxed to two episodes, which allows for the inclusion of less frequently recurring disorders. The two main predictors of a switch from depressive to bipolar episodes are an early age of onset, and a family history of bipolar disorder. Other predictive factors include retardation, hypersomnia, hypomania precipitated by antidepressants, melancholia, delusions and hallucinations, and occurrence in the year after childbirth (Jablensky, 1987).

Differences in course and outcome between unipolar and bipolar disorders

There are surprisingly few differences, but those which exist are clear cut. Bipolar disorders tend to begin at an earlier age, and have shorter illnesses (with a median duration of four months) but more frequent recurrences. There appear to be no differences in rates of recovery, chronicity, suicide or overall mortality. After onset, the average proportion of lifetime spent ill has been estimated as 20% for both bipolar and unipolar patients (Angst, 1988). Outcomes amongst bipolar patients tend to be either very good or very poor. Mixed episodes and rapidly cycling disorders (four or more episodes in a year) are more likely to develop very poor outcomes, but otherwise there are no reliable predictors amongst bipolar patients.

Prognosis for the individual patient

The best predictions of future course are often based on knowledge of the individual's past illnesses. Clinicians will also weigh the predictive factors outlined above, and consider the personal strengths and vulnerabilities of their patients alongside the continuing supports and stresses in their environment. Maintaining factors and further life events will contribute to delays in recovery. Vulnerability factors such as unemployment and lack of a confiding relationship will increase the risk of recurrence. Therapeutic factors are also very important. Delays in adequate treatment are strongly associated with chronicity. Outcome may very much depend on the depressed person's compliance, and on whether adequate biomedical and psychosocial measures are available, both for immediate treatment, and for prophylaxis in recurrent disorders. One consistent finding of recent follow-up studies has been the discovery of many chronically depressed people who have been severely disabled for many years but who no longer seek or receive psychiatric help. The recognition of this need and its extent may well present psychiatric services with one of the major public health challenges for the future.

Bereavement

"The chambers of the mansion of my heart, in every one whereof thine image dwells, are black with grief eternal for thy sake." (James Thomson, 1932)

Human grief is universal, and many experiences which are familiar to the bereaved overlap with clinical features of depression. In *Mourning and Melancholia* (1917) Sigmund Freud based an aetiological theory of depression on these similarities. This was the first of many models of the processes of mourning which have drawn on such diverse perspectives as psychoanalysis, behaviourism, ethology, social anthropology and developmental psychology. Of these, attachment theory (Bowlby, 1982) has proved to have an exceptional degree of explanatory power. Bowlby's work has been very influential in shaping thinking about the extremely painful process of adjusting to the death of a loved person.

There are few widely agreed criteria or definitions, but a useful distinction can be made between the situation of bereavement, the process of mourning and the experiences of grief. Bereavement describes the situation of having lost someone significant through their death. Mourning is the process of adjusting to bereavement. Grief refers to the personal experience of mourning. Amongst the bereaved there are very wide cultural variations in the practices and rituals of mourning. These are both derived from, and serve to reinforce, existing religious and social conventions. By contrast, many of the phenomena of grief are ubiquitous, for example weeping and feelings of painful sadness occur throughout the world.

Uncomplicated mourning

Many authors have attempted to describe stages in the mourning process. These have varied in emphasis depending on theoretical assumptions. One very influential account has been that of Lindemann (1944), who described the phenomenology of normal grief in 101 bereaved subjects.

Robertson & Bowlby's (1952) observations of two- to three-year-old children temporarily separated from their mothers has also been widely quoted, so that many accounts of mourning invoke a progression from preoccupation and protest, through despair towards detachment.

One of the best syntheses of different models is that of Brown and Stoudemire (1983) who combine the work of Lindemann, Bowlby, Parkes and Greenblatt. Three phases are distinguished, characterised by (1) shock, (2) preoccupation with the deceased, and (3) resolution. In the first phase of shock, intense mental and somatic distress is defended against by mechanisms of numbing, denial and disbelief, with associated feelings of depersonalisation and derealisation. Those affected may appear dazed or immobile. They will often describe intermittent feelings of intensely distressing mental pain, tension and anxiety, which may be experienced as tightness in the throat, choking with shortness of breath, a need for sighing, empty feelings in the abdomen or a lack of muscular power.

After a period of usually between one and 14 days, the first stage of shock evolves into a second stage of intense preoccupation with the deceased. More structured phenomena of separation occur, such as pining and yearning, searching behaviours in the hope of reunion, and anger directed at third parties, the self and the deceased. The bereaved person will spend long periods thinking about the deceased and will dream frequently of them. One person in ten will report brief hallucinatory experiences. Past conflicts will be reviewed and intense guilt will be experienced by at least one person in three. Mechanisms of identification may be evidenced by the appearance of traits and activities of the deceased.

The second phase is also characterised by social withdrawal and a range of fluctuating depressive symptoms including sadness, anhedonia, fatigue, insomnia and anorexia. The tasks of this second phase of the mourning process have been described as reliving memories, working through feelings, reparation, and gradually restructuring the representation of the lost person from one of reality to one of memory. This process of internalisation involves a freeing of the self from the bondage of the deceased, and the formation of a new adjustment to the environment.

Over a period of months to years, this process gradually merges into a third and final phase characterised by a subjective feeling of acceptance, the capacity to remember the deceased without excessive pain, and a reorganisation of life towards the possibility of new attachments. Phenomena from the second phase may sometimes re-emerge, and these are often more sharply focused at times of significant anniversaries.

Relationship with depressive disorders

Although clinical depression and mourning share many phenomena, and the boundary between them is not always clear, this does not imply that they are the same syndrome. Clayton & Darvish (1979) found that 42% of bereaved spouses examined at one month showed sufficient depressive symptoms to meet Feighner Criteria for a depressive episode. By one year this figure had fallen to 15%. There are many who believe that those who meet criteria for a depressive episode are better understood and treated in the same way as others whose depressive episodes have been precipitated by different major life events. Others feel that they may be better understood and managed using models of the mourning process. There is continuing controversy surrounding this issue. Parkes (1985) and others have described features which may distinguish normal mourning and secondary depressive disorders. Pangs of grief, angry pining, anxiety when confronted by reminders of loss, brief hallucinations, somatic symptoms and identification-related behaviours all point to normal mourning. The presence of retardation, generalised guilt and suicidal thoughts after the first month all suggest a secondary depressive disorder. DSM–IV criteria advise against the diagnosis of a depressive episode in the first two months unless there is marked functional impairment or severe symptoms including worthlessness, suicidal ideation, psychotic symptoms, or retardation.

Complicated mourning

The development of a depressive episode is only one of the ways in which mourning can be complicated. Compared with normal cultural patterns, mourning can be absent, delayed or abnormally prolonged, and may show unusual behaviours such as extreme preoccupation with the deceased. There may be excessive identification with, or idealisation of, the lost person. Patterns of extreme denial, avoidance, and compulsive self-reliance can emerge. Health related behaviours such as smoking and drinking alcohol may increase to pathological levels. Mourning may be further complicated by secondary physical and other psychological disorders which in turn may modify and colour the experience of grief. Several studies have shown widowers to have increased risks of death, particularly from cardiovascular disorders, in the year following bereavement.

Risk factors for complicated mourning

Freud (1917) predicted that mourning would be complicated by depression in those with a harsh superego, those who had chosen their loved ones on the basis of narcissism, and those whose relationships were marked by intense ambivalence. Bowlby (1982) observed that the loss of ambivalently loved persons was often consistent with healthy mourning. Bowlby's theory stressed the role of anxious attachments to parents as precursors of insecure adult relationships and subsequent difficulties in negotiating mourning. In this way overdependence might lead to chronic grief whilst patterns of compulsive self-reliance would result in the denial of loss and the delayed onset of grief. Parkes (1985) identified clinging behaviours and inordinate pining as early signs of prolonged grief.

Other factors which have been suggested as increasing the risks of complicated grief include a sudden, unexpected or untimely bereavement, potentially stigmatised losses such as abortions, suicides and deaths from AIDS, and deaths where the bereaved may be held to be to blame. Violent or severely traumatic deaths may induce symptoms in the bereaved which resemble those of post traumatic stress disorder. Multiple losses and deaths resulting from negligence appear to be very hard to negotiate. Mourning may also be complicated if previous losses remain unresolved, and in the presence of pre-existing physical and mental health problems. Low socio-economic status, lack of social support, absence of contact with organised religion and the need to care for dependent children are also risk factors.

The loss of a child has been shown to result in more intense levels of grief, greater somatisation and an increased risk of secondary depressive disorders. Feelings of guilt and powerlessness are common. The outcome may be increasing marital stresses, overprotection of other children, idealisation of the lost child or unreal expectations of a replacement child.

The loss of a spouse may bring with it many practical problems. These include increased responsibilities for dependent children, financial hardship, and social isolation. Persisting sexual feelings can cause frustration, conflict and guilt. Elderly people who lose their partners may be particularly vulnerable to social isolation and the loss of support and care. Those bereaved after a lifetime together commonly experience extremely prolonged feelings of grief.

The death of an elderly parent seems to be the least likely form of bereavement to result in complicated mourning. Painful but healthy grief is often followed by a period of increased creativity and fruitful reparation.

Appendix

A practical scheme for diagnosing and describing depression

The convergence of ICD–10 and DSM–IV has made the task of clinicians much easier. It is now possible to diagnose and classify depressive disorders in a way which is descriptive, authoritative, and yet which makes clinical sense.

Firstly, do the clinical phenomena amount to depressive symptoms?

If they do, then are they sufficient to constitute a depressive syndrome?

Can one then exclude other disorders and bereavement, so that one can say that a depressive episode is present?

Is the episode mild, moderate or severe?

Are there psychotic features?

If so are they mood congruent or mood incongruent?

Does the episode show melancholic features (somatic symptoms)?

Are there any other very prominent features (agitation, retardation, panic attacks, obsessional or histrionic features)?

Does the episode show chronicity, having lasted for more than two years?

Is this the only episode, or is the episode part of a recurrent depressive disorder or a bipolar disorder? Is there evidence of a seasonal pattern, rapid cycling or a postpartum onset?

If the depressive symptoms do not amount to a depressive syndrome or episode, is the patient suffering from dysthymia or cyclothymia, or recurrent brief depressive disorder? Or is one seeing a depressive episode in partial remission?

References

Akiskal, H. S. (1983) Dysthymic disorder: psychopathology of proposed chronic depressive subtypes. *American Journal of Psychiatry,* **140,** 11–20.

American Psychiatric Association (1980) *Diagnostic and Statistical Manual of Mental Disorders (3rd edn)* (DSM–III). Washington, DC: APA.

—— (1987) *Diagnostic and Statistical Manual of Mental Disorders (3rd edn, revised)* (DSM–III–R). Washington, DC: APA.

—— (1994) *Diagnostic and Statistical Manual of Mental Disorders (4th edn)* (DSM–IV). Washington, DC: APA.

Angst, J. (1966) *Zur Atiologie und Nosolgie Endogener Depressiver Psychosen.* Monographien aus dem Gesamtgebiete der Neurologie und Psychiatrie. Berlin: Springer.

—— (1988) Clinical course of affective disorders. In *Depressive Illness: Prediction of Course and Outcome* (eds T. Hegalson & R. J. Daly). Berlin: Springer-Verlag.

——, Merikangas, K., Scheidegger, P. *et al* (1990) Recurrent brief depression: a new subtype of affective disorder. *Journal of Affective Disorders,* **19,** 87–98.

Baillarger, J. F. (1854) De la folie a double-forme. *Annales Medico-Psychologiques,* **6,** 367–391.

Beck, A. T., Ward, C. H., Mendelson, M., *et al* (1961) An inventory for measuring depression. *Archives of General Psychiatry,* **4,** 561–571.

Berrios, G. E. (1992) History of the affective disorders. In *Handbook of Affective Disorders* (2nd edn). (ed E. S. Paykel). Edinburgh: Churchill Livingstone.

Bertelsen, A., Harvald, B. & Hauge, M. (1977) A Danish twin study of manic depressive disorders. *British Journal of Psychiatry,* **130,** 330–351.

Bowlby, J. (1982) Attachment and loss: retrospect and prospect. *American Journal of Orthopsychiatry,* **52,** 664–678.

Bright, T. (1586) *A Treatise of Melancholie.* London: Vautrollier.

Brown, J. T. & Stoudemire, G. A. (1983) Normal and pathological grief. *Journal of the American Medical Association*, **250**, 378–382.

Burton, R. (1621) *The Anatomy of Melancholy*. Oxford: Cripps.

Carney, M. W. P., Roth, M. & Garside, R. F. (1965) The diagnosis of depressive syndromes and the prediction of ECT response. *British Journal of Psychiatry*, **111**, 659–674.

Clayton, P. J. & Darvish, H. S. (1979) Course of depressive symptoms following the stress of bereavement. In *Stress and Mental Disorder* (eds J. Barret, R. M. Rose & G. L. Klerman). New York: Raven Press.

Cotard, M. (1882) Du delire de negations. *Archives de Neurologie, Paris*, **4**, 152–170 and 282–296. Translated into English by M. Rohde in *Themes and Variations in European Psychiatry* (eds S. R. Hirsch & M. Shepherd), 353–373. Bristol: Wright.

Crowe, T. J. (1991) The failure of the Kraepelinian binary concept and the search for the psychosis gene. In *Concepts of Mental Disorder* (eds A. Kerr & H. McClelland). London: Gaskell.

Dunner, D. L., Gershon, E. S. & Goodwin, F. K. (1976) Heritable factors in the severity of affective illness. *Biological Psychiatry*, **11**, 31–42.

Falret, J. P. (1854) Memoire sur la folie circulaire. *Bulletin de l'Academie de Medicine* **19**, 382–415. Translated into English by M. J. Sedler & E. C. Dessain (1983). Falret's discovery: the origin of the concept of bipolar affective illness. *American Journal of Psychiatry*, **140**, 1227–1233.

Freud, S. (1917) Mourning and melancholia. *The Standard Edition of the Complete Psychological Works* **14**, 243–258. London: Hogarth Press.

Griesinger, W. (1861) *Die Pathologie und Therapie der Psychischen Krankheiten fur Aerzte und Studierende*. Stuttgart: Adolphe Krabbe.

Guze, S. B. & Robins, E. (1970) Suicide and primary affective disorders. *British Journal of Psychiatry*, **117**, 437–438.

Hamilton, M. (1960) A rating scale for depression. *Journal of Neurology, Neurosurgery and Psychiatry*, **23**, 56–62.

—— (1982) Symptoms and assessment of depression. In *Handbook of Affective Disorders* (1st edn) (ed E. S. Paykel). Edinburgh: Churchill Livingstone.

Holy Bible. Authorised King James Version. (1967) London: Oxford University Press.

Hunter, R. & Macalpine, I. (1963) *Three Hundred Years of Psychiatry 1535–1860*. London: Oxford University Press.

Jablensky, A. (1987) Prediction of the course and outcome of depression. *Psychological Medicine*, **17**, 1–9.

Jaspers, K. (1963) *General Psychopathology*. Translated into English by J. Hoenig & M. W. Hamilton from *Allgemeine Psychopathology*, (7th edn). Manchester: University Press.

Keller, M. B. & Shapiro, R. W. (1983) Double depression: superimposition of acute depressive episodes on chronic depressive disorders. *American Journal of Psychiatry*, **139**, 438–442.

——, Lavorie, W., Rice, J., *et al* (1986) The persistent risk of chronicity in recurrent episodes of nonbipolar major depressive disorder: a prospective follow-up. *American Journal of Psychiatry*, **143**, 24–28.

Kendell, R. E. (1968) *The Classification of Depressive Illnesses*. Maudsley Monograph, No. 18. London: Oxford University Press.

Kendler, K. S. (1991) Mood incongruent psychotic affective illness: a historical and empirical review. *Archives of General Psychiatry*, **48**, 362–369.

Kiloh, L. G., Andrews, G. & Neilson, M. (1988) The long-term outcome of depressive illness. *British Journal of Psychiatry*, **153**, 752–757.

Kraepelin, E. (1921) *Manic Depressive Insanity and Paranoia*. Translated into English by R. M. Barclay from the 8th edn. of *Lehrbuch der Psychiatrie, Vols. III and IV*. Edinburgh: E. & S. Livingstone.

Lee, A. S. & Murray, R. M. (1988) The long-term outcome of Maudsley depressives. *British Journal of Psychiatry*, **153**, 741–751.

Leonhard, K. (1979) *The Classification of Endogenous Psychoses*. Translated into English by R. Berman from the 8th edn. of *Aufteiling der Endogenen Psychosen*. New York: Irvington (1979).

Lewis, A. J. (1934) Melancholia: a clinical survey of depressive states. *Journal of Mental Science*, **80**, 277–278.

—— (1938) States of depression: their clinical and aetiological differentiation. *British Medical Journal*, **ii**, 875–878.

Lindemann, E. (1944) Symptomatology and management of acute grief. *American Journal of Psychiatry*, **101**, 141–148.

Martin, R. L., Cloninger, C. R., Guze, S. B., *et al* (1985) Mortality in a follow-up of 500 psychiatric out-patients. *Archives of General Psychiatry*, **42**, 47–54.

Montgomery, S. A. & Asberg, M. (1979) A new depression scale designed to be sensitive to change. *British Journal of Psychiatry*, **134**, 382–389.

Parkes, C. M. (1985) Bereavement. *British Journal of Psychiatry*, **146**, 11–17.

Paykel, E. S., Rao, B. M. & Taylor, C. N. (1984) Life stress and symptom pattern in out-patient depression. *Psychological Medicine*, **14**, 559–568.

Perris, C. (1966) A study of bipolar (manic depressive) and unipolar recurrent depressive psychoses. *Acta Psychiatrica Scandinavica*, **42**, Suppl. 194.

Poort, R. (1945) Catamnestic investigations on manic-depressive psychoses with special reference to the prognosis. *Acta Psychiatrica et Neurologica*, **20**, 59–74.

Robertson, J. & Bowlby, J. (1952) Responses of young children to separation from their mothers. *Courrier de la Centre Internationale de l'Enfance*, **2**, 131–142.

Scott, J. (1988) Chronic depression. *British Journal of Psychiatry*, **35**, 287–297.

Sedman, G. (1970) Theories of depersonalisation: a re-appraisal. *British Journal of Psychiatry*, **117**, 1–14.

Snaith, R. P. (1987) The concept of mild depression. *British Journal of Psychiatry*, **150**, 387–393.

——, Ahmed, S. N., Mehta, S., *et al* (1971) The assessment of the severity of primary depressive illness. Wakefield Self-Assessment Inventory. *Psychological Medicine*, **1**, 143–149.

——, Bridge, G. W. K. & Hamilton, M. (1976) The Leeds Scales for the self-assessment of anxiety and depression. *British Journal of Psychiatry*, **128**, 156–165.

Spitzer, R. L., Endicott J. & Robins, E. (1978) Research diagnostic criteria: rationale and reliability. *Archives of General Psychiatry*, **35**, 773–782.

Stengel, E. (1945) A study of some clinical aspects of the relationship between obsessional neurosis and psychotic reaction types. *Journal of Mental Science*, **91**, 166–187.

Styron, W. (1991) *Darkness Visible*. London: Jonathan Cape.

Thomson, J. (1932) *The City of the Dreadful Night*. London: Methuen.

Tsuang, M. T. & Woolson, R. F. (1977) Mortality in patients with schizophrenia, mania, depression and surgical conditions: a comparison with general population mortality. *British Journal of Psychiatry*, **130**, 162–166.

Wehr, T. A. & Rosenthal, N. E. (1989) Seasonality and affective illness. *American Journal of Psychiatry*, **146**, 829–839.

Wing, J. K., Cooper, J. E. & Sartorius, N. (1974) *Measurement and Classification of Psychiatric Symptoms*. Cambridge: University Press.

Winokur, G., Cardoret, R., Dorzab, J., *et al* (1971) Depressive disease: a genetic study. *Archives of General Psychiatry*, **24**, 135–144.

World Health Organization (1978) *Mental Disorders: Glossary and Guide to their Classification in Accordance with the Ninth Revision of the International Classification of Diseases*. Geneva: WHO.

—— (1992) *The Tenth Revision of the International Classification of Diseases and Related Health Problems (ICD–10)*. Geneva: WHO.

Zealley, A. K. & Aitken, R. C. P. (1969) Measurement of Mood. *Proceedings of The Royal Society of Medicine*, **62**, 993–996.

Zung, W. W. K. (1965) A self-rating depression scale. *Archives of General Psychiatry*, **12**, 63–70.

2 Mania, bipolar disorder and treatment

John Cookson

Diagnostic criteria • *Classification* • *Course* • *Psychosocial factors* •
Treatment of mania • *Lithium* • *Carbamazepine* • *Other treatments* •
Prophylaxis of bipolar disorder • *Alternatives to lithium* • *The
psychology of mania*

The writers of ancient Greece used the terms mania and melancholia
to include what we now regard as mania, but also a broader grouping
of mental disorders. Hippocrates (4th to 5th century BC) argued that
such disorders were due to physical (humoral) imbalance and not
to supernatural forces. Aretaeus of Cappodocia (2nd century AD)
was probably the first to see mania and depression as manifestations
of the same disorder. With the dominance of the monasteries in
Europe in the Middle Ages, mental illness was attributed to sin or
supernatural forces, until clinical science began to re-emerge in the
17th century.

Falret who described *folie circulaire* and Baillarger who described
folie a double forme in 1854 recognised that mania and depression could
occur in the same episode of illness. Kahlbaum (1874) described
cyclothymia, and the association between states of excitement resembling
mania, and catatonia. Kraepelin, basing his views upon both the pattern
of symptoms and the longitudinal course, evolved the concept of manic-
depressive insanity (1889), and distinguished it from dementia praecox
(1921). Bleuler (1920) used the term 'affective illness' to describe the
condition.

Diagnostic criteria

The manic syndrome is one of the most clearly defined in psychiatry, but
the diagnosis is frequently missed, or mistaken for schizophrenia or
personality disorder (see Horgan, 1981). Box 2.1 shows the inclusion
criteria for the diagnosis according to DSM–IV (American Psychiatric
Association, 1994).

The majority of patients exhibit all the listed symptoms, although hyper-
sexuality, flight of ideas, and distractibility are less frequent, and fewer
patients have delusions or hallucinations.

Box 2.1   DSM–IV diagnostic criteria for mania

(i)   Distinct period of elation, irritability or mood disturbances lasting at least one week (or for any period of hospital-isation)

(ii)   Three of the following:
inflated self-esteem or grandiosity (which may be delusional)
decreased need for sleep
increased talkativeness or pressure of speech
flight of ideas or racing thoughts
distractibility
increase in goal-directed activity (e.g. social, at work) or psychomotor agitation
indiscreet behaviour with poor judgement (sexual, financial etc.)

(iii)   Symptoms do not meet criteria for mixed episode

(iv)   Marked impairment in occupational or social function

(v)   Not due to a drug of abuse (or other medication) or a physical illness such as hyperthyroidism

Adapted with permission from DSM–IV. Copyright 1994 American Psychiatric Association.

Clinical features

Mood

The essential criterion for the diagnosis of mania is elevation of mood in the form of elation or irritability. The elation is described by the patient in terms such as "never felt better", "full of energy", "marvellous". It may be accompanied by a sense of limitless optimism, exaltation or religious revelation. Often there is an infectious quality to the good humour which cheers other people and leads to laughter.

However the sustained elation is wearing on those around the patient. Any frustration of their ambitious plans provokes anger and a sense of persecution which may lead to abuse and aggression. Often the mood is labile and capricious. Tearful swings of mood occur, especially when the patient is confronted with personal problems. These swings of depression or hostility tend to be fleeting, but in some cases the irritability or depression can effectively mask the elation. Some patients report that their excitement is unpleasant.

Appearance

The patient often appears over-dressed or garish. Those with more severe illnesses may look untidy and neglected. They may appear in bare feet often with signs of infection, especially of the chest. Fluid retention and peripheral oedema may develop. Excessive consumption of alcohol may also complicate the picture (see below).

Over-activity

This is apparent in an excessive use of gestures, and the patient's tendency to leave the chair during the interview. Sometimes this excessive energy is used effectively in purposeful activities, but in more severe phases their actions are hurried and clumsy and ultimately can be repetitive and stereotyped. General over-activity tends to diminish if the environment is calm and not too stimulating but offers distractions. Extreme over-activity, continuing for days with little sleep or food, can lead to exhaustion and physical debility.

Behaviour

Indiscreet behaviour may result from a loss of normal social inhibitions leading them to be over-familiar, out-spoken, abusive or assaultative. They may have over-spent either on excessive quantities of everyday items, or on luxuries. One patient whose first episode followed the death of his father, a greengrocer, purchased hundreds of crates of apples with the aim of relieving starvation in India.

The effects on patients and their families may be ruinous with all savings spent and debts accumulated within the space of a few days or weeks. Those in sensitive jobs may have behaved with such poor judgement in planning, finance or in relation to their superiors as to jeopardise their careers. A junior manager, in a well-known theatre, used the ward telephone to invite international figures to a conference which he planned to hold at his theatre, without the knowledge of his director.

Vegetative signs

There is a decreased need for sleep, the patient awakening from a short sleep, feeling energetic. The patient in mild mania takes longer to go to sleep and wakes earlier than usual. Increased appetite occurs but is not necessarily accompanied by increased food intake or weight gain because the patient may be too distracted to complete their meal. Likewise there may be an increased interest and enjoyment of sexual activity, leading to flirtatiousness, and new or promiscuous relationships. In more severe states the patient is too easily distracted to consummate the relationship.

Speech

Many patients appear to feel a great need to seek out other people and to talk to them at length. They talk excessively, at an increased rate and it is difficult to interrupt them (pressure of speech). Their voice is often raised, leading to hoarseness. Others demonstrate such pressure by voluminous writings.

With 'flight of ideas' the association of thoughts proceeds in a fast and lively, but usually understandable way, and puns and other sorts of word-play are common. It differs from schizophrenic thought disorder in that connections can be seen as the patient jumps from one topic to another. The links may be in the content, where it appears as if a connecting thread has been left out, probably because the patient is thinking faster than they can speak.

Alternatively the links may be through sounds as in clang associations, rhymes or puns. The patient may describe their own thoughts as being fast or racing. The term 'prolixity' is used to describe milder abnormalities of speech in mania. In severe mania, flight of ideas may degenerate into incoherent speech.

> A West Indian woman named Samuels, who was transferred to an Intensive Therapy Unit, introduced herself to the doctor as follows: "I'm Samuel, I'm not a mule. I'm a new parent. I pay rent. I can just whisk myself off to Dominica, I'm a woman of leisure. When I came up here, I didn't want to come to England at the age of three. I didn't want to go to school, the intense therapy of developing from 11 to 13. At the age of 16 I burst out of school uniform into chiffon and lace, 'cos I'm a teenager, young lady, and I went to work."

Increased self-esteem, grandiosity

The thought content reflects the mood and displays increased self-esteem and ambitiousness. They have an increased estimation of their abilities, wealth or status.

Delusions

The grandiosity may become delusional, with the conviction that they have great wealth, some special mission, are of royal descent or have some special relationship or identity with a great leader, politician, religious figure or even a deity. Patients may falsely believe that they are pregnant, and perhaps bearing a prophet or Messiah.

In keeping with the mood state, the content of delusions in mania are, typically, grandiose or persecutory. Such delusions are congruent with altered mood. Persecutory ideas develop from when their grandiose plans are frustrated, although in other cases the clinical picture is dominated by paranoia. Sometimes, the ideas are over-valued rather than delusional and seem to be metaphorical or exaggerated expressions of the patient's wishes or frustrations.

Hallucinations

Auditory hallucinations may occur in the form of voices addressing the patient with a content that is either reassuring or exciting, for example the comforting voices of dead relatives or God's voice encouraging them to religious acts.

Cognition

The patients' thoughts and behaviour are easily distracted by changes in the environment, such as extraneous noises. Distractibility may lead to forgetfulness, for example with the suspicion that others are taking their belongings. Patients are correctly oriented for time and place except at the height of a severe manic episode.

Insight

Mania is the most insightless form of mental illness and patients not only believe but also behave in accordance with their increased self-esteem.

> A manic female introduced herself to the doctor as the Queen of England. She responded to his friendly but informal return of greetings by slapping his face. It was no way to speak to the Queen.

Only a small proportion of patients being admitted with mania recognise that they are ill, but others will sometimes acknowledge that there has been a change in their behaviour or that they might benefit from a 'rest'. As their condition improves in hospital, the patient is usually amenable to explanations about their condition and the need for treatment, but this insight can soon be lost if their manic state re-emerges.

Types of mania

Kraepelin divided manic states into hypomania, acute mania, delirious mania and chronic mania. The term hypomania has been used inconsistently; if it is to be used at all it should probably be reserved for conditions which would only be recognised as pathological by those who are familiar with the patient or with psychiatry (Hare, 1976).

Carlson & Goodwin (1973) described three stages of mania through which an episode may develop, corresponding to mild, moderate and severe levels of symptoms. At moderate severity the euphoric mood is increasingly interrupted by periods of irritability and depression, and thinking becomes delusional. In the severe stage, there is frenzied over-activity, mood is experienced by the patient as unpleasant or even terrifying, delusional thinking becomes bizarre and they have hallucinations, and in some cases disorientation. Beigel & Murphy (1971) found that patients with repeated manic attacks tended to exhibit similar behaviour and mood patterns during subsequent episodes.

Dysphoric mania

This term has been used to describe patients in whom classical manic symptoms are accompanied by marked anxiety, depression or anger (Post *et al*, 1989). Although these symptoms tend to emerge in more severe stages of the illness, some patients present throughout with a 'destructive-paranoid' pattern rather than the classic 'elated-grandiose' type.

Delirious mania

Occasionally manic patients become disorientated or have other symptoms, suggestive of a confusional state including visual hallucinations. These are more likely to occur in severe mania or where self-neglect and physical exhaustion develop. Evidence of chest infection and cardiac failure should be sought. If left untreated such patients become increasingly ill and may die.

The term 'delirious mania' or Bell's mania is used for cases with confusional symptoms without evidence of underlying physical illness, usually developing with a rapid onset.

Chronic mania

In rare cases mania runs an unremitting course. This seems to have occurred more commonly in the 19th century. Kraepelin described the chronic form as showing some intellectual and emotional blunting compared to acute mania. Hare (1981) has attributed the decline of this condition to improvements in general health and public hygiene. Some cases of chronic mania seen today may be secondary to organic brain disease.

Mixed affective states

Depression occurs as an integral part of bipolar disorder, and often either precedes or succeeds an episode of mania (Kotin & Goodwin, 1972; Morgan, 1972). The switch between mania and depression may occur suddenly, but it is usually more gradual with an intervening mixed state or period of normality. Sometimes the whole affective episode contains a mixture of manic and depressive symptoms.

It appears that three areas of functioning (mood, activity and thinking) can be altered independently to produce 'mixed states'. The best recognised are manic stupor (in which the patient is retarded but appears elated and later describes having experienced racing thoughts) and depression with flight of ideas. Transient depression in mood is very common in mania but the term 'mixed state' is best reserved for cases in which symptoms of both mania and depression are consistently present.

Mood-incongruent psychotic features

Some patients with symptoms fulfilling the inclusion criteria for the diagnosis of mania have in addition one or more of the 'first rank symptoms' of schizophrenia described by Schneider (Brockington *et al*, 1980). Disagreement can arise about the diagnosis. According to the Research Diagnostic Criteria, the diagnosis is "schizo-affective disorder" (schizomania). According to DSM–IV the diagnosis is "mania with psychotic features", if the content of the delusions or hallucinations is congruent with raised mood; otherwise the diagnosis is "mania with mood-incongruent psychotic features". Delusions of control and other first rank symptoms occur in 10–20% of manic patients. Catatonic symptoms (e.g. stereotypies, mannerisms, posturing, negativism, mutism) were originally described by Kahlbaum (1874) in association with mania.

Mania should not be diagnosed if psychotic features are present before the manic syndrome has developed or after it has remitted; such patients have schizoaffective disorder, according to DSM–IV.

Self-reports of mania

Several writers have described their experiences after a manic episode and some of these seem generally applicable. The main features of the subjective experience are an intense sense of well-being, a heightened sense of reality, a sense of communion and of mystical revelation, inhibition of the sense of repulsion, loss of normal sexual and social inhibitions, and grandiose ideas (see Lerner, 1980).

> "The intense sense of well-being which is physical as well as mental is not wholly illusory. My digestive system works particularly well, without the slightest hint of constipation or diarrhoea and I have an inordinate appetite."
> "The sense of communion extends to all fellow creatures with whom I come into contact."
> "When in a manic state I have no objection to being more or less herded together – as is inevitable in public Mental Hospitals – with men of all classes and conditions."
> "The question of selecting an attractive girl, which normally plays a large part in sexual adventures, did not trouble me in the least. I was quite content to leave it to chance". "I have no repulsion to excreta, urine and so on. I have no distaste of dirt. I do not care in the least whether I am washed or not."
> "The condition of my mind for many months is beyond all description. My thoughts ran with lightning-like rapidity from one

subject to another. I had an exaggerated feeling of self-importance.
All the problems of the universe came crowding into my mind,
demanding instant discussion and solution."
"And now it is that as your goodness grows and your happiness
increases, your eyes are unblinded more and more and your ears
are undeafened more and more."

An American psychoanalyst said that a person who has not experienced
mania "has not lived". Whereas a British psychiatrist recalled, "You learn
who your friends are in mania; they arrange a compulsory treatment order
if necessary".

Classification

Kraepelin's concept of manic-depressive illness was too broad, and in
1957 Leonard proposed a distinction between bipolar patients (those
with a history of mania) and unipolar depressives. Some patients with
recurrent depression have hypomanic episodes (not requiring
hospitalisation), especially on recovery from depression, and these were
described as BP (Bipolar)–II; those with a history of mania as BP–I (Dunner
et al, 1976*b*). DSM–IV defines BP–I disorder as episodes of mania (with
or without depression) and BP–II disorder as recurrent episodes of major
depression with hypomanic episodes. ICD–10 (World Health Organization,
1992) merely classifies BP–II disorders under the heading of "other bipolar
affective disorders". Unipolar mania accounts for 5–10% of bipolar disorder
but has not been established as being different in any way from BP–I
disorder. Because of the different combinations of severity of manic and
depressive episodes, Angst (1985) proposed four categories:
(i)   MD (in which both manic and depressive episodes are severe
      enough to require hospitalisation)
(ii) Md (recurrent mania with only mild depression)
(iii) mD (BP–II) (hypomania with severe depression)
(iv) md (cyclothymia).
Unipolar depressives with a family history of mania are sometimes called
BP–III or pseudo-unipolar.

Kukopulos *et al* (1985) has used the sequence of mood changes, to
distinguish patients in whom mania is followed by depression, followed
by a well interval (MDI), from those with depression followed by mania
(DMI), those with a continuously circular pattern (CC) and those with
completely separate affective swings.

Post *et al* (1981) distinguished patients who switched rapidly (within
24 hours) into mania from those in whom the change was more gradual.
The former had been ill longer and had experienced more affective
episodes.

Hypomania is a less severe condition than mania. Criteria are similar to those for mania but DSM–IV specifies a minimum duration of four days as compared to one week for mania. Both DSM–IV and ICD–10 exclude the presence of delusions for hypomania, thus if delusions are present the diagnosis is mania. Hypomania impairs social function to a lesser degree than mania, but more than cyclothymia.

DSM–IV also describes 'mixed episodes', where the patient fulfils criteria both for mania as described above and major depression; the condition should last for at least one week (two weeks in ICD–10).

Bipolar affective disorder in DSM–IV and ICD–10

In DSM–IV the minimum criteria for bipolar affective disorder is a single episode of mania (or mixed disorder). ICD–10 specifies at least two separate episodes, one of which must have been hypomanic, manic or mixed, but the other episode may be depression. Both schemes require that the current episode is also classified. ICD–10 has different subtypes but DSM–IV has a slightly different terminology and uses the word 'specifiers' instead.

ICD–10 describes bipolar affective disorder with the current episode being: hypomanic; manic without psychotic symptoms, manic with psychotic symptoms; mild or moderate depression; severe depression without psychotic symptoms; severe depression with psychotic symptoms; mixed episode; or in remission.

DSM–IV has three groups of specifiers, the first describing severity, the second the clinical type, and thirdly the longitudinal course. Thus bipolar affective disorder may be: mild; moderate; severe without psychotic features; severe with psychotic features, in partial remission, in full remission; with catatonic features; with a postpartum onset. If the most recent episode is depressive it may be: chronic; melancholic; or with atypical features. Longitudinal course specifiers are: with or without full inter-episode recovery; with a seasonal pattern; or with rapid cycling. All of the above specifiers may be associated with either bipolar I or bipolar II disorder.

Mania in childhood and adolescence

Mania is rare before puberty and it is doubtful if it ever occurs before the age of nine. This suggests a hormonal interaction with the brain that occurs around puberty among those with a predisposition to mania.

Adolescents show similar symptom profiles in mania to those of adults, except that psychotic symptoms may be more common in patients with an earlier age of onset. An onset before the age of 20 has not been found consistently to affect the prognosis by comparison with an older onset.

There is no evidence of a deleterious effect upon their later maturity but their education and training is liable to be interrupted and impaired.

High risk studies

Studies of children at high risk of developing bipolar disorder by virtue of their family history, have found associations with increased aggressiveness and greater affective expression; the children also demonstrated some positive strengths such as more involvement in activities (Kron *et al*, 1982). Cyclothymia was much more common in the high risk group, developing at the age of 12–14, and a large proportion of these presented within 3 years with bipolar disorder (Akiskal *et al*, 1985; Klein *et al*, 1985).

Mania among those with learning disabilities

Mania occurs with the usual frequency in persons with learning disabilities. In those with severe learning disability, verbal expressions are fewer but the diagnosis can be based upon the cyclical nature of the disorder, changes in mood and irritability, activity, sleep and the family history. Among those with mild and moderate degrees of learning disability the manifestations of mania are similar to those without such disabilities (Carlson, 1980).

Measurement

The measurement of mania must be by observer ratings, as self-ratings are unreliable. The first validated rating scale for mania was that of Beigel *et al* (1971). Specially trained nurses scored 26 items for intensity and frequency. Blackburn *et al* (1977) modified this scale for use by doctors, rating 28 items for severity on six-point scales, but without defined anchor points. This scale is comprehensive but time-consuming, and its reliability depends on a structured interview. Young *et al* (1978) provided a scale consisting of 11 items, each with five-point subscales and defined anchor points. Completion of the scale requires a 15–30 minute interview. This instrument is convenient for following the progress of mania in an individual patient during treatment.

Course

Age of onset

The peak age of first hospitalisation is in the late teens, the median in the mid twenties and the mean age of first hospitalisation about 26. There have often been earlier affective episodes sufficient to cause some impairment or to receive treatment outside hospital. There is a greater prevalence of affective illness among the first degree relatives of those whose first episode of mania occurred by the age of 20, than those occurring later (Pauls *et al*, 1992). There is a slight secondary peak of onset in women aged 45–50, and first episodes of mania continue to be seen in late life (Takei *et al*, 1992). An onset over the age of 60 is more likely to be associated with organic brain disease (Stone, 1989). The literature on mania in late life was reviewed by Young & Klerman (1992).

Number and duration of episodes

The great majority of patients have more than one episode, confirming the view that bipolar disorder is a recurrent illness.

The duration of manic episodes in the pre-treatment era was usually 3–12 months with a mean of 6 months. Treatment shortens this duration. In an individual, the episode duration tends to be stable through the course of the illness but the onset may become more rapid in later episodes.

Frequency of episodes

The interval from one episode to the next tends to decrease during the first five episodes. For instance, in Kraepelin's series the average time between the first and second episode was 5 years, whereas this had fallen to 2 years between the fifth and sixth episode. However in an individual there is great variability in the length between episodes, and a tendency for episodes to be clustered at particular times in the patient's life (Cutler & Post, 1982), for instance when they have difficulties coping with children, or when relationships are ending. It is possible that antidepressant treatments increase the tendency to switch from depression to mania, and have altered the natural course of the illness towards more frequent episodes. The work of Angst (1985) is cited in support of this; he found an increase in the incidence of manic switches, when the era before treatment was compared with that after the introduction of ECT and antidepressant drugs.

Rapid-cycling

If the patient has four or more affective episodes in a year, they are said to be in a phase of rapid-cycling. This can occur at the onset of illness but is more common later in its course. It is also more common in women. Antidepressant medication can increase the frequency of cycling, and withdrawal of antidepressants can restore normal cycling in such patients (Wehr & Goodwin, 1979). Some cases of rapid-cycling are associated with clinical or subclinical hypothyroidism although a causal relationship has not been proved; lithium treatment might also contribute to this (Bauer *et al*, 1990). Rapid-cycling has been described in secondary mania associated with organic brain disease and among those with learning disabilities (Glue, 1989). Rare cases exist – about 20 in the world literature – of patients who oscillate from mania to depression and back again every 48 hours (ultra rapid-cycling).

Seasonal pattern

There is a slight excess of manic episodes in summer months in temperate climates. There is rarely evidence of a regular seasonal pattern in individual patients with BP–I illness (Hunt *et al*, 1992*b*). Patients with 'seasonal affective disorder' are more commonly of BP–II type (Rosenthal *et al*, 1984).

Outcome

Before effective treatment was available, about 20% of hospitalised manic patients died, many from exhaustion. With modern treatment, increased mortality from natural causes occurs only in those with a concurrent physical illness. However, death by suicide occurs in about 15–20% of cases (Black *et al*, 1987*a*).

A proportion of patients become socially and economically disadvantaged. In an American study of tertiary referrals, less than half returned to their previous jobs (Carlson *et al*, 1974). In a Canadian study patients lost 11% of their productive time in the 15–20 years after their index admission (Bland & Orn, 1982). However, in a study from Belgium comparing bipolar with unipolar patients and normal controls, bipolar patients in remission showed only mild social maladjustment (Bauwens *et al*, 1991). There can be a considerable social and economic burden on the family (Fadden *et al*, 1987). A study in India revealed greater burden on the relatives of bipolar than unipolar depressive patients; prolonged illness, number of episodes and the degree of dysfunction in the patients correlated with the degree of burden (Chakrabarti *et al*, 1992).

Psychosocial factors

Life events and expressed emotion

Episodes of mania may develop following major life events such as bereavement, personal separation, work-related problems or loss of role (Ambelas, 1987). An interesting example of an 'independent' event precipitating mania was described after a hurricane; the only patients in a lithium clinic who relapsed were those who had been less stable prior to the event (Aronson & Shukla, 1987). A recent prospective study showed an increased rate of life events in the month before mania, but the proportion of patients affected was small (Hunt *et al*, 1992*a*). It has been suggested that the first episode is more likely to be triggered by life events than later episodes (Sclare & Creed, 1987). This view is in keeping with the suggestion that a process of 'kindling' occurs facilitating the development of subsequent episodes (see below), and Post (1992) has reviewed the possible biochemical substrates for the progressive effects of stress in recurrent affective disorders.

Psychological stress may also arise from 'high expressed emotion' in the environment in which the patient lives. Bipolar patients returning to such environments show an increased rate of relapse (Miklowitz *et al*, 1988).

Insomnia or sleep deprivation has been suggested as an important factor that may trigger a manic episode (Wehr *et al*, 1987).This may be relevant to the observation that flying overnight from west to east is more likely to lead to mania than travel in the opposite direction (Jauhar & Weller, 1982), and in cases of mania in fathers following childbirth. A short course of sedative antipsychotic may be helpful in bipolar patients with transient sleep disturbance to reduce the risk of developing mania.

Marriage and parenting

Manic symptoms tend to be destructive to existing relationships. Although spouses may at first be attracted by mildly manic behaviour, such as increased sociability and sexual activity, a full-blown manic episode is embarrassing and frightening. There is evidence of assortative mating in bipolar disorder, the choice of marital partner being an individual with a matching or complementary temperament. During depression the patient may seem excessively dependent on the spouse but in mania they may assert their independence and humiliate the spouse. Although marriages often survive single episodes of mania, the divorce rate in bipolar disorder is very high – 57% in one series compared to 8% in unipolar patients (Brodie & Leff, 1971). Very few of the spouses of bipolar patients have seen the patient during a manic episode prior to marriage. Fortunately treatment with lithium often improves the quality of the marriage. Bipolar disorder in the mother may adversely affect attachment patterns with younger children. However, the development of abnormal patterns is less if there is a father in the household (Radke-Yarrow *et al*, 1985).

Alcohol and drug misuse in bipolar disorder

Some patients increase and some decrease alcohol or drug use when manic compared to euthymic (Bernadt & Murray, 1986). Alcohol and stimulants, such as amphetamine and cocaine, are used by patients to restore hypomania during a dysphoric phase, or to heighten existing states of elation (Gawin & Kleber, 1986).

These drugs can alter the course of bipolar disorder by triggering mania; they diminish impulse control and impair judgement and are serious risk factors for suicide. Therefore the recognition and treatment of alcohol or drug misuse in bipolar patients is a matter of urgency.

Cannabis has been associated with an increase in psychotic symptoms in mania (Harding & Knight, 1973), and with the induction of mania (Rottanburg *et al*, 1982).

Secondary mania

A manic state may develop following a physical disturbance by drugs or disease. When this occurs in clear consciousness, in patients without any past history of affective disorder, it is called secondary mania (Krauthammer & Klerman, 1978). Box 2.2 shows the commonest causes of secondary mania.

Drugs

Psychostimulants

Low doses of amphetamines in normal subjects produce a state resembling mild mania but with reduced hunger and appetite and anomalous endocrine effects (Jacobs & Silverstone, 1986). Dopamine agonists, such as bromocriptine, used in the treatment of pituitary tumours or to suppress lactation can lead to psychotic states including mania (Turner *et al*, 1984). The dopamine precursor L-dopa can trigger mania but this is far more likely to occur in individuals with a bipolar predisposition. Likewise a manic episode may be triggered by amphetamine in pre-disposed individuals (Gerner *et al*, 1976). Anticholinergics, such as benzhexol and procyclidine are liable to be misused for their psychostimulant effects, and can produce a state resembling mania (Coid & Strang, 1982) or a confusional state. In addition to their anticholinergic properties, these drugs also block dopamine reuptake (Horn *et al*, 1971), and this may be relevant to their stimulant properties.

Endocrine causes

Cortico-steroids in high doses can produce elated psychotic states resembling mania (Ling *et al*, 1981), although Cushing's disease is more associated with depression (in 40% of cases) and with mania in only 2%. Anabolic steroids can produce character changes resembling mania (Freinhar & Alvarez, 1985).

Thyrotoxicosis is often accompanied by hyperactivity and irritability. The main diagnostic similarity is with anxiety states, rather than mania,

---

Box 2.2   Causes of secondary mania

Drugs
Psychostimulants
   Amphetamines
   Cocaine
Recreational drugs
   Cannabis
   Alcohol
Medication
   Dopamine agonists (bromocriptine etc)
   L-dopa
   Cortico-steroids
   Anabolic steroids
   Thyroid hormone
   Anticholinergics (benzhexol and procyclidine)
Endocrine/metabolic conditions
   Thyrotoxicosis
   Cushing's disease
   Childbirth: puerperal psychosis

Drug withdrawal
   Fenfluramine
   Baclofen
   Clonidine

Organic brain disease
   Cerebrovascular disease
   Head injury
   Cerebral tumour
   Epilepsy
   Multiple sclerosis
   Dementia

---

although mania can be precipitated in pre-disposed individuals (Corn & Checkley, 1983). The commencement of treatment of myxoedema with thyroid hormone leads in some cases to a worsening of pre-existing psychotic symptoms and to the emergence of mania (Josephson & Mackenzie, 1980). There are also neuroendocrine changes during mania (Cookson, 1985).

Brain injury

Reports of mania and bipolar disorder following brain injury have been reviewed by Jeste *et al* (1988).

Stroke

Following vascular lesions, in contrast to secondary depression, mania is associated with right-sided cerebral lesions and is more likely to occur if there is a family history or past history of affective disorder (Starkstein & Robinson, 1989). The brain areas most often involved are the frontal and temporal regions.

Head injury

Patients in whom mania follows head injuries, tend to have damage to the right hemisphere rather than the left. In contrast to post-stroke mania, a positive family history is not more likely; the mania tends to be characterised by irritability rather than euphoria (Shukla *et al*, 1987).

Treatment of mania

The need for admission

While milder cases may be treated in out-patients, mania requires admission when associated with aggressive behaviour, and also when overspending, grandiosity, sexual indiscretion or substance misuse threaten health or safety.

The loss of insight, grandiosity and hyperactivity often preclude voluntary admission. Compulsory admission should be considered before the situation deteriorates. Whatever the means of admission, the patient should always be reassured that admission will enable them to rest and have relief from their excessive activities, personal conflicts and their 'over-excitement'.

Milieu management

There should be stable external control and administrative issues should be handled in a firm and non-negotiable manner. Firm and consistent limits should be set in order to prevent behaviour that is dangerous or disruptive to the patient or others. All the staff should be consistent in this. The patient will often require either individual attention or nursing in a (locked) intensive care setting to prevent them leaving the ward. The emphasis should be on calming the patient. Restrictions on visiting, and time spent alone help to reduce stimulation. Argument about the content of delusions should be avoided. When speaking with the patient the voice should be lowered with slightly slower cadence than usual.

A structured timetable may be helpful, and writing or colouring materials should be available if the patient can concentrate sufficiently to use them. Other reality-based diversionary activities should be provided. The patient should be addressed tactfully, avoiding provocation or pressure.

Specific issues to be addressed are the alienation of family members, the progressive testing of limits by the patient, the over-involvement with other patients and the tendency to dominate the ward. Janowsky *et al* (1974) described these tendencies as 'the manic game' and implied that the manic patient demands care without having to admit their need for it. Staff need to understand these manoeuvres in order to avoid becoming too personally involved, for example in angry exchanges. Community meetings are helpful as they allow the responses of other patients to the manic's behaviour to be recognised and guided.

As the patient's condition improves, individual work should be aimed at identifying factors that may have contributed to the present episode, and helping the patient to tolerate feelings of depression or distress that may emerge. They may need help to re-establish personal and occupational relationships. Empathic meetings between a member of the ward team and relatives can prepare them to understand explanations that the patient's condition is a treatable illness which in the long term needs their support and may benefit from prophylactic medication.

Drug treatment

A physical examination and tests of the blood and urine should precede drug treatment or take place soon after the patient is sedated. These tests will elucidate any intercurrent physical illness, especially infection, and any causes of secondary mania (e.g. drugs), and to determine baseline renal, hepatic and thyroid function.

Antipsychotic drugs

Mild mania may be treated with antipsychotic drugs such as haloperidol 5–10mg daily; lithium treatment may also be useful, but improvement takes up to two weeks. Moderate or severe mania is usually most rapidly controlled by antipsychotic drugs. Phenothiazines (e.g. chlorpromazine) and thioxanthines (e.g. zuclopenthixol) are effective but the butyrophenone, haloperidol, is often particularly useful in a dose of 5–10mg three times a day. The more disturbed patient may be given haloperidol (5–10mg) intramuscularly at hourly intervals until they are calm. Haloperidol (5–10mg) may also be given intravenously. Larger intramuscular doses (e.g. 30mg) are discouraged because they are excessive in some patients and their effects may last for several days, obscuring the diagnosis and making further management difficult. The patient may no longer appear very disturbed but is likely to deteriorate unless treatment is continued. Large doses of antipsychotic drugs have been associated with sudden deaths in disturbed young patients probably through cardiac dysrhythmias.

Haloperidol tends to produce initial sedation which wears off after a day or so during continued treatment (Cookson *et al*, 1983). If the patient remains very behaviourally disturbed, chlorpromazine may be more useful because, having anti-histaminic properties, it is more sedative than haloperidol. However many manic patients resent being made to feel drowsy and this limits the dose of chlorpromazine that they will accept. Chlorpromazine is hypotensive and should be used cautiously in the elderly.

Extra-pyramidal side-effects seem less of a problem with larger doses of haloperidol, but may emerge as the dose is reduced or a few days after it is discontinued. Anti-parkinsonian medication should therefore be continued for up to seven days after haloperidol is stopped.

Rapid improvement in mania occurs for one to three days after medication is commenced; the manic states tend then to improve more gradually over the next two weeks. There is no evidence that increasing the dose of haloperidol above 30mg per day achieves greater improvement (Rifkin *et al*, 1994).

For manic patients whose failure to improve is due to poor compliance, depot antipsychotic medication including haloperidol or zuclo-penthixol decanoates can be used. Zuclopenthixol acetate is a depot formulation, which has a duration of action of up to three days, and a more rapid onset of action than the decanoates; it is useful in disturbed patients who persistently refuse oral medication during the first few days of treatment.

Mechanism of action

The mechanism of the anti-manic effect of these drugs is thought to be largely through blockade of dopamine (D) receptors, since the relatively specific D blocker, pimozide, is as effective as chlorpromazine in reducing the manic syndrome, although it is not as sedative as chlorpromazine (Cookson *et al*, 1981). It is possible that the D pathways and receptor sub-types relevant to the anti-manic effect are different from those involved in the anti-schizophrenic effect of these drugs. Thus some drugs may be relatively more potent in mania than in schizophrenia (Janicak *et al*, 1988). Pimozide is a less sedative antipsychotic drug but its use requires a normal ECG as it can lengthen the QT interval and cause cardiac dysrhythmia in higher doses. Blockade of histamine H_1 and noradrenaline alpha$_1$ receptors may contribute to the initial effects including sedation (Cookson *et al*, 1985).

Other sedative drugs

For manic patients who are not adequately sedated by antipsychotic drugs, or to avoid prescribing such drugs, sedation may be achieved by diazepam (10–20mg intravenously or 30mg orally). For intramuscular use the benzodiazepine midazolam is absorbed faster, causes less local pain and is useful in the control of acutely agitated patients (Wyant *et al*, 1990). The anti-convulsant benzodiazepine, clonazepam (4–16mg a day) is sedative and may improve mania (Chouinard, 1987). However, in a double-blind comparison, manic patients on clonazepam alone showed little improvement, whereas those on lorazepam alone (6–24mg/day) showed marked improvement (Bradwejn *et al*, 1990). Lorazepam has also been used as an adjunct to other anti-manic drugs (Modell *et al*, 1985). Behavioural disinhibition, depersonalisation and disassociation are potential problems during treatment with benzodiazepines, and dependence and symptoms of withdrawal occur during longer-term treatment.

Neuroleptic-resistant mania

A proportion of manic patients show only partial improvement or initial improvement followed by partial relapse with antipsychotic drugs. There is little evidence that increasing the dose will produce further improvement. It is thought that clozapine exerts antipsychotic effects though an action on a different sub-type of D_2 receptors, and this drug may prove to be useful in resistant mania as in resistant schizophrenia. However at the present time the main alternatives or adjuncts to the antipsychotic drugs are lithium and the anticonvulsants, carbamazepine and valproate.

Lithium

History

Amdisen (1984) has described two eras of lithium's medicinal use. The earlier included the use of lithium salts in the 19th century for 'gouty diseases', among which Garrod in 1876 included mania; Hammond in 1871 recommended the use of lithium salts in mania. However by 1920 this notion was rejected and with it the use of lithium. The toxicity of lithium salts received prominence in 1949 when, following several deaths, they were banned in the USA for use as salt substitutes in heart disease.

The modern era of lithium began in 1949 with the re-investigation by Cade in Australia of the use of lithium in severe psychosis. Working first with guinea pigs and later with psychotic patients, he found that in ten patients with mania there was a positive response. Problems with toxicity remained, until by the late 1960s the importance of serum monitoring below specific levels became established. Cade's findings were confirmed and extended, particularly by Schou in Denmark.

Studies

In a review of ten open studies, 81% of 443 patients showed some improvement on lithium, usually beginning within a week of starting treatment (Goodwin & Ebert, 1973). There have been four placebo-controlled studies (using a cross-over design). These were conducted in Denmark by Schou *et al* (1954), later in England by Maggs *et al* (1963), and in the USA (Goodwin *et al*, 1969; Stokes *et al*, 1971). There was an overall response rate of 78% from a total of 116 patients on lithium, much greater than with placebo. More recent reviews put the figure at 60%. Lithium usually takes two to four weeks to achieve its full effect on mania. Bowden et al (1994) showed lithium to be superior to placebo in mania, in the first parallel-group trial, while also studying valproate.

Prediction of anti-manic response to lithium

Used alone, lithium is more useful in mild than in severe cases (Prien *et al*, 1972; Swann *et al*, 1986). Patients who respond tend to have classical mania rather than mixed or schizoaffective disorders (Himmelhoch *et al*, 1976; Swann *et al*, 1986). There is no data to confirm whether a family history of bipolar disorder predicts an acute anti-manic response as it does for prophylaxis. Patients in a rapid-cycling phase tend not to respond to lithium (Dunner & Fieve, 1974). Elated-grandiose mania showed a better response than destructive-paranoid mania in Murphy & Beigel's study (1974), but not in Swann *et al's* (1986). Dysphoric mania was less likely to improve (Post *et al*, 1989). Patients who have benefited previously from lithium are more likely to do so again.

Doses in acute mania

The narrow gap or overlap between therapeutic and toxic blood levels of lithium necessitates careful monitoring of lithium levels, usually based on samples taken 12 hours after the last dose. The pharmacokinetics of lithium involve rapid absorption with a peak at 4 hours followed by distribution in body fluids and slow penetration of the intracellular space and brain. Elimination is largely by the kidney, and the plasma half-life varies from 7–20 hours in physically healthy individuals but is longer in the elderly or physically unwell. Thornhill & Field (1982) found it to range from 15–55 hours in euthymic psychiatric patients. Thus on a regular dose steady-state blood levels would be reached after a period of between 2 and 9 days. Many of the features of toxicity may reflect high intracellular rather than extracellular levels; hence, in assessing toxicity and efficacy, clinical judgement rather than blood levels should be paramount.

In acute mania, salt metabolism is altered so that lithium is distributed in bone and other sites (Almy & Taylor, 1973) and higher doses are needed for a given blood level (Kukopulos *et al*, 1985). Increasing plasma levels of lithium up to 1.4mmol/l are associated with higher rates of response in mania but levels above 1.2 require special care in monitoring to avoid toxicity (Stokes *et al*, 1976).

Mode of action of lithium

Lithium has numerous effects on biological systems, especially at high concentrations. It is unclear which of these are relevant to its therapeutic effects (see Wood & Goodwin, 1987).

Ionic mechanisms

As the smallest alkaline cation, lithium can substitute for sodium, potassium, calcium and magnesium in several ways. It penetrates cells via sodium and other channels, but is extruded less efficiently than sodium by the sodium-potassium active transport system and other transporters. Thus the cell:plasma ratio for lithium (about 0.5 in red blood cells) is much higher than that for sodium. Within the cell, lithium can interact with systems, which normally involve other cations, including transmitter release and second messenger systems.

Adenylate cyclase – Many neurotransmitters and hormones (LH, TSH, vasopressin at V_2 receptors, dopamine at D_1 receptors, nordrenaline at beta receptors etc) interact with receptors that use cyclic-AMP as the second (intracellular) messenger. Lithium is known to inhibit c-AMP production in these systems. In humans, therapeutic levels of lithium have been shown to inhibit the adrenaline-induced rise in plasma c-AMP. The inhibition by lithium of ADH-linked adenylate cyclase is thought to contribute to the polyuria and polydipsia (nephrogenic diabetes insipidus) which is a side-effect. Goitre and hypothyroidism are due in part to interference with the action of TSH at its receptors in the thyroid. Noradrenaline beta receptors and dopamine D_1 receptors are also linked to adenylate cyclase and lithium inhibits these, although it is not certain that this occurs at therapeutic concentrations.

Phosphoinositide turnover – This second messenger system involves the release and uptake of inositol phosphates which control intracellular calcium levels. The phosphoinositide cycle is the second messenger for several neurotransmitters including TRH in the pituitary, acetyl choline at muscarinic M_1 receptors, noradrenalin at alpha-one, and 5-HT at 5-HT$_2$ receptors. Lithium inhibits inositol monophosphatase and has an inhibitory or stabilising effect on responses for instance to acetyl choline.

Effects on 5-HT

Lithium can potentiate the uptake of L-tryptophan, the precursor of 5-HT. It can also potentiate the release of 5-HT in some synapses and can potentiate 5HT$_1$ responses; for instance in man the rise in prolactin levels induced by L-tryptophan but not that induced by d-fenfluramine is potentiated by lithium.

Receptor up-regulation

Lithium can block the development of dopamine receptor super-sensitivity that normally occurs during prolonged treatment with dopamine-blocking (antipsychotic) drugs. It has been suggested that lithium might reduce the development of tardive dyskinesia (TD) in bipolar patients on antipsychotic drugs. Although in two studies TD was more common in patients who had a briefer exposure to lithium, in a third study the opposite was found (Dinan & Kohen, 1989).

Side-effects

Lithium has actions on many bodily systems even at therapeutic doses. These are important, as some require intervention and they contribute to non-compliance. The majority of patients on lithium will experience at least one side-effect (Vestergaard *et al*, 1980). All patients should be informed about side-effects and signs of toxicity.

Thyroid

Lithium tends to reduce thyroid function. The most sensitive laboratory index, increased TSH, occurs in 23% of patients (Transbol *et al*, 1978). Thyroid enlargement (goitre) develops in about 5% (Myers *et al*, 1985), and clinical hypothyroidism in 5–10% of patients depending upon the dose and duration of treatment (Yassa *et al*, 1988). Patients with pre-existing thyroid antibodies or a family history of thyroid disease are at greater risk of developing hypothyroidism (Lazarus *et al*, 1981), and lithium treatment can increase antibody levels (Calabrese *et al*, 1985; Myers *et al*, 1985).
The development of hypothyroidism is often signalled by weight gain and lethargy, and should be distinguished from depression. Treatment with L-thyroxine is usually straightforward. The occurrence of thyrotoxicosis during lithium treatment has also been described, and there may be a rebound exacerbation when lithium is discontinued.

Kidneys

Polyuria and excessive thirst with polydipsia are noted by about one third of patients on lithium. The condition is usually reversible but sometimes not after long-term treatment (Bucht *et al*, 1980). Giving lithium once daily as opposed to divided doses was associated with lower daily urine volumes in some studies although others found no difference (Bowen *et al*, 1991). For patients in whom a reduction in dose is not appropriate in order to avoid polyuria, the loop diuretic frusemide, or amiloride may be helpful. Alternatively a combination with carbamazepine may be tried as this tends to have an opposing effect and may allow a lower dose of lithium to be used.

In 1977, Hestbech *et al* reported histological changes in patients on lithium including glomerular damage, interstitial fibrosis and tubular atrophy (focal interstitial nephrophy). However similar findings were later made in patients who had received no lithium treatment. Further work has shown that during long-term treatment with lithium, monitored at therapeutic doses, no deterioration occurs in glomerular filtration rate in the vast majority of patients. However, occasional cases of chronic renal failure have been reported and attributed by nephrologists to lithium, even in patients whose lithium levels have been monitored carefully; this is thought to be a rare idiosyncratic reaction to lithium (Waller & Edwards, 1989).

Central nervous system

A fine tremor of the hands, similar to that in anxiety, occurs in about 25% of patients. It may be worsened by tricyclic antidepressants. Beta-blockers such as propranolol (starting at 10mg b.d.) reduce this and are probably best taken intermittently. Lithium can increase extra-pyramidal (parkinsonian) side-effects in patients on antipsychotic drugs (Tyrer *et al*, 1980), and can itself produce cog-wheel rigidity in a small minority of patients (Asnis *et al*, 1979). In contrast to neuroleptic-induced parkinsonism, this does not improve with anticholinergic drugs. Cerebellar tremor and uncoordination are signs of toxicity, as are more severe forms of fine tremor and parkinsonism.

Mental and cognitive effects

There is some objective evidence of an effect of therapeutic levels of lithium upon memory, but not all studies show this. Memory problems are frequently affirmed by patients interviewed about possible side-effects.

The possible effect of lithium upon creativity was explored by Schou (1979) who interviewed 24 successful artists and professionals taking lithium. Some did not want to continue lithium because of this effect, but the majority, although missing some hypomanic swings, considered that their long-term productivity and creativity were higher under lithium treatment. Only six thought they were diminished.

In therapeutic doses lithium does not impair psychomotor coordination and is not a bar to driving private motor vehicles, although a diagnosis of manic-depressive illness excludes patients from driving certain public service vehicles (Cookson, 1989).

Cardiovascular effects

Lithium can produce benign reversible T-wave flattening or inversion, a pattern similar to that with hypokalaemia. Cardiac dysrhythmias are rare with therapeutic doses especially in younger patients (Mitchell & MacKenzie, 1982). Caution should be exercised in using lithium in patients with cardiac failure and the elderly.

Skin

Lithium can produce or exacerbate acne and psoriasis. Tetracyclines should be used with caution because of their possible interaction with lithium but retinoids can be used. Hair loss and altered texture may also occur in about 6% of patients. Hair loss is sometimes associated with thyroid impairment but can occur in the presence of normal thyroid function. There may also be golden discolouration of the distal nail plates.

Parathyroid, bones and teeth

Lithium produces mild increases in parathyroid hormone level and serum calcium. Stancer & Forbath (1989) reported cases of clinical hyper-parathyroidism in patients on lithium but some may have been coincidental. No long-term effects on bone have been found in animals or man (Birch *et al*, 1982). It is unknown whether this applies to the growing bones of children. There is no evidence of a direct effect of lithium upon the teeth, but increased consumption of sweet drinks will lead to caries. Lithium produces a benign reversible leucocytosis probably by an effect on marrow growth factors.

Metabolic effects and weight gain

About 25% of patients gain more than 10 pounds in weight. The mechanism is unknown and an attempt to replicate the weight gain in volunteers was unsuccessful (Chen & Silverstone, 1990). Although increased consumption of sweet drinks is cited, an increase in food intake and altered metabolism are also possible. Lithium produces subtle alterations in glucose and insulin metabolism and can increase glucose tolerance. It may occasionally worsen control of diabetes. Fluid retention and oedema may occur especially with higher doses. Lithium may antagonise aldosterone and increase angiotensin levels (Stewart *et al*, 1988).

Gastro-intestinal

About one third of patients experience mild abdominal discomfort, sometimes with loose motions during the first few weeks of treatment, especially with higher doses. By using divided doses, these side-effects can usually be avoided. Sometimes a slow release preparation is tolerated better, but occasionally these irritate the lower bowel. Severe or persistent diarrhoea suggests toxicity.

Sexual function

Impairment of sexual drive, arousal and ejaculation have been attributed to lithium, but are thought to be rare (Blay *et al*, 1982). The LH response to LHRH is potentiated by lithium treatment, as is the TSH response to TRH.

Neuromuscular junction

Lithium reduces acetyl choline release and impairs neuromuscular transmission. Normally the safety factor in neuromuscular transmission is sufficient to overcome these effects. Lithium potentiates neuromuscular blocking agents including succinyl choline, and exacerbates myasthenia gravis.

Respiratory effects

Lithium can produce respiratory depression in patients with chronic obstructive airways disease, especially at toxic blood levels (Lawler & Cove-Smith, 1986).

Contraindications

There are no absolute contraindications to lithium treatment but caution is required in people with renal failure, heart failure, recent myocardial infarction, electrolyte imbalance, the elderly and in patients who are unreliable in taking medication. It should be avoided in the first months of pregnancy, as it carries a risk of cardiac malformations, such as Ebstein's anomaly, in the foetus. This risk was thought to be as high as 10%, but a recent small case-control study suggests it may be lower (Jacobson *et al*, 1992).

Lithium toxicity

Clinical features

Lithium toxicity is indicated by the development of three groups of symptoms: gastro-intestinal; motor, especially cerebellar, and cerebral (see Table 2.1). Nausea and diarrhoea progress to vomiting and incontinence. Marked fine tremor progresses to a coarse (cerebellar or parkinsonian) tremor, giddiness, cerebellar ataxia, and slurred speech, and to gross incoordination with choreiform movements and muscular twitching (myoclonus), upper motor neuron signs (spasticity and extensor plantar reflexes), EEG abnormalities and seizures.

In mild toxicity there is impairment of concentration but this deteriorates into drowsiness and disorientation, and in more severe toxicity there is marked apathy and impaired consciousness leading to coma. A Creutzfeldt-Jakob-like syndrome with characteristic EEG changes, myoclonus and cognitive deterioration has been described, and was in these cases reversible (Smith & Kocen, 1988).

Diagnosis of toxicity

Lithium toxicity should be assumed in patients on lithium with vomiting or severe nausea, cerebellar signs or disorientation. Lithium treatment should be stopped immediately, and serum lithium, urea and electrolyte levels measured. However, the severity of toxicity bears little relationship to serum lithium levels (Hansen & Amdisen, 1978), and neurotoxicity can occur with serum levels in the usual therapeutic range (West & Meltzer, 1979). Diagnosis should be based upon clinical judgement and not upon the blood level. Lithium should only be re-started, at an adjusted dose, when the patient's condition has improved, or an alternative cause of the symptoms has been found.

Treatment of lithium toxicity

Often, cessation of lithium and provision of adequate salt and fluids, included in saline infusions, will suffice. In patients with high serum levels (greater than 3 mmol/l) or coma, haemodialysis can speed the removal of lithium and reduce the risk of permanent neurological damage (Johnson, 1984).

Outcome

Patients who survive episodes of lithium toxicity will often make a full recovery. However, a proportion have persistent renal or neurological damage with cerebellar symptoms, spasticity and cognitive impairment. This outcome is more likely if patients are continued on lithium while showing signs of toxicity, or during intercurrent physical illnesses (Schou, 1984). Those patients who develop persistent neurological damage had more severe signs of toxicity within the episode (Hansen & Amdisen, 1978). Signs of toxicity develop gradually over several days during continued lithium treatment, and, in some cases, continue to develop for days after treatment is stopped. Serum lithium levels may also continue to rise after treatment is stopped, probably because of the release of lithium from intracellular stores (Sellers *et al*, 1982).

Table 2.1   Symptoms of lithium toxicity

	Gastro-intestinal	Motor/cerebellar	Mental
Mild	Nausea Diarrhoea	Severe fine tremor	Poor concentration
Moderate	Vomiting	Coarse tremor Cerebellar ataxia Slurred speech	Drowsiness Disorientation

Severe	Vomiting
	Incontinence
		Choreiform/Parkinsonian
		  movements
		General muscle
		twitching (myoclonus)
		Spasticity & cerebellar
		  dysfunction
		EEG abnormalities and
		  seizures
			Apathy
			Coma

Factors predisposing to lithium toxicity

Conditions of salt depletion (diarrhoea, vomiting, excessive sweating during fever or in hot climates) can lead to lithium retention. Drugs which reduce the renal excretion of lithium include thiazide diuretics (but not frusemide or amiloride), certain non-steroidal anti-inflammatory drugs (indomethacin, piroxicam, naproxen, ibuprofen and phenylbutazone, but not aspirin, paracetamol or sulindac), and certain antibiotics (erythromycin, metronidazole and probably tetracyclines). These drugs should be avoided if possible, but if they are used, the dose of lithium should be reduced and blood levels monitored.

In patients with serious intercurrent illnesses especially infections, lithium should be stopped or reduced in dose, and carefully monitored until the patient's condition is stable. Gastro-enteritis is particularly liable to lead to toxicity. In the elderly renal function is decreased, lower doses are required and toxicity can develop more readily (Stone, 1989).

Lithium–neuroleptic combination

Combinations of high levels of lithium with high doses of antipsychotics including haloperidol have been associated with severe neurological symptoms, hyperthermia, impaired consciousness and irreversible brain damage (Cohen & Cohen, 1974; Loudon & Waring, 1976). The conditions reported resemble both lithium toxicity and neuroleptic malignant syndrome. Antipsychotic drugs can increase intracellular lithium levels suggesting a possible mechanism for this interaction (Von Knorring, 1990).

Subsequent series have demonstrated the safety of combining haloperidol (up to 30mg per day) with lithium at levels of up to 1mmol/l (see Johnson *et al*, 1990).

In practice, when combining lithium with antipsychotics, the blood levels should generally be maintained below 1 mmol/l, staff should be advised to observe and report the development of neurological symptoms, and lithium should be temporarily discontinued if they develop. The combination of antipsychotics and lithium in bipolar patients can also lead to somnambulism requiring dosage reduction (Charney *et al*, 1979).

Carbamazepine

The mood stabilising effect of carbamazepine was initially recognised in epilepsy. Japanese psychiatrists were the first to report that carbamazepine improved acute mania, even in patients who were resistant to other drugs (Okuma *et al*, 1973). Ballenger & Post (1980) studied carbamazepine in bipolar disorder; they developed the theory that affective illness might involve a 'kindling' process in limbic brain areas, such as they had found with cocaine-induced behavioural changes in animals.

Small placebo-controlled studies have confirmed the anti-manic efficacy of carbamazepine, and studies comparing carbamazepine with antipsychotic drugs or lithium show it approximately as effective as lithium with about 60% of patients doing well. There is some delay in its action, but less so than with lithium.

Predicting response to carbamazepine

Patients who respond differ somewhat from those responding to lithium, and a history of non-response to lithium does not reduce the chances of responding to carbamazepine. Severely ill patients, including dysphoric manics, can benefit from carbamazepine as can patients with mixed states. Patients with no family history of mania may have a greater chance of responding to carbamazepine (Post *et al*, 1987). Patients with mania secondary to brain damage can also benefit.

The dose of carbamazepine used in acute mania in most studies was similar to that used for epilepsy except that the starting dose has to be higher if considerable delay is to be avoided. A starting dose of 400mg daily can then be increased, according to response and side-effects, to a maximum of 1600mg daily.

Carbamazepine side-effects

The commonest side-effects are nausea, dizziness, ataxia and diplopia. A maculopapular itchy rash develops within two weeks in up to 10% of patients and requires great caution and usually cessation of the drug. The incidence is less if the dose is increased gradually. Serious toxic side-effects are agranulocytosis, aplastic anaemia, Stevens-Johnson syndrome and water intoxication. Carbamazepine regularly lowers the white cell count by a pharmacological effect on the marrow. Agranulocytosis and aplastic anaemia can develop suddenly, and occur in about eight patients per million treated. Hyponatraemia and water intoxication may occur due to potentiation of ADH; this may lead to malaise, confusion and fits.

Pharmacokinetics and drug interactions

Carbamazepine induces liver enzymes. This results in the lowering not only of its own blood levels after three weeks of treatment, but also increasing the metabolism of other drugs such as haloperidol and oral contraceptives. On the other hand, the blood level of carbamazepine is increased by drugs including erythromycin, verapamil, dextropro-poxyphene and cimetidine. Thyroid hormone metabolism is increased and blood levels lowered; particularly in combination with lithium, carbamazepine may precipitate hypothyroidism.

Blood tests – Serum levels are sometimes helpful in monitoring carbamazepine therapy but, as in epilepsy, clinical judgement is generally more useful in deciding changes in dose. No clear relationship between plasma level and antimanic effect was found by Post *et al* (1987). The differential blood count and electrolyte levels should be monitored.Carbamazepine should be discontinued if hyponatraemia develops, or if the total white cell count is less than 3000 per cubic millimetre or the neutrophil count falls to less than 1500.

Mechanism of action

An anti-kindling effect may underlie some of the actions of carbamazepine, but the pharmacological mechanism of action in acute mania is unknown. Carbamazepine potentiates central 5-HT transmission in normal subjects, as judged by the prolactin response to L-tryptophan (Elphick *et al*, 1990).

Valproate in acute mania

Valproate is also effective in a proportion of manic patients including non-responders to antipsychotic drugs and lithium. Patients who respond to valproate do not necessarily respond to carbamazepine and vice versa. Two placebo-controlled studies have demonstrated the efficacy of valproate, about 50% of manic patients showing marked improvement (Pope et al, 1991; Bowden et al, 1994). The time course appeared similar to that with lithium, and the therapeutic levels appeared to be 15–100mg/l. The drug is generally well tolerated but side-effects include tremor, weight gain, rash, transient hair loss and, potentially, acute liver damage. Liver function tests should be monitored. The starting dose is 600mg daily, rising to 2000mg according to clinical response.

Combination treatment

Many patients who fail to improve when taking carbamazepine alone do so when lithium is added (Kramlinger & Post, 1989). This combination may – as with neuroleptics – increase the risk of lithium neurotoxicity (Shukla *et al*, 1984).

Other treatments

Patients not improving on a combination of lithium and antipsychotics may improve when reserpine is added (Bacher & Lewis, 1979; Telner *et al*, 1986). The calcium channel blocker verapamil has been found effective in acute mania although few controlled studies have been conducted (Dinan *et al*, 1988; Hoschl & Kozeny, 1989). Nifedipine and diltiazem have also been reported to have anti-manic effects.

While it is of theoretical interest that the cholinesterase inhibitor physostigmine has anti-manic properties, its side-effects preclude clinical use (Janowsky *et al*, 1973). Likewise the addition of lecithin (a precursor of acetyl choline) may potentiate other anti-manic medication but its value in clinical practice is doubtful.

L-tryptophan may have anti-manic properties (Prange *et al*, 1974) but placebo-controlled trials have not consistently supported this. Serotonin antagonists such as methysergide exacerbate mania (Coppen *et al*, 1969). The use of clonidine in neuroleptic-resistant mania has been reported (Maguire & Singh, 1987) but placebo controlled studies have not confirmed its value (Janicak *et al*, 1989).

Dopamine agonists with preferential pre-synaptic effects are sedative and may improve mania, but dopamine agonists may also cause secondary mania, presumably by stimulation of post-synaptic receptors. Paradoxically single doses of amphetamine may improve mania in some cases (see Chiarello & Cole, 1987).

ECT in mania

The earlier reports of the use of ECT in mania, showed that about two-thirds of the patients responded. More recently in a retrospective study, 78% of patients treated with ECT showed marked improvement compared to 62% on lithium (Black *et al*, 1987*b*). In a double-blind trial, ECT was superior to lithium during the first eight weeks especially for severe mania and mixed states (Small *et al*, 1988). Many clinicians reserve ECT for only the most severe and drug-resistant manic patients and it is possible that more widespread use would be justified. Lithium should be administered cautiously if ECT is to be used because neurotoxic complications have been reported, but not confirmed, in a case-control study (Jha *et al*, 1986).

Leucotomy in bipolar disorder

Patients with intractable bipolar disorders, operated upon by stereotactic subcaudate tractotomy appeared to have a good result (Poynton *et al*, 1988).

Prophylaxis of bipolar disorder

Selection of patients

Maintenance treatment should be considered after a second major episode of bipolar disorder, especially if the interval between episodes is less than five years. Because the intervals between the first and second episode tends to be longer than between subsequent episodes, maintenance treatment should only be used after a first episode if the dangers of a subsequent episode are thought to justify it – for instance if the episode was severe and disruptive, had a relatively sudden onset and was not precipitated by external factors, or if the person's job is very sensitive, or there is a suicide risk.

Lithium prophylaxis

Predicting response to lithium

Patients with typical bipolar disorder and complete recovery between episodes are more likely to benefit (Grof *et al*, 1979). A family history of bipolar disorder is so strongly predictive of prophylactic efficacy as to question whether 'secondary' bipolar disorder ever responds to lithium; indeed neurological signs predict a poor response to lithium (Himmelhoch *et al*, 1980). Patients whose first episode was manic rather than depressive also do better on lithium (Prien *et al*, 1984), and the MDI pattern predicts a better response than the DMI pattern (Faedda *et al*, 1991). It is assumed, although unproven, that a good response to lithium in acute mania or depression predicts prophylactic efficacy. Patients with a rapid-cycling phase of illness are less responsive to lithium (Dunner & Fieve, 1974). Other factors mitigating strongly against prophylactic efficacy are poor adherence to treatment, and drug abuse.

In the prophylaxis of unipolar depressive disorder, a good response to lithium is predicted by a family history of mania or of response to lithium, stable premorbid personality, low neuroticism and good inter-episode functioning.

Blood levels and monitoring

Recent studies have indicated that blood levels lower than those formerly used are sufficient in prophylaxis (Coppen *et al*, 1983). Thus, efficacy was preserved until levels were below 0.6 mmol/l. For some patients lower levels than this would suffice, although Gelenberg *et al* (1989) found that a group with levels of 0.8–1.0 mmol/l had a better outcome than a group with levels of 0.4–0.6 mmol/l. In the elderly, a level of 0.5 mmol/l is recommended (Hardy *et al*, 1987).

Recommendations vary about monitoring lithium, renal and thyroid function tests, but even in the most stable patient these tests should be performed at least once a year, and during less stable phases lithium levels should be done more frequently.

Open studies

The first major report of the prophylactic efficacy of lithium in recurrent affective disorders (Baastrup & Schou, 1967) was a retrospective analysis of the course of illness in 88 patients. While on lithium, affective morbidity was reduced from an average of 13 weeks a year, to 2 weeks. These observations were widely confirmed, but the study design was criticised by Blackwell & Shepherd (1968); the natural course of the illness might have been improvement after a period of frequent episodes, and a double-blind design would be needed to eliminate the effect of bias in the observer and patient.

Trial design in studies of prophylaxis

The methodology for demonstrating the efficacy of a drug such as lithium in long-term prophylaxis is the double-blind placebo-controlled trial with random allocation. Open studies should have been performed first, to explore possible efficacy and side-effects. The trial should select patients with known bipolar disorder, who may be stratified according to the number and pattern of previous episodes, for example rapid-cyclers or older patients would be assigned equally to the two treatments.

The patients should be in remission and receiving no other medication, or steps should be taken to avoid the possibility of withdrawal problems complicating the commencement of the trial – either by weaning off before or tapering the medication after the start of the trial. The patients should be sufficient in numbers to avoid the possibility of a type II statistical error (false negative result). Each patient should give informed consent and the trial should have the approval of the local Ethics Committee and be conducted according to the national and European Community (1991) requirements for Good Clinical Practice, with the possibility of external audit. If an effective treatment already exists, patients can only be admitted ethically to the trial if they are non-responding, or have unacceptable side-effects with existing treatment, or if they recognise the risk of relapse on placebo and agree to this.

The patients should be assigned randomly, to receive either placebo or the study medication (lithium). The dosage may be variable according to blood levels, perhaps within pre-set limits. Dose changes should be made without revealing the nature of the medication to the rating doctor; this can be achieved by making adjustments to the dose in patients in each treatment group. The use of more than one dose range of the active treatment allows dose–response relations to be explored, and compared with side-effect incidence. The blood tests serve also to confirm the patients' adherence to treatment. The trial should be of sufficient duration to show the benefit of the active treatment compared to placebo.

The patients should be assessed regularly using validated clinical rating skills for depression and mania. The criteria for relapse should be defined before the study commences. Patients who relapse during the study should be withdrawn and given treatment appropriate to their condition. During the study other medication should be avoided, although special arrangements may be made for the treatment of intercurrent illnesses not related to the side-effects of the medication under study. In a study of a new treatment, enquiries should be made throughout the study about possible side-effects, but in the case of a medication with a well-established side-effect profile this procedure may undermine the trial by revealing (to the blinded rater) the nature of the patient's medication.

All data should be collected, before the trial code, showing which patient received which medication, is broken. Patients who drop out of the study through side-effects rather than relapse, should be included in the analysis only up to the time of withdrawal. The results should be analysed using appropriate statistical methods preferably by a statistician independent of the investigators. A sequential method of analysis should be considered, to minimise the number of patients exposed to placebo.

Placebo-controlled studies of lithium prophylaxis

There have been ten major double-blind comparative trials of lithium versus placebo in bipolar patients. Three types of design have been used. Two studies used double-blind discontinuation, patients already on lithium being assigned randomly either to continue on lithium or to switch to placebo (Baastrup *et al*, 1970). Twenty-one out of the 39 patients who switched to placebo, and none of the 45 on lithium, relapsed within five months. However this design is weakened by the occurrence of lithium withdrawal mania (see below). One study used a cross-over design which also involved a lithium withdrawal phase (Cundall *et al*, 1972).

A prospective design was used by Coppen *et al* (1971) in the UK and by Prien *et al* (1973) in the USA and in five other studies. Overall in 251 patients on lithium, 34% relapsed in the study period, which varied from

4 months to 3 years, compared to 81% of 263 patients on placebo (see Goodwin & Jamison, 1990). In these studies the efficacy of lithium was more apparent for manic than for depressive relapses. However, retrospective mirror-image studies designed to clarify this suggested that the efficacy in preventing depression may even be greater than that in preventing mania (Poole *et al*, 1978). Lithium reduces both the severity and frequency of episodes. Usually it also stabilises the mood between major episodes.

Antidepressants and lithium

Depression occurring during lithium treatment can be treated with monoamine reuptake inhibitors. In patients with BP–I disorder, the course of antidepressant treatment should be gradually discontinued as the depression improves, in order to reduce the risk of triggering a manic episode (Quitkin *et al*, 1981), and to avoid the induction of rapid-cycling (Wehr & Goodwin, 1979). For patients with a predominantly depressive pattern of bipolar disorder (BP–II) the combination of lithium and a monoamine reuptake inhibitor may be more effective in preventing depression than either drug alone (Shapiro *et al*, 1989).

Pregnancy

In the first trimester lithium can cause cardiac malformations in the foetus, and anti-convulsants are also associated with brain and developmental defects. Because of the possible developmental effects upon the child, pregnancy (in bipolar patients) should if possible be managed without psychotropic drugs. Antipsychotics are probably the safest, if antimanic medication is needed. A woman who becomes pregnant while on lithium or anticonvulsants should be counselled about the risks and offered screening including ultrasound at 18 weeks to detect cardiac defects with a view towards termination.

Withdrawal of lithium

Symptoms of anxiety, irritability and emotional lability can occur following sudden discontinuation of lithium (King & Hullin, 1983). In a double-blind placebo-controlled cross-over study, sudden cessation of lithium in bipolar patients led to the development of mania two to three weeks later in seven out of 14 patients (Mander & Loudon, 1988). A review of all published studies suggests that half the bipolar patients who discontinued lithium had a recurrence within 5 months, usually of mania (Suppes *et al*, 1991). In some patients, discontinuation of lithium leads to recurrent affective swings which cannot be controlled by the reintroduction of lithium (Post, 1990). Discontinuation of lithium should therefore be gradual. Patients whose mood has been stable are less likely to relapse on stopping lithium than those who have continued to show mild mood swings. Lithium may be reduced at the rate of one-quarter to one-eighth of the original dose every two months, to minimise the risk of precipitating withdrawal mania.

Natural outcome on lithium

Dickson & Kendell (1986) reported a three-fold increase in admissions for mania in Edinburgh during the period 1970–1981 when the use of lithium increased. This highlights the difficulty of delivering an effective treatment to a community. A large proportion of patients at risk do not seek treatment, and many who do, adhere poorly to lithium. In addition there is the risk of withdrawal mania in those who stop treatment too abruptly, for instance during a mild upswing of mood when subjects feel they do not need any medication. A naturalistic follow-up in the USA found no difference in outcome over 18 months between bipolar patients discharged on or off lithium (Harrow *et al*, 1990). However, these patients were not randomly assigned. The mortality rate among a group of patients on lithium studied between 1969–1976 was similar to that of manic-depressives before lithium was introduced (Norton & Whalley, 1984).

Under circumstances where special steps are taken to encourage and check adherence, relapse rates and affective morbidity on lithium can be as low as those in controlled trials (McCreadie & Morrison, 1985; Coppen & Abou-Saleh, 1988). This is part of the rationale for specialist lithium or affective disorder clinics. A case-record study of 827 manic-depressive or schizo-affective patients treated with lithium for more than 6 months showed that mortality was reduced to the same level as the general population (Mueller-Oerlinghausen *et al*, 1992). A similar finding was reported by Coppen *et al* (1991).

Adherence to treatment

In the UK the use of lithium is only about 0.8 per 1000 population, even in centres with active lithium clinics (McCreadie & Morrison, 1985); about half the patients who commenced lithium discontinued it within one year, but a quarter remained on it for over 10 years.

The patients who are less likely to adhere tend to be younger, male and to have had fewer previous episodes of illness. The reasons they give for stopping are drug side-effects, missing periods of elation, feeling well and in no need of treatment, feeling depressed or less productive, or not wanting to depend on medication. The side-effects most often given as reasons for non-adherence are excessive thirst and polyuria, tremor, memory impairment, weight gain and hair loss.

In order to increase adherence, the doctor should take side-effects seriously, keep lithium levels as low as possible, educate the patients and their families about their illness and the use of lithium, and discuss adherence with the patient. For non-adherent patients, the regular contact provided by counselling or psychotherapy can be useful and has been shown to improve compliance and affective morbidity (Glick *et al*, 1985). It may be helpful to plot a 'life chart' with the patient and Squillace *et al* described a method for doing this (1984).

Alternatives to lithium

Even in favourable clinical trials, lithium prophylaxis was unsuccessful in over 30% of patients and more recent studies put the average failure rate at 40%. Alternative treatments are clearly needed (for references see Prien & Gelenberg, 1989; Post, 1990).

Carbamazepine

The first controlled studies of the use of carbamazepine in prophylaxis were those of Okuma *et al* (1981) and Post *et al* (1983). This drug has now been shown to be superior to placebo in one study and to be of similar efficacy to lithium in at least seven studies (Coxhead *et al*, 1992). Approximately 65% of bipolar patients showed a good response. In contrast to lithium, rapid-cycling patients benefit as much from carbamazepine as do other bipolar patients. In longer-term use there may be partial loss of efficacy by the third year of treatment, although it is not clear to what extent poor adherence to medication is responsible. The trials of carbamazepine have been reviewed critically by Prien & Gelenberg (1989); further controlled studies are needed to define its place in clinical practice.

Side-effects

These can be minimised by commencing treatment with low doses (100–200mg at night), and increasing every few days to the maximum dose that is well tolerated (usually 400–600mg, maximum 1600mg daily). The patients should be informed of the risk of side-effects including blood disorders (see above), and told to report to the doctor possible symptoms such as sore throat, rash or fever.

Lithium and carbamazepine combination

Some patients appear to benefit more from the combination than from either drug alone. There have been reports of reversible neurological side-effects, characterised mainly by confusional states and cerebellar signs (Shukla *et al*, 1984).

Valproate

Sodium valproate has been studied less but it may be useful for prophylaxis in those who are resistant to lithium or carbamazepine. The combination of lithium with valproate produces less neurological problems than the combination of lithium with carbamazepine. The drug is effective in a large proportion of patients during the rapid-cycling periods of their illness. The efficacy against mania appears greater than against depression (Calabrese & Delucchi, 1990).

Antipsychotic drugs

Because of sedative effects and long-term neurological side-effects, antipsychotic drugs should be avoided if possible for long-term use in bipolar patients. However, for those who have frequently recurring episodes, and either do not benefit from or do not adhere to oral medication, depot formulations of antipsychotic drugs can provide a period of stability (Lowe & Batchelor, 1991; Littlejohn *et al*, 1994).

It has been suggested that patients with bipolar disorder are particularly susceptible to developing tardive dyskinesia (Hamra *et al*, 1983). Other authors have found a prevalence, about 20%, similar to that among patients with chronic schizophrenia (Hunt & Silverstone, 1991). However tardive dyskinesia may be more preventable in bipolar patients since they have less need for long-term antipsychotic drug treatment.

Adjunctive thyroid hormone

There is evidence from placebo-controlled studies that L-thyroxine or tri-iodothyronine in replacement doses can potentiate the antidepressant effect of monoamine reuptake inhibitors in patients with resistant depression. However in long-term prophylaxis this treatment eventually loses efficacy (Wehr *et al*, 1988). High dose thyroid hormone treatment has also been advocated for resistant bipolar patients, especially rapid-cyclers, but prospective placebo-controlled studies are required (Bauer & Whybrow, 1990).

The psychology of mania

Psychoanalytical views

Freud (1917) saw the psychological precipitant of mania (and depression) as the loss of an ambivalently regarded 'object'. Instead of depressive anxiety and guilt, mania is the 'festival of the ego' released from its domination by the super-ego with which it now becomes fused.

Astute clinical observations led Karl Abraham (1924) to regard the basis of all manic symptoms as increased oral drives with accompanying fantasies of cannibalistic incorporation. Manic patients seem to identify with what is incorporated, including both parents. This leads symbolically to phallic identification which can be viewed as a central feature of the psychology of mania.

Winnicott (1935) and Klein (1935), who had herself been analysed by Abraham, introduced the idea of the 'manic defence' against depressive anxiety. The manic defences (omnipotent control, triumph and contempt) protect the ego against despair, but interrupt the process of reparation, and produce a vicious circle by further attacks upon the 'object'. However a manic form of reparation can occur and some of the identifications made in mania can be seen as potential advances in individual development.

Lewin (1951) wrote of the 'oral triad' of the wishes to eat, be 'eaten'(or taken in) and to sleep. In mania the second component is resisted because of a dread of phallic rivalry; oral devouring is prolonged and sleep postponed.

These ideas are sometimes helpful in understanding the content of the manics ideas. However their aetiological significance is less clear, a fact recognised by Freud who referred to the 'economic problem' of the libido in mania and depression.

Dependence

Fromm-Reichmann emphasised the contrast between the dependence of the depressive, and the assertiveness, rivalry and independence of the manic state (Cohen *et al*, 1954). These changes in feelings of dependence are relevant to the marital difficulties and the tendency to substance misuse in bipolar patients.

Beliefs

Religious and other beliefs can be altered by pathological mood states and can become important parts of the individual's identity. Martin Luther, the leader of the Reformation in Germany, experienced marked depressive and hypomanic swings. He composed hymns of joy and strength and revived the doctrine of justification by the faith of the individual. The mechanisms behind his ambivalent rejection of the Pope's authority are open to psychoanalytical interpretation. His life was the subject of a book by Erikson (1958).

Leadership and creativity

There has been a view held at periods in history that madness and genius are related. Much of the evidence is based on individual biographical accounts, but recent work has investigated the association critically (Goodwin & Jamison, 1990).

Leadership

Among military leaders Achilles in legend, Alexander the Great and Napoleon have all showed features of cyclothymia. Oliver Cromwell's biographer, Christopher Hill (1970) describes explicitly the evidence of hypomanic phases as well as depression. Among war-time political leaders, Churchill, Roosevelt and Mussolini exhibited features of hypomania, and Churchill was prone also to periods of depression which he called "black dog". Driving energy, sense of purpose and right, confidence and the ability to convey this to others, are relevant traits, together with varying degrees of grandiosity. In peacetime leaders these traits tend to be less important or even disadvantageous. Even in war it is likely that they lead to rash or catastrophic decisions, for instance the destruction of whole cities or civilisations.

Artistic creativity

Among visual artists Michelangelo, Van Gogh, and many others showed severe mood swings and some died by suicide. The composers Schumann, Bruckner, Tchaikovsky and Mahler were cyclothymic or manic-depressive. Schumann's creative output was greatly increased during two hypomanic periods and diminished during depression, and he died of self-starvation in an asylum. In these individuals the intense feelings associated with mood swings may have increased a desire to express themselves in art. Freedom from normal restraints and heightened sensory perceptions may have contributed to their originality.

The poets Shelley, Byron, and Chatterton were manic-depressive, Robert Lowell had BP-I disorder, Sylvia Plath had BP-II disorder and committed suicide. The novelists and playwrights Balzak, Ruskin, Hemingway, Scott Fitzgerald and Virginia Woolf were cyclothymic or manic-depressive. In the case of Virginia Woolf the writing of her most original, 'stream of conciousness', novels usually led into a psychotic breakdown. In the interval between these novels she wrote less original 'novels of fact' or 'holiday books'. Her nephew and biographer Quentin Bell described her imagination as being "furnished with an accelerator but no brakes", an admirable description of a manic trait (Lehmann, 1987). Caramagno (1992) has studied the links between her cycles of mood and creativity in depth.

In Churchill's case, Storr (1969) emphasised the creative use of words and ideas; his writing, painting and oratory were 'manic defences' against the depressive tendencies which could be traced in the family to the first Duke of Marlborough. His daughter however has stated that her mother "very largely kennelled the black dog" except in his old age (Soames, 1993). Among performing artists, comedians seem particularly likely to have bipolar conditions, and this association has been described in detail in one case (Milligan & Clare, 1993). In some cases the long intervals between major works suggests a link with affective swings. Joseph Conrad considered writing "a sort of mental revulsion" and described his completion of Nostromo as a "recovery from a dangerous illness".

Critical studies

Andreasen (1987) found a lifetime prevalence of bipolar disorder of 43% among a group of American writers compared to 10% among matched controls. Alcoholism was also more prevalent in the writers. In their first-degree relatives, affective disorder had occurred in 18% of writers and 2% of controls, usually in the form of major depression. Jamison (1989) investigated the link between creativity and affective swings in 47 outstanding British artists and writers. 38% had been treated for an affective illness, 6% for BP–I disorder. Poets were the most commonly treated with medication, and were the only group to have BP–I disorder (17%). Playwrights were the most commonly treated with psychotherapy. Biographers and visual artists had somewhat lower rates than the other writers, though greater than in the general population. Ninety per cent of all the subjects reported intense creative episodes; these usually lasted about two weeks but a quarter lasted more than a month and were characterised by many of the features of hypomania though not usually by increased talkativeness or sociability.

Conclusion

Mania can affect people of all social and occupational groups and is usually a phase in a recurring bipolar illness. Hypomanic traits and episodes can be associated with successful leadership, productivity and creativity but can also be disruptive. Manic episodes are very disruptive and there is a high rate of divorce and successful suicide in bipolar patients. Treatment will often minimise or allow such disruptions to be avoided, and reduce the suicide risk. Sufferers from these conditions are now able to choose such treatments, and doctors and relatives should encourage them to make this choice.

References

Abraham, K. (1924) A short study of the development of the libido, viewed in the light of mental disorders: mania. In *Selected papers of Karl Abraham* (Trans. D. Bryan & A. Strachey, 1949), pp. 470–475. London: Hogarth.

Ahlfors, U. G., Baastrup. P. C., Dencker, S. J., *et al* (1981) Flupenthixol decanoate in recurrent manic depressive illness: a comparison with lithium. *Acta Psychiatrica Scandinavica*, **64**, 226–237.

Akiskal, H. S., Downs, J., Jordan, P., *et al* (1985) Affective disorder in referred children and younger siblings of manic-depressives: Mode of onset and prospective course. *Archives of General Psychiatry*, **42**, 996–1003.

Almy, G. L. & Taylor, M. A. (1973) Lithium retention in mania. *Archives of General Psychiatry*, **29**, 232–234.

Ambelas, A. (1987) Life events and mania: a special relationship? *British Journal of Psychiatry*, **150**, 235–240.

Amdisen, A. (1984) In *Depression and Mania: Modern Lithium Therapy* (ed. N. Johnson), pp. 24–28. Oxford: IRL Press.

American Psychiatric Association (1994) *Diagnostic and Statistical Manual of Mental Disorders* (4th edn) (DSM–IV). Washington, DC: APA.

Andreasen, N. C. (1987) Creativity and mental illness: prevalence rates in writers and their first-degree relatives. *American Journal of Psychiatry*, **144**, 1288–1292.

Angst, J. (1985) Switch from depression to mania: a record study over decades between 1920 and 1982. *Psychopathology*, **18**, 140–155.

Aronson, T. A. & Shukla, S. (1987) Life events and relapse in bipolar disorder: the impact of a catastrophic event. *Acta Psychiatrica Scandinavica*, **75**, 571–576.

Asnis, G. M., Asnis, D., Dunner, D. L., *et al* (1979) Cogwheel rigidity during chronic lithium therapy. *American Journal of Psychiatry*, **136**, 1225–1226.

Baastrup, P. C. & Schou, M. (1967) Lithium as a prophylactic agent: its effect against recurrent depression and manic-depressive psychosis. *Archives of General Psychiatry*, **16**, 162–177.

——, Poulsen, J. C., Schou, M., *et al* (1970) Prophylactic lithium: double-blind discontinuation in manic-depressive and recurrent-depressive disorder. *Lancet*, **2**, 326–330.

Bacher, N. M. & Lewis, H. A. (1979) Lithium plus reserpine in refractory manic patients. *American Journal of Psychiatry*, **136**, 811–814.

Ballenger, J. C. & Post, R. M. (1980) Carbamazepine in manic-depressive illness: A new treatment. *American Journal of Psychiatry*, **137**, 782–790.

Bauer. M. S. & Whybrow, P. C. (1990) Rapid-cycling bipolar affective disorder. II. Treatment of refractory rapid-cycling with high dose levothyroxine: a preliminary study. *Archives of General Psychiatry*, **47**, 435–440.

——, —— & Winokur, A. (1990) Rapid-cycling bipolar affective disorder. Association with Grade I hypothyroidism. *Archives of General Psychiatry*, **47**, 427–432.

Bauwens, F., Tracy, A., Pardoen, D., *et al* (1991) Social adjustment of remitted bipolar and unipolar out-patients. *British Journal of Psychiatry*, **159**, 239–244.

Bech, P., Kastrup, M. & Rafaelsen, O. J. (1986) Mini-compendium of rating scales for states of anxiety, depression, mania and schizophrenia with corresponding DSM–III syndromes. *Acta Psychiatrica Scandinavica*, **326** (Suppl.), 1–37.

Beigel, A. & Murphy, D. L. (1971) Assessing clinical characteristics of the manic state. *American Journal of Psychiatry*, **128**, 688–694.

——, —— & Bunney, W. E. (1971) The Manic-State Rating Scale: Scale construction, reliability, and validity. *Archives of General Psychiatry*, **25**, 256–262.

Bernadt, M. W. & Murray, R. M. (1986) Psychiatric disorder, drinking and alcoholism. *British Journal of Psychiatry*, **148**, 393–400.

Birch, N. J., Horsman, A. & Hullin, R. P. (1982) Lithium, bone and body weight studies in long-term lithium-treated patients and in the rat. *Neuropsychobiology*, **8**, 86–92.

Black, D. W., Winokur, G. & Nasrallah, M. A. (1987*a*) Suicide in sub-types of major affective disorder: A comparison with general population suicide mortality. *Archives of General Psychiatry*, **44**, 878–880.

——, —— & —— (1987*b*) Treatment of mania. A naturalistic study of electroconvulsive therapy versus lithium in 438 patients. *Journal of Clinical Psychiatry*, **48**, 132–139.

Blackburn, I. M., Loudon, J. B. & Ashworth, C. M. (1977) A new scale for measuring mania. *Psychological Medicine*, **7**, 453–458.

Blackwell, B. & Shepherd, M. (1968) Prophylactic lithium. Another therapeutic myth? *Lancet*, **1**, 968–971.

Bland, R. C. & Orn, H. (1982) Course and outcome of affective disorders. *Canadian Journal of Psychiatry*, **27**, 573–578.

Blay, S. L., Toledo Ferraz, M. P. & Calil, H. M. (1982) Lithium-induced male sexual impairment: two case reports. *Journal of Clinical Psychiatry*, **43**, 497–498.

Bowden, C. L., Brugger, A. M., Swann, A. C., et al (1994) Efficacy of Divalproex vs lithium and placebo in the treatment of mania. *Journal of the American Medical Association*, **271**, 918–924.

Bowen, R. C., Grof, P. & Grof, E. (1991) Less frequent lithium administration and lower urine volume. *American Journal of Psychiatry*, **148**, 189–192.

Bradwejn, J., Shriqui, C., Koszycki, D., *et al* (1990) Double-blind comparison of the effects of clonazepam and lorazepam in acute mania. *Journal of Clinical Psychopharmacology*, **10**, 403–408.

Brockington, I. F., Wainwright, S. & Kendell, R. E. (1980) Manic patients with schizophrenic or paranoid symptoms. *Psychological Medicine*, **10**, 73–83.

Brodie, H. K. H. & Leff, M. J. (1971) Bipolar depression – a comparative study of patient characteristics. *American Journal of Psychiatry*, **127**, 1086–1090.

Bucht, G., Wahlin, A., Wentzel, T., *et al* (1980) Renal function and morphology in long-term lithium and combined lithium-neuroleptic treatment. *Acta Medica Scandinavica*, **208**, 381–385.

Cade, J. F. J. (1949) Lithium salts in the treatment of psychotic excitement. *Medical Journal of Australia*, **36**, 349–352.

Calabrese, J. R. & Delucchi, G. A. (1990) Spectrum of efficacy of valproate in 55 patients with rapid-cycling bipolar disorder. *American Journal of Psychiatry*, **147**, 431–434.

——, Gulledge, A. D., Hahn, K., *et al* (1985) Autoimmune thyroiditis in manic-depressive patients treated with lithium. *American Journal of Psychiatry*, **142**, 1318–1321.

Caramagno, T. C. (1992) *The Flight of Mind. Virginia Woolf's Art and Manic-Depressive Illness*. Oxford: University of California Press.

Carlson, G. A. (1980) Manic-depressive illness and cognitive immaturity. In *Mania: An Evolving Concept* (eds R. H. Belmaker & H. M. van Praag), pp. 281–289. New York: Spectrum Books.

—— & Goodwin, F. K. (1973) The stages of mania: a longitudinal analysis of the manic episode. *Archives of General Psychiatry*, **28**, 221–228.

——, Kotin, J., Davenport, Y. B., *et al* (1974) Follow-up of 53 bipolar manic-depressive patients. *British Journal of Psychiatry*, **124**, 134–139.

Chakrabarti, S., Kulhara, P. & Verma, S. K. (1992) Extent and determinants of burden among families of patients with affective disorder. *Acta Psychiatrica Scandinavica*, **86**, 247–252.

Charney, D. S., Kales, A., Soldatos, C., *et al* (1979) Somnambulistic-like episode, secondary to contained lithium-neuroleptic treatment. *British Journal of Psychiatry*, **135**, 418–424.

Chen, Y. & Silverstone, T. (1990) Lithium and weight gain. *International Clinical Psychopharmacology*, **5**, 217–225.

Chiarello, R. J. & Cole, J. O. (1987) The use of psychostimulants in general psychiatry. *Archives of General Psychiatry*, **44**, 286–295.

Chouinard, G. (1987) Clonazepam in acute and maintenance treatment of bipolar affective disorder. *Journal of Clinical Psychiatry*, **48** (Suppl.), 29–36.

Cohen, M. B., Baker, G., Cohen, R. A., *et al* (1954) An intensive study of twelve cases of manic-depressive psychosis. *Psychiatry*, **17**, 103–137.

Cohen, W. J. & Cohen, N. H. (1974) Lithium carbonate, haloperidol, and irreversible brain damage. *Journal of the American Medical Association*, **230**, 1283–1287.

Coid, J. & Strang, J. (1982) Mania secondary to procyclidine (Kemadrin) abuse. *British Journal of Psychiatry*, **141**, 81–84.

Cookson, J. C. (1985) The neuroendocrinology of mania. *Journal of Affective Disorder*, **8**, 233–241.

—— (1989) Manic-depressive illness and driving. *Travel Medicine International*, **7**, 105–108.

——, Silverstone, T. & Wells, B. (1981) A double-blind comparative clinical trial of pimozide and chlorpromazine in mania: a test of the dopamine hypothesis. *Acta Psychiatrica Scandinavica*, **64**, 381–397.

——, Moult, P. J. A., Wiles, D., *et al* (1983) The relationship between prolactin levels and clinical ratings in manic patients treated with oral and intravenous test doses of haloperidol. *Psychological Medicine*, **13**, 279–285.

——, Silverstone, T., Williams, S., *et al* (1985) Plasma corticol levels in mania: Associated clinical ratings and change during treatment with haloperidol. *British Journal of Psychiatry*, **146**, 498–502.

Coppen, A., Prange, A. J., Whybrow, P. C., *et al* (1969) Methysergide in mania: A controlled trial. *Lancet*, **2**, 338–340.

——, Noguera, R., Bailey, J., *et al* (1971) Prophylactic lithium in affective disorders: controlled trial. *Lancet*, **2**, 275–279.

——, Abou-Saleh, M. T., Milln, P., *et al* (1983) Decreasing lithium dosage reduces morbidity and side-effects during prophylaxis. *Journal of Affective Disorders*, **5**, 353–362.

—— & —— (1988) Lithium therapy. From clinical trials to practical management. *Acta Psychiatrica Scandinavica*, **78**, 754–762.

——, Standish-Barry, H., Bailey, J., *et al* (1991) Does lithium reduce the mortality of recurrent mood disorders? *Journal of Affective Disorders*, **23**, 1–7.

Corn, T. H. & Checkley, S. A. (1983) A case of recurrent mania with recurrent hyperthyroidism. *British Journal of Psychiatry*, **143**, 74–76.

Coxhead, N., Silverstone, T. & Cookson, J. C. (1992) Carbamazepine versus lithium in the prophylaxis of bipolar affective disorder. *Acta Psychiatrica Scandinavica*, **85**, 114–118.

Cundall, R. L., Brooks, P. W. & Murray, L. G. (1972) A controlled evaluation of lithium prophylaxis in affective disorders. *Psychological Medicine*, **2**, 308–311.

Cutler, N. R. & Post, R. M. (1982) Life course of illness in untreated manic-depressive patients. *Comprehensive Psychiatry*, **23**, 101–115.

Dickson, W. E. & Kendall, R. E. (1986) Does maintenance lithium therapy prevent recurrences of mania under ordinary clinical conditions? *Psychological Medicine*, **16**, 521–530.

Dinan, T. G., Silverstone, T. & Cookson, J. C. (1988) Cortisol, prolactin and growth hormone levels with clinical ratings in manic patients treated with verapamil. *International Clinical Psychopharmacology*, **3**, 151–156.

—— & Kohen, D. (1989) Tardive dyskinesia and bipolar affective disorder: relationship to lithium therapy. *British Journal of Psychiatry*, **155**, 55–57.

Dunner, D. L. & Fieve, R. R. (1974) Clinical factors in lithium prophylaxis failure. *Archives of General Psychiatry*, **30**, 229–233.

——, Fleiss, J. L. & Fieve, R. R. (1976a) Lithium carbonate prophylaxis failure. *British Journal of Psychiatry*, **129**, 40–44.

——, Gershon, E. S. & Goodwin, F. K. (1976b) Heritable factors in the severity of affective illness. *Biological Psychiatry*, **11**, 31–42.

Elphick, M., Yang, J. D. & Cowen, P. H. (1990) Effects of carbamazepine on dopamine and serotonin-mediated neuroendocrine responses. *Archives of General Psychiatry*, **47**, 135–143.

Erikson, E. H. (1958) *Young Man Luther*. New York: W. W. Norton.

Fadden, G., Bebbington, P. & Kuipers, L. (1987) Caring and its burdens: a study of spouses of depressed patients. *British Journal of Psychiatry*, **151**, 660–667.

Faedda, G. L., Baldessarini, R. J., Tohen, M., *et al* (1991) Episode sequence in bipolar disorder and response to lithium treatment. *American Journal of Psychiatry*, **148**, 1237–1239.

Freinhar, J. P. & Alvarez, W. H. (1985) Androgen-induced hypomania (Letter). *Journal of Clinical Psychiatry*, **46**, 354–355.

Freud, S. (1917) *Mourning and Melancholia*. Standard Edition of the Complete Works. Volume XIV. (ed. J. Strachey). London: Hogarth Press.

Gawin, F. H. & Kleber, H. D. (1986) Abstinence symptomatology and psychiatric diagnosis in cocaine abusers. *Archives of General Psychiatry*, **43**, 107–113.

Gelenberg, A. J., Kane, J. M., Keller, M. B., *et al* (1989) Comparison of standard and low serum levels of lithium for maintenance treatment of bipolar disorder. *New England Journal of Medicine*, **321**, 1489–1493.

Gerner, R. H., Post, R. M. & Bunney, W. E. (1976) A dopaminergic mechanism in mania. *American Journal of Psychiatry*, **133**, 1177–1180.

Glick, I. D., Clarkin, J. F., Spencer, J. H., *et al* (1985) A controlled evaluation of in-patient family intervention: preliminary results of the six-month follow-up. *Archives of General Psychiatry*, **42**, 882–886.

Glue, P. (1989) Rapid-cycling affective disorders in the mentally retarded. *Biological Psychiatry*, **26**, 250–256.

Goodwin, F. K., Murphy, D. C. & Bunney, W. F. (1969) Lithium carbonate treatment in depression and mania: a longitudinal double-blind study. *Archives of General Psychiatry*, **21**, 486–496.

—— & Ebert, M. (1973) Lithium in mania. Clinical trials and controlled studies. In *Lithium: Its Role in Psychiatric Research and Treatment* (eds S. Gershon & B. Shopsin) pp. 237–252. New York: Plenum Press.

—— & Jamison, K. R. (1990) *Manic-Depressive Illness*. Oxford: Oxford University Press.

Grof, P., Angst, J., Karasek, M., *et al* (1979) Patient selection for long-term lithium treatment in clinical practice. *Archives of General Psychiatry*, **36**, 894–897.

Hamra, B., Nasrallah, H., Clancy, J., *et al* (1983) Psychiatric diagnosis and risk for tardive dyskinesia. *Archives of General Psychiatry*, **40**, 346–347.

Hansen, H. E. & Amdisen, A. (1978) Lithium intoxication (report of 23 cases and a review of 100 cases from the literature). *Quarterly Journal of Medicine*, **47**, 123–144.

Harding, T. & Knight, F. (1973) Marijuana-modified mania. *Archives of General Psychiatry*, **29**, 635–637.

Hardy, B. G., Shulman, K. I., Mackenzie, S. E., *et al* (1987) Pharmacokinetics of lithium in the elderly. *Journal of Clinical Psychopharmacology*, **7**, 153–158.

Hare, E. H. (1976) Hypomania. *Bethlem and Maudsley Gazette*. Summer Number, 3–5.

—— (1981) The two manias: A study of the evolution of the modern concept of mania. *British Journal of Psychiatry*, **138**, 89–99.

Harrow, M., Goldberg, J. F., Grossman, L. S., *et al* (1990) Outcome in manic disorder: a naturalistic follow-up study. *Archives of General Psychiatry*, **47**, 665–671.

Hestbech, J., Hansen, S. E., Amdisen, A., *et al* (1977) Chronic renal lesions following long-term treatment with lithium. *Kidney International*, 12, 205–213.

Hill, C. (1970) *God's Englishman*. London: Weidenfeld and Nicholson.

Himmelhoch, J. M., Mulla, D., Neil, J. F., *et al* (1976) Incidence and significance of mixed affective states in a bipolar population. *Archives of General Psychiatry*, **33**, 1062–1066.

——, Neil, J. F., May, S. J., *et al* (1980) Age, dementia, dyskinesias, and lithium response. *American Journal of Psychiatry*, **137**, 941–945.

Horgan, D. (1981) Change of diagnosis to manic-depressive illness. *Psychological Medicine*, **11**, 517–523.

Horn, A. S., Coyle, J. T. & Snyder, S. H. (1971) Catecholamine uptake by synaptosomes from rat brain. Structure-activity relationships of drugs with differential effects on dopamine and norepinephrine neurones. *Molecular Pharmacology*, **7**, 66–80.

Hoschl, C. & Kozeny, J. (1989) Verapamil in affective disorders. A controlled, double-blind study. *Biological Psychiatry*, **25**, 128–140.

Hunt, N. & Silverstone, T. (1991) Tardive dyskinesia in bipolar affective disorder: A catchment area study. *International Clinical Psychopharmacology*, **6**, 45–50.

——, Bruce-Jones, W. & Silverstone, T. (1992a) Life events in bipolar affective disorder. *Journal of Affective Disorders*, **25**, 13–20.

——, Sayer, H. & Silverstone, T. (1992b) Season and manic relapse. *Acta Psychiatrica Scandinavia*, **85**, 123–126.

Jacobs, D. & Silverstone, T. (1986) Dextroamphetamine-induced arousal in human subjects as a model for mania. *Psychological Medicine*, **16**, 323–329.

Jacobson, S. J., Jones, K., Johnson, K., *et al* (1992) Prospective multi-centre study of pregnancy outcome after lithium exposure during first trimester. *Lancet*, **339**, 530–533.

Jamison, K. R. (1989) Mood disorders and seasonal patterns in British writers and artists. *Psychiatry*, **52**, 125–134.

Janicak, P. G., Bresnahan, D. B., Sharma, R., *et al* (1988) A comparison of thiothixine with chlorpromazine in the treatment of mania. *Journal of Clinical Psychopharmacology*, **8**, 33–37.

——, Sharma, R. P., Easton, M., *et al* (1989) A double-blind, placebo controlled trial of clonidine in the treatment of acute mania. *Psychopharmacology Bulletin,* **25**, 243–245.

Janowsky, D. S., El-Yousef, M. K., Davis, J. M., *et al* (1973) Parasympathetic suppression of manic symptoms by physostigmine. *Archives of General Psychiatry,* **28**, 542–547.

——, —— & —— (1974) Interpersonal manoeuvers of manic patients. *American Journal of Psychiatry,* **131**, 250–255.

Jauhar, P. & Weller, M. P. I. (1982) Psychiatric morbidity and time zone changes: a study of patients from Heathrow Airport. *British Journal of Psychiatry,* **140**, 231–235.

Jeste, D. V., Lohr, J. B. & Goodwin, F. K. (1988) Neuroanatomical studies of major affective disorders. A review and suggestions for further research. *British Journal of Psychiatry,* **153**, 444–459.

Jha, A. K., Stein, G. S. & Fenwick, P. (1996) Negative interaction between lithium and electroconvulsive therapy. A case-control study. *British Journal of Psychiatry,* **168**, 241–243.

Johnson, D. A. W., Lowe, M. R. & Batchelor, D. H. (1990) Combined lithium-neuroleptic therapy for manic-depressive illness. *Human Psychopharmacology,* **5** (suppl.), 262–297.

Johnson, G. (1984) Lithium. *Medical Journal of Australia,* **141**, 595–601.

Josephson, A. M. & Mackenzie, T. B. (1980) Thyroid-induced mania in hypothyroid patients. *American Journal of Psychiatry,* **137**, 222–228.

Kahlbaum, K. L. (1874) *Catatonia* (translated from the German, 1974). Baltimore: Johns Hopkins University Press.

King, J. R. & Hullin, R. P. (1983) Withdrawal symptoms from lithium. Four case reports and a questionnaire study. *British Journal of Psychiatry,* **143**, 30–35.

Klein, D. N., Depue, R. A. & Slater, J. F. (1985) Cyclothymia in the adolescent offspring of parents with bipolar affective disorder. *Journal of Abnormal Psychology,* **94**, 115–129.

Klein, M. (1935) See Segal, H. (1975) *Introduction to the works of Melanie Klein* (ed. M. M. P. Khan) International Psychoanalytical Library. London: Hogarth Press.

Kotin, J. & Goodwin, F. K. (1972) Depression during mania: clinical observations and theoretical implications. *American Journal of Psychiatry,* **129**, 679–686.

Kramlinger, K. G. & Post, R. M. (1989) Adding lithium carbonate to carbamazepine: anti-manic efficacy in treatment-resistant mania. *Acta Psychiatrica Scandinavica,* **79**, 378–385.

Krauthammer, C. & Klerman, G. L. (1978) Secondary mania: manic syndromes associated with antecedent physical illness or drugs. *Archives of General Psychiatry,* **35**, 1333–1339.

Kron, L., Decina, P., Kestenbaum, C. J., *et al* (1982) The offspring of bipolar manic-depressives: clinical features. In *Adolescent Psychiatry, Vol. 10.* (eds S. C. Feinstein, J. G. Looney & A. Z. Schwartzbert), pp. 273–291. Chicago: University Press.

Kukopulos, A., Minnai, G. & Muller-Oerlinghausen, B. (1985) The influence of mania and depression on the pharmacokinetics of lithium: a longitudinal single-case study. *Journal of Affective Disorders,* **8**, 159–166.

Lawler, P. G. & Cove-Smith, J. R. (1986) Acute respiratory failure following lithium intoxication. *Anaesthesia,* **41**, 623–627.

Lazarus, J. H., John, R., Bennie, E. H., *et al* (1981) Lithium therapy and thyroid function: a long-term study. *Psychological Medicine*, **11**, 85–92.

Lehmann, J. (1987) *Virginia Woolf*. London: Thames and Hudson Literary Lives.

Lerner, Y. (1980) The subjective experience of mania. In *Mania: An Evolving Concept* (eds R. H. Belmaker & H. M. van Praag), pp. 77–88. Jamaica, NY: Spectrum Publications.

Lewin, B. (1951) *The Psychoanalysis of Elation*. London: Hogarth Press.

Ling, M. H. M., Perry, P. J. & Tsuang, M. T. (1981) Side-effects of corticosteroid therapy. *Archives of General Psychiatry*, **38**, 471–477.

Littlejohn, R., Leslie, F. & Cookson, J. C. (1992) Depot anti-psychotics in the prophylaxis of bipolar affective disorder. *British Journal of Psychiatry*, **165**, 827–829.

Loudon, J. B. & Waring, H. (1976) Toxic reactions to lithium and haloperidol. *Lancet*, **2**, 1088.

Lowe, M. R. & Batchelor, D. H. (1990) Lithium and neuroleptics in the management of manic-depressive psychosis. *Human Psychopharmacology*, **5**, 267–274.

Maguire, J. & Singh, A. N. (1987) Clonidine. An effective antimanic agent. *British Journal of Psychiatry*, **150**, 863–864.

McCreadie, R. G. & Morrison, D. P. (1985) The impact of lithium in south-west Scotland. *British Journal of Psychiatry*, **146**, 70–74.

Mander, A. J. & Loudon, J. B. (1988) Rapid recurrence of mania following abrupt discontinuation of lithium. *Lancet*, ii, 15–17.

Maggs, R. (1963) Treatment of manic illness with lithium carbonate. *British Journal of Psychiatry*, **109**, 56–65.

Miklowitz, D. J., Goldstein, M. J., Neuch Terlein, K. H., *et al* (1988) Family factors and the course of bipolar affective illness. *Archives of General Psychiatry*, **45**, 225–231.

Milligan, S. & Clare, A. (1993) *Depression and How to Survive it*. London: Ebury Press.

Mitchell, J. E. & Mackenzie, T. B. (1982) Cardiac effects of lithium therapy in man: a review. *Journal of Clinical Psychiatry*, **43**, 47–51.

Modell, J. G., Lenox, R. H. & Weiner, S. (1985) In-patient clinical trial of lorazepam for the management of manic agitation. *Journal of Clinical Psychopharmacology*, **5**, 109–113.

Morgan, H. G. (1972) The incidence of depressive symptoms during recovery from hypomania. *British Journal of Psychiatry*, **120**, 537–539.

Muller-Oerlinghausen, B., Ahren, B., Grof, E., *et al* (1992) The effects of long-term lithium treatment on the mortality of patients with manic-depressive and schizo-affective illness. *Acta Psychiatrica Scandinavica*, **86**, 218–222.

Murphy, D. L. & Beigel, A. (1974) Depression, elation, and lithium carbonate responses in manic patient sub-groups. *Archives of General Psychiatry*, **31**, 643–648.

Myers, D. H., Carter, R. A., Burns, B. H., *et al* (1985) A prospective study of the effects of lithium on thyroid function and on the prevalence of thyroid antibodies. *Psychological Medicine*, **15**, 55–61.

Norton, B. & Whalley, L. J. (1984) Mortality of a lithium-treated population. *British Journal of Psychiatry*, **145**, 277–282.

Okuma, T., Kishimoto, A., Inoue, K., *et al* (1973) Antimanic and prophylactic effects of carbamazepine (Tegretol) on manic depressive psychosis: a preliminary report. *Folia Psychiatrica Neurology Japan*, **27**, 283–297.

——, Inanaga, K., Otsuki, S., *et al* (1981) A preliminary double-blind study of carbamazepine in prophylaxis of manic-depressive illness. *Psychopharmacology*, **73**, 95–96.

Pauls, D. L., Morton, L. A. & Egeland, J. A. (1992) Risks of affective illness among first degree relatives of bipolar I old-order Amish probands. *Archives of General Psychiatry*, **49**, 703–708.

Poole, A. J., James, H. D. & Hughes, W. C. (1978) Treatment experience in the lithium clinic at St. Thomas' Hospital. *Journal of Royal Society of Medicine*, **71**, 890–894.

Pope, H. G., McElroy, S. L., Keck, P. E., *et al* (1991) Valproate in the treatment of acute mania: a placebo-controlled study. *Archives of General Psychiatry*, **48**, 62–68.

Post, R. M. (1990) Prophylaxis of bipolar disorders. *International Review of Psychiatry*, **2**, 227–320.

—— (1992) Transduction of psychosocial stress into the neurobiology of recurrent affective disorder. *American Journal of Psychiatry*, **149**, 999–1010.

——, Ballenger, J. C., Rey, A. C., *et al* (1981) Slow and rapid onset of manic episodes: implications for underlying biology. *Psychiatry Research*, **4**, 229–237.

——, Uhde, T. W., Ballenger, J. C., *et al* (1983) Prophylactic efficacy of carbamazepine in manic-depressive illness. *American Journal of Psychiatry*, **140**, 1602–1604.

——, ——, Roy-Byrne, P. P., *et al* (1987) Correlates of antimanic responses to carbamazepine. *Psychiatry Research*, **21**, 71–83.

——, Rubinow, D. R., Uhde, T. W., *et al* (1989) Dysphoric mania: clinical and biological correlates. *Archives of General Psychiatry*, **46**, 353–358.

Poynton, A., Bridges, P. & Bartlett, J. R. (1988) Resistant bipolar affective disorder treated by stereotactic subcaudate tractotomy. *British Journal of Psychiatry*, **152**, 354–358.

Prange, A. J., Wilson, I. C., Lynn, C. W., *et al* (1974) L-tryptophan in mania: Contribution to a permissive hypothesis of affective disorders. *Archives of General Psychiatry*, **30**, 56–62.

Prien, R. F., Caffey, E. M. & Klett, C. J. (1972) Comparison of lithium carbonate and chlorpromazine in the treatment of mania. *Archives of General Psychiatry*, **26**, 146–153.

——, —— & —— (1973) Prophylactic efficacy of lithium carbonate in manic-depressive illness. *Archives of General Psychiatry*, **28**, 337–341.

——, Kupfer, D. J., Mansky, P. A., *et al* (1984) Drug therapy in the prevention of recurrences in unipolar and bipolar affective disorder: Report of the NIMH Collaborative Study Group comparing lithium carbonate, imipramine, and a lithium carbonate-imipramine combination. *Archives of General Psychiatry*, **41**, 1096–1104.

—— & Gelenberg, A. J. (1989) Alternatives to lithium for preventive treatment of bipolar disorder. *American Journal of Psychiatry*, **146**, 840–848.

Quitkin, F. M., Kane, J., Rifkin, A., *et al* (1981) Prophylactic lithium carbonate with and without imipramine for bipolar 1 patients: a double-blind study. *Archives of General Psychiatry*, **38**, 902–907.

Radke-Yarrow, M., Cummings, E. M., Kuczynski, L., *et al* (1985) Patterns of attachment in two and three year olds in normal families and families with parental depression. *Child Development*, **56**, 884–893.

Rifkin, A., Doddi, S., Borenstein, M., *et al* (1994) Dosage of haloperidol for mania. *British Journal of Psychiatry*, **165**, 113–116.

Rosenthal, N. E., Sack, D. A., Gillin, J. C., *et al* (1984) Seasonal affective disorder. *Archives of General Psychiatry*, **4**, 72–80.

Rottanburg, D., Robins, A. H., Ben-Arie, O., *et al* (1982) Cannabis-associated psychosis with manic features. *Lancet*, **ii**, 1364–1366.

Schou, M. (1979) Artistic productivity and lithium prophylaxis in manic-depressive illness. *British Journal of Psychiatry*, **135**, 97–103.

—— (1984) Long-lasting neurological sequelae after lithium intoxication. *Acta Psychiatrica Scandinavica*, **70**, 594–602.

——, Juel-Nielson, N., Stromgren, E., *et al* (1954) The treatment of manic psychoses by administration of lithium salts. *Journal of Neurology, Neurosurgery and Psychiatry*, **17**, 250–260.

Sclare, P. & Creed, F. (1987) Life events and the onset of mania. *British Journal of Psychiatry*, **156**, 508–514.

Sellers, J., Tyrer, P., Whiteley, A., *et al* (1982) Neurotoxic effects of lithium with delayed rise in serum lithium levels. *British Journal of Psychiatry*, **140**, 623–625.

Shapiro, D. R., Quitkin, F. M. & Fleiss, J. L. (1989) Response to maintenance therapy in bipolar illness: effect of index episode. *Archives of General Psychiatry*, **46**, 401–405.

Shukla, S., Godwin, C. D., Long, L. E. B., *et al* (1984) Lithium-carbamazepine neurotoxicity and risk factors. *American Journal of Psychiatry*, **141**, 1604–1606.

——, Cook, B. L., Mukherjee, S., *et al* (1987) Mania folowing head trauma. *American Journal of Psychiatry*, **144**, 93–96.

Small, J. G., Klapper, M. H., Kellams, J. J., *et al* (1988) Electroconvulsive treatment compared with lithium in the management of manic states. *Archives of General Psychiatry*, **45**, 727–732.

Smith, S. J. M. & Kocen, R. S. (1988) A Creutzfeldt-Jakob like syndrome due to lithium toxicity. *Journal of Neurology, Neurosurgery and Psychiatry*, **51**, 120–123.

Soames, M. (1993) *Life with my father Winston*. The Observer, Feb 14, 49–50.

Squillace, K., Post, R. M., Savard, R., *et al* (1984) Life charting of the longitudinal course of recurrent affective illness. In *Neurobiology of Mood Disorders* (eds R. M. Post & J. C. Ballenger), pp. 38–59. Baltimore: Williams & Wilkins.

Stancer, H. C. & Forbath, N. (1989) Hyperparathyroidism, hypothyroidism, and impaired renal function after 10 to 20 years of lithium treatment. *Archives of Internal Medicine*, **149**, 1042–1045.

Starkstein, S. E. & Robinson, R. G. (1989) Affective disorders and cerebral vascular disease. *British Journal of Psychiatry*, **154**, 170–182.

Stewart, P. M., Atherden, S. M., Stewart, S. E., *et al* (1988) Lithium carbonate – a competitive aldosterone antagonist? *British Journal of Psychiatry*, **153**, 205–207.

Stokes, P. E., Shamoian, C. A., Stoll, P. M., *et al* (1971) Efficacy of lithium as acute treatment of manic-depressive illness. *Lancet*, **1**, 1319–1325.

——, Kocsis, J. H. & Arcuni, O. J. (1976) Relationship of lithium chloride dose to treatment response in acute mania. *Archives of General Psychiatry*, **33**, 1080–1084.

Stone, K. (1989) Mania in the elderly. *British Journal of Psychiatry*, **155**, 220–224.

Storr, A. (1969) Churchill: the man. In *Churchill's Black Dog and other Phenomena of the Human Mind*, pp. 3–51. (Reprinted 1989.) London: Flamingo, Harper Collins.

Suppes, T., Baldessarini, R., Faedda, G. L., *et al* (1991) Risk of recurrence following discontinuation of lithium treatment in bipolar disorder. *Archives of General Psychiatry*, **48**, 1082–1088.

Swann, A. C., Secunda, S. K., Katz, M. M., *et al* (1986) Lithium treatment of mania: clinical characteristics, specificity of symptom change, and outcome. *Psychiatry Research*, **18**, 127–141.

Takei, N., O'Callaghan, E., Sham, P., *et al* (1992) Seasonality of admissions in the psychoses: effect of diagnosis, sex and age at onset. *British Journal of Psychiatry*, **161**, 506–511.

Telner, J. I., Lapierre, Y. D., Horn, E., *et al* (1986) Rapid reduction of mania by means of reserpine therapy. *American Journal of Psychiatry*, **143**, 1058.

Thornhill, D. P. & Field, S. P. (1982) Distribution of lithium elimination in a selected population of psychiatric patients. *European Journal of Clinical Pharmacology*, **21**, 351–354.

Transbol, I., Christiansen, C. & Baastrup, P. C. (1978) Endocrine effects of lithium: I. Hypothyroidism, its prevalence in long-term treated patients. *Acta Endocrinology*, **87**, 759–767.

Turner, T., Cookson, J. C., Wass, J. A. H., *et al* (1984) Psychotic reactions during treatment of pituitary tumours with dopamine agonists. *British Medical Journal*, **289**, 1101–1103.

Tyrer, P., Alexander, M. S., Regan, A., *et al* (1980) An extrapyramindal syndrome after lithium therapy. *British Journal of Psychiatry*, **136**, 191–194.

Vestergaard, P., Amdisen, A. & Schou, M. (1980) Clinically significant side-effects of lithium treatment. A survey of 237 patients in long-term treatment. *Acta Psychiatrica Scandinavica*, **62**, 193–200.

Von Knorring, L. (1990) Possible mechanisms for the presumed interaction between lithium and neuroleptics. *Human Psychopharmacology*, **5**, 287–292.

Waller, D. G. & Edwards, J. G. (1989) Lithium and the kidney: an update. *Psychological Medicine*, **19**, 825–831.

Wehr, T. A. & Goodwin, F. K. (1979) Rapid cycling in manic-depressives induced by tricyclic antidepressants. *Archives of General Psychiatry*, **36**, 555–559.

——, Sack, D. A. & Rosenthal, N. E. (1987) Sleep reduction as a final common pathway in the genesis of mania. *American Journal of Psychiatry*, **144**, 201–204.

——, ——, ——, *et al* (1988) Rapid cycling affective disorder: Contributing factors and treatment responses in 51 patients. *American Journal of Psychiatry*, **145**, 179–184.

West, A. P. & Meltzer, H. Y. (1979) Paradoxical lithium neurotoxicity: a report of five cases and a hypothesis about risk for neurotoxicity. *American Journal of Psychiatry*, **136**, 963–966.

Winnicott, D. W. (1935) In *Through Paediatrics to Psychoanalysis*. Chapter 9. London: Hogarth Press.

Wood, A. J. & Goodwin, G. M. (1987) A review of the biochemical and neuropharmacological actions of lithium. *Psychological Medicine*, **17**, 579–600.

World Health Organization (1992) T*he Tenth Revision of the International Classification of Diseases and Related Health Problems* (ICD–10). Geneva: WHO.

Wyant, M., Diamond, B. I., O'Neal, E., *et al* (1990) The use of midazolam in acutely agitated psychiatric patients. *Schizophrenia Bulletin*, **26**, 126–129.

Yassa, R., Saunders, A., Nastase, C., *et al* (1988) Lithium induced thyroid disorders: A prevalence study. *Journal of Clinical Psychiatry*, **49**, 14–16.

Young, R. C., Biggs, J. T., Ziegler, V. E., *et al* (1978) A rating scale for mania: reliability, validity and sensitivity. *British Journal of Psychiatry*, **133**, 429–435.

—— & Klerman, G. L. (1992) Mania in late life: Focus on age at onset. *American Journal of Psychiatry*, **149**, 867–876.

3 The causes of depression

Nicol Ferrier & Jan Scott

Epidemiology ● Genetic aspects ● Biological factors ● Psychosocial factors ● Conclusions

---

Descriptions of the core features of affective disorders are recognisable in the scientific and poetic literatures dating back to antiquity. Aetiological theories demonstrated wide diversity with many writers proposing supernatural or magical influences (for a review see Goodwin & Jamison, 1990). As early as 400 BC, Hippocrates produced a treatise, *The Nature of Man*, which identified mania and melancholia as two of six forms of 'madness'. Hippocrates suggested that mental disorders were psychological manifestations of underlying biological dysfunction, namely a disturbance in the four humours (blood, black bile, yellow bile and phlegm). Melancholia was attributed to an excess of black bile, while mania was associated with an excess of yellow bile. Later writers such as Aristotle (although suggesting the heart was the dysfunctional organ) were credited with introducing the notion of 'predisposition'. He suggested that black bile was present in everyone in small amounts, but that an excess of this humour increased individual vulnerability to melancholia.

Goodwin & Jamison (1990) note that over the centuries the mentally ill increasingly became the responsibility of the monasteries rather than of medical doctors. Perhaps as a reflection of this, writers in the middle ages showed a tendency to attribute the cause of depression to magical forces or possession by the devil. Such ideas changed only gradually, but from the 17th century onwards empirical observations regained ascendancy. These views were augmented by the more recent works of Kraepelin who is acknowledged as being among the first of the modern day clinicians to apply the four stage 'medical illness model' (comprising aetiology, pathology, signs and symptoms, course and outcome) to psychiatric disorders. While Kraepelin's writings largely focused on biological models of illness, the post-war era of the 1950s saw increasing attention given to psychosocial theories of the causes of depression. To an extent, biological and psychosocial hypotheses then developed in isolation, and competing rather than complementary models were promulgated. In the last decade, it has been acknowledged that integrated psychobiosocial models are required as a multifactorial aetiology provides the most plausible explanation of the phenomena observed.

This chapter reviews biological, psychological and social factors associated with the onset of depressive disorders. It begins with an overview of the epidemiology of affective disorders and concludes with brief comments on integrated models of causality.

Epidemiology

The importance of epidemiological data rests not just with the enumeration of rates of a disorder, but with the analysis of patterns of distribution leading to the identification of putative risk factors. Only tentative inferences can be drawn about aetiology from survey data, as the association of a variable with a particular disorder does not establish causation. However, such studies represent a critical first step in developing illness models. Epidemiological surveys will be reviewed first, followed by a discussion of associated socio-demographic factors.

Epidemiological surveys

Two key areas will be reviewed in this section: treatment/admission studies, and community based studies of affective disorders. The former are distorted by non-illness influences on help-seeking behaviour and referral practices, while until recently, the latter (although offering a more complete picture) were hampered by problems of case definition.

Treatment/admission studies

Paykel (1989a) has provided a succinct review of epidemiological data from primary care and hospital studies of affective disorders. About 30 per 1000 of the general population are treated by their GP for depression annually (HMSO, 1986). It is estimated that an equivalent number of depressives also visit their GP during the course of a year, but that the disorder remains undetected (Goldberg & Huxley, 1980; Freeling *et al*, 1985). Two per 1000 of the general population present with psychotic depression (HMSO, 1986) of whom most are referred on to hospital services (Grad de Alarcon *et al*, 1975). About three per 1000 of the general population are referred annually to out-patient clinics, with one per 1000 being admitted for depression (Bebbington, 1978). It is not yet known how the shift towards more community orientated services has affected these rates. As long ago as 1966, Rosenthal pointed out that changes in service accessibility in the USA led to hospital clinics treating an increasing proportion of less severe cases. Although hospital studies have largely been superseded by community surveys, treatment/admission reviews confirm the considerable morbidity associated with depression: the median prevalence of chronicity (symptoms persisting for 2 or more years) in hospital-treated depressives is 16% (Scott, 1988), and 5–15% of new long stay patients have a primary diagnosis of affective disorder (McCreadie *et al*, 1983).

Community studies

A major problem in community studies of depressive syndromes relates to difficulties in distinguishing distress from illness. Depression may be regarded as a mood state, a symptom or a specific disorder. Given that the entire population will probably suffer from transiently depressed affect at some time, this phenomenon can hardly be regarded as an abnormal experience. Boyd & Weissman (1982) reviewed the reporting of depressive symptoms in community studies and identified a prevalence rate of 13–20%. Methodological diversity and the use of different diagnostic criteria and thresholds for 'caseness' led to considerable variation in the results obtained by earlier community studies of affective syndromes. However, the advent of structured clinical interviews for ICD–9 (the Present State Examination (PSE); Wing *et al*, 1974) and for DSM–III (the Diagnostic Interview Schedule (DIS); Robins *et al*, 1981), allowed more reliable and valid cross-national comparisons to be undertaken. Results indicate a degree of agreement with prevalence rates for bipolar disorder of about 1% and unipolar disorder (including the different depressive syndromes) of about 5–8%. A brief review of community studies using recognised criteria for diagnosis and caseness is provided below, but attention is focused on the most important of these: the Epidemiological Catchment Area (ECA) study undertaken in the USA.

The ECA study.   Regier *et al* (1984) provide an overview of the methodology and aims of the ECA study. Representative community and institutional population sampling was undertaken at five sites across the USA, recruiting about 18 000 people. The study had two phases, the first established the prevalence of DSM–III disorders, while the second comprised a follow-up phase to determine relapse/remission rates as well as incidence data. As pointed out by Eaton *et al* (1981) the latter offers a greater opportunity for exploring aetiology than prevalence data alone.

Reviewing the published ECA results on affective disorders (Weissman *et al*, 1988*a,b*; Smith & Weissman, 1992), the annual and lifetime prevalence rates for bipolar disorder were 1% and 1.2% respectively (clearly reflecting the chronic nature of the illness). The mean age of first onset was 21 years and no significant gender differences were found in the estimated rates.

With regard to major depression, the annual incidence rate was 1.8%. The annual and lifetime prevalence rates were 2.7% (range 1.7–3.4) and 4.4% (2.9–5.8) respectively. The mean age of onset was 27 years and the lifetime female to male ratio was 2.7:1.

The exploration of rates for dysthymia were limited to lifetime prevalence (as it is by definition a chronic disorder); the ECA rate was 3%. While the overall female to male ratio was about 2:1, there was a gender by age interaction such that gender differences were particularly accentuated between the ages of 45–64 years (female:male ratio 4:1).

Dysthymia was also found to have a high prevalence of comorbidity with 65–70% individuals reporting a lifetime experience of another mental illness – in 42% this was of major depression.

Other community studies. Smith & Weissman (1992) reviewed other national studies using the DIS. Although these surveys were undertaken as far afield as New Zealand and Taiwan, the authors suggest that the similarities in the epidemiological data on affective disorders are more striking than the differences. The PSE has also been used extensively and results from other countries show similar trends with the London study of Bebbington *et al* (1981). The prevalence rates for PSE depression were 4.8% in men and 9% in women (overall rate 7%). While these rates are higher than those established for major depression in the ECA study, the results are comparable when neurotic depressions are excluded (Smith & Weissman, 1992); matched samples from Edinburgh and St Louis demonstrated similar rates of major depression (Surtees & Sashidaran, 1986). Brown & Harris (1978) report a prevalence rate for chronic depression of about 8% in their study of Camberwell women.

Two other epidemiological studies are particularly noteworthy because of their long-term prospective nature. The Lundby study (Rorsman *et al*, 1990) from Sweden followed a cohort of over 2500 subjects for 15 years and described annual age-standardised incidence rates per 1000 person years for 'definite depression' of 4 and 8 for males and females respectively. More recognisable diagnostic criteria were employed by Angst and colleagues (Angst & Dobler-Mikola, 1985; Angst *et al*, 1990). So far, this group have followed a cohort of 19–20-year-olds for 10 years. The one year prevalence rate of bipolar disorder was 0.8% and of major depression was 7%. In addition, Angst *et al* (1990) described the phenomenon of brief recurrent depression. In the young adult population studies, the prevalence rate was about 10%. Although the clinical validity of this concept is still being debated (Anon, 1991), it was notable that half of the subjects with this diagnosis had sought treatment for the condition and, when compared to those with major depression, suicide attempts were reportedly twice as frequent.

Associated socio-demographic factors

As noted above, young adulthood represents a high risk period for bipolar disorder and major depressive disorder, with a residual state of dysthymia more frequently associated with middle and old age (Weissman *et al*, 1988*b*). The age of first onset identified for major depression is earlier than suggested by previous research, and the rise in lifetime risk also challenges conventional wisdom about this disorder (Smith & Weissman, 1992). Both period effects (rate changes associated with time of onset of the disorder; in the ECA study 1960–1970s) and birth cohort effects (period of time during which the proband was born; in the ECA study 1935–45) may be implicated in the development of these trends (Klerman & Weissman, 1989).

Gender

One of the most robust socio-demographic associations is the significant gender differences in rates of unipolar disorders. As these differences are evident in community studies, are consistent across cultures and persistent over time, the results are unlikely to represent biases in help-seeking behaviour (Paykel, 1989*a*). Explanations of the gender differences have predominantly focused on social hypotheses relating to womens' role and status in society (Weissman & Klerman, 1977), through to biological models relating differences to hormonal effects. Recent research on first admission rates for affective disorders by Gater *et al* (1989) suggested that female parity accounted for the gender differences in relative risk, with non-parous females having a lower risk of admission than males. However, others have argued (Paykel, 1989*a*) that the gender differences are not restricted to the postpartum period and that this explanation is too limited. Data from a two stage general population survey of minor affective disorders (Bebbington *et al*, 1991) suggested a possible role for parity in explaining the increased female prevalence, but largely favoured the adverse effect of marriage rather than childbearing on these women.

Marital status

The association between marital status and depression is complex and will be explored further in the section on interpersonal relationships. However, it is noteworthy that recent research suggests that marital history (not current status *per se*) is a powerful influence on depression rates, with continuously married subjects, cohabitees and never married subjects demonstrating the lowest morbidity (Smith & Weissman, 1992).

Social class and economic status

Previous notions about the association between social class and affective disorders have been hampered by a number of confounding variables such as treatment biases (those of lower social class are less likely to obtain treatment) and difficulties in accurately defining social class. Community studies of milder depressions and dysthymia confirm an inverse relationship between depression and social disadvantage (Surtees *et al*, 1983; Weissman *et al*, 1988*b*) and a review by Smith & Weissman (1992) suggested that higher level of education, employment and financial independence were associated with lower rates of depression. The link between unemployment and depression is explored later in the chapter.

Race and ethnicity

When socio-economic and education variables are controlled for, there is minimal evidence of racial or ethnic differences in the prevalence of depression (Somerville *et al*, 1989). It is suggested that previously reported differences related more to biases in sample selection (Jones *et al*, 1988) or misdiagnosis of individuals from black or other ethnic minorities (Horgan, 1981). There is limited evidence that unipolar probands are significantly more likely to emigrate than control subjects (Grove *et al*, 1986).

Geographical location

Trends in depression rates between urban and rural locations are largely in the expected direction, with several studies in Britain, the USA and other countries (e.g. Puerto Rico) showing significantly greater prevalences of depression in urban areas. Brown & Prudo (1981) demonstrated a 15% prevalence of PSE depression in Camberwell and an 8% prevalence in the Hebrides. There is some evidence that areas in transition from rural to more industrialised environments show particularly high morbidity rates (Hwu *et al*, 1989). Other psychosocial and biological variables associated with depression are discussed below.

Genetic aspects

Enough convincing genetic work has been carried out to confirm the hypothesis that genetic factors play a role in the causation of certain subtypes of the affective disorders. The strongest evidence for the role of genes is for bipolar affective disorder. The evidence that genes play an important role in the less severe subtypes of depression is weak although many have not been studied in detail.

There have been many recent advances in our knowledge of genes, their effects and relationship with brain function. It seems likely that we are on the threshold of identifying pathogenetic mechanisms for the more strongly genetic affective disorders. The traditional approach in behavioural genetics has consisted of twin, family, adoption and half-sib studies. Recombinant DNA technology is likely to produce major advances in psychiatric genetics because of the systematic approach that can be utilised to screen chromosomes for susceptible genes. These techniques (details of which are beyond the scope of this chapter) are particularly useful for studying pedigrees, and bring the promise of the identification of gene defects at the level of abnormal nucleotide sequencing. These advances offer the prospect of elucidating the interplay between genes and the environment and have the potential for identifying new preventative and therapeutic strategies.

There are a number of problems with which genetic studies of affective disorders must contend. The most prominent of these is diagnostic uncertainty and the related shortcomings of classification. The problems of clinical heterogeneity and the lack of any objective validation of diagnosis cause great problems for genetic studies. For example if an individual has a non-genetic form of affective disorder within (say) a family of severe unipolar depression, then the inclusion of that individual as a 'genetic' case in linkage analysis will weaken the evidence for linkage.

There is also the problem that diagnosis is essentially based on a retrospective history and can be inaccurate or misleading because of colouring from the present affective state or rigid concepts. Furthermore the original diagnosis may have to be changed at a future date leading to a need for re-analysis of data.

All of the methods suffer from the limitation that the effects of genes and the environment may not be separated in the experimental design. For example adoption studies are generally carried out on small numbers and the circumstances are often unusual within both the biological family and the adopted family. Twin studies have similar limitations exacerbated by the special environment of twins which can produce unsuspected correlations. Analyses of family data which seek to estimate genetic effects by correlating relatedness with the presence or absence of a disorder may also be misleading if the rate of assortative mating or disputed paternity in the family is not known or taken into account. All of these problems (and their cumulative effect) must be considered when interpreting results of genetic studies.

Family studies

Much of the early evidence for the importance of genetic factors in the affective disorders is derived from family studies. The morbid risk (adjusted prevalence) of the illness is determined within families and rates of occurrence in the different classes of relative are compared with those of the general population.

The distinction between bipolar (BP) and unipolar (UP) illness made by Leonhard (1959) has underpinned most of this work. McGuffin & Katz (1989) have re-analysed the pooled results from a large number of studies examining the morbid risk of BP illness in the relatives of BP and UP probands. The risk of developing BP illness in the first degree relatives of BP probands is elevated (approximately 7%) while the first degree relatives of UP probands have a risk for BP illness no higher than the general population (0.7%). The morbid risk of UP illness in the first degree relatives of BP and UP probands was 11.5% and 9.1% respectively. It is noteworthy that the combined rates for affective disorder are higher in the relatives of BP probands than in relatives of UP probands. Andreason *et al* (1987) demonstrated that while 1.1% of relatives of bipolar II probands have bipolar I type illness, a much greater frequency (8.2%) have bipolar II type disorder suggesting that these disorders are independent.

Family studies have another useful purpose in that, because large numbers are studied, subgroups and 'risk factors' can be identified. Weissman *et al* (1988*c*) reported that an early age of onset of depression or major depression with an anxiety disorder or secondary alcoholism were associated with an increased risk of major depression in relatives. The evidence for an increased morbid risk in relatives of early onset probands applies both to unipolar affective illness (where Hopkinson & Ley (1969) showed a higher risk in the families of patients with an onset under 40) and bipolar illness (Strober *et al*, 1988). Schizo-affective disorder has the highest genetic loading with 37% of relatives having affective illness at some point in their lives (Gershon *et al*, 1982).

In the past it has been assumed that depression arising for no apparent reason ('endogenous') was more 'genetic' than that following stress or adverse life-events. However, this has not been supported by recent research (Andreason *et al*, 1986; Weissman *et al*, 1986). It is established that relatives of patients with endogenous types of illness do not have higher rates of depression than their non-endogenous counterparts. Indeed McGuffin & Katz (1989) found no difference in the frequency of depression in the relatives of probands who had significant life events compared with those who did not. This links to the observation that there is an increase in the morbid risk for affective disorder in the relatives of probands with depressive neurosis. A wide range (5 to 25%) of morbid risk has been found (the divergent rates no doubt explicable by methodological differences and difficulties). Some family studies have shown evidence for comorbidity of depression and alcoholism and raised the possibility that, in some families, depression presents in female family members and that the male relatives of depressed probands present with an increased frequency of alcoholism and antisocial behaviour.

Twin studies

The central assumption of twin studies is that monozygotic (MZ) twins share the same genes whereas dizygotic twins have an average of 50% of genes in common, thus affording the possibility of dissecting the role of genes from that of the environment in a way which cannot be easily done in family studies. Unfortunately there are a number of problems which make twin studies less clear cut than they first appear. For example, exposure to the same family environment may have different effects on MZ as opposed to DZ twins, and MZ twins share the same intrauterine environment where adverse factors may operate.

Bertelsen (1979) using the Danish Twin Study Register to study BP and UP disorder found a concordance rate of 67% for MZ twins and 20% for DZ twins. The hereditability of affective disorders has been calculated to be 59%, comparable to that for schizophrenia, diabetes and hypertension. The concordance rates for BP disorder were much higher than those for UP disorder. There is a need to follow up such cohorts over a prolonged period of time to take age-related risk into account. If this is done the concordance rates for MZ twins rises, particularly for BP disorder (where it approaches 100%). However, there are several recorded instances of pairs of MZ twins with BP in one twin and UP disorder in the other. On the basis of published twin studies, Baron (1980) proposed that an autosomal single major locus provided an acceptable fit to the data and that a polygenic model was unlikely. The concordance rate for MZ and DZ twins with neurotic depression is roughly equal but the overall concordance is greater than that of the population, which suggests that familial rather than genetic factors are operating. Hereditability for minor depression has not been demonstrated in twin studies. McGuffin & Katz (1989) concluded, on the basis of twin studies, that BP illness is largely determined by genetic factors, UP illness occupies an intermediate position and that the familial clustering in neurotic depression is predominantly environmental and non-genetic in origin.

Adoption studies

Adoption studies are advanced as a method of separating biological and environmental factors but suffer from a number of drawbacks. The biological parents of adopted children tend to be more deviant and suffer from a higher rate of psychiatric disturbances than ordinary parents whereas adoptive parents are usually carefully screened so that such problems are avoided. Most, but not all, adoption studies of affective disorders have shown a role for genetic factors with little evidence for family associated environmental factors. As in the family and twin studies the evidence for genetic factors is strongest for BP disorder, but there is a highly significant increase in the prevalence of a range of affective illnesses in the biological parents of adoptees, who suffer from a spectrum of affective disturbance when compared to the rates in the adoptive parents.

Segregation analyses

Segregation analysis compares the likelihood for the observed frequency of illness in a pedigree containing many cases of affective disorder with those that can be predicted by different models of transmission. Most studies have indicated that a single major locus which is dominant with a multifactorial background variance is the likeliest mode of transmission of UP and BP disorder, although a large number of assumptions have to be made in such studies (Rifkin & Gurling, 1991).

Genetic linkage and association analyses

Studies of association can be undertaken between markers and the disorder compared with a control group. Classical marker studies have focused on the association between disease and the human leucocyte antigen (HLA) system and ABO blood groups. Studies of affective disorders using this approach have produced contradictory and inconsistent results (Berretini *et al*, 1984).

Another approach is to study 'candidate' genes which, on *a priori* basis, may genetically predispose to the disorder under study. For example, many of the serotonin, noradrenaline and dopamine receptor subtype genes have been cloned as have the genes for tyrosine hydroxylase (TH) and pro-opiomelanocortin (POMC). There have been reports of non-significant linkage to unipolar affective disorders with such markers. The genes for TH and the D1 receptor are on chromosome 11 and some studies of families with psychiatric disorders including affective illness have revealed cytogenetic abnormalities related to this chromosome. The question of whether these changes are of significance outside these pedigrees remains to be determined. In 1987 Egeland and co-workers reported linkage between BP illness and two markers on the tip of chromosome 11 in the old Order Amish religious community in Pennsylvania. There are several large pedigrees with a high incidence of affective disorders within this community and there is a low incidence of drug or alcohol abuse. However, when the pedigrees were extended and re-evaluated individuals previously unaffected showed recent onset of affective disorders so that when the data were re-analysed the significance of the linkage fell. Further studies of pedigrees from North America, Iceland and Europe have failed to demonstrate linkage to the gene markers reported by Egeland *et al* (1987) or to the TH or D2 genes (located in the same region of chromosome 11). The possibility remains that chromosome 11 abnormalities may be important in some pedigrees with BP disorder, suggesting that there is genetic heterogeneity for the affective disorders.

This notion is strengthened by research investigating the possibility of X-linkage in BP illness. In some early studies linkage between colour blindness, other X-chromosome markers and BP disorder was shown with evidence of reduced frequency of male to male transmission. However, these findings are disputed and the weight of evidence now suggests that approximately one-third of BP illness, and a lower proportion of UP illness, is X-linked. It is of interest that, in some studies, linkage is greater if people with cyclothymia are included in the pedigree as cases. In further studies Mendlewicz *et al* (1987) showed linkage between the subterminal end of the long arm of the X-chromosome and affective disorder. No clinical features differentiating those BP patients with probable X-linkage and those without have been identified.

Conclusions

There is strong evidence for a genetic component to BP disorder and evidence for a single major gene locus on the X-chromosome in a proportion of BP patients. In BP disorder there is genetic heterogeneity and it is likely that this also applies to UP affective disorder and its many subtypes. Multivariate models of gene/environment effects offer a way forward to disentangle the subtle interplay between genetic and multifactorial environmental influences. It is apparent that even where genetic factors are strong, environmental influences are important in terms of whether (and when) illness occurs and in the form it takes. Genetic research affords the possibility of identifying biological markers which will greatly enhance the ascertainment of the role of specific genes and environmental factors in the aetiology of individual affective disorders.

Biological factors

Neurotransmitter function

During the last 25 years the biogenic amine hypothesis of affective disorders has dominated research in biological psychiatry. Results from neuropsychopharmacological studies have, by and large, provided data to support this hypothesis.

Origins of the monoamine hypothesis of depression

In the 1950s it was noted that reserpine, given for the treatment of hypertension, was associated with the development of severe depression in a proportion of cases. Around the same time, patients with tuberculosis being treated with iproniazid developed euphoria prompting the use of this drug which has monoamine oxidase (MAO) inhibitor properties as an antidepressant. Shortly thereafter, the tricyclic drug imipramine was found to be an effective antidepressant. These clinical observations came at the time that great strides were being made in understanding the neurochemistry and function of central monoamine systems. This research led to an elucidation of the pharmacological properties of reserpine (depletion of catecholamines and serotonin) and of MAO inhibitors (MAOIs) and tricyclics (TCAs) (increased availability of noradrenaline (NA) and/or serotonin (5HT) either through the blocking of MAO or the neuronal uptake of amines). This information, in turn, provided the scientific basis for the catecholamine and serotonin hypotheses of affective disorder (see below). Later these hypotheses were modified and the 'receptor sensitivity hypothesis' proposed. Behind the latter were the observations that (a) the function of a CNS neurotransmitter could alter following changes in presynaptic or postsynaptic receptor sensitivity with no change in the amount of neurotransmitter itself and (b) despite rapid changes in neurotransmitter levels the therapeutic response to antidepressants was delayed for several weeks. These observations also led to the formulation of the linked receptor sensitivity hypothesis of antidepressant action: that the benefits of antidepressant action are related to time-dependent alterations in NA and 5-HT receptors.

Catecholamine hypotheses of affective disorder

Schildkraut (1965) credits Jacobson for giving the earliest formulations of the catecholamine hypothesis of depression. In his seminal paper, Schildkraut (1965) concluded that both MAOIs and TCAs could reverse the effects of reserpine by increasing NA at brain adrenergic receptors, and formulated the noradrenergic hypothesis of affective illness which postulated that depression was due to deficiency and mania to an excess of brain noradrenaline. In pioneer studies, it was found that there was a reduced urinary excretion of the NA metabolite 3-methoxy-4 hydroxy-phenyl glycol (MHPG) in depression. Originally urinary MHPG was thought to derive mostly from brain, but it is now clear that true contribution of brain MHPG to the total MHPG excretion is approximately 30%. The finding of reduced MHPG in urine and cerebrospinal fluid (CSF) have not been replicated in subsequent studies. Any such changes are inconsistent and more likely to relate to non-specific stress, abnormal diets etc. The hope that some patients who were demonstrated as being NA deficient would specifically respond to TCAs with major effects on neuronal NA uptake has not been fulfilled. Recent evidence suggests that depressed patients excrete disproportionately greater amounts of NA relative to total catecholamine synthesis (Potter *et al*, 1992). Studies in post-mortem brains of depressed patients and/or suicide victims have failed to show consistent evidence of a major perturbation in NA or its related enzymes.

However, as emphasis began to shift to receptor function (as described above) some interesting observations were made. It was discovered that chronic antidepressant treatments caused sub-sensitivity of NA receptor-coupled adenylate cyclase (the second messenger) and that virtually all effective antidepressant treatments (including TCAs, atypical anti-depressants and ECT) induce a decrease in the density of β-receptors in the brain. This effect is shared by some, but not all, of the newer selective serotonin reuptake inhibitors (SSRIs) (Sulser, 1986; Pryor & Sulser, 1991). There have been reports of increased numbers of β-receptors in the brains of unmedicated suicide victims (Bigeon & Israel, 1988; Arango *et al*, 1990) but also contradictory reports (Ferrier *et al*, 1986; de Parmentier *et al*, 1990). Increasing attention is being paid to the α_2 pre-synaptic autoreceptor which modulates the release of NA. There is evidence that some antidepressants down-regulate central α autoreceptors thus inducing increased NA release by reduced α_2-receptor-mediated autoinhibitory control (Garcia-Sevilla *et al*, 1990). Some drugs with selectivity for α_2 autoreceptors are antidepressants (e.g. mianserin, idazoxan – although the potency of the latter is a matter of dispute) and there is evidence that α_2 adrenoreceptors are increased in various brain regions of depressed suicide victims (Meana *et al*, 1992). It is noteworthy that blockade of α_2 receptors also facilitates 5-HT neurotransmission in the hippocampus.

It is important to recognise that clinically effective antidepressants may have very different ranges of activities on NA and 5-HT systems and that there is strong evidence of interaction between the two systems (see below). A plausible hypothesis put forward by Siever & Davis (1985) is that in affective disorders regulatory or homeostatic mechanisms controlling neurotransmitter function are dysregulated (the 'dysregulation hypothesis') and that effective pharmacological agents restore normal regulation to these systems.

Serotonin (5-HT) hypothesis of affective illness

The 5-HT (indolamine) hypothesis postulates that a deficit brain 5-HT (serotonin) is responsible for depression since drugs which increase synaptic 5HT relieve depression (Coppen, 1967).

There is a wealth of indirect evidence for a perturbation in 5-HT function in depression. This has been reviewed in detail elsewhere (Meltzer, 1989) but a brief account is given below. It is known that the 5-HT system has an important role in the regulation of sleep, appetite, sexual function, pain and circadian rhythms, all of which are disrupted in depression. There is an extensive and widespread innervation of the cerebral cortex and limbic system by ascending projections of 5-HT neurons whose cell bodies are located in brain-stem raphe nuclei and each of which is linked to over half a million terminals to the cerebral cortex.

Manipulation of plasma tryptophan (the precursor of 5-HT) has significant effects on mood in both normal and depressed subjects. There is evidence that depressed patients have lower levels of plasma tryptophan, a lower ratio of plasma tryptophan to neutral amino acids and lower levels of 5-hydroxy-indole-acetic acid (5-HIAA – the major metabolite of 5-HT) after L-tryptophan infusion (Cowen *et al*, 1989; Meltzer, 1989). L-tryptophan is a weak antidepressant in its own right but there is evidence that it complements the antidepressant response to MAOIs (Eccleston, 1993). Shopsin *et al* (1976) showed that the antidepressant effect of MAOIs could be reversed by parachlorophenyalanine - a compound that inhibits the synthesis of 5-HT.

More recently, Delgado *et al* (1990) showed an increase in the severity of depression when tryptophan was removed from the diet of recovered depressives. This effect was most marked in the patients on MAOIs and was reversed on replacing L-tryptophan in the diet. A number of severe chronic depressives on MAOIs or TCAs relapsed when L-tryptophan was withdrawn from the market (Ferrier *et al*, 1990).

The platelet is considered to be a model for neuronal 5-HT uptake and for neurotransmitter receptor activity. A number of abnormalities of platelet 5-HT mechanisms have been found in depression e.g. reduced 5-HT 'uptake sites' (also reported in the brain in depression (Leake *et al*, 1991)), increased 5-HT$_2$ receptors and reduced 5-HT uptake most of which normalise on recovery (Meltzer, 1989; Boyer & Feighner, 1991).

Neuroendocrine studies show that the prolactin response to L-tryptophan and fenfluramine is blunted when patients are depressed, suggesting that pre-synaptic 5-HT dysfunction is a state marker in depression (Uppadhyaya *et al*, 1990; Delgado & Charney, 1991): these changes normalise with antidepressants suggesting that they reverse the deficit (Delgado & Charney, 1990). 5-HIAA in CSF is reported as being reduced in major depression – a change which normalises on recovery. A group of depressed patients with low 5-HIAA were more prone to attempt suicide by violent means (Asberg *et al*, 1976), an observation which led to a series of studies. The evidence now indicates that low CSF 5-HIAA is not a marker for depression itself but a marker of impulsivity (Coccaro, 1989).

In view of the delay in the specific therapeutic response to antidepressants – a delay which is concordant with the time taken for 5-HT receptor adaptation in animal experiments with TCAs – attention has been centred on the pathophysiology of 5-HT receptors in depression. There is evidence for increased numbers of post-synaptic (5-HT$_2$) receptors in the brains of drug-free depressives and unmedicated suicide victims (Arora & Meltzer, 1989; Arango *et al*, 1990; Yates *et al*, 1990). Most, but not all, antidepressant treatments reduce the number of 5-HT$_2$ receptors in the brain (Charney *et al*, 1981). However, specific 5-HT$_2$ antagonists are weak antidepressants. The pathophysiology of the change in 5-HT$_2$ receptors in depression is uncertain but it seems unlikely to follow from underactivity of presynaptic 5-HT function, since the deficits in 5-HIAA in post-mortem depressed cases and suicide victims are not large (Ferrier *et al*, 1986; Cheetham *et al*, 1991). There is considerable current interest in the notion that the function of a subtype of the 5-HT$_1$ receptor – the 5-HT$_{1A}$ receptor – is abnormal in depression (Giral *et al*, 1988; Deakin, 1989; Cheetham *et al*, 1990).

Antidepressants produce changes in this receptor so that net 5-HT neurotransmission is increased particularly in the hippocampus (Cowen, 1991). Depression occurs in a variety of neuropsychiatric conditions such as Alzheimer's disease and Parkinson's disease and there is evidence that in both of these conditions depression is associated with low 5-HT turnover (Mayeux *et al*, 1988; Zubenko *et al*, 1990).

Thus there is much circumstantial evidence that 5-HT function is abnormal in depression. However, it is likely that changes in this system in depression are only one part of a complex chain of events. It is probable that 5-HT abnormalities are a mechanism whereby recurrent or abnormal stress leads to depressive symptomatology in a predisposed individual rather than being the 'cause' of depression.

Antidepressants and depression

Antidepressant drugs are of proven efficacy both in the treatment of depression (Nelson, 1991) and in its prophylaxis (Frank *et al*, 1990). Tricyclics have a number of neurochemical effects among the most prominent of which are blockade of NA and 5-HT uptake by neurones. The advent of selective 5-HT uptake inhibitors (SSRIs) which have antidepressant properties could be seen as strengthening the notion for the importance of 5-HT in depression. However, it is important to note that SSRIs are not totally selective for 5-HT (Johnson, 1991) and because they are only as effective as TCAs it is likely that the changes in 5-HT system induced by these drugs are important but not sufficient to produce optimal treatment of this condition (Ferrier *et al*, 1992). Furthermore it is clear that SSRIs are not specific for depression but are effective in the treatment of other conditions including obsessive–compulsive disorder, panic disorder and anxiety states even when depression is not evident in these conditions (Montgomery & Fineberg, 1989). Taken together, the evidence of 5-HT abnormalities in psychiatric disorders and the changes induced on the 5-HT system by drugs leads to the conclusion that 5-HT has an important bearing on behaviour and mood and that 5-HT is altered in a dimensional rather than a categorical way in depression. Finally it is clear that a number of effective antidepressants have low potency of activity at 5-HT synapses. This suggests that manipulation of the 5-HT system is not essential for successful treatment of depression. However, there is good evidence for an interaction between the 5-HT and NA system, particularly with respect to the effects of antidepressants, so that changes in one system induced by drugs cause changes in the other (Pryor & Sulser, 1991). The precise mechanism of action of antidepressants remains uncertain. It may be that their neurochemical effects are of secondary importance and alteration of gene expression, resetting of biological clocks or altering the organism's response to stress (Kitayami *et al*, 1988; Pfeiffer *et al*, 1991) may prove to be of greater importance.

Other neurotransmitters

Although antidepressants have profound effects on NA and/or 5-HT neurotransmission there is no convincing evidence that these effects link directly to changes in clinical state and the role of other neurotransmitters in depression has therefore been examined. The cholinergic, dopaminergic and GABAergic systems have all been implicated in depression and there are a number of circumstantial pieces of evidence to support each of these hypotheses (see Meltzer, 1987).

The cholinergic hypothesis of depression was postulated by Janowsky *et al* (1972) and states that excess cholinergic activity is involved in depression. Some cholinomimetic drugs are associated with depression in normal subjects and the cholinergic agonist arecoline worsens depressive symptoms in depressed patients (Nurnberger *et al*, 1989). Furthermore evidence has been adduced from neuroendocrine (Janowsky *et al*, 1988) and sleep studies (Nurnberger *et al*, 1989) of normal and depressed subjects that there is postsynaptic cholinergic supersensitivity in depression. However, there is no evidence that anticholinergic drugs are effective antidepressants and, while most tricyclics are potent cholinergic receptor blockers, the rank order of the potency of TCAs as anticholinergics and as antidepressants differs.

The proposal that underactivity of the dopamine (DA) system is important in the aetiology of depression, first put forward by Randrup & Braestrup (1977), continues to receive support. There is some evidence that drugs which increase dopamine function have effects on mood. For example the psychostimulants amphetamine and methylphenidate have transient mood-elevating properties. The direct dopamine agonists bromocriptine and peribedil have antidepressant properties although they are clinically disappointing in long-term use. MAOI drugs may be clinically effective by enhancing the amount of DA released per impulse. Low CSF homovanillic acid (HVA) (a measure of DA turnover) has been reported consistently in a proportion of depressed patients (particularly those with retardation). Animal models of depression and antidepressant action indicate an important role for dopamine and a clinically relevant linkage to noradrenergic and serotonergic systems (Wilner, 1983). Psychotic depression responds poorly to TCAs alone but the addition of neuroleptics (DA antagonists) is often effective. ECT is the treatment of choice for this disorder and there is good evidence that ECT selectively effects dopaminergic function (Kapur & Mann, 1992).

There is little direct evidence for a disturbance of GABA or GABA binding in depression but increasing evidence that antidepressants affect GABA receptors and that $GABA_B$ agonists enhance monoaminergic neuro-transmission. These findings suggest that $GABA_B$ agonists, either alone or in combination with antidepressants may be useful treatments for depression (Enna *et al*, 1986).

Neuroendocrine function

Depressed patients frequently exhibit disturbed sleep, reduced appetite, reduced libido and disruption of circadian rhythms. These observations have led to the notion that the hypothalamus functions abnormally in depression. The increased frequency of depression in endocrine diseases such as hypothyroidism and Cushing's syndrome has further stimulated interest in neuroendocrine function in depression.

The regulation of pituitary hormones and their control by neuro-transmitters is complex and the myriad of neuroendocrine studies in affective illness are beyond the scope of this text. An outline of the main aspects of neuroendocrine research in affective disorders is given below.

Thyroid hormones

The relevance of thyroid abnormalities to the aetiology and treatment of affective disorders remains unresolved. Approximately one-third of depressed patients show blunting of the TSH response to the hypothalamic tripeptide TRH – a smaller proportion show an exaggerated response. Basal TSH levels are elevated (probably indicating sub-clinical hypothyroidism) in approximately 15% of affectively disordered patients and thyroid autoantibodies are found in a similar percentage – both frequencies higher than the normal population (Haggerty *et al*, 1987). There is evidence that the frequency of these thyroid abnormalities is further increased in depressed patients unresponsive to treatment and this observation may link with the reports that the addition of T_3 to antidepressants is of clinical benefit in some resistant depressives (Joffe & Singer, 1993), and that abnormal thyroid function is associated with the development of treatment refractory depression (Scott, 1988). The pathophysiological basis of these observations remains obscure. However, TRH is increased in the CSF of depressed patients suggesting that the thyroid disturbance in these patients is due to a disturbance at the pituitary or thyroid gland level (Banki *et al*, 1988).

Corticosteroids

About 60% of patients with major depression have evidence of raised glucocorticoid secretion with disruption of the normal circadian rhythm and failure to suppress with the synthetic glucocorticoid dexamethasone ('DST non-suppression') (Arana *et al*, 1985; Charlton & Ferrier, 1989). Patients with depression may also have enlarged pituitary and adrenal glands (Amsterdam *et al*, 1987; Krishnan *et al*, 1991). It is likely that the pathophysiology of these changes relates to increased secretion of corticotrophin releasing hormone (CRH) from the hypothalamus. This is of interest since CRH appears to a mediator of behavioural, cardiovascular and hormonal responses to stress (Nemeroff, 1988). Cortisol secretion is elevated by stress but there is evidence that the elevations seen in depression relate more to depression than anxiety (Evans & Nemeroff, 1987). Elevated cortisol secretion and DST non-suppression in depression are related to poor prognosis and cognitive failure, but are not indicators of successful drug treatment (Rubinow *et al*, 1984; Charles *et al*, 1989; Siegel *et al*, 1989).

There is a considerable interest in whether the hypercortisolaemic state found in many depressives has any influence on the neurochemical, neuroendocrinological or clinical changes seen in depression. Corticosteroids have effects on 5-HT, noradrenaline and dopamine function in rats (Nausieda *et al*, 1982; Dickinson *et al*, 1985; Lesch & Lerer, 1991) but whether the levels of corticosteroids seen in depressed patients are related to putative changes in central monoamine function described above remains conjectural. Hypercortisolaemia in depression does not seem to influence the blunting of the TSH response to TRH but may affect the hormonal response to 5-HT agonists (see below). The lowering of plasma cortisol by metapyrone in patients with Cushing's syndrome is associated with an improvement in the severity of the associated depression (Jeffcoate *et al*, 1979; Kramlinger *et al*, 1985). A number of investigations are underway to elucidate whether metapyrone or glucocorticoid receptor antagonists are of clinical benefit in depressed patients.

A plausible hypothesis, that corticosteroids may provide a neuro-biological basis for the interaction between the genetic predisposition to depression and the effects of life events and stress, has been put forward by Bebbington & McGuffin (1989). Repeated stress, particularly if initiated in early life, leads to hyper-responsive pituitary-adrenal responses and eventually to chronically raised corticosteroid secretion at levels which may have adverse consequences on structure and function of vulnerable areas within the central nervous system (Thoman *et al*, 1968; Restrepo & Armario, 1987; Orr *et al*, 1990; McEwan *et al*, 1992). The discovery of the hypercortisolaemia of depression lead to the false hope that this was the biological marker of the condition. However, there is increasing evidence that continued research into the mechanisms and consequence of hypercortisolaemia in depression will prove fruitful in terms of our understanding of the aetiology of depression and in the development of novel, perhaps, protective, therapies.

Prolactin (PRL)

Most studies now agree that PRL levels and rhythms are normal in depression. The PRL response to tryptophan and to 5-HT agonists is reduced in depression (and increased with treatment with TCAs or lithium) and this has been adduced as evidence of altered 5-HT receptor function in depression (Cowen *et al*, 1991).

Growth hormone (GH)

GH levels are probably normal in major depression and any perturbations in the rhythm of its secretion secondary to the disruption of the sleep wake cycle seen in depression. The GH response to α_2-adrenoreceptor agonists is reduced but this may be part of a generalised reduction in GH responsiveness in depression (perhaps related to cortisol hypersecretion).

Melatonin

There has been much interest in this pineal hormone as it is under the control of both 5-HT and β-receptors and a marker for diurnal and other rhythms. However, most evidence indicates that in unipolar depression and in seasonal affective disorder melatonin levels and rhythms are normal.

A summary of the biological research discussed so far would indicate that the neurochemical and neuroendocrine changes are variable in extent and duration. They are unlikely to be primary events but rather the mechanism whereby genetic and/or environmental factors lead to enhanced vulnerability, behavioural change and symptoms.

Organic aspects

It is apparent that depression is a heterogeneous disorder and there appear to be a number of routes to the final common pathway of depressive symptomatology. An interplay of genes and environment is evident in most cases but depression may also be directly related to physical/medical disorders and to cease when these are treated. Some of the medical conditions causing depression may do this as a result of general debility (e.g. chronic cardiac failure) or as a consequence of disability. Other conditions seem to have effects on mood through a direct biological process. Brief examples are given below.

Neurological disease and neuropathological changes

A wide variety of neurological conditions are associated with depression and appear to cause the problem in different ways. For example, affective changes are common in multiple sclerosis but it seems these problems arise either as a consequence of disability or (particularly when euphoria is a feature) where cognitive decline is evident. Cerebrovascular accidents (CVA) are often associated with depression and this could be seen as a consequence of the devastating effects of such an incident, although biological factors may be operating in some cases. The CVA is more likely to cause affective disturbance if the lesion is in close proximity to either the left frontal pole or the right parieto-temporal cortex (Robinson *et al*, 1987; House *et al*, 1990). In general, lesions on the right side of the brain are related to affective disturbance and this is particularly the case with secondary mania (Starkstein *et al*, 1991). The temporal lobe may be implicated in depression since lesions in the temporal lobe are often associated with depression.

At the same time, there has been increasing research into organic changes in major affective disorder. In some patients these organic changes have been identified but their role, particularly in causation, is uncertain. The drive behind this research is to understand more about the role of neuroanatomical substrates in depression, to investigate the nature of cognitive failure in depression and to examine whether the aetiology of depression in some patients, particularly the elderly, has a neuro-pathological basis.

The seminal work of Post (1968) indicated that subtle cerebral changes may make ageing persons increasingly liable to affective illness. Jacoby *et al* (1981) found a trend for late onset depressives to have enlarged ventricles on CT scan and that there was a subgroup with strikingly enlarged ventricles who, in a follow-up study, had an increased mortality rate. These findings have largely been confirmed in subsequent studies (Alexopoulos *et al*, 1991). Studies of younger patients have been more contradictory. Most studies show small subgroups with cortical atrophy and enlarged ventricles (Dolan *et al*, 1992). These changes are more prominent in groups of patients who have cognitive failure and have a bipolar disorder. The nature of these changes and their role in aetiology, clinical symptoms and course of illness is unknown. However, in general, patients with organic cerebral changes respond poorly to antidepressants (see Ferrier & McKeith, 1991, for review).

More recently, depressed patients have been studied using sophisticated neuroradiological techniques. Magnetic resonance imaging (MRI) has advantages compared to CT particularly in its power to image parenchymal changes. There have been several reports of high rates of patchy white matter hyperintensities, particularly in frontal and temporal subcortical areas, in patients with depression. These are particularly found in the elderly, those with late onset and those with bipolar disorder (Diecken *et al*, 1991; Swayze *et al*, 1992). The nature of these lesions and their role in the causation of symptoms is unknown – they may represent an interplay between cerebrovascular factors and depression first suggested by Kay (1962). Other structural changes are also reported on MRI scan studies and there is a need for combined neuroradiological and neuropathological studies (Jeste *et al*, 1988; Baldwin, 1993).

Single photon emission tomography (SPET) has shown reduced uptake in the majority of sub-cortical and cortical structures, particularly temporal and inferior frontal areas. This result is taken to represent decreased blood flow, and by implication decreased activity, in these areas (Austin *et al*, 1992). Using positron emission tomography (PET) and oxygen-15, Bench and co-workers (1992) have shown decreased regional cerebral blood flow in left anterior cingulate and dorsolateral frontal cortex. In patients with cognitive failure the changes were more pronounced in the left medial frontal gyrus and cerebral blood flow was increased in the cerebellar vermis. These findings suggest that pre-frontal and limbic areas may be functionally abnormal in major depression. The role of changes in blood flow in depression has not been established – it is not even clear if they are state or trait phenomena – and the relationship of these changes to structural abnormalities or putative neurochemical dysfunction has not been determined. The areas involved are those which appear to be involved in mood and its regulation. The temporal lobe is of particular interest – further fuelled by the finding of abnormal EEG temporal lobe foci in unipolar and bipolar patients with refractory depression (Levy *et al*, 1988).

It seems plausible that in some cases, particularly the elderly, organic change has a role to play in the genesis of symptoms and it may be that neurochemical change in these cases follows on from neuronal fall-out. Such mechanisms have been implicated in the depression associated with Alzheimer's and Parkinson's diseases.

Endocrine conditions

Cushing's syndrome and hypothyroidism are associated with depression and in severe cases the depression can be psychotic in form (Ferrier, 1991). It is noteworthy that rapid and usually complete resolution of the depression is seen when the underlying disorder is treated. Considerable research on a possible hormonal basis to postpartum mood disorder has been undertaken but few clearcut findings have emerged (see chapter 21). It seems likely that within the aetiology of these syndromes there is a profound interaction between the sufferer (genetic or family influences), the environment (hormonal changes postpartum, other illnesses etc.) and the social circumstances. There is limited evidence that 'maternity blues' links to progesterone withdrawal following delivery and that a few cases of postnatal depression may be associated with the presence of postpartum thyroiditis (see Harris (1994) for review). Puerperal psychosis, usually an affective disorder, may be linked to the sudden fall in oestrogen which causes increased dopamine receptor sensitivity (Wiek *et al*, 1991). The hormonal basis, if any, of premenstrual tension is similarly obscure. However, if this disorder is associated with affective symptoms the whole condition may be improved by antidepressant medication.

Drugs

There are a number of drugs which are associated with depression. Examples include antihypertensives (including calcium channel blockers), antituberculosis drugs, steroids and long-term use of certain psychotropics. Mechanisms of these effects are ill-understood.

Infections

Viral and (to a lesser extent) bacterial infections are often associated with depression. On occasions the infection appears to induce a specific depressive state. It seems likely that the infection acts a trigger for an episode which appears indistinguishable from other episodes. Mechanisms remain speculative. It is however, noteworthy that interferon which is raised in viral infections is associated with feelings of lethargy, lassitude and dysphoria.

Other factors

Finally there are a whole series of unexplained facts about affective illness. For example, it is not at all clear why depression, suicide and affective swings in bipolar patients are more common in the spring. It may be that part of the biological disturbance in depression may be close (physiologically and/or anatomically) to the supra-chiasmatic nucleus of the hypothalamus which entrains both circadian and circannual rhythms.

Psychosocial factors

Psychological factors feature prominently in 'stress-diathesis' models of the onset of depressive disorders. The factors can be divided into three key areas: intrapersonal issues (psychodynamic and cognitive hypotheses, premorbid personality); interpersonal issues (interactions with others, social support networks); and environmental issues (early adversity, recent life events). Although such factors may precipitate (e.g. recent life events) or predispose (e.g. lack of a confidant) an individual to the development of depression, the effects probably operate through other mechanisms (Brown, 1989). For example, early loss of mother or current unemployment may affect the development or maintenance of self-esteem.

Intrapersonal aspects

Psychodynamic models

It is difficult to simply summarise psychoanalytic models of depression, partly because of the complexities of the different theories put forward and partly because of the intricacies of the 'metaphoric' language used (Ryle, 1991). While brief descriptions of the most relevant contributions will be provided, Ryle has pointed out that the most important concept to grasp is the notion that intrapsychic structure is interpersonally derived. Thus, adult personality bears traces of both the infant and the internalised parent. It is hypothesised that problems in early life lead to defects in development that render the individual vulnerable to depression.

Psychodynamic models of depression have largely developed from the basic paradigm postulated by Freud (1917) in his classic work *Mourning and Melancholia*. It should be noted that Freud clearly stated that not all depressive disorders had a psychological aetiology, but he observed a resemblance between grief and psychotic depression. Freud suggested that melancholia also occurred following object loss (either a real loss or the loss of 'some abstraction'). The model proposed that the hostility felt towards the lost object (which was largely denied) became directed against the self, explaining some of the classic features of depression as demonstrated in this quote:

> 'If one listens patiently to a patient's many and various self-accusations, one cannot in the end avoid the impression that often the most violent of them are hardly applicable to the patient himself, but that with insignificant modifications they do fit someone else, someone whom the patient loves or has loved or should love.'

Like Abraham (1911), Freud believed that the individuals ambivalent relationship with the object (the simultaneous presence of feelings of love and hostility) predisposed to the development of depression. Freud argued that identification of the ego with the lost object was accompanied by regression to the oral phase of psychosexual development when sadistic feelings were at their most powerful. Abraham's (1911) belief that neurotics resorted to oral gratification to prevent or relieve depression has been viewed by some as an explanation of the phenomenon of comfort eating.

As highlighted in the excellent reviews by Mendelson (1990, 1992), important modifications or alternatives to Freud's model were proposed by Bibring (1953), Jacobson (1953) and object relations theorists (particularly Klein (1934)). Bibring and Jacobson both gave primacy to the role of loss of self-esteem in the development of depression whereas the Kleinians focused on the quality of the mother–infant relationship (Pedder, 1982). Object relations theory describes the 'depressive position', as a developmental phase during which a child learns to modify ambivalence and retain self-esteem during periodic loss of the 'good mother' (Mendelson, 1990). It is proposed that if the infant does not acquire confidence that its mother will return and be loving, despite hostile feelings toward the parent during separation, the child becomes fixated at this level of development and will be more prone to depression in adulthood.

Bibring's work highlighted two key concepts. Firstly, that while loss of self-esteem was frequently experienced in the oral phase, it could also occur in other developmental phases when narcissistic aspirations (such as the desire to be good or to be strong) were frustrated. Secondly, Bibring suggested that depression was an ego phenomenon and resulted from inner system tensions within the ego rather than from inter-system conflicts (between ego and superego, or ego and id). This notion was used to explain why not all depressions are characterised by guilt (which is believed to derive from inter-system conflict).

Although Jacobson agreed with Bibring that self-esteem was affected by many variables, her model is particularly noted for its exposition of the development of self and object representations, and its distinction of the ego (a psychic structure) from the self (one's person as distinct from others). Low self-esteem was seen as the central psychological problem in depression, but was not regarded as an ego phenomenon. It was suggested that optimal levels of self-esteem were determined by the individuals' self-representations, superego, ego ideal and self-critical ego functions. A less positive self-image, a more primitive superego, a less attainable ego-ideal or unrealistic expectations and goals, the more vulnerable the self-esteem and the greater the risk of depression. Jacobson proposed that in 'regressive identification' there was a loss of the boundaries between self and object representations which explained why hostility directed at the object was turned inward. Jacobson saw aggression as critical to the development of depression through its impact on self-esteem. However, it is important to understand that the term aggression in this model refers to psychic energy rather than hostile behaviours.

Cognitive models

Mendelson (1990) commented that psychoanalytic models of depression represent art more than science and rarely produce testable hypotheses. This may be one of the reasons for the increasing interest in cognitive–behavioural models of depression as the two prominent theories, promulgated by Seligman and co-workers (Seligman, 1975, Seligman *et al*, 1978) and Beck and colleagues (Beck, 1976; Beck *et al*, 1983), are partly supported by empirical data (Twaddle & Scott, 1991). The former model was derived from laboratory experiments with animals, while the latter originated from Beck's observations of the thoughts and ideas expressed by depressed patients.

Learned helplessness.   Seligman's (1975) original 'learned helplessness' model suggested that animals exposed to inescapable shock later failed to learn to avoid escapable stimuli in similar situations. The central issue in this hypothesis is that rewards (or punishments) are non-contingent with actions. The model in its original form was an inadequate explanation of the laboratory observations and was reformulated (Abramson *et al*, 1978) into a more comprehensive theory with four premises. It was suggested that the 'depression prone' individual:

  (a) perceives that highly aversive outcomes are likely to happen
  (b) perceives that these events will be uncontrollable
  (c) possesses a maladaptive attributional style such that negative events are attributed to internal, stable global causes and positive events to external, unstable and specific causes

(d) the greater the certainty of the aversive state of affairs and the expected uncontrollability, the greater the severity of the motivational and cognitive deficits; the greater the importance of the uncontrollable event to the individual, the greater the affective and self-esteem disruption.

The majority of research has focused on attributional style, but the results of such studies have been contradictory (Twaddle & Scott, 1991). Alloy *et al* (1988) were critical of the research methodologies employed and also suggested a further modification to the model (this has been called the 'hopelessness model') which requires the matching of a stressor with the attributional style relating to that specific domain of functioning. For example, a depressive reaction may occur following social rejection in someone with a maladaptive attributional style for interpersonal events. As yet this development has not been researched in detail, but it parallels recent modifications of Beck's cognitive model of depression discussed below.

Beck's cognitive model of depression.   In its most succinct form, Beck's model of depression suggests that three elements of psychological functioning are implicated in the development or maintenance of depression: depressogenic schemata (underlying beliefs), negative automatic thoughts and systematic logical errors of reasoning. Those at risk of depression are believed to have developed (as a result of certain types of negative early experiences) dysfunctional cognitive structures (schemata) which determine how the individual interprets their subjective reality. These underlying beliefs may be conditional (e.g. 'In order to be happy, I must be successful in everything I do') or unconditional (e.g. 'I am unlovable'). It is hypothesised that these schemata are latent for long periods, but become activated when the individual is exposed to negative events in later life. The reactivation of the schemata leads to the generation of repetitive, unintended and largely uncontrolled 'negative automatic thoughts' characterised in terms of the cognitive triad (negative thoughts about the self, the world and the future). These negative cognitions are sustained through information processing biases (systematic errors in thinking such as overgeneralisation, selective abstraction etc.) and a vicious cycle is generated in which increases in the intensity of depressed mood lead to increases in the intensity of negative thinking, which further increase the severity of mood and behavioural disturbance. Beck *et al* (1983) later clarified components of the model and suggested that while it may represent a causal theory for some unipolar non-biological depressions, in other depressives it was largely a model to explain the maintenance of the disorder.

Beck *et al* (1983) also reviewed the stress-diathesis hypothesis and suggested that the matching of events to certain personality modes may explain why the same experience can have a different impact on different individuals. Beck suggested that 'sociotropic' individuals (those placing high value on positive interchanges with others) may react negatively to experiences such as personal rejection. However, 'autonomous' individuals (who place high value on independent functioning) may become depressed in response to events such as failure to achieve a personal goal.

Explorations of Beck's model suggest that, regardless of clinical subtype, the descriptions of the cognitive content of a depressive's thinking and of information processing biases accurately reflect clinical experience of the acute presentation. However, there is limited empirical data to support the view that latent dysfunctional schemata predispose to the onset of depression (Williams, 1992), as there are difficulties in trying to measure structures deemed latent during depression-free intervals (Twaddle & Scott, 1991). It is not clear whether this is a problem with the model or the research techniques employed.

Personality and personality disorder

The relationship between premorbid personality and vulnerability to depression is complex. Despite the vast literature on the topic there is little in the way of premorbid personality traits or disorder that predicts the vast majority of cases. Earlier suggestions regarding premorbid vulnerability to affective disorders being increased in those with 'pyknic' body build (Kretshner, 1936), or those with a cyclothymic personality (Kraepelin, 1921) have not been substantiated (Tellenbach, 1975; von Zerssen, 1976). Cognitive–behavioural models of depression suggest the presence of premorbid personality vulnerability (characterised by maladaptive attributional style or the presence of depressogenic schemata) while the psychoanalytic literature highlights the relationship between orality, obsessionality and depression (Abraham, 1911). However, these concepts are not systematically assessed in day to day clinical practice.

There is a great deal of evidence that personality may affect the course of an affective disorder (Weissman & Klerman, 1976; Duggan *et al*, 1990; Scott *et al*, 1992). However, no personality characteristics have been found to be specifically associated with onset of depression (as opposed to any other disorder). The reliability and validity of measures of personality made during an episode of depression are questionable and any measures made after recovery may be measuring personality features evolving as a consequence of the illness. The ideal research method in this situation is to undertake prospective longitudinal studies but these are difficult to mount and expensive to run. Current theories largely relate to vulnerability models where certain traits predispose to depression and spectrum models, which view certain traits as a milder manifestation of the disorder.

Research by Hirschfeld and colleagues (1977, 1987, 1990, 1992), suggests that recovered depressives differ from never psychiatrically ill controls

(Hirschfeld *et al*, 1986). Assessment of a cohort of 438 adults (Hirschfeld *et al*, 1989) before anyone became a case showed significant differences in premorbid traits only in individuals aged 31–41 years who developed a first episode of depression compared with those who did not. Those who became depressed were shown to have higher levels of premorbid neuroticism, lower levels of emotional stability, less resilience and more interpersonal dependency. However, these case-control differences did not emerge in the 17–30-year-old cohort. These age-group differences have not been explained, although one hypothesis is that it may be due to a cohort effect or a change in psychosocial risk factors over time with, for example, a decrease in emotional strength between age groups (Hirschfeld & Shea, 1992).

In the Swiss cohort study, Angst & Clayton (1986) identified an increased risk of first episode of depression in individuals with increased aggression and autonomic lability. The latter construct is regarded as being similar to neuroticism. Interestingly, neuroticism has been the focus of recent work by Martin (1985) and Teasdale (1988). Cognitive constructions of neuroticism are provided (particularly relating to 'global negative affectivity and 'negative self-reference') which may explain the possible role of this trait in predisposing to depression. Hopefully, future research will integrate the cognitive psychology and clinical psychopathology literature to allow a clearer definition of premorbid characteristics that increase vulnerability to depression.

A different approach was advocated by Winokur (1974) who has written widely on the concept of 'depressive spectrum disease'. The model suggests that antisocial personality disorder (ASPD) and alcoholism form part of a spectrum with depression. Support for the model came from familial studies which demonstrated an increased prevalence of ASPD and alcoholism in the first degree relatives of unipolar probands. The latter were regarded as having 'depressive spectrum disease' and often showed some character disturbance along with their affective disorder. Those with no such family history were regarded as having 'pure depressive disease'. Attempts to replicate this model show varying degrees of support for the proposed characteristics of depressive spectrum disease such as early age of onset of depression, female gender, marital instability and biological differences (e.g. lower DST non-suppression rates).

Akiskal *et al* (1981) identify two other subgroups: 'character spectrum disorder' and 'subaffective disorders'. The former are similar to Winokur's depressive spectrum group while the latter (the cyclothymic–bipolar II group) are distinguished by the fact that the personality disorder is regarded as arising secondary to the affective disorder. Other researchers argue that cyclothymia and bipolar disorder (Klein & Depue, 1984) or borderline personality disorder and depression are genetically linked (Hirschfeld & Shea, 1992). Comorbidity between depressive and borderline personality disorder and the other personality disorders is also discussed in chapter 18.

Interpersonal issues

Marriage

Previous research has suggested that with regard to depressive disorders, marriage was protective for men, but detrimental for women (Gove, 1972; Der & Bebbington, 1987). However, it is difficult to retrospectively disentangle cause and effect; marital status may change as a result of depression rather than being associated with its onset. The ECA study suggested that even when controlling for gender and age, continuously married subjects demonstrated the lowest depression rates and divorced or separated subjects the highest, with a threefold increase in risk (Smith & Weissman, 1992). The prevalence of depression in never married subjects was closest to that of the continuously married or cohabiting subjects. To try to explain these apparently conflicting results, the researchers postulated that earlier studies were undertaken at a time when divorce was less socially acceptable. It was suggested that for women, remaining in an unsatisfactory marriage may have particularly predisposed toward the development of depression. This hypothesis clearly requires exploration. Evidence from Hickie *et al* (1991) suggests that the risk of non-endogenous depression in both men and women is increased five-fold if the current intimate partner is perceived as dysfunctional. The ratings of dysfunctional characteristics (identified as low care and high control) did not appear to be state dependent. Hickie *et al* (1990) also noted that individuals reporting markedly deficient care in childhood were more likely to report very poor current intimate relationships.

Presence of a confidant

Of the vulnerability/protective factors identified by Brown & Harris (1978), the role of a confidant in reducing depression among women experiencing adversity, has received the most robust support. Lack of intimacy may independently increase the risk of depression (Tennant & Bebbington, 1978) and women in a relationship demonstrating coldness and indifference have three times the risk of depression following a major life event (35% *v.* 10%) than those in a more positive partnership (Brown *et al*, 1986). Cooper's (1990) literature review also indicates that a confiding relationship, particularly one in which reciprocity exists, may protect an individual against recurrence of depression. Interestingly, Champion (1990) found a positive relationship between lack of intimacy and the occurrence of adverse events. However, it must be remembered that this association may be apparent rather than real as the life events experienced can involve the loss of a 'significant other' from the support network.

A community study by Brown *et al* (1986) further extended our knowledge of the role of a confidant. It was noted that many women with apparently supportive partners were still at risk of developing depression when followed prospectively. This led to the suggestion that it is the level of effective support provided by the confidant in crisis situations that is critical in preventing the onset of depression. Furthermore, it was found that the presence of other forms of support did not attenuate the effect of being let down by the confidant. It is currently hypothesised that the confidant protects against depression by modifying the impact of adversity on self-esteem.

Expressed emotion

Expressed emotion (EE) assesses the quality of close family relationships, particularly between the depressed individual and their spouse. The studies of Vaughn & Leff (1976), and Hooley *et al* (1986), found that level of EE in a key relative at the time of an index depressive episode was a significant predictor of further relapse. Leff & Vaughn (1980) found a link between high levels of EE and onset of depression, but noted that the depressed individuals studied also reported high rates of life events. It was suggested that the conjunction of life events and a critical relative may play a causal role in depression onset, but this theory has yet to be proven (Cooper, 1990).

Social networks

Cobb (1976) viewed social support as information that helped an individual believe they are cared for, loved, esteemed, valued and belonged to a network. Current conceptualisations of social support are multidimensional (Thoits, 1985), and incorporate both structural and functional components. Structural aspects relate to the size and interconnectedness of the primary and secondary groups, while functional aspects describe the practical help and emotional support available. There is evidence of an association between social support and depression (Paykel & Cooper, 1992), but its role in onset is as yet unclear. Recent reviews by Brugha (1988,1989) suggested that perceived numerical and qualitative deficiencies in close personal relationships may predict onset of depression. However, it has been shown that individuals prone to developing depression may demonstrate premorbid deficits in making and sustaining relationships, highlighting the possible confounding role of personality.

The majority of studies have explored two theories: the 'buffer theory' (which suggests that the presence of social support reduces risk of depression by modifying the impact of adversity) and the 'main effect' hypothesis (which suggests that lack of social support directly predisposes to depression). Alloway & Bebbington (1987) reviewed 23 cross-sectional and 12 longitudinal studies on the relationship between depression and social support. The evidence for the 'buffer theory' was inconsistent and when present was not of dramatic proportions. Longitudinal prospective studies may shed some light on the relationship between social support and depression. One of the most important was undertaken by Henderson *et al* (1978). It was found that the 'buffer theory' could only be substantiated if the perceived adequacy rather than simply the extent of the social support was assessed. This finding suggested that subjective views of the existing network were important and it was hypothesised that as premorbid personality may influence perceptions of the available support, it may be an important intervening variable. There is some data suggesting that lack of social support is directly associated with minor affective disorders (Henderson *et al*, 1978; Brugha *et al*, 1982), whether this relationship is causal is not yet established.

Environmental issues

Life events and illness

The aftermath of natural or man-made disasters has provided clear evidence of the impact of extreme stress on the psychological wellbeing of previously healthy individuals. While such disasters are rare, the study of these situations provided a possible theoretical model for the investigation of the relationship between life events and somatic or psychiatric disturbance. As pointed out by Dohrenwend & Dohrenwend (1979), given the prevalence of these disorders, if stressful situations do have a causal role, the events must be relatively ordinary and frequently experienced within a given population. Early questionnaire studies therefore began by focusing on events that happened to most people at some time or another. Holmes & Rahe (1967) believed that if the clustering of events in an individual's life reached a sufficient magnitude this would provide a necessary if not sufficient cause of the onset of disorder. They explored the events recorded in the life charts of naval ratings who developed physical illness and derived a list of 43 frequently reported life events. To try to measure the magnitude of the effect of the event on an individual, Holmes & Rahe (1967) then developed the Social Readjustment Rating Scale (see Table 3.1). The list of events was presented to general population samples and each individual was asked to rate the degree of adjustment required regardless of the desirability of the event. Marriage was chosen as the 'modulus' and individuals then gave quantitative judgements of the amount of change or readjustment required (measured in life change units; LCU) relative to this arbitrary standard. As seen in Table 3.1, many events given high scores were socially undesirable but positive experiences may also be regarded as stressful.

Holmes & Rahe (1967) initally argued that the risk of illness in any individual was directly related to the magnitude of LCU score. However, others commented on deficiencies of this model, and questionnaire

Table 3.1 Social Readjustment Rating Scale (reprinted with permission from Holmes & Rahe, 1967)

Rank	Life event	Mean value
1	Death of spouse	100
2	Divorce	73
3	Marital separation	65
4	Jail term	63
5	Death of close family member	63
6	Personal injury or illness	53
7	Marriage	50
8	Sacked at work	47
9	Marital reconciliation	45
10	Retirement	45
11	Change in health of family member	44
12	Pregnancy	40
13	Sex difficulties	39
14	Gain of new family member	39
15	Business readjustment	39
16	Change in financial state	38
17	Death of close friend	37
18	Change to different line of work	36
19	Change in number of arguments with spouse	35
20	Mortgage over £10 000	31
21	Foreclosure of mortgage or loan	30
22	Change in responsibilities at work	29
23	Son or daughter leaving home	29
24	Trouble with in-laws	29
25	Outstanding personal achievement	28
26	Wife begins or stops work	26
27	Begin or stop school	26
28	Change in living conditions	25
29	Revision of personal habits	24
30	Trouble with boss	23
31	Change in work hours or conditions	20
32	Change in residence	20
33	Change in schools	20
34	Change in recreation	19
35	Change in church activities	19
36	Change in social activities	18
37	Mortgage or loan less than £10 000	17
38	Change in sleeping habits	16
39	Change in number of family get-togethers	15
40	Change in eating habits	15
41	Vacation	13
42	Christmas	12
43	Minor violations of the law	11

surveys have lost favour as more sophisticated research tools have been developed. Hudgens (1974) suggested that many events listed on questionnaires (29 of the 43 on the readjustment scale) could occur as a consequence of illness rather than precede it (representing dependent rather than independent events). Brown (1974) also noted that there was considerable variability in the LCU ratings obtained from individuals with different social or cultural backgrounds. Brown also demonstrated that the use of an interview rather than a questionnaire approach to life events showed that 'contextual threat' (the circumstances surrounding the event) had an important influence on the impact of the event on the individual.

Frequency of life events and chronic difficulties

A large body of research has since explored the potential role of recent stress in precipitating the onset of depressive episodes. Life events can be viewed as sudden changes in an individual's social world, while chronic difficulties may represent a lack of change (for > 4 weeks) in a stressful situation. Both factors have been implicated in the onset of disorder (Brown & Harris, 1978). Chronic difficulties rated as threatening and persistent (> 2 years) are independently associated with an increased risk of depression, but in general the coexistence of life events and difficulties together do not significantly alter the level of risk associated with the occurrence of one or other experience alone (Brown & Harris, 1978).

About 30 retrospective case-control studies have compared depressed and non-depressed adults on interview rated life event schedules (for reviews see Brown & Harris (1989) and Paykel & Cooper (1992)). The results of this research demonstrate that depressed individuals report more independent undesirable life events in the six months prior to episode onset than population controls, assessed for the same time period. This association does not appear to be coincidental, nor to be a function of 'effort after meaning' (the retrospective reinterpretation of an event as stressful in an attempt to explain the origins of the depression). In studies comparing depressed individuals to other patient populations, only subjects attempting suicide reported more preceding life events than depressives (Paykel *et al*, 1975). Medical patients (Hudgens *et al*, 1967) and patients with schizophrenia report fewer life events preceding episode onset (Brown *et al*, 1973; Leff & Vaughn, 1980).

Types of life event

Paykel (1982) suggests that overall there is only weak evidence for any specific hypothesis relating type of event and type of disorder, although there is a trend for depression to be preceded by loss events or separations (Paykel & Cooper, 1992). In an earlier study of nearly 200 depressed patients (Paykel *et al*, 1969) found that in the six months prior to illness onset, undesirable events were reported about three times more frequently in depressed as opposed to general population control subjects. If the events were reclassified as exit/entrance events, exit events showed the same pattern of occurrence with about the same frequency. In contrast desirable events or entrance events occurred as often in control and depressed populations. Tennant & Bebbington (1978) demonstrated an association between the threatfulness of events and the level of emotional distress experienced (as measured on the GHQ), but the association was not deemed specific to depression.

Even allowing for the considerable overlap between the symptoms of grief and depressive disorder, bereavement shows a high rate of association with depression. A prospective study by Clayton & Darvish (1979) showed that 42% of recently bereaved spouses met research criteria for depression one month after the death and 15% still met criteria at 12 months. The life events study of Paykel *et al* (1969) showed that the loss of an immediate family member was four times as common in the depressed (n=16) as in the control subjects, with loss of a child (n=5) being reported only in the depressed group. Many studies suggest that loss of a child is the most significant and traumatic form of bereavement.

Life events and depressive symptom profile

Bebbington *et al* (1981) noted that life events were recalled more frequently by depressives seen in the community compared to those seen in the out-patient setting. While it might be hypothesised that the more severe depressions seen in hospitals are less likely to be preceded by life events, the data available does not confirm this. Only about 30% of depressives report no preceding events (Paykel & Cooper, 1992) and studies attempting to demonstrate differential rates of life events in endogenous and non-endogenous depressions show that (when symptoms and events are rated independently) there is only a low correlation between experience of an event and symptom profile (Paykel *et al*, 1984; Bebbington *et al*, 1981). Although these associations were in the expected direction, it seems that symptom profile is determined by other factors.

Impact of life events

The trend for depressives to experience more events in the months prior to episode onset, must be understood in the context of variations in individual susceptibility to the impact of such events. Paykel (1974) demonstrated hypothetically that only about 10% of individuals in the community who experienced an exit life event actually developed a clinical depression. Furthermore, a follow-up of depressed subjects found that, although the number of events they experienced fell over time, the occurrence rate continued to exceed that of other members of the general population (Paykel, 1974). Thus, life events research has explored factors mediating the effects of the event on the individual and tried to define the magnitude of the effect. As discussed earlier, mediating factors may operate at a personality or cognitive level, or may be a function of the presence or absence of vulnerability factors such as level of social support.

The magnitude of effect has predominantly been assessed through prospective event-centred research using one of three techniques, the concept of 'brought forward time' (Brown *et al*, 1973) , or the measurement of 'relative risk' (Paykel, 1978), or of 'population attributable risk' (Cooke, 1987). Brown and colleagues suggested that the occurrence of life events brought forward the onset of depression (which may otherwise have occurred spontaneously) by about two years. This concept has been less widely applied than the epidemiological measures proposed. Paykel showed that there was a sixfold increase in the relative risk of developing depression in the six months following the occurrence of stressful events. Cooke demonstrated that the development of depression in 40% of the cases recorded in any study sample could be (on average) attributed to the effects of life alone, while about 60% could be attributed to life events in the absence of a confidant. The latter calculation suggests that while life events and social support may play a significant role in the onset of depression, other parameters are still important and a multifactorial aetiological model still offers the most plausible explanation.

Life events and the outcome of depression

The role of life events in the course and outcome (relapse, recurrence and chronicity) of depression has been less well researched. There is evidence that adverse events occurring during the course of treatment may lead to exacerbation of depressive symptoms (Brown & Harris, 1978) while 'neutralising' (Tennant *et al*, 1981) or 'fresh start' events (Brown *et al*, 1988) may be associated with remission. Paykel & Tanner (1976) found that adverse events occurring during the prophylactic treatment phase were associated with increased risk of relapse, while Scott *et al* (1988) showed that chronicity in major depression was associated with an increased rate of independent undesirable life events after the onset of the index depressive episode. Interestingly, Ghaziuddin *et al* (1990) showed that subjects suffering from a recurrent episode of depression were significantly less likely to experience adversity than subjects suffering their first episode of depression. If later illness episodes are likely to occur in the absence of a precipitant, this will need to be taken into account in future life events research.

Employment status

As noted earlier, it is suggested that employment and financial independence are associated with lower rates of depression. Smith &

Weissman (1992) reported that the risk of depression in unemployed people shows a threefold increase. British studies tend to suggest that unemployment is associated with an increase in psychiatric morbidity, particularly anxiety and depression (Banks & Jackson, 1982; Melville *et al*, 1985) and that this trend is reversed by gaining employment (Jenkins *et al*, 1982). Jenkins *et al* (1982) also found that the severity of symptoms was greater in young unemployed women than in men. The explanation is not entirely clear, but concurs with Brown & Harris's (1978) study of the social origins of depression in women which clearly linked vulnerability with lack of employment outside of the home. There is a non-specific increase in rates of depression in retired individuals (Martin & Doran, 1966).

While the link between unemployment and depression may arise directly because of the adverse influence on socioeconomic status, indirect mechanisms may also be relevant. Jahoda (1982) identifies that, beside providing income, employment has several functions including providing the individual with status, a sense of purposefulness and control, a social network, and structure and activity. Recent research supports the importance of these latent functions demonstrating the negative impact of unemployment on social supports and self-esteem (Bolton & Oakley, 1987; Scott, 1992).

Maternal separation and death during childhood

A major theme in psychoanalytic writings on depression suggested that deficiencies in or loss of the early mother–child relationship predisposed to adult depression. While analysts used the recollections of their adult patients to explore the 'deprivation hypothesis', Bowlby (1951) observed the behaviour of young children to develop his views on the consequences of early adversity. He suggested that the disruption to bonding (rather than the meaning of the event) was critical in predisposing to depression or other types of dysfunction (e.g. antisocial behaviour)(Bowlby's views are also discussed in chapter 13). Rutter (1972, 1985) extended the argument, suggesting that the loss may lead to a range of other adverse events (producing a cascade-like effect) and that the latter are more pathogenic than the loss itself in leading to adult psychopathology. The well-documented community studies of Brown *et al* (1987) suggested that loss of mother before the age of 11 years was associated with increased risk of adult depression in the presence of a provoking agent. Harris *et al* (1986) proposed a mechanism for this effect, believing that early loss increased future vulnerability to depression because of its adverse effect on self-esteem.

Refinements of the research have looked at loss as a consequence of parental death, loss due to parent–child separations and the effects of parental style on early development. There are at least 80 recent papers on these topics and the association with adult depression. However, a critical review of the literature suggests that the results of many studies may be undermined because of methodological inadequacies (e.g. failure to match experimental and control groups). Assessment of the remaining research has been undertaken previously (Crook & Eliot, 1980; Tennant *et al*, 1980; Tennant, 1991; Parker, 1992) and clearly reveals that when loss is divided into that due to parental death and that due to parent–child separation, there is no evidence childhood bereavement specifically predisposes to adult depression. It appears that the negative effects are probably a consequence of the inadequate mothering occurring after the loss (Birtchnell, 1980). The data on parent–child separation suggest that this may contribute to adult depression, particularly if it occurs in the context of family discord, unless family break-up does not adversely affect the quality of parenting (Tennant, 1991). Two studies by Brown's research group (Harris *et al*, 1986; Bifulco *et al*, 1987) also established that parental loss *per se* did not predict later depression unless post-loss parental care was also assessed.

Parker (1992) points out that the above findings may be a function of higher order effects relating to two constructs, namely parental attitudes and behaviours. Measuring parenting is problematic, but the use of the 'Parental Bonding Instrument' (Parker *et al*, 1979) has allowed subjects to reliably rate their parents' attributes on two subscales: 'care' and 'protection'. Low scores on the 'care' scale and high scores on the 'protection' scale (a combination termed 'affectionless overcontrol') were associated with increased risk of development of neurotic disorders, particularly depression, in adult life (Parker *et al*, 1987). While this relationship holds for less severe depression, Parker (1979, 1992) reported no association between anomalous parenting and melancholia.

Childhood sexual abuse

There appears to be an increased risk of depression and other psychiatric disorders in women who were sexually abused in childhood. The true prevalence of childhood abuse in males and females is unknown, but of nearly 300 women interviewed in a three year community study in Islington, 9% reported childhood sexual abuse. Two-thirds of these women developed at least one episode of depression during the study period (Bifulco *et al*, 1991).

Conclusions

In order to review the extensive literature on causal models of depression, this chapter was subdivided into sections focusing on specific research fields. However, this should not be taken to imply any support for unitary models of depression. It is quite clear that depression is a heterogeneous disorder and that multifactorial stress-diathesis models offer a more coherent explanation of the phenomena observed in clinical practice (Akiskal & McKinney, 1975). Interesting results are beginning to emerge from such approaches. A study of 680 female-female twins examined prospectively suggested that at least four major and interacting risk factor domains are needed to understand the aetiology of major depression. These were traumatic experiences, genetic factors, temperament and interpersonal relations (Kendler *et al*, 1993).

The practical difficulties and the financial cost of large scale prospective studies of the causes of depression has meant that most of our hypotheses regarding aetiology are derived from case-control studies. Such investigations require the researchers to proceed retrospectively from effect (depression) to cause. Schlesselman (1982) points out that to prove cause and effect it is necessary to specify the mechanism by which the effect is produced. Unfortunately, retrospective studies can only make inferences and the clear identification of direct or indirect effects of specific variables is rarely feasible.

The term psychosocial obviously implies that an individuals' psychological perception of social factors is important. The latter may be proximal to the onset of depression (recent life events, chronic difficulties) or distal (early adversity). The interaction of recent stress with personality or cognitive style may explain why a particular individual develops depression at a particular moment in time. For example, Brown & Harris (1978) described the development of depression in women in Camberwell occurring when predisposed individuals (identified as those who described early loss of a parent, three or more young children, unemployment and lack of a confidant) experienced a major life event. Teasdale's (1988) cognitive model of onset and persistence of depression (termed the 'differential activation hypothesis') showed that in certain individuals the development and maintenance of depression was determined by the increased accessibility of negative memories occurring after a transient negative mood shift had occurred in response to the stress. Interestingly, high N score individuals are particularly at risk of showing such cognitive processing biases.

Social and cognitive models of depression (Beck, 1976; Brown, 1989) are now beginning to address how the matching of events with intrapersonal factors may determine the impact of an event on a particular subject. It is likely that the effects of early adversity on any individual differs not only according to their childhood temperament but also in its later effect on adult personality development, particularly influencing self-esteem and attributional style. Thus distal factors such as early learning experiences increase individual vulnerability to the impact of specific stressors in adult life.

Psychosocial and biological factors can also be clearly linked. While explorations of underlying mechanisms are in the early stages, it is well-recognised that psychological perceptions have their substrates and concomitants in brain functioning (Paykel & Cooper, 1992). Animal experiments have shown that the behavioural changes of the learned helplessness paradigm may be associated with NA depletion in the locus coerulus and with specific changes in the hippocampal β-receptors (Henn & McKinney, 1987). These changes are reminiscent of those postulated to operate in the CNS in major depression. Furthermore glucocorticoids in excess may enhance these learned 'negative' behaviours (Veldhuis *et al*, 1985). While the behaviours seen in this particular animal model of depression responded specifically to antidepressants, it must be remembered that there are obvious dangers in extrapolating animal behaviour to human behaviour and in linking effects of antidepressants in normal animals to depressed humans.

There is growing evidence that both adverse and positive stimuli to young animals alter their subsequent response to stress in a predictable direction. One neural substrate of these adaptations appears to be central glucocorticoid receptor numbers (Meaney *et al*, 1991). These observations link to research done on normal controls and depressed patients which have examined the mechanisms involved in the transduction of psychosocial stress (Post, 1992). These studies have, in turn, led to clinical interest in the phenomenon of 'kindling' (a term to describe spontaneous changes in neuronal excitability in the presence of sub-threshold stimulation). In a simplistic form, this mechanism may be one explanation of why early depressive episodes are preceded by significant stress events, but later episodes occur in the absence of any obvious precipitant (as described by Ghaziuddin *et al* (1990)). It could be postulated that experiences of psychosocial stress may lead to changes in neuronal excitability so that the individual shows increased sensitivity to lower levels of stress at a later date. Of course these changes may parallel changes in self-esteem or personality functioning occurring as a consequence of repeated episodes of depression. Hence biological and psychological factors may operate concurrently. This is further borne out by family studies. Recent research has not supported the notion that genetic and psychosocial vulnerability are inversely related. Bipolar patients were studied by Patrick *et al* (1978), while McGuffin *et al* (1988) investigated unipolar disorders in probands and their families. Interestingly the latter study concluded that the tendency to experience adversity and to experience depression were familial.

The apparent complexities of multifactorial models should not disarm clinicians. The reasons for seeking models of causation are to inform our preventative efforts. While no model of depression is robust enough to make primary prevention an option, some attempts have been made to

Table 3.2 Outline of causes of depression

Predisposition	Stimulus	Intermediate changes	Outcome
Genes	'Stress'	Cognitive	Dysphoria
Family	Adversity	Psychodynamic	Dysthmia
Personality	Physical factors	Neurochemical	Major depression
		Neuroendocrine	with biological features
			with psychotic features
		Neuropathological	with cognitive features

target high risk groups. For example, Newton (1988) describes a project aimed at offering social support to young, isolated, unemployed mothers potentially at risk from depression. The women appeared to benefit in terms of subjective well-being and, importantly, their ability to care for their children was enhanced. An alternative approach is described by Parkes (1981), who used an event-centred approach, targeting recently bereaved adults at high risk of abnormal grief reactions. Support and counselling appeared to reduce psychiatric morbidity in this group to the same levels as individuals identified as being at 'low risk' of abnormal grief reactions. Such approaches help elucidate why it is beneficial to take a psychobiosocial approach to causality. While it may not be feasible to prevent certain life events occurring, the occurrence can be used to signal a time of increased vulnerability. It may be possible to manipulate social support to modify the impact of events on certain individuals, reducing the likelihood that they reach the pathological end state of depression.

In summary it is likely that there is no one cause of depression but rather a series of overlapping vulnerability factors which operate in different ways and with differing force throughout life. In the majority of cases, a stimulus of some sort acts on those people predisposed to depression (by virtue of their genetic makeup or early environmental experiences or some combination of these). Depending on the nature and strength of the stimulus and on predisposition, a variety of intermediate changes occur which lead to the development of a variety of clinical symptoms and syndromes (see Table 3.2).

References

Abraham, K. (1911) Notes on the psychoanalytic investigation and treatment of manic-depressive insanity and allied conditions. In *Selected Papers on Psychoanalysis*, pp.137–156. London: Hogarth Press, 1927.

Abramson, L. Y., Seligman, M. E. P. & Teasdale, J. D. (1978) Learned helplessness in humans: critique and reformulation. *Journal of Abnormal Psychology*, **87**, 49–74.

Akiskal, H. S. & McKinney, W. T. (1975) Overview of recent research in depression. Integration of ten conceptual models into a comprehensive clinical frame. *Archives of General Psychiatry*, **32**, 285–305.

——, King, D., Rosenthal, L., *et al* (1981) Chronic depression: Part I. Clinical and familial characteristics of 137 probands. *Journal of Affective Disorders*, **3**, 297–315.

Alexopoulos, G. S., Young, R. C. & Shindledecker, R. D. (1992) Brain computed tomography findings in geriatric depression and primary degenerative dementia. *Biological Psychiatry*, **31**, 591–599.

Alloway, R. & Bebbington, P. E. (1987) The buffer theory of social support: a review of the literature. *Psychological Medicine*, **17**, 91–108.

Alloy, L. B., Abramson, G. & Hartlage, S. (1988) The helplessness theory of depression: attributional aspects. *British Journal of Clinical Psychology*, **27**, 5–21.

Amsterdam, J. D., Marinelli, D. L., Arger, P., *et al* (1987) Assessment of adrenal gland volume by computed tomography in depressed patients and healthy volunteers: a pilot study. *Psychiatric Research*, **21**, 189–197.

Andreason, N. C., Rice, J., Endicott, J., *et al* (1987) Familial rates of affective disorder. *Archives of General Psychiatry*, **44**, 461–469.

——, Scheftner, W., Reich, *et al* (1986) The validation of the concept of endogenous depression – a family study approach. *Archives of General Psychiatry*, **43**, 246–251.

Angst, J. & Clayton, P. (1986) Premorbid personality of depressive, bipolar, and schizophrenic patients with special reference to suicidal issues. *Comprehensive Psychiatry*, **27**, 511–532.

—— & Dobler-Mikola, A. (1985) The Zurich Study. A prospective epidemiological study of depressive, neurotic and psychosomatic syndromes. IV. Recurrent and nonrecurrent brief depression. *European Archives of Psychiatry and Neurological Sciences*, **234**, 408–416.

——, Merikangas, K., Scheidegger, P., *et al* (1990) Recurrent brief depression: a new subtype of affective disorder. *Journal of Affective Disorders*, **19**, 87–89.

Anon (1991) Recurrent brief depression and anxiety. *Lancet*, **337**, 586–587.

Arana, G. W., Baldessarini, R. J. & Ornsteen, M. (1985) The dexamethasone suppression test for diagnosis and prognosis in psychiatry. Commentary and review. *Archives of General Psychiatry*, **42**, 1193–1204.

Arango, V., Ernsberger, P., Marzuk, P. M., *et al* (1990) Autoradiographic demonstration of increased serotonin 5-HT2 and β-adrenergic receptor binding sites in the brains of suicide victims. *Archives of General Psychiatry*, **47**, 1038–1047.

Arora, R. C. & Meltzer, H. Y. (1989) Serotonergic measures in the brains of suicide victims: $5HT_2$ binding sites in the frontal cortex of suicide victims and control subjects. *American Journal of Psychiatry*, **146**, 730–736.

Asberg, M., Thoren, P. & Traskman, L. (1976) "Serotonin depression" – a biochemical sub-group within the affective disorders? *Science*, **191**, 478–480.

Austin, M. P., Dougall, N., Ross, M., *et al* (1992) Single photon emission tomography with 99Tc-examtazine in major depression and the pattern of brain activity underlying the neurotic/psychotic continuum. *Journal of Affective Disorders*, **26**, 31–44.

Baldwin, R. C. (1993) Late life depression and structural brain changes: a review of recent magnetic resonance imaging research. *International Journal of Genetic Psychiatry*, **8**, 115–123.

Banki, C. M., Bissette, G., Arato, M., *et al* (1988) Elevation of immunoreactive CSF TRH in depressed patients. *American Journal of Psychiatry*, **145**, 1524–1531.

Banks, M. H. & Jackson, P. R. (1982) Unemployment and the risk of minor psychiatric disorders in young people; cross-sectional and longitudinal evidence. *Psychological Medicine*, **12**, 789–798.

Baron, M. (1980) Genetic models of sex effect in unipolar affective illness: Application to twin data. *Acta Geneticae Medicae et Gemellologiae (Roma)*, **29**, 289–294.

Bebbington, P. E. (1978) The epidemiology of depressive disorders. In *Culture, Medicine and Psychiatry* (ed. A. M. Kleinman), pp. 297–341. Reidel: Dordrecht.

—— (1981) The epidemiology of affective disorders. In *Social Psychiatry: Theory, Methodology and Practice* (ed. P. Bebbington), pp. 265–304. London: Transaction Publishers.

——, Dean, C., Der, G., *et al* (1991) Gender, parity and the prevalence of minor affective disorder. *British Journal of Psychiatry*, **158**, 40–45.

——, Hurry, J., Tennant, C., *et al* (1981) Epidemiology of mental disorders in Camberwell. *Psychological Medicine*, **11**, 561–579.

—— & McGuffin, P. (1989) Interactive models of depression: the evidence. In *Depression, An Integrative Approach* (eds. K. R. Herbst & E. S. Paykel). Oxford: Heinemann Medical.

Beck, A. T. (1976) *Cognitive Therapy and the Emotional Disorders*. New York: International Universities Press.

——, Epstein, N. & Harrison, R. (1983) Cognitions, attitudes and personality dimensions in depression. *British Journal of Cognitive Psychotherapy*, **1**, 1–16.

Bench, C. J., Friston, K. J., Brown, R. G., *et al* (1992) The anatomy of melancholia – focal abnormalities of cerebral blood flow in major depression. *Psychological Medicine*, **22**, 607–615.

Berretini, W., Goldin, W., Nurnburger, J., *et al* (1984) Genetic factors in affective illness. *Journal of Psychiatric Research*, **18**, 329–350.

Bertelsen, A. (1979) *Origin, Prevention and Treatment of Affective Disorders* (eds M. Schou & E. Stomgren), pp. 227–239. Orlando: Academic Press.

Bibring, E. (1953) The mechanism of depression. In *Affective Disorders* (ed. P. Greenacre), pp. 14–47. New York: International Universities Press.

Bifulco, A., Brown, G. W. & Adler, Z. (1991) Early sexual abuse and clinical depression in adult life. *British Journal of Psychiatry*, **159**, 115–122.

——, —— & Harris, T. O. (1987) Childhood loss of parent and adult psychiatric disorder: the Islington study. *Journal of Affective Disorders*, **12**, 115–128.

Bigeon, A. & Israel, M. (1988) Regionally selective increases in β-adrenergic receptor density in the brains of suicide victims. *Brain Research*, **442**, 199–203.

Birtchnell, J. (1980) Women whose mothers died in childhood: an outcome study. *Psychological Medicine*, **10**, 699–713.

Bolton, W. & Oakley, K. (1987) A longitudinal study of social support and depression in unemployed men. *Psychological Medicine*, **17**, 453–460.

Bowlby, J. (1951) *Maternal Care and Mental Health.* Monograph No 2. Geneva: World Health Organization.

Boyd, J. H. & Weissman, M. M. (1982) Epidemiology. In *Handbook of Affective Disorders* (ed. E. S. Paykel). Edinburgh: Churchill-Livingstone.

Boyer, W. F. & Feighner, J. P. (1991) The serotonin hypothesis: necessary but not sufficient. In *Selective Serotonin Re-uptake Inhibitors* (eds J. P. Feighner & W. F. Boyer), pp. 71–80. Chichester: John Wiley.

Brown, G. W. (1974) Meaning, measurement and stress of life events. In *Stressful Life Events: Their Nature and Effect* (ed. B. S. Dohrenwend & B. P. Dohrenwend), pp. 217–243. New York: Wiley.

—— (1989) Depression: a radical social perspective. In *Depression: An Integrative Approach* (eds K. Herbst & E. S. Paykel), pp. 21–44. Oxford: Heinemann.

——, Adler, Z. & Bifulco, A. (1988) Life events, difficulties and recovery from chronic depression. *British Journal of Psychiatry,* **152,** 487–498.

——, Andrews, B., Harris, T. O., *et al* (1986) Social support, self-esteem and depression. *Psychological Medicine,* **16,** 813–831.

——, Bifulco, A. & Harris, T. O. (1987) Life events vulnerability and onset of depression – some refinements. *British Journal of Psychiatry,* **150,** 30–42.

—— & Harris, T. O. (1978) *Social Origins of Depression: a Study of Psychiatric Disorder in Women.* London: Tavistock Publications; New York: Free Press.

——, —— & Peto, J. (1973) Life events and psychiatric disorders: Part 2; nature of causal link. *Psychological Medicine,* **3,** 159–176.

Brown, G. W. & Prudo, R. (1981) Psychiatric disorder in a rural and an urban population: 1. Aetiology of depression. *Psychological Medicine,* **11,** 581–599.

Brugha, T. S. (1988) Social support. *Current Opinion in Psychiatry,* **1,** 206–211.

—— (1989) Social support and social networks. *Current Opinion in Psychiatry,* **2,** 278–282.

——, Conroy, R., Walsh, N., *et al* (1982) Social networks, attachments and support in minor affective disorders: a replication. *British Journal of Psychiatry,* **141,** 249–255.

Champion, L. (1990) The relationship between social vulnerability and the occurrence of severely threatening events. *Psychological Medicine,* **20,** 157–161.

Charles, G. A., Schittecatte, M., Rush, A. J., *et al* (1989) Persistent cortisol non-suppression after clinical recovery predicts symptomatic relapse in unipolar depression. *Journal of Affective Disorders,* **17,** 271–278.

Charlton, B. G. & Ferrier, I. N. (1989) Hypothalamo-pituitary-adrenal axis abnormalities in depression: a review and a model. *Psychological Medicine,* **19,** 331–336.

Charney, D. S., Menkes, D. B. & Heninger, G. R. (1981) Receptor sensitivity and the mechanism of action of antidepressant treatment: implications for the etiology and the therapy of depression. *Archives of General Psychiatry,* **38,** 1160–1180.

Cheetham, S. C., Crompton, M. R., Katona, C. L. E., *et al* (1990) Brain 5-HT, binding sites in depressed suicides. *Psychopharmacology,* **102,** 544–548.

———, Katona, C. L. E. & Horton, R. W. (1991) Postmortem studies of neurotransmitters biochemistry in depression and suicide. In *Biological Aspects of Affective Disorders* (eds R. Horton & C. Katona), pp. 191–221. London: Academic Press.

Clayton, P. J. & Darvish, H. S. (1979) Course of depressive symptoms following the stress of bereavement. In *Stress and Mental Disorder* (eds J. Barret, R. M. Rose & G. L. Klerman), pp. 121–136. New York: Raven Press.

Cobb, S. (1976) Social support as a moderator of life stress. *Psychosomatic Medicine*, **38,** 300–315.

Coccaro, E. F. (1989) Central serotonin and impulsive aggression. *British Journal of Psychiatry*, **155** (suppl. 8), 52–62.

Cooke, D. J. (1987) The significance of life events as a cause of psychological and physical disorder. In *Psychiatric Epidemiology: Progress and Prospects* (ed. B. Cooper), pp. 67–80. London & Sydney: Croom Helm.

Cooper, Z. (1990) Psychosocial factors in onset and course of depressive disorders. In *Prediction and Treatment of Recurrent Depression* (eds J. Cobb & N. Goeting), pp. 12–20. Southampton: Duphar Laboratories.

Coppen, A. (1967) The biochemistry of affective disorders. *British Journal of Psychiatry*, **113,** 1137–1164.

Cowen, P. J. (1991) 5HT receptor subtypes: implications for psychopharmacology. *British Journal of Psychiatry*, **159** (suppl.12), 7–14.

——, McCance, S. L., Ware, C. J., *et al* (1991) Lithium in tricyclic resistant depression: correlation of increased brain 5-HT function with clinical outcome. *British Journal of Psychiatry* **159**, 341–346.

——, Parry-Billings, M. & Newsholme, E. A. (1989) Decreased plasma tryptophan levels in major depression. *Journal of Affective Disorders*, **16**, 27–31.

Crook, T. & Eliot, J. (1980) Parental death during childhood and adult depression: A critical review of the literature. *Psychological Bulletin*, **87**, 252–259.

Deakin, J. F. W. (1990) 5HT receptor subtypes in depression. In *Behavioural Pharmacology of 5HT* (eds T. Archer, P. Bevan & A. Cools), pp. 179–204. New York: Lawrence Erlbaum.

Deicken, R. F., Reus, V. I., Manfredi, L., *et al* (1991) MRI deep white matter hyperintensity in a psychiatric population. *Biological Psychiatry*, **29**, 918–922.

Delgado, P. L., Charney, D. S., Price, L. H., *et al* (1990) Serotonin function and the mechanism of antidepressant action. *Archives of General Psychiatry*, **47**, 411–418.

—— & —— (1991) Neuroendocrine challenge tests in affective disorders: implications for future pathophysiological investigations. In *Biological Aspects of Affective Disorders* (eds R. Horton & C. Katona), pp.145–190. London: Academic Press.

De Parmentier, F., Cheetham, S. C., Crompton, M. R., *et al* (1990) Brain β adrenoceptor binding sites in antidepressant free suicides. *Brain Research*, **52**, 71–77.

Der, G. & Bebbington, P. E. (1987) Depression in inner London: a register study. *Social Psychiatry*, **22**, 73–84.

Dickinson, S. L., Kennett, G. A. & Curzon, G. (1985) Reduced 5-hydroxytryptamine-dependent behaviour in rats following chronic corticosterone treatment. *Brain Research*, **345**, 18–19.

Dohrenwend, B. I. & Dohrenwend, B. S. (1979) The conceptualisation and measurement of stressful life events: An overview of the issues. In *The Psychology of Depressive Disorders: Implications for the Effects of Stress* (ed. R.A. Depue), pp. 105–121. New York: Academic Press.

Dolan, R. J., Bench, C. J., Brown, R. G., *et al* (1992) Regional cerebral blood flow abnormalities in depressed patients with cognitive impairments. *Journal of Neurology, Neurosurgery and Psychiatry*, **55**, 768–773.

Duggan, C. F., Lee, A. S. & Murray, R. M. (1990) Does personality predict long-term outcome in depression? *British Journal of Psychiatry*, **157**, 19–24.

Eaton, W. W., Reiger, D. A., Locke, B. Z., *et al* (1981) The epidemiological catchment area programme of the National Institute of Mental Health. *Public Health Reports*, **96**, 319–325.

Eccleston, D. (1993) L-tryptophan and depressive illness – a valuable adjunct to therapy? *Psychiatric Bulletin*, **17**, 223–224.

Egeland, J., Gertard, D. S., Pauls, D. L., *et al* (1987) Bipolar affective disorder linked to DNA marker on chromosome II. *Nature*, **325**, 783–787.

Enna, S. J., Karbon, E. W. & Duman, R. S. (1986) GABA$_B$ agonists and imipramine-induced modifications in rat brain B adrenergic receptor binding and function. In *GABA and Mood Disorders* (eds G. Barthdini, G. Lloyd & P. L. Marselli), pp. 23–31. New York: Raven Press.

Evans, D. L. & Nemeroff, C. B. (1987) The clinical use of the dexamethasone suppression test in DSM–III affective disorders: correlation with the severe depressive subtypes of melancholia and psychosis. *Journal of Psychiatric Research*, **21**, 185–194.

Ferrier, I. N. (1991) Neuroendocrine changes in psychotic disorders (excluding ACTH). *Clinical Endocrinology and Metabolism*, **5**, 1–13.

Ferrier, I. N. & McKeith, I. G. (1991) Neuroanatomical and neurochemical changes in affective disorders in old age. *International Journal of Geriatric Psychiatry*, **6**, 445–451.

——, Eccleston, D., Moore, P. B., *et al* (1990) Relapse of chronic depressives on withdrawal of L-tryptophan. *Lancet*, **336**, 380–381.

——, McKeith, I. G., Cross, A. J., *et al* (1986) Postmortem neurochemical studies in depression. *Annals of New York Academy of Science*, **487**, 128–142.

Ferrier, I. N., Silverstone, T. & Eccleston, D. (1992) Selective serotonin re-uptake inhibitors: use in depression. *Psychiatric Bulletin*, **16**, 737–739.

Frank, E., Kupfer, D. J., Perel, J. M., *et al* (1990) Three-year outcomes for maintainance therapies in recurrent depression. *Archives of General Psychiatry*, **47**, 1093–1099.

Freeling, P., Rao, B., Paykel, E. S., *et al* (1985) Unrecognised depression in general practice. *British Medical Journal*, **290**, 1880–1883.

Freud, S. (1917) *Mourning and Melancholia. Standard Edition, Vol.14* (1957), pp. 243–258. London: Hogarth Press.

Garcia-Sevilla, J. A., Padro, D., Giratt, M., *et al* (1990) x2-adrenoceptor-mediated inhibition of platelet adenylate cyclase and induction of aggregation in major depression: effect of long term cyclic antidepressant drug treatment. *Archives of General Psychiatry*, **47**, 125–132.

Gater, R. A., Dean, C. & Morris, J. (1989) The contribution of childbearing to the sex difference in first admission rates for affective psychosis. *Psychological Medicine*, **19**, 719–724.

Gershon, E. S., Hamovit, J., Guroff, J. J., *et al* (1982) A family study of schizoaffective, bipolar I, bipolar II, unipolar and normal control probands. *Archives of General Psychiatry*, **39**, 1157–1167.

Ghaziuddin, M., Ghaziuddin, M. B. & Stein, G. S. (1990) Life events and the recurrence of depression. *Canadian Journal of Psychiatry*, **35**, 239.

Giral, P., Martin, P., Soubrit, P., *et al* (1988) Reversal of helpless behaviour in rats by putative 5HT$_A$ agonists. *Biological Psychiatry*, **23**, 237–242.

Goldberg, D. & Huxley, P. (1980) In *Mental Illness in the Community: The Pathway to Psychiatric Care*, pp. 57–107. London: Tavistock Publications.

Goodwin, F. K. & Jamison, K. R. (1990) *Manic-Depressive Illness*. Oxford: Oxford University Press.

Gove, W. R. (1972) The relationship between sex roles, marital status, and mental illness. *Social Forces*, **51**, 34–44.

Grad de Alarcon, J., Sainsbury, P. & Costain, W. R. (1975) Incidence of referred mental illness in Chichester and Salisbury. *Psychological Medicine*, **5**, 32–54.

Grove, W. M., Clayton, P., Endicott, J., *et al* (1986) Immigration and major affective disorder. *Acta Psychiatrica Scandinavica*, **74**, 548–552.

Haggerty, J. J., Simon, J. S., Evans, D. L., *et al* (1987) Relationship of serum TSH concentration and antithyroid antibiotics to diagnosis and DST response in psychiatric patients. *American Journal of Psychiatry*, **144**, 1491–1493.

Harris, B. (1994) Biological and hormonal aspects of postpartum depressed mood. *British Journal of Psychiatry*, **164**, 288–292.

Harris, T., Brown, G. W. & Bifulco, A. (1986) Loss of parent in childhood and adult psychiatric disorder: the role of lack of adequate parental care. *Psychological Medicine*, **16**, 641–659.

Henderson, S., Duncan-Jones, P., McAuley, H., *et al* (1978) The patient's primary group. *British Journal of Psychiatry*, **132**, 74–86.

Henn, F. A. & McKinney, W. T. (1987) Animal models in psychiatry. In *Psychopharmacology. The Third Generation of Progress* (ed. H.Y. Meltzer), pp. 687–695. New York: Raven Press.

Hickie, I., Parker, G., Wilhelm, K., *et al* (1991) Perceived interpersonal risk factors of non-endogenous depression. *Psychological Medicine*, **21**, 399–412.

——, Wilhelm, K. , Parker, G., *et al* (1990) Perceived dysfunctional intimate relationships: a specific association with the non-melancholic depressive subtype. *Journal of Affective Disorders*, **19**, 99–107.

Hirschfeld, R. M. A. (1990) Personality and dysthymia. In *Dysthymic Disorder* (eds S. W. Burton & H. S. Akiskal), pp. 69–77. London: Gaskell.

——, Klerman, G. L., Gough, H. G., *et al* (1977) A measure of interpersonal dependency. *Journal of Personality Assessment*, **41**, 610–618.

——, ——, Andreasen, N. C., *et al* (1986) Psychosocial predictors of chronicity in depressed patients. *British Journal of Psychiatry*, **148**, 648–654.

—— & Cross, C. K. (1987) The measurement of personality in depression. In *The Measurement of Depression* (eds A. J. Marsella, R. M. A. Hirschfeld & M. M. Katz), pp. 319–345. Chichester: John Wiley.

——, Klerman, G. L., Lavoria, P., *et al* (1989) Premorbid personality assessments of first onset of major depression. *Archives of General Psychiatry*, **46**, 345–350.

—— & Shea, M. T. (1992) Personality. *In Handbook of Affective Disorders* (ed. E. S. Paykel), pp. 185–194. Edinburgh: Churchill Livingstone.

HMSO (1986) *Morbidity Statistics from General Practice: Third National Study*. London: HMSO.

Holmes, T. H. & Rahe, R. H. (1967) The social readjustment rating scale. *Journal of Psychosomatic Research*, **11**, 213–218.

Hooley, J. M., Orley, J. & Teasdale, J. (1986) Levels of expressed emotion and relapse in depressed patients. *British Journal of Psychiatry*, **148**, 642–647.

Horgan, D. (1981) Change of diagnosis to manic-depressive illness. *Psychological Medicine*, **11**, 517–523.

Hopkinson, G. & Ley, P. (1969) A genetic study of a affective disorder. *British Journal of Psychiatry*, **115**, 917–922.

House, A., Dennis, M., Warlow, C., *et al* (1990) Mood disorders after stroke and their relation to lesion location. *Brain*, **13**, 1113–1129.

Hudgens, R. W. (1974) Personal catastrophe over depression. In *Stressful Life Events: Their Nature and Effects* (ed. R. A. Depue), pp. 119–134. New York: Academic Press.

——, Morrison, J. R. & Barchka, R. (1967) Life events and onset of primary affective disorders. A study of 40 hospitalised patients and 40 controls. *Archives of General Psychiatry*, **16**, 134–145.

Hwu, H.-G., Yeh, E.-K. & Chang, L.-Y. (1989) Prevalence of psychiatric disorders in Taiwan defined by the Chinese Diagnostic Interview Schedule. *Acta Psychiatrica Scandinavica*, **79**, 136–147.

Jacobson, E. (1953) Contribution to the metapsychology of cyclothymic depression. In *Affective Disorders* (ed. P. Greenacre), pp. 49–83. New York: International Universities Press.

Jacoby, R. J., Levy, R. & Bird, J. M. (1981) Computed tomography and the outcome of affective disorder. *British Journal of Psychiatry*, **138**, 288–292.

Jahoda, M. (1982) *Employment and Unemployment*. Cambridge: Cambridge University Press.

Janowsky, D., El-Yousef, M. & Davis, J. (1972) A cholinergic-adrenergic hypothesis of mania and depression. *Lancet*, **ii**, 632–635.

——, Golden, R. N. & Risch, S. C. (1988) Cholinergic mechanisms in mood: neuroendocrine aspects. In *Neuroendocrinology of Mood* (eds D. Ganeta & D. Pfaff), pp. 211–229. Berlin: Springer-Verlag.

Jeffcoate, W. J., Silverstone, J. T., Edwards, C. W. R., *et al* (1979) Psychiatric manifestations of Cushing's syndrome: response to lowering of plasma cortisol. *Quarterly Journal of Medicine*, **48**, 465–472.

Jenkins, R., MacDonald, A., Murray, J., *et al* (1982) Minor psychiatric morbidity and the threat of redundancy in a professional group. *Psychological Medicine*, **12**, 799–807.

Jeste, D. V., Lohr, J. B. & Goodwin, F. K. (1988) Neuroanatomical studies of major affective disorders. *British Journal of Psychiatry*, **153**, 444–459.

Joffe, R. T. & Singer, W. (1993) A placebo-controlled comparison of lithium and tri-iodothyronine augmentation of tricyclic antidepressants in unipolar refractory depression. *Archives of General Psychiatry*, **50**, 387–393.

Johnson, A. M. (1991) The comparative pharmacological properties of selective serotonin re-uptake inhibitors in animals. In *Selective Serotonin Re-uptake Inhibitors* (eds J. P. Feighner & W. F. Boyer), pp. 37–70. Chichester: John Wiley.

Jones, B. E., Gray, B. A. & Parson, E. B. (1988) Major affective disorders in blacks: a preliminary report. *Integrated Psychiatry*, **6**, 131–140.

Kapur, S. & Mann, J. J. (1992) Role of dopaminergic system in depression. *Biological Psychiatry*, **32**, 1–17.

Kay, D. W. K. (1962) Outcome and cause of mental disorders of old age. *Acta Psychiatric Scandinavica*, **38**, 249–276.

Kendler, K. S., Kessler, R. C., Neale, M. C., *et al* (1993) The prediction of major depression in women: toward an integrated etiologic model. *American Journal of Psychiatry*, **150**, 1139–1148.

Kitayami, I., Cintra, A. M., Fuxe, K., *et al* (1988) Effects of chronic imipramine treatment on glucocorticoid receptor immunoreactivity in various regions of the rat brain. *Journal of Neural Transmission*, **73**, 191–203.

Klein, D. N. & Depue, R.A. (1984) Continued impairment in persons at risk for bipolar affective disorder: results of a 19-month follow-up study. *Journal of Abnormal Psychology*, **93**, 345–347.

Klein, M. (1934) A contribution to the psychogenesis of manic-depressive states. In *Contributions to Psychoanalysis 1921*, pp. 282–310. London: Hogarth Press.

Klerman, G. & Weissman, M. (1989) Increasing rates of depression. *Journal of the American Medical Association*, **261**, 2229–2235.

Kraepelin, E. (1921) *Manic-Depressive Insanity and Paranoia* (ed. G. M. Robertson). Edinburgh: E. & S. Livingstone.

Kramlinger, K. G., Peterson, G. C. & Watson, P. K. (1985) Metyrapone for depression and delirium secondary to Cushing's syndrome. *Psychosomatics*, **26**, 67–71.

Kretschner, E. (1936) *Physique and Character, 2nd Edition* (translated by V. & W. Baskin). London: P. Owen.

Krishnan, K. R. R., Doraiswamy, P. M., Lurie, S. N., *et al* (1991) Pituitary size in depression. *Journal of Clinical Endocrinology and Metabolism*, **72**, 256–259.

Leake, A., Fairbairn, A. F., McKeith, I. G., *et al* (1991) Studies on the serotonin uptake binding site in major depressive disorder and control postmortem brain: neurochemical and clinical correlates. *Psychiatry Research*, **39**, 155–165.

Leff, J. & Vaughn, C. (1980) The interaction of life events and relatives' expressed emotion in schizophrenia and depressive neurosis. *British Journal of Psychiatry*, **136**, 246–253.

Leonhard, K. (1959) *Aufteilung der Endogenem Psychosen*. Berlin: Verlag.

Lesch, K. P. & Lerer, B. (1991) The 5-HT receptor-G-protein-effector system complex in depression. I. Effect of glucocorticoids. *Journal of Neural Transmission*, **84**, 3–18.

Levy, A. B., Drake, M. E., Shy, K. E., *et al* (1988) EEG evidence of epileptiform paroxysms in rapid cycling bipolar patient. *Journal of Clinical Psychiatry*, **49**, 232–234.

Martin, J. & Doran, A. (1966) Evidence concerning the relationship between health and retirement. *Sociological Review*, **14**, 329.

Martin, M. (1985) Neuroticism as a predisposition towards depression: a cognitive mechanism. *Personality and Individual Differences*, **6**, 353–365.

Mayeux, R., Stern, Y., Sano, M., *et al* (1988) The relationship of serotonin to depression in Parkinson's disease. *Movement Disorders*, **3**, 237–244.

McCreadie, R. G., Wilson, A. O. & Burton, L. (1983) The Scottish survey of 'new chronic' in-patients. *British Journal of Psychiatry*, **143**, 564–571.

McEwan, B. S., Gould, E. A. & Sakai, R. R. (1992) The vulnerability of the hippocampus to protective and destructive effects of glucocorticoids in relation to stress. *British Journal of Psychiatry*, **16**, 85–103.

McGuffin, P. & Katz, R. (1989) The genetics of depression and manic-depressive disorder. *British Journal of Psychiatry*, **155**, 294–304.

——, —— & Bebbington, P. (1988) The Camberwell Collaborative Depression Study. III. Depression and adversity in the relatives of depressed probands. *British Journal of Psychiatry*, **152**, 775–782.

Meana, J. J., Barturen, F. & Garcia-Sevilla, J. A. (1992) a$_2$ adrenoceptors in the brain of suicide victims: increased receptor density associated with major depression. *Biological Psychiatry*, **31**, 471–490.

Meaney, M. J., Mitchell, J. B., Aitken, D. H., *et al* (1991) The effects of neonatal handling on the development of the adrenocortical response to stress.

Implications for neuropathology and cognitive deficits in later life. *Psychoneuroendocrinology*, **16**, 85–103.

Meltzer, H. Y. (1987) *Psychopharmacology: The Third Generation of Progress.* New York: Raven Press.

—— (1989) Serotonergic dysfunction in depression. *British Journal of Psychiatry*, **155** (suppl. 8), 25–31.

Melville, D. I., Hope, D., Bennison, D., *et al* (1985) Depression among men made involuntarily redundant. *Psychological Medicine*, **15**, 789–793.

Mendelson, M. (1990) Psychoanalytic views on depression. In *Depressive Disorders* (eds B. B. Wolman & G. Strickler), pp. 22–37. New York: John Wiley.

—— (1992) Psychodynamics. In *Handbook of Affective Disorders* (ed. E. S. Paykel), pp. 295–308. Edinburgh: Churchill Livingstone.

Mendlewicz, J., Simon, P., Sevy, S., *et al* (1987) Polymorphic DNA marker on X chromosome and manic depression. *Lancet*, **i**, 1230–1231.

Montgomery, S. A. & Fineberg, N. (1989) Is there a relationship between serotonin receptor subtypes and selectivity of response in specific psychiatric illnesses? *British Journal of Psychiatry*, **155** (suppl. 8), 63–70.

Nausieda, P. A., Carvey, P. M. & Weiner, W. J. (1982) Modification of central serotonergic and dopaminergic behaviours in the course of chronic corticosteroid administration. *European Journal of Pharmacology*, **78**, 335–343.

Nelson, C. J. (1991) Current status of tricyclic antidepressants in psychiatry: their pharmacology and clinical applications. *Journal of Clinical Psychiatry*, **52**, 193–200.

Nemeroff, C. B. (1988) The role of corticotrophin-releasing factor in the pathogenesis of major depression. *Pharmacopsychiatry*, **21**, 76–82.

Newton, J. (1988) *Preventing Mental Illness.* London: Routledge & Kegan Paul.

Nurnberger, J. J., Berrettini, W., Mendelson, W., *et al* (1989) Measuring cholinergic sensitivity. 1. Arecoline effects in bipolar patients. *Biological Psychiatry*, **25**, 610–617.

Orr, T. E., Meyerhoff, J. L., Mougery, E. H., *et al* (1990) Hyper-responsiveness of the rat neuroendocrine system due to repeated exposure to stress. *Psychoneuroendocrinology*, **15**, 317–328.

Parker, G. (1992) Early environment. In *Handbook of Affective Disorders* (ed. E. S. Paykel), pp. 171–184. Edinburgh: Churchill Livingstone.

——, Kiloh, L. & Hayward, L. (1987) Parental representations of neurotic and endogenous depressives. *Journal of Affective Disorders*, **13**, 75–82.

——, Tupling, H. & Brown, L. B. (1979) Parental bonding instrument. *British Journal of Medical Psychology*, **52**, 1–10.

Parkes, C. M. (1981) Evaluation of a bereavement service. *Journal of Preventative Psychiatry*, **1**, 179–188.

Patrick, V., Dunner, D. L. & Fieve, R. R. (1978) Life events and primary affective illness. *Acta Psychiatrica Scandinavica*, **58**, 48–55.

Paykel, E. S. (1974) Life stress and psychiatric disorder: application of the clinical approach. In *Stressful Life Events: their Nature and Effects* (eds B. S. Dohrenwend & B. P. Dohrenwend), pp. 135–149. New York: John Wiley.

—— (1978) Contribution of life events to causation of psychiatric illness. *Psychological Medicine*, **8**, 245–253.

—— (1982) Life events and early environment. In *Handbook of Affective Disorders* (ed. E. S. Paykel), pp. 146–161. Edinburgh: Churchill Livingstone.

—— (1989*a*) The background: extent and nature of the disorder. In *Depression, An Integrative Approach* (eds K. R. Herbst & E. S. Paykel), pp. 3–20. Oxford: Heinemann Medical Books.

—— (1989*b*) Treatment of depression: The relevance of research for clinical practice. *British Journal of Psychiatry*, **155**, 754–763.

——, Myers, J. & Dienelt, M. (1969) Life events and depression: a controlled study. *Archives of General Psychiatry*, **21**, 753–760.

——, Prusoff, B. A. & Myers, J. K. (1975) Suicide attempts and recent life events: a controlled comparison. *Archives of General Psychiatry*, **32**, 327–333.

—— & Tanner, J. (1976) Life events, depressive relapse and maintenance treatment. *Psychological Medicine*, **6**, 481–485.

——, Rao, B. M. & Taylor, C. N. (1984) Life stress and symptom pattern in outpatient depression. *Psychological Medicine*, **14**, 559–568.

—— & Cooper, Z. (1992) Life events and social stress. In *Handbook of Affective Disorders* (ed. E. S. Paykel), pp. 149–170. Edinburgh: Churchill Livingstone.

Pedder, J. R. (1982) Failure to mourn and melancholia. *British Journal of Psychiatry*, **141**, 329–337.

Pfeiffer, A., Veilleux, S. & Barden, N. (1991) Antidepressant and other centrally acting drugs regulate glucocorticoid receptor messenger RNA levels in rat brain. *Psychneuroendocrinology*, **16**, 505–515.

Post, F. (1968) The factor of ageing in affective disorders. In *Recent Developments in Affective Disorders* (eds A. Coppen & A. Walk), pp. 105–116. Kent: Headley Bros.

Post, R. M. (1992) Transduction of psychosocial stress into the neurobiology of recurrent affective disorder. *American Journal of Psychiatry*, **149**, 999–1010.

Potter, W. Z., Manji, K., Dawkins, K., *et al* (1992) Combined measures of noradrenergic output and receptor responsivity in depression. *Clinical Neuropharmacology*, **15** (Suppl. 1A), 319.

Pryor, J. C. & Sulser, F. (1991) Evolution of the monoamine hypotheses of depression. In *Biological Aspects of Affective Disorders* (eds. R. Horton & C. Katona), pp. 77–94. London: Academic Press.

Randrup, A. & Braestrup, C. (1977) Uptake inhibition of biogenic amines by newer antidepressant drugs: relevance to the dopamine hypothesis of depression. *Psychopharmacology*, **53**, 309–314.

Regier, D. A., Myers, J. K., Kramer, M., *et al* (1984) Epidemiologic catchment area program: historical context, major objectives, and study population characteristics. *Archives of General Psychiatry*, **41**, 934–941.

Restrepo, C. & Armario, A. (1987) Chronic stress alters pituitary-adrenal function in prepubertal rats. *Psychoneuroendocrinology*, **12**, 393–398.

Rifkin, L. & Gurling, H. (1991) Genetic aspects of affective disorders. In *Biological Aspects of Affective Disorders* (eds R. W. Horton & C. L. K. Katona), pp. 305–334. London: Academic Press.

Robins, I. N., Helzer, J. E., Croughan, J., *et al* (1981) National Institute of Mental Health Diagnostic Interview Schedule. *Archives of General Psychiatry*, **38**, 381–389.

Robinson, R. G., Bolduc, P. L. & Price, T. R. (1987) Two-year longitudinal study of post stroke mood disorders: diagnosis and outcome at one and two years. *Stroke*, **18**, 837–843.

Rorsman, B., Grasbeck, A., Hagnell, O., *et al* (1990) A prospective study of first-incidence depression. The Lundby Study, 1957–72. *British Journal of Psychiatry*, **156**, 336–342.

Rosenthal, S. H. (1966) Changes in a population of hospitalised patients with affective disorders. *American Journal of Psychiatry*, **6**, 671–681.

Rubinow, H. R., Post, R. M., Savard, R., *et al* (1984) Cortisol hypersection and cognitive impairment in depression. *Archives of General Psychiatry*, **41**, 279–283.

Rutter, M. (1972) *Maternal Deprivation Reassessed*. London: Penguin.

—— (1985) Psychopathology and development: links between childhood and adult life. In *Child and Adolescent Psychiatry* (eds M. Rutter & L. Hersov). London: Blackwell Scientific Publications.

Ryle, A. (1991) Depression. In *Textbook of Psychotherapy in Psychiatric Practice* (ed J. Holmes), pp. 265–286. Edinburgh: Churchill Livingstone.

Schildkraut, J. J. (1965) The catecholamine hypothesis of affective disorders: a review of the supporting evidence. *American Journal of Psychiatry*, **122**, 509–522.

Schlesselman, J. (1982) *Case Control Studies*. Oxford: Oxford University Press.

Scott, J. (1988) Chronic depression. *British Journal of Psychiatry*, **153**, 287–297.

—— (1992) Social and community approaches. In *Handbook of Affective Disorders* (ed E. S. Paykel) , pp. 525–538. Edinburgh: Churchill Livingstone.

——, Barker, W. A. & Eccleston, D. (1988) The Newcastle chronic depression study: patient characteristics and factors associated with chronicity. *British Journal of Psychiatry*, **152**, 28–33.

——, Eccleston, D. & Boys, R. (1992) Can we predict the persistence of depression? *British Journal of Psychiatry*, **161**, 633–637.

Seligman, M. E. P. (1975) *Helplessness: On Depression, Development and Death*. San Francisco: W.H. Freeman.

——, Abramson, L. Y., Semmel, A., *et al* (1978) Depressive attributional style. *Journal of Abnormal Psychology*, **88**, 242–247.

Shopsin, B., Friedman, E. & Gershon, S. (1976) Parachlorphenylalanine reversal of tranylcypromine effects in depressed patients. *Archives of General Psychiatry*, **33**, 811–819.

Siegel, B., Gurevich, D. & Oxenbrug, G. F. (1989) Cognitive impairment and cortisol resistance to dexamethasone suppression in elderly depression. *Biological Psychiatry*, **25**, 229–234.

Siever, L. J. & Davis, K. L. (1985) Overview: toward a dysregulation hypothesis of depression. *American Journal of Psychiatry*, **142**, 1017–1031.

Smith, A. L. & Weissman, M. M. (1992) Epidemiology. In *Handbook of Affective Disorders* (ed. E. S. Paykel), pp. 111–130. Edinburgh: Churchill Livingstone.

Somerville, P. D., Leaf, P. J., Weissman, M. M., *et al* (1989) The prevalence of major depression in black and white adults in five United States communities. *American Journal of Epidemiology*, **130**, 725–735.

Starkstein, S. E., Fedoroff, P., Berthier, M. L., *et al* (1991) Manic depressive and pure manic states after brain lesions. *Biological Psychiatry*, **29**, 149–158.

Strober, M., Morrell, W., Burroughs, J., *et al* (1988) A family study of bipolar 1 disorder in adolesence: early onset of symptoms linked to increased familial loading and lithium resistance. *Journal of Affective Disorders*, **15**, 255–268.

Sulser, F. (1986) Update of neuroreceptor mechanisms and their implications for the pharmacotherapy of affective disorders. *Journal of Clinical Psychiatry*, **10** (Suppl.), 13–18.

Surtees, P. G., Dean, C., Ingham, J. G., *et al* (1983) Psychiatric disorder in women in an Edinburgh community: associations with demographic factors. *British Journal of Psychiatry*, **142**, 238–246.

—— & Sashidharan, S.P. (1986) Psychiatric morbidity in two matched community samples: a comparison of rates and risks in Edinburgh and St. Louis. *Journal of Affective Disorder*, **10**, 101–113.

Swayze, V. W., Andreason, N. C., Alliger, R. J., *et al* (1992) Subcortical and temporal structures in affective disorder and schizophrenia: a magnetic resonance imaging study. *Biological Psychiatry*, **31**, 221–240.

Teasdale, J. D. (1988) Cognitive vulnerability to persistent depression. *Cognition and Emotion*, **2**, 247–274.

Tellenbach, R. (1975) Typologische untersuchunger zur pramorbiden Personlichkeit. *Confinia Psychiatrica*, **18**, 1–15.

Tennant, C. (1991) Parental loss in childhood: Its effect in adult life. In *Social Psychiatry: Theory, Methodology and Practice* (ed. P. E. Bebbington), pp. 305–324. New Brunswick & London: Transaction Publishers.

—— & Bebbington, P. (1978) The social causation of depression: a critique of the work of Brown and his colleagues. *Psychological Medicine*, **8**, 565–575.

——, —— & Hurry, J. (1980) Parental death in childhood and risk of adult depressive disorders: a review. *Psychological Medicine*, **10**, 289–299.

——, —— & —— (1981) The short-term outcome of neurotic disorders in the community: the relation of remission to clinical factors and to 'neutralising' life events. *British Journal of Psychiatry*, **139**, 213–220.

Thoits, P. A. (1985) Dimensions of life events that influence psychological distress: An evaluation and synthesis of the literature. In *Psychosocial Stress: Trends in Theory and Research* (ed. H. B. Kaplan), pp. 33–103. New York: Academic Press.

Thoman, E. B., Levine, S. & Arnold, W. J. (1968) Effects of maternal deprivation and incubator rearing on adrenocortical activity in the adult rat. *Developmental Psychobiology*, **1**, 21–23.

Twaddle, V. & Scott, J. (1991) Depression. In *Adult Clinical Problems: a Cognitive-Behavioural Approach* (eds W. Dryden & R. Rentoul), pp. 56–85. London & New York: Routledge.

Uppadhyaya, A. K., Pennell, I., Cowen, P. J., *et al* (1990) Blunted growth hormone and prolactin responses to L-tryptophan in depression: a state dependent abnormality. *Journal of Affective Disorders*, **21**, 213–218.

Vaughn, C. E. & Leff, J. P. (1976) The influence of family and social factors on the course of psychiatric illness. *British Journal of Psychiatry*, **129**, 125–137.

Veldhuis, H. D., De Korte, C. C. M. M. & De Kloet, E. R. (1985) Glucocorticoids facilitate the retention of acquired immobility during forced swimming. *European Journal of Pharmacology*, **115**, 211–217.

Von Zerssen, D. (1976) Physique and personality. In *Human Behaviour Genetics* (ed. A. R. Kaplan), pp. 230–278. Springfield: Thomas.

Weissman, M. M. & Klerman, G. L. (1977) The chronic depressive in the community: unrecognised and poorly treated. *Comprehensive Psychiatry*, **18**, 523–532.

——, Merikangas, K. R., Wickramaratne, P., *et al* (1986) Understanding the clinical heterogeneity of major depression using family data. *Archives of General Psychiatry*, **43**, 430–434.

—, Leaf, P. J. , Bruce, M. L., *et al* (1988*a*) The epidemiology of dysthymia in five communities: rates, risks, comorbidity, and treatment. *American Journal of Psychiatry*, **145**, 815–819.

—, —, Tischler, G. L., *et al* (1988*b*) Affective disorders in five United States communities. *Psychological Medicine*, **18**, 141–153.

—, Warner, V., Wickramaratne, P., *et al* (1988*c*) Early onset major depression in parents and their children. *Journal of Affective Disorders*, **15**, 269–277.

Wiek, A., Kumar, R. & Hirst, A. D., *et al* (1991) Increased sensitivity of dopamine receptors and recurrence of affective psychosis after childbirth. *British Medical Journal*, **363**, 613–616.

Williams, J. M. G. (1992) *The Psychological Treatment of Depression: a Guide to the Theory and Practice of Cognitive–Behaviour Therapy.* London & New York: Routledge.

Wilner, P. (1983) Dopamine and depression: a review of recent evidence. *Brain Research Review*, **6**, 237–246.

Winokur, G. (1974) The division of depressive disease into depressive spectrum disease and pure depressive disease. *International Pharmacopsychiatry*, **9**, 5–13.

Wing, J. K., Cooper, J. E. & Sartorius, N. (1974) *Measurement and Classification of Psychiatric Symptoms: an Instruction Manual for the PSE and CATEGO Program.* New York: Cambridge University Press.

Yates, M., Leake, A., Candy, J. M., *et al* (1990) 5HT$_2$ receptor changes in major depression. *Biological Psychiatry*, **27**, 489–496.

Zubenko, G. S., Moossy, J. & Koop, U. (1990) Neurochemical correlates of major depression in primary dementia. *Archives of Neurology*, **47**, 209–214.

4 Drug treatment of depression

Morris Bernadt

---

*Tricyclic antidepressants • Selective serotonin reuptake inhibitors •
Monoamine oxidase inhibitors • Other drugs • Treating a depressive
episode • Long-term treatment of depression • Treatment-resistant
depression*

Canst thou not minister to a mind diseas'd,
Pluck from the memory a rooted sorrow,
Raze out the written troubles of the brain,
And with some sweet oblivious antidote
Cleanse the stuff'd bosom of that perilous stuff
Which weighs upon the heart?
Macbeth, Act V, Scene 1.

Four fundamental advances in psychopharmacology occurred in the nine-
year period between 1948 and 1957. These concerned imipramine, iproniazid,
chlorpromazine and lithium. Imipramine was introduced by the Swiss drug
company, Geigy, which had been investigating anti-histamine substances
similar to chlorpromazine as potential antipsychotic drugs. Geigy arranged
for the Zurich professor of psychiatry Roland Kuhn to test imipramine on
patients with schizophrenia. Kuhn treated more than 300 patients with various
mental illnesses and he noticed that a few patients suffering from endogenous
depression made a pronounced improvement. He wrote:

> "G22355 (imipramine) is a substance with markedly antidepressive
> properties. Its mode of action remains completely unknown. The
> effect is striking in patients with depression. The patients get up in
> the morning of their own accord, speak louder and more rapidly,
> their facial expression becomes more vivacious, they begin to
> entertain themselves and take part in games, become more cheerful
> and are once more able to laugh" (Kuhn, 1958).

Using a drug as an antidepressant was a momentous development
because as Kuhn pointed out in his classic paper the only other treatments
for depression available at the time were ECT and psychoanalysis.

Serendipity also led to the discovery of the therapeutic effects of
iproniazid, chlorpromazine and lithium. The two hydrazine derivatives of
isonicotinic acid, isoniazid and iproniazid, had been developed by another
Swiss drug company Hoffman-La-Roche for the treatment of tuberculosis.
During clinical trials of these drugs in 1951 and 1952 physicians noted that
patients on iproniazid but not isoniazid became cheerful, exuberant and
even manic (Bloch *et al*, 1954). The psychiatrists who examined these
patients diagnosed the mania, attributed it to the drug and yet failed to

follow up on the antidepressant potential of iproniazid. Only later did laboratory studies show that iproniazid was a much more potent inhibitor of monoamine oxidase (MAO) than isoniazid. The initial clinical trials in psychiatry were with chronically apathetic patients with schizophrenia but in 1957 Nathan Kline in New York arranged a small trial in depressed patients and reported that iproniazid had a stimulating and mood-elevating effect on them.

Lithium salts had been widely used during the 19th century and the early part of the 20th century for the treatment of gout, epilepsy, arthritis and a variety of other disorders (Merck's Index, 1930), but their use fell into disrepute because of severe toxic reactions (blood lithium estimations were unavailable). In 1949, the US Food and Drugs Administration issued a stern warning on the risks of lithium salts. It was in the same year that the Australian psychiatrist John Cade published his remarkable findings in the *Medical Journal of Australia* (Cade, 1949). His theory was that mania was due to poisoning with some endogenous substance, while depression was associated with a deficiency of the same substance. He made an analogy with thyrotoxicosis and myxoedema. Cade injected the urine of patients with mania into guinea pigs and found this was more toxic than the urine of healthy subjects and those with schizophrenia. He next examined the separate effects of urea, uric acid and creatinine. Because of the comparative insolubility of uric acid in water he chose the most soluble urate: lithium urate. He noticed that the animals became lethargic and unresponsive. He then tried lithium carbonate. When the guinea pigs were laid on their backs, instead of displaying a frantic righting response they calmly gazed back at him (Cade,1970). In 1948 he gave it to 10 manic patients and reported a good result. Cade's publications were later overshadowed by the development of chlorpromazine and lithium was almost forgotten, but in the late 1950s it again attracted interest, in particular from the Danish psychiatrist Mogens Schou of the University of Aarhus.

This chapter considers the different classes of antidepressant drugs followed by a description of the management of depressive episodes.

Tricyclic antidepressants

The number of drugs available for treating depression is rapidly increasing. The first-generation antidepressants include many of the tricyclic antidepressants (TCAs) and MAO inhibitors (MAOIs). In the latter half of the 1970s newly introduced TCAs and antidepressants with novel chemical structures were termed second-generation antidepressants.

The chemical structures of some tricyclics are shown in Fig. 4.1. Slight modifications in the ring structure and side chain identify the different TCAs. These chemical alterations result in pharmacological differences. In the first row of the figure, the nitrogen atoms in the side chains have three carbon atoms attached. Such tricyclics are called tertiary amine TCAs and include imipramine, amitriptyline, dothiepin, doxepin, clomipramine and trimipramine (the latter three are shown lower down in the figure). In the second row of the figure are side chains where the nitrogen atom is linked to two carbon atoms – this is characteristic of the secondary amine TCAs. The columns of Fig. 1 show a TCA grouping according to the middle ring structure.

Pharmacokinetics

A working knowledge of pharmacokinetics is essential for safe and effective practice. TCAs are relatively homogeneous with regard to their pharmacokinetics, unlike the selective serotonin reuptake inhibitors (SSRIs). Antidepressant pharmacokinetics have been reviewed by Preskorn (1993).

Absorption and first-pass metabolism

TCAs are lipid-soluble and therefore well absorbed from the gastro-intestinal tract. Because of first-pass metabolism only 50–60% of an orally

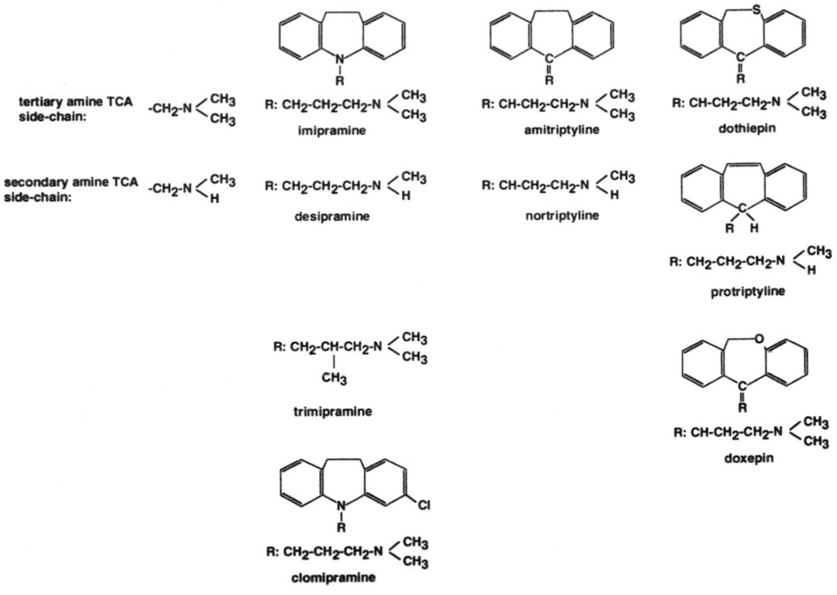

Fig. 4.1 Chemical structure of some TCAs.

administered dose reaches the systemic circulation. The rest is metabolised by the liver and excreted in the bile, from which metabolites pass back into the gut. A substantial proportion of these metabolites are re-absorbed. Thus both active and inactive metabolites are involved in an enterohepatic circulation.

The extent of first-past metabolism is affected by genetic factors as well as being decreased by liver disease and by right heart failure, due to resultant hepatic congestion. Alcohol has a triphasic effect on the first-pass metabolism of TCAs. The acute ingestion of sufficient alcohol can substantially impair first-pass metabolism resulting in a doubling or tripling of the amount of the drug that reaches the systemic circulation (Weller & Preskorn, 1984); thus overdoses of TCAs in conjunction with alcohol are more likely to be lethal. With more long-term alcohol administration hepatic isoenzymes are induced, which increases first-pass metabolism. However, if cirrhosis and portacaval shunting occur, the TCA may pass directly into the systemic circulation having a more rapid and greater effect.

Time to reach maximum plasma concentration

The tertiary amine TCAs have a maximum plasma concentration 1–3 hours after ingestion. By contrast, the secondary amine TCAs are more slowly absorbed reaching their peak concentration 4–8 hours after ingestion. This difference may contribute to better tolerability and safety of secondary amine TCAs in comparison with tertiary amine TCAs. Tricyclics may delay their own absorption (and that of other drugs) because their anticholinergic effect decreases the rate of gastric emptying and intestinal peristalsis.

Peak plasma levels of TCAs are associated with a number of effects which can be discomforting, and occasionally serious, such as sedation, postural hypotension and a quinidine-like effect on the heart. The peak effect can be used to advantage, for example obtaining a maximum sedative effect at night by prescribing the total daily dose of a tertiary amine TCA two hours before going to sleep. Plasma drug levels will have fallen substantially by the next morning so daytime sedation is reduced. During the night the patient lies flat which means that the risk of postural hypotension is reduced. However, for the elderly who visit the toilet more frequently at night, postural hypotension may lead to falls. A divided administration would lower peak levels, lessening the risk of a fall, as would a reduction in the total daily dose. It is the peak plasma concentration that varies with the number of daily doses, not the average steady-state plasma drug level. The latter is what is measured by a plasma drug sample which should be taken approximately 12 hours after the last dose. The steady-state plasma drug concentration is itself an important determinant of adverse drug reactions. The effect of the maximum plasma concentration is superimposed on that of the steady-state concentration and is more pronounced in the early phase of drug treatment.

Metabolism and excretion

TCAs are extensively metabolised before their eventual elimination from the body. The initial liver biotransformations are either hydroxylation of the ring structure or demethylation of the side chain terminal nitrogen. Demethylation involves converting a tertiary amine TCA to a secondary amine TCA and then to a primary amine TCA. Thus imipramine becomes desipramine, and amitriptyline is demethylated to nortriptyline (see Fig. 4.1). The secondary amine but not the primary amine metabolites are antidepressant in their own right. Hydroxylated metabolites also inhibit amine re-uptake but their potency as antidepressants in relation to tertiary and secondary amine TCAs is unknown. Genetic factors determine the extent of hydroxylation and demethylation.

TCA metabolites are generally more polar and therefore more water-soluble; they are eliminated directly by filtration through the kidney, or conjugated with glucuronic acid, which makes them even more polar, before being cleared by the kidney. Diseases which decrease glomerular filtration can result in an accumulation of polar metabolites causing toxicity in some patients. The same applies to the age-related decrease in renal function. For example, plasma levels of 10-hydroxynortriptyline in the elderly may be three times higher than plasma levels of nortriptyline itself (Young *et al*, 1987). Laboratories measure the main demethylated metabolite, but not the plasma level of these polar metabolites.

Individual variability in metabolism

Among physically healthy individuals there can be as much as a 30-fold variation in plasma TCA levels after administration of the same dose of a TCA. The main rate-limiting step in the elimination of TCAs is the biotransformation mediated by one of the hepatic cytochrome P450 isoenzymes, usually 2D6 (Preskorn, 1993). Five to ten per cent of Caucasian populations have an inherited deficiency in the functional integrity of this isoenzyme. Other populations carry this deficiency to varying extents. TCA clearance rates in individuals with this deficiency are substantially prolonged; four-fold higher plasma TCA levels compared with those in non-affected individuals may occur. Thus conventional doses in these individuals may result in toxic concentrations with the possibility of confusion, seizures and cardiac arrythmias. The P450 isoenzymes are discussed in more detail on page 178. Left heart failure will impair clearance rates of TCAs by decreasing hepatic arterial blood flow.

Half-lives

For the tertiary amine TCAs, the following half-lives are given: doxepin 6–8 hours, amitriptyline 9–25 hours and clomipramine 19–37 hours. The demethylated secondary amine TCAs have half-lives of about 24 hours. Protriptyline, a secondary amine, has the longest half-life of all the TCAs, of approximately 80 hours. Considering the parent drug and its active metabolites, the half-lives of the TCAs are long enough for once-daily administration to result in the same average steady state plasma drug concentration throughout the day as a twice daily or three times daily schedule. Assuming a half-life of approximately 24 hours, TCAs reach a steady state in about five days (i.e. five times the half-life). When the dose is changed a new steady state is reached in another five days. If a drug is discontinued, near complete washout to about 3% of the original level will take approximately five days. Slow metabolisers whose TCA half-life is increased will take longer to reach a steady state and to achieve a washout.

Plasma drug levels

Asberg *et al* (1971) reported on a curvilinear relationship between nortriptyline plasma levels and therapeutic efficacy. Nortriptyline showed best effects at concentrations from 50 to 150 ng/ml and its therapeutic action was less above and below this range. This study gave rise to the hope that a 'therapeutic window' could be defined for other antidepressants. Many studies were carried out with amitriptyline, imipramine, desipramine, maprotiline, doxepin and others but the results were conflicting. A critical review (APA Task Force, 1985) concluded that adequate data were available for only four products: for nortriptyline the curvilinear relationship with an optimal concentration range was confirmed; for imipramine and desipramine the relationship was linear with minimum effective plasma levels of 200 and 125 ng/ml, respectively; for amitriptyline there was no clear correlation between plasma levels and clinical efficacy, possibly because amitriptyline is degraded into numerous other active metabolites.

Because of wide individual differences in the metabolism of TCAs a fixed dose schedule (for example, amitriptyline 150 mg daily) may not constitute a therapeutic trial. For some patients the dose may be too large and for others too small and in these circumstances monitoring plasma antidepressant concentrations may be helpful. Plasma levels can also be used as a check on compliance; an unexpectedly low plasma level has obvious implications. Non-response to treatment may simply be a consequence of low plasma levels due to rapid metabolism. Similarly for those who are genetically deficient in the hepatic cytochrome isoenzyme P450 2D6, high plasma levels on an average starting dose of a tricyclic may explain severe side-effects. Most laboratories report the levels of the teritary and secondary TCA as well as the sum of the two. Therapeutic total plasma levels for a tertiary TCA range from 100 to 300 ng/ml.

Drug interactions

A variety of drugs interact with TCAs, for example by interfering with TCA metabolism or interfering at the site of action (reviewed by Bernstein, 1995*a*).

Smoking, and most anticonvulsants, may increase TCA metabolism by enzyme induction, and this results in a lowering of TCA plasma levels and hence decreased antidepressant effects. Drugs which inhibit TCA metabolism may lead to raised levels in the plasma and brain, a greater antidepressant effect and increased toxicity. These include stimulants (such as dexamphetamine, methylphenidate and cocaine), disulfiram, isoniazid, cimitidene, beta blockers, calcium channel blockers, some antipsychotic drugs such as chlorpromazine and the SSRIs, particularly fluoxetine and paroxetine which inhibit the breakdown of TCAs by inhibiting the cytochrome P450 isoenzymes. In addition TCAs lower seizure threshold and the likelihood of fits is increased. Antipsychotic drugs also have anticholinergic effects (and these are often used in conjunction with other anticholinergic drugs such as benztropine or procyclidine) so that their use with TCAs may lead to an anticholinergic toxicity resulting in agitation, confusion or delirium. The risk is greater in the elderly (see page 1125).

TCAs may be inadvertently combined with catecholamines such as adrenaline and noradrenaline in dentistry, and when local anaesthesia at other sites is used. The TCA inhibition of neuronal uptake of adrenaline and noradrenaline may result in these catecholamines having an enhanced effect, causing hypertension. TCAs also inhibit the neuronal uptake of anti-hypertensive drugs such as guanethidine, bethanidine, clonidine and debrisoquine and through this mechanism decrease the antihypertensive effect of these drugs. TCAs have dopaminergic effects and so their use in Parkinsonian patients can be beneficial, but when combined with L-dopa they may cause agitation, tremor and rigidity. Additive sedative interactions may occur with alcohol, barbiturates, benzodiazepines and neuroleptics, causing excessive drowsiness.

At the cell membrane level quinidine-like effects occur and so the co-administration of anti-arrythmic drugs such as quinidine, procainamide, lidocaine and propranolol may result in ECG changes, arrhythmias and myocardial depression. Occasionally in patients with diminished cardiac reserve, this may trigger cardiac failure. Anaesthetics may also interact leading to an increased risk of arrhythmias and hypotension.

Efficacy of TCAs

To combat various forms of bias and error that arise in the assessment of drug efficacy a comprehensive technology of drug evaluation has developed. This is based on the need for randomised controlled double-blind trials. Their methodology is discussed in detail in *College Seminars in Clinical Psychopharmacology* (Harrison *et al*, 1995).

An early meta-analysis of placebo-controlled studies of TCAs found that 61 (65%) of 93 studies favoured the TCA (Morris & Beck, 1974). A more recent summary is provided by Davis & Glassman (1989). Imipramine has been the most frequently studied TCA and 30 (68%) of 44 studies have shown it to be better than placebo. In these studies there were 1334 patients of whom 65% improved substantially on imipramine compared with 30% who improved substantially on a placebo, giving a drug–placebo difference of 35% (Davis & Glassman, 1989). There are no studies reporting a placebo producing more improvement than imipramine.

The alternative to a placebo comparison is a comparison with a reference drug. With imipramine as the reference drug, Davis & Glassman (1989) found that in 26 (84%) of 31 studies another tricyclic was equal to imipramine in efficacy. Because imipramine is the best studied of the TCAs it is often used for comparison with newer antidepressants.

Tertiary amine TCAs

Amitriptyline

This used to be advocated as the first-line antidepressant to be used in nearly all depressed patients; some authorities still state this and it may be the preferred drug in psychotic depression. Figure 4.2 shows the selectivity of antidepressants in respect of serotonin and noradrenaline. The parent compound amitriptyline lies about midway. Once metabolites are taken into account the picture becomes more complicated. For example, amitriptyline's metabolite nortriptyline is more noradrenergic, so precisely where on the noradrenaline–serotonin scale the combined effect of amitriptyline and its metabolites lie will depend on the proportions of the different compounds which vary from individual to individual. Amitriptyline is one of the most sedative and anticholinergic of the tricyclics. Doses are in the range 25–300 mg per day.

Clomipramine

Clomipramine has a chemical structure similar to imipramine with a chlorine atom attached to one of the benzene rings (see Fig. 4.1). The parent compound is the most serotonergic of the TCAs (Fig. 4.2). However its demethylated metabolite chlordesipramine, which has antidepressant activity, is more active at noradrenergic reuptake sites. During its early development clomipramine was approved for intravenous administration, but this had no advantage over oral administration. Very occasionally it is used intramuscularly, for example, in severely depressed patients refusing to take fluids, food or medication by mouth and for whom ECT may be inadvisable. Clomipramine has been found to reduce morbidity in obsessive–compulsive neurosis and this effect appears to be independent of whether there is comorbid depression. Its effect in obsessive–compulsive disorder may be related to its serotonin reuptake activity as other serotonin-specific antidepressants such as fluvoxamine have similar effects. The manufacturers advise starting at a low dose such as 10 mg daily, and the maximum recommended dose is 250 mg daily.

Dothiepin and doxepin

These two antidepressants are identical in chemical structure to amitriptyline except that dothiepin has a sulphur substitution and doxepin an oxygen substitution in the central ring (see Fig. 4.1). A reputed ranking of anticholinergic side-effects runs, from most to least: amitriptyline, dothiepin, doxepin. Dothiepin is one of the most widely prescribed antidepressants in the UK. For dothiepin, doses range from 25 mg to a maximum of 225 mg per day, while for doxepin the maximum dose is 300 mg daily in divided doses (the manufacturers recommend that no more than 100 mg should be taken as a single dose).

Imipramine

The first tricyclic shown to have antidepressant activity, imipramine is demethylated to desipramine, an active metabolite. At steady-state the amount of desipramine usually exceeds that of the parent compound. Imipramine blocks reuptake of both noradrenaline and serotonin (Fig. 4.2); desipramine

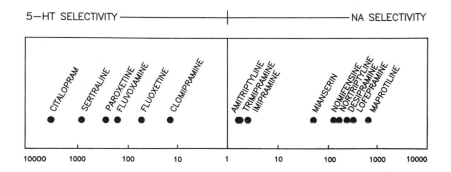

Fig. 4.2 *In vitro* selectivity ratios for parent (non-metabolised) antidepressant compound. On the x-axis the measure is a ratio: to the left, $IC_{50}NA/IC_{50}5\text{-HT}$; to the right, $IC_{50}5\text{-HT}/IC_{50}NA$. IC_{50} represents 50% inhibition of uptake of noradrenaline (NA) or serotonin (5-HT) into rat brain synaptosomes. (The lower the IC_{50} the more potent is the drug effect on uptake). For further explanation see Hyttel (1994).

is a more specific noradrenaline reuptake inhibitor. There are moderate sedative, anticholinergic and alpha-adrenoreceptor blocking actions, the latter leading to postural hypotension. The daily dose range is 25–300 mg.

Lofepramine

Although lofepramine is metabolised in the liver to desipramine, there is evidence that lofepramine itself has some antidepressant activity (Leonard, 1987). It is relatively safe in overdose. The mortality from suicide for those prescribed lofepramine is among the lowest for all the antidepressants (Isacsson *et al*, 1994*a*; Henry *et al*, 1995; Jick *et al*, 1995; see also Table 4.4). There may be an artefact in the fatal poisoning studies (Isacsson *et al*, 1994*b*; Henry *et al*, 1995) because the metabolite (desipramine) screened for in toxicology studies is present in low concentrations at recommended doses of lofepramine. However, this would not account for the low mortality from all causes of suicide (Jick *et al*, 1995). The recommended dose range is 140 to 210 mg daily in divided doses but the elderly may respond to lower doses.

Trimipramine

Trimipramine has a similar structure to imipramine, the only difference being an additional methyl group attached to the side chain (Fig. 4.1). It is the most sedative of the TCAs. It is sometimes used together with an MAOI in combined antidepressant treatment, in cases of refractory depression. Doses range from 25 mg to a maximum of 300 mg daily (for no more than four to six weeks), and the usual maintenance dose is 75–150 mg daily.

Secondary amine TCAs

Amoxapine

Amoxapine has a tricyclic structure with a fourth ring attached by an -N bond; some authorities have classified it as a secondary amine TCA, others as a tetracyclic. It is the N-desmethyl derivative of the antipsychotic drug loxapine. Amoxapine has weak dopamine blocking activity and this is associated with occasional extrapyramidal side-effects, menstrual irregularities, breast enlargement and galactorrhoea. It has some anti-cholinergic activity but negligible effect on alpha-1 and histamine receptors. Doses range from 100 to 300 mg daily.

Desipramine

This metabolite of imipramine can be prescribed separately. Desipramine has fewer sedative, anticholinergic and alpha-adrenoreceptor blocking actions than the tertiary amine TCAs. Doses are similar to those of imipramine. Only 25 mg tablets are available, so if a high dose is prescribed, there is the disadvantage of the patient having to swallow many tablets. The dose range is 25–200 mg daily; in resistant depression a maximum of 300 mg daily may be used with plasma drug level monitoring.

Nortriptyline

This metabolite of amitriptyline is available for prescription. Nortriptyline's position in relation to serotonin–noradrenaline selectivity is shown in Fig. 4.2. Its effect on dopaminergic reuptake is weak. The 10-hydroxy metabolite is more abundant than the parent compound and is probably more selective for noradrenergic neurones, so there is a predominance of noradrenergic effects. Nortriptyline has fewer sedative, alpha-1 blocking and anticholinergic effects than amitriptyline. The usual dose range is 75–100 mg daily.

Protriptyline

Protriptyline has a stimulant action. For those with insomnia, the last dose should not be taken after 4 p.m. It has some anticholinergic effects. Doses are lower than for other tricyclics, generally 10–40 mg per day.

Related antidepressants

Maprotiline

This tetracyclic was introduced as one of a 'new generation' of antidepressants. The parent compound is the most noradrenergic antidepressant (Fig. 4.3). There seem to be no advantages in relation to tricyclics. It is particularly prone to cause convulsions. The dose range is 25–150 mg daily.

Mianserin

Mianserin, another tetracyclic (Fig. 4.3), does not block reuptake of serotonin, noradrenaline or dopamine. It blocks pre-synaptic alpha-2 adrenoreceptors, which are inhibitory, thereby increasing synaptic availability of noradrenaline. Mianserin also blocks post-synaptic 5-HT$_2$ receptors. It is sedative which is helpful for insomnia associated with depression and has fewer anticholinergic side-effects than the tricyclics. Bone marrow depression presenting as granulocytopenia or agranulo-cytosis has been reported during treatment with mianserin. These effects have occurred most commonly after four to six weeks of treatment and were usually reversible on stopping treatment. A full blood count is recommended every four weeks during the first three months of treatment. This adverse reaction has been observed in all age groups but appears to be more common in the elderly. The usual dose range is 30–90 mg daily.

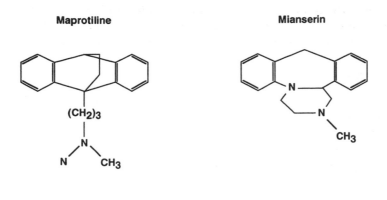

Fig. 4.3 Chemical structure of some non-tricyclic antidepressants.

Trazodone

This antidepressant, which is neither a tricyclic nor a tetracyclic, is chemically related only to nefazodone. The parent compound antagonises the 5-HT$_{2A}$ post-synaptic receptor; blockade at this site may stimulate other receptor responses to 5-HT, in particular the 5-HT$_{1A}$ response. A trazodone metabolite is an agonist at other 5-HT receptors. It also increases the release of noradrenaline via pre-synaptic alpha-2 receptor blockade. Its weak serotonin reuptake blockade is probably clinically insignificant. It is sedative but with little anticholinergic effect. Priapism, a prolonged painful engorgement of the penis, has been reported with an incidence of one per 6000 males treated (Warner *et al*, 1987). The dose range is 100–600 mg per day, usually given at night.

Nefazodone

Nefazodone is an analogue of trazodone but its pharmacological profile is different. Like trazodone it has 5-HT$_{2A}$ antagonist activity and this is the more potent of its effects but it also inhibits serotonin reuptake It has a benign side-effect profile because it lacks anticholinergic, anti-adrenergic and antihistamine activity. Nausea, drowsiness and asthenia have been reported, but so far priapism has not. When used to treat depressive episodes there is a suggestion of a therapeutic window with optimum doses in the range 300–500 mg per day, and the drug is usually administered twice daily.

Venlafaxine

The structure of this phenethylamine (Fig. 4.3) is unrelated to other antidepressants listed above. It inhibits the reuptake of both noradrenaline and serotonin but unlike amitriptyline it has little affinity for muscarinic, histaminic or alpha-1 adrenergic receptors. (The acronym SNRI stands for serotonin and noradrenaline reuptake inhibitor.) The most common adverse effect is nausea; anticholinergic effects may also occur, although less frequently than with TCAs. Hypertension has been reported and may be dose-dependent: 0% at 75 mg per day,1% at 225 mg per day and 3% at 375 mg per day (Preskorn,1995). It should not be used with an MAOI. The usual starting dose is 37.5 mg twice daily; if necessary the dose can be increased to a maximum recommended dose of 375 mg per day, which, if possible, should be reduced gradually.

Viloxazine

Viloxazine, originally developed as a beta blocker, has a bicyclic structure like venlafaxine and fluoxetine (Figs 4.3 and 4.4). It selectively inhibits noradrenaline reuptake at central and peripheral sites and may facilitate release of neuronal stores of serotonin. It has very limited anticholinergic, antihistamine and quinidine-like effects. Viloxazine inhibits liver enzymes associated with the metabolism of carbamazepine and phenytoin; increased plasma concentrations of these two anti-epileptic drugs have been associated with consequent neurotoxicity. The most common unwanted effect is nausea.

The recommended daily dose is 300 mg taken as 200 mg in the morning and 100 mg midday, with a maximum daily dose of 400 mg. The manufacturers suggest the last dose should not be taken after 6.00 p.m.

Withdrawn new antidepressants

Nomifensine was introduced in 1978. It blocks noradrenaline and dopamine reuptake systems. The Committee for the Safety of Medicines (CSM) Yellow Card scheme detected the occurrence of haemolytic anaemia and nomifensine was withdrawn after eight years. Zimelidine, introduced in 1981, was one of the first SSRIs. It was withdrawn after a year, because of an association with the Guillain–Barré syndrome.

Adverse tricyclic reactions

An adverse drug reaction (ADR) is defined as "a noxious and unintended response in man to a drug administered at a dose appropriate for prophylaxis, diagnosis, or therapy" (Karch & Lasagna, 1975). ADRs, also known as side-effects, are obviously important; whenever one prescribes, one has to anticipate likely ADRs, recognise their occurrence, differentiate them from unrelated phenomena such as the depression itself and deal effectively with them.

The prevalence of ADRs depends on a variety of factors, for example on the way the ADR is defined; thus an arbitrary measure of severity may decide whether an ADR is present or not. Patient variables, drug dosages, and how long the drug has been on the market (more critical scrutiny being directed towards newer drugs) affect the prevalence. Large-scale surveillance of antidepressants in hospitals in Germany has provided information on the overall prevalence rate of ADRs; rates per hundred exposures were as follows: clomipramine 10.3%, maprotiline 9.1%, amitriptyline 7.1%, mianserin 3.0% and doxepin 1.3%, and the most common ADRs were autonomic, CNS and cardiac (Schmidt *et al*, 1986).

Anticholinergic effects

Anticholinergic effects include dry mouth, blurred vision, urinary retention, constipation, memory impairment and confusion. Some tolerance to these effects usually develops after a few days. Table 4.1 shows antidepressant affinities for muscarinic acetylcholine receptors of human brain. There are a number of difficulties in extrapolating from *in vitro* to *in vivo* studies. Thus a two- to three-fold difference in potency of muscarinic receptor blockade found *in vitro* may reflect no clinical difference, but drugs at the extremes of the table will show clinical differences (El-Fakahany & Richelson, 1983).

Dry mouth.   Diminished parasympathetic stimulation decreases salivation. This may be exacerbated by anxiety and depression. Dental caries and stomatitis may develop. A persistently dry mouth is usually treated by a reduction in dose, or the use of a tricyclic with a low anticholinergic profile such as desipramine. Some authors advocate using sugarless sweets or gum to stimulate salivary flow but foods containing sugar should be avoided because of the risk of dental caries.

Blurred vision.   This is associated with mydriasis, sluggish pupillary reaction to light, cycloplegia (paresis of the ciliary muscle acting on the lens) and presbyopia (disturbed near vision). Narrow angle glaucoma is a contraindication to TCAs but open angle glaucoma is not. For patients with glaucoma who are maintained on a tricyclic, regular ophthalmologic consultation with tonometry is required. SSRIs have neglible anticholinergic effects and are therefore usually the antidepressants of choice in patients with glaucoma.

Urinary retention.   The detrusor muscle of the bladder is under parasympathetic control and serves to propel the stream of urine. The internal and external bladder sphincters are likewise affected by anticholinergic activity. This side-effect may lead to urinary slowness, dribbling, decreased flow and retention. An atonic bladder with urinary tract infection secondary to urine stasis and, rarely, renal failure may follow. Patients with enlarged prostate glands are particularly at risk of developing these complications because of the mechanical obstruction to outflow. In children with nocturnal enuresis small doses of imipramine are sometimes helpful.

Constipation.   Anticholinergic effects on the gastro-intestinal tract lead to decreased intestinal motility and consequently increased water absorption from the bowel. In the elderly this may cause faecal impaction and paralytic ileus. An osmotic or bulk laxative will enlarge and soften the stool, but stimulant laxatives are best avoided.

Neurological ADRs

As previously noted the anticholinergic effects of TCAs may overlap with neurological ADRs.

Memory impairment.   Cognitive function has a cholinergic contribution and the anticholinergic effect of TCAs is associated with poor memory. Even young adults taking TCAs may notice difficulty in remembering, but this effect is more marked among the elderly. A complaint of poor memory may also be symptomatic of depression itself and improve with TCA treatment.

Confusional states.   This anticholinergic effect of TCAs is more prevalent in the elderly, presenting with evening restlessness, sleep disturbance, disorientation, illogical thoughts and sometimes delusional states. Delirium is more likely with higher plasma TCA levels. In one study nine of 16 patients with a plasma TCA level greater than 450 ng/ml developed cognitive or behavioural disturbance compared with only one of 15 patients in whom the plasma TCA was below this value (Meader-Woodruff *et al*, 1988).

Tremor.   The underlying mechanism of the fine tremor is uncertain. Blockade of noradrenaline reuptake at post-ganglionic sympathetic receptors may contribute and noradrenaline also has a weak stimulating effect on beta-receptors. Adrenaline may play a role as it stimulates both alpha and beta sympathetic receptors. Propranolol, a beta blocker, reduces this tremor. There may be a contribution from serotonergic receptors since 10–13% of patients on SSRIs develop a fine tremor.

Sedation. This is probably associated with blockade of histamine receptors. It can be used to advantage in alleviating depressive insomnia. Sedative effects are greatest at the start of TCA therapy or when the dose is increased. Morning drowsiness after a nocturnal TCA dose may pass after a few days. The tertiary amines (amitriptyline, doxepin and trimipramine) are more sedative than the secondary amines (nortriptyline, protriptyline and desipramine). Imipramine is a less sedative tertiary amine.

Convulsions. The mechanism underlying TCA-induced fits is unknown, although this effect is dose dependent and more likely with higher doses. Recent studies suggest an incidence lying between 0.5 and 2.2% (Rouillon *et al*, 1992). The risk is greatest for maprotiline; this drug accounted for 63% of all reported convulsions due to antidepressants (Schmidt *et al*, 1986).

Myoclonus. This is defined as an involuntary, irregular contraction of a muscle or a group of muscles. Garvey & Tollefson (1987) reported that 30% of patients treated with imipramine suffered from a mild degree of myoclonus but in 9% it was sufficiently troublesome to require a medication change. The phenomenon includes jaw-jerking, intermittent arm myoclonus causing patients to drop objects, and nocturnal myoclonus consisting of a relatively continuous sequence of single myoclonic jerks of various muscles throughout the night. Myoclonus usually develops in the first few weeks of treatment and may be dose related. The biological basis of myoclonus is unknown although there are hypotheses suggesting

Table 4.1 Antidepressant affinities for muscarinic acetylcholine receptors of human brain (from El-Fakahany & Richelson, 1983)

Drug	Affinity[1]
Amitriptyline	5.5
Protriptyline	4.0
Clomipramine	2.7
Trimipramine	1.7
Doxepin	1.3
Imipramine	1.1
Nortriptyline	0.7
Desipramine	0.5
Maprotiline	0.2
Amoxapine	0.1
Trazodone	0.0003
Atropine[2]	48

1. Affinity = $10^{-7}/Kb$ where Kb is the equilibrium dissociation constant in moles.
2. Listed for comparison.

increased serotonergic activity induced by TCAs as well as alterations in the balance between serotonin and acetylcholine (see page 440).

Extrapyramidal signs.   Choreoathetoid movements are rare and may be related to a TCA-induced hyperdopaminergic state. Depression itself may constitute a risk factor for the onset of tardive dyskinesia. Akathisia has been reported in women taking conjugated oestrogens as oral contraceptives and TCAs. Oestrogens affect dopamine-sensitive adenylate cyclase and modulate dopamine receptors.

Sleep disturbance, nightmares, hypnagogic hallucinations and hypnopompic hallucinations have a frequency of 0.2 to 1.6% (Schmidt *et al*, 1986). Reduced sleep time and increased wakefulness may be found in antidepressants acting selectively on serotonin receptors. Impaired speech may be related to high plasma levels of antidepressants. Speech problems consist of difficulty in finding words, stuttering, or increased verbal pauses, and usually respond to a lowering of the dose. Paraesthesia, a 'pins and needles' feeling in the extremities, has also been described.

Cardiovascular effects of antidepressants

Antidepressants can affect blood pressure, cardiac conduction and cardiac contractility (reviewed by Warrington *et al*, 1989). The most common cardiovascular side-effect of TCAs is postural hypotension, which is probably due to alpha-adrenergic blockade.

The constriction of veins in the legs is mediated by the activation of alpha-adrenoceptors and a receptor antagonist such as a TCA will result in alpha-adrenergic blockade, a consequent 'pooling' of blood in the major veins on standing and so postural hypotension. Patients complain of dizziness, unsteadiness, and sometimes falls which may occasionally be complicated by fractures. Predictive factors include a large pretreatment postural drop, being older and having a higher plasma TCA concentration.

Imipramine causes more postural hypotension than nortriptyline (Roose *et al*, 1981) and amitriptyline more than lofepramine (Marneros & Philipp, 1979). Although mianserin has alpha-adrenergic blocking activity, it causes less postural hypotension than typical TCAs. Venlafaxine does not have alpha adrenergic blocking activity and is thought not to be associated with postural hypotension.

TCAs can cause abnormalities of cardiac conduction and arrythmias. These effects are uncommon at therapeutic doses, affecting less than 5% of patients, and are mostly clinically insignificant (Warrington *et al*, 1989). The anticholinergic TCA effect may cause some degree of tachycardia. However the most important effect of TCAs is membrane stabilisation by a quinidine-like effect due to inhibition of the enzyme Na^+/K^+ ATPase. This produces slowing of cardiac conduction, that is, slowing of atrial and ventricular depolarisation and prolongation of conduction time in the bundle of His.

ECG manifestations include increased PR, QRS and QT intervals and a decrease in T wave amplitude. The changes appear to be dose related; thus at very high plasma levels, that is, greater than 350 µg/l, 70% of physically healthy young depressed adults will develop first-degree heart block compared with only 3% with levels below 350 µg/l (Preskorn & Fast, 1991).

Long QT intervals are thought to predict the onset of fatal ventricular arrythmias. When corrected for heart rate, the QT_c interval ($QT_c = QT/$ the square root of the RR interval) is the best ECG measure of a quinidine-like effect, and modern ECG machines now print out QT and QT_c values. Lofepramine has little quinidine-like activity, but its main metabolite desipramine may have. Mianserin has less effect on cardiac conduction than amitriptyline (Pete *et al*, 1977).

Amitriptyline and imipramine werc implicated in reports of a few individuals who died suddenly and unexpectedly, but the Boston Collaborative Drug Surveillance Programme (1972) failed to confirm any causal link between sudden death and TCA therapy. Case reports of patients occasionally developing congestive cardiac failure while on TCAs are of uncertain significance, but probably occurred only in patients with diminished reserves of cardiac function (Warrington *et al*, 1989).

After an overdose the clinical manifestations of TCA intoxication are seen in the CNS (coma, convulsions and respiratory depression) and cardiovascular system (tachycardia, blood pressure changes, conduction disturbances and dysrhythmias). Fatalities are associated with ventricular tachycardia because this may progress to ventricular fibrillation or asystole. After an overdose, QRS duration and TCA plasma concentrations are strongly correlated (Petit *et al*, 1977). QRS duration has also been evaluated as a predictive measure as ventricular arrythmias are only seen with a QRS of 160 ms or longer.

Hypertension itself does not increase the hazards of treatment with antidepressant drugs, and TCAs may decrease blood pressure. Because of their anticholinergic and quinidine-like effects, TCAs are probably best avoided in patients with angina pectoris, recent myocardial infarction, arrythymias and cardiac failure.

Sexual dysfunction

Doctors often do not routinely enquire about sexual dysfunction and patients may be reluctant to report it, yet it may be distressing and an important cause of non-compliance. Both depression and medication may decrease libido. Depressive loss of libido is associated with a generalised loss of interest but the TCA mechanism is unclear.

Erection may be impaired. Kowalski *et al* (1985) compared the effects of amitriptyline 150 mg, mianserin 60 mg and placebo on nocturnal sexual arousal as measured by penile plethysmography in a cross-over trial of men with no previous psychiatric history. Both active compounds significantly decreased the change in penile circumference with erection and the total duration of nocturnal erections. Mianserin increased the latency time to the first erection. Retarded or absent ejaculation, which may represent a more minor form of impairment than failure of erection, has been reported, as has painful ejaculation. Anorgasmia may occur in both men and women. Priapism has been reported with trazodone. It requires immediate cessation of treatment, and may be a surgical emergency.

Increased appetite and body weight

Harris *et al* (1986) studied 168 depressed out-patients on seven antidepressant regimes (amitriptyline, trimipramine, phenelzine, isocarboxazid, trimipramine plus phenelzine, trimipramine plus isocarboxazid, and flupenthixol). All produced an increase in appetite and weight. The two tricyclics resembled the non-tricyclic flupenthixol. The combination of trimipramine and isocarboxacid produced the greatest increase in both appetite and weight. The mechanism by which increases in appetite and weight occur is unknown. An effect on the hypothalamus, a change in expenditure of energy, an alteration of metabolic rate, changes in glucose metabolism, fluid retention and increased energy efficiency have been postulated. Carbohydrate craving with a preference for sweet foods such as chocolate is commonly reported, but precise mechanisms are unclear.

Management of weight gain includes advising the patient to stick to previous eating patterns both as regards type and quantity of food, to resist craving for sweet foods, and to take exercise.

Gastro-intestinal and hepatic effects

Although nausea and vomiting are more common with SSRIs, gastro-intestinal ADRs occur with TCAs. Schmidt *et al* (1986) reported an overall incidence of 5.4% and for individual drugs the rates were: mianserin 10.5%, clomipramine 6.9%, amitriptyline 5.4% and doxepin 1.9%. By contrast the withdrawn SSRI zimelidine had an incidence of 27.3%. Impaired liver function was found in less than 1% of patients and the rates for individual drugs were clomipramine 0.9%, amitriptyline 0.6% and mianserin 0.6%.

Skin reactions

Two to four per cent of patients on antidepressants develop skin reactions, usually in the first two weeks of treatment. Of these, the most common are exanthematous (46%), urticarial (23%) and, less commonly, erythema multiforme (5.4%), exfoliative dermatitis (3.7%) and photosensitivity (2.8%).

Endocrine and metabolic effects

TCAs may stimulate prolactin secretion, but galactorrhoea and secondary amenorrhoea are rare. Hyponatraemia via the syndrome of inappropriate antidiuretic hormone secretion is uncommon, but has been reported with all classes of antidepressants. It is more common in the elderly and should be considered in any patient taking an antidepressant who develops drowsiness, confusion or convulsions (CSM advice in the *BNF*, 1996).

Blood dyscrasias

Mianserin use has been associated with an increased rate of leucopenia, agranulocytosis, aplastic anaemia and idiopathic thrombocytopenia. A few of these cases have been fatal. In the UK 34 cases of blood dyscrasias were noted following 1.2 million mianserin prescriptions, but the rate of under-reporting is unknown. In Germany, Schmidt *et al* (1986) found a rate of blood dyscrasia of 15.8% for mianserin compared with 3.9% for doxepin, 3.1% for amitriptyline and 0.0% for clomipramine. However, Inman (1988) using UK data found no difference in the rates for mianserin and amitriptyline (both 0.3%).

A pharmacodynamic classification of ADRs

Cookson (1993) has proposed an alternative classification of ADRs based on the pharmacodynamic action of antidepressants, predominantly of their effects on neurotransmitters.

(1) *Blockade of serotonin reuptake.* Apart from the therapeutic effect, there may be gastro-intestinal disturbances such as loss of appetite, nausea and diarrhoea, and anxiety. The latter may be associated with a mild form of the serotonin syndrome (see page 183).

(2) *Blockade of noradrenaline reuptake.* As well as the therapeutic effect, increased noradrenaline at post-ganglionic sympathetic receptors may cause tremor, tachycardia and a hypertensive effect in certain circumstances.

(3) *Blockade of dopamine reuptake.* Increased dopamine at post-synaptic receptors may alleviate Parkinsonism. However there may also be blockade of dopamine receptors resulting in the opposite effect, causing extrapyramidal movements. Dopamine is the prolactin inhibitory factor and there may be hyperprolactinaemia.

(4) *Blockade of alpha-1 adrenergic receptors.* This is probably the cause of postural hypotension with associated dizziness and a reflex tachycardia. This mechanism may also contribute to impotence and ejaculatory delay.

(5) *Blockade of muscarinic receptors.* The well-known anticholinergic effects are dry mouth, constipation, urinary retention, blurred vision, sinus tachycardia and memory impairment. In the elderly the anticholinergic effect may cause confusion and a paralytic ileus.

(6) *Blockade of histamine receptors.* This causes sedation and may be associated with weight gain.

(7) *Membrane stabilising effect.* A–V block,other dysrrhythmias and asystole.

(8) *Poorly understood side-effects.* Excessive sweating, epileptic fits, myoclonus and inappropriate secretion of antidiuretic hormone.

Selective serotonin reuptake inhibitors

The biogenic amine theory of depression had proponents who at different times emphasised the relative importance of serotonin, noradrenaline and dopamine. The evidence in favour of serotonin served as an impetus for the development of drugs which enhanced serotonergic neural transmission. After receiving product licences, zimelidine had to be withdrawn because of adverse effects particularly the Guillain–Barré syndrome. At the time of writing, citalopram, fluvoxamine, fluoxetine, paroxetine and sertraline are available for prescription in the UK.

To receive a product licence a minimum requirement is that a drug has been shown to have been as good as a reference antidepressant such as imipramine, and in at least two studies, better than placebo. Most of the available SSRIs have been the focus of considerably more studies.

Pharmacokinetics

In contrast to the TCAs members of this class of drug have dissimilar chemical structures (Fig. 4.4) and pharmocokinetics. Their prolonged half-lives and non-linear pharmocokinetics (for example, flat dose–response curves) need to be taken into account when prescribing (reviewed by Preskorn, 1993).

Absorption, first-pass metabolism and distribution

The SSRIs are extensively absorbed from the gastro-intestinal tract. More than 90% of the orally administered dose reaches the systemic circulation. Fluoxetine, paroxetine and sertraline are highly protein-bound (>90%) with a large volume of distribution; citalopram and fluvoxamine are less protein-bound (82 and 77% respectively) and have a smaller volume of distribution.

Time to reach peak plasma levels

Fluoxetine, fluvoxamine, paroxetine and sertraline reach peak plasma levels after 4–8 hours, whereas citalopram takes 2–4 hours. The occurrence of gastro-intestinal distress within 30 minutes of drug ingestion suggests a direct effect on the gastro-intestinal mucosa. For patients who complain of a stimulating effect in relation to sleep, or sedation, the time taken to reach peak plasma levels is a guide as to the best times to take the drugs. With sustained treatment and the attainment of plasma steady-state levels, this variable becomes less important.

Active metabolites

SSRIs differ with regard to active metabolites. The two demethylated metabolites of citalopram (demethylcitalopram and didemethylcitalopram) are themselves selective serotonin reuptake inhibitors *in vitro*, but are much less potent. The demethylated metabolite norfluoxetine is three times more selective for serotonin uptake than fluoxetine and is essentially equipotent to fluoxetine in terms of serotonin reuptake inhibition. After a few weeks plasma levels of norfluoxetine are two to three times higher than fluoxetine levels and so norfluoxetine is likely to be a major determinant of the pharmacological response. By contrast, desmethylsertraline is only one-tenth as potent as sertraline and as desmethylsertraline levels are only about 1.5 times higher than those of sertraline it probably has negligible effects. The metabolites of fluvoxamine and paroxetine are thought to have no effect on serotonin reuptake inhibition. The SSRIs slow their own metabolism by inhibiting the hepatic cytochrome P450 isoenzymes; this effect is greatest for paroxetine and fluoxetine.

Individual variability in metabolism

As with the TCAs there is wide individual variability in SSRI metabolism. Hence for some rapid metabolisers the usually effective dose may be inadequate for an antidepressant response. None of the five SSRIs demonstrates a correlation between steady-state plasma levels and therapeutic response in depressed patients. However, the adverse effects of SSRIs such as nausea, anxiety, restlessness, fatigue and sexual dysfunction are dose dependent although they tend to lessen with time. The fact that the average antidepressant response rate is achieved regardless of dose escalation is compatible with the presumed mechanism of action since the minimum effective dose of all five SSRIs produces approximately 80% inhibition of platelet serotonin uptake in most patients. This degree of inhibition appears to be required for an antidepressant response, while higher levels produce more serotonin-mediated adverse effects.

The metabolism of each of the five SSRIs becomes slower with increasing age. Steady-state plasma levels after citalopram 20 mg once daily were up to four times higher in elderly subjects than in younger patients or volunteers (Baldwin & Johnson, 1995). Compared with the young on similar doses, fluoxetine plus norfluoxetine levels may be double in the elderly, paroxetine levels are about 70% higher and the clearance of sertraline is about 40% less (Wilde *et al*, 1993).

Half-lives

Substantial differences among the SSRIs in terms of their half-lives are shown in Table 4.2.

As fluoxetine and paroxetine inhibit their own metabolism, their half-lives are dose dependent and increase with higher doses; that is, their pharmacokinetics are non-linear. This is not the case with the other SSRIs over their clinically relevant dose ranges. In spite of the figures in the table,

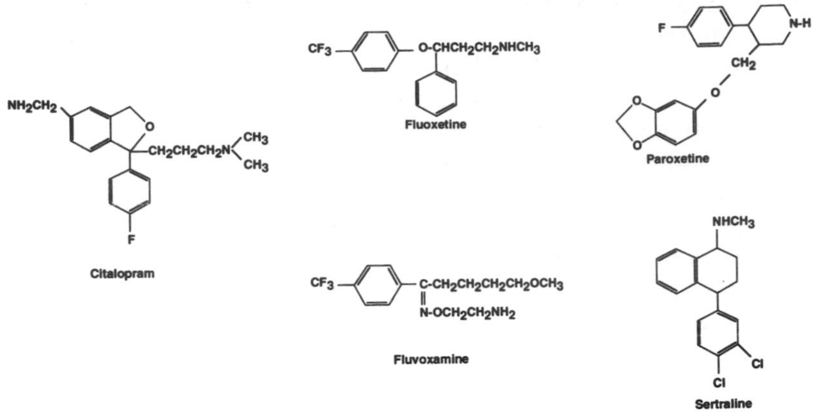

Fig. 4.4 Chemical structure of the SSRIs.

paroxetine's half-life at higher doses becomes longer than those of citalopram, fluvoxamine and sertraline. The extended half-life of fluoxetine and its metabolites increases the risk of late emergent concentration-dependent adverse effects. It also results in prolonged carryover effects such as delayed recovery of hepatic cytochrome isoenzyme 2D6 function after withdrawal of fluoxetine. Because of the wide range of therapeutic plasma levels, plasma monitoring is not done on a routine basis for any of the SSRIs.

Excretion

SSRI metabolites are mainly excreted in the urine and to only a small extent in the faeces. For example, 75–80% of ^{14}C-labelled fluoxetine given to volunteers was recovered in the urine and 10% in the faeces. Fluoxetine itself accounted for only 10% of excreted products, the rest having been metabolites. With fluvoxamine 94% of a single dose was recovered in the urine as metabolites and none appeared as the parent compound. Only 2% of paroxetine is excreted unchanged, with metabolites found in both urine and faeces. Both sertraline and desmethylsertraline are metabolised to the ketone and further hydroxylated to the major excretory metabolites with only a small amount of unchanged sertraline appearing in the urine. For patients who have achieved a steady state on citalopram about 32% of a daily dose is excreted in the urine over 24 hours as citalopram and its metabolites.

Drug interactions

Many SSRI interactions can now be explained by the effect SSRIs have on the liver cytochrome P450 isoenzymes. There are two major classes of P450 isoenzymes. Those involved in the synthesis of endogenous substances such as steroids, prostaglandins and fatty acids are located in the mitochondria; those which catabolise foreign substances such as drugs are located on the smooth endoplasmic reticulum of the liver cells. Their name arises from their having an absorption peak on the spectrometer at 450 nm. When the cytochrome P450 isoenzyme oxidises a drug, oxygen incorporation is associated with electron transfer by reduced flavoprotein and NADPH (Benet *et al*, 1996). More than 30 isoenzymes have been identified in man. The nomenclature of the P450 isoenzyme, for example 2D6, is that the first numeral (2) refers to the gene family, the letter (D) refers to a sub-family and the second numeral (6) refers to an individual gene within the sub-family. The topic has been reviewed by Preskorn & Magnus, (1994), Nemeroff *et al* (1996) and Taylor & Lader (1996).

The catalytic specificity of the P450 isoenzymes can range from being quite non-discriminatory to very exacting (Guengerich, 1992). Thus P450 isoenzyme-mediated reactions are often the rate-limiting step and may be dependent on the functional activity of a single enzyme. If the enzyme is not functional because of a genetic deficiency or because of its inhibition, toxicity may result. The combination of a drug which is metabolised by this system together with one which inhibits it such as an SSRI may lead to a significant drug interaction. SSRI inhibition is competitive and reversible. The hepatic 2D6 isoenzyme may be the rate-limiting enzyme for the clearance of drugs such as TCAs. High TCA levels caused by SSRIs are due to the inhibition of demethylation and hydroxylation in the breakdown of TCAs and the putative enzyme subtypes involved in the inhibition of these reactions are shown in Table 4.3. Toxicity may be associated with delirium, seizures, heart block and sudden death.

Drugs vary in the degree to which they inhibit this enzyme system. Crewe *et al* (1992) reported on the inhibition constants (K_i) for different drugs for cytochrome P450 2D6 activity in human liver microsomes (a small K_i indicates a greater inhibitory effect). The descending order of inhibitory activity, with K_i values shown, was: paroxetine 0.15, paroxetine's M2 metabolite 0.50, norfluoxetine 0.43, fluoxetine 0.60, thioridazine 0.52, sertraline 0.70, clomipramine 2.2, desipramine 2.3, amitriptyline 4.0, citalopram 5.1, fluvoxamine 8.2. Although paroxetine is a more potent inhibitor of cytochrome P450 2D6 *in vitro* than fluoxetine, *in vivo* each produce approximately the same degree of inhibition because on the same dose (20 mg per day) fluoxetine has a much higher plasma concentration associated with its longer half-life.

Citalopram, fluvoxamine and sertraline produce much weaker cytochrome P450 2D6 inhibition (Preskorn & Magnus, 1994). However, fluvoxamine has an important effect on the cytochrome isoenzyme 1A2 (see Table 4.3). Grapefruit juice is a powerful inhibitor of cytochrome isoenzyme P450 3A4 (Guengerich, 1992). The health consequences of a long-term and substantial reduction in hepatic isoenzyme function require further study (Preskorn & Magnus, 1994).

The SSRIs are a heterogeneous class of chemical compounds, and so drug interactions which occur with one SSRI may not necessarily occur with another. Particular drug interactions are mentioned in the section dealing with individual SSRIs, but pharmacodynamic interactions common to the SSRIs are described below.

A hypertensive reaction occurs if an SSRI is combined with an MAOI, and this may also cause the serotonin syndrome (see page 183). As MAOIs (with the exception of moclobemide) irreversibly inhibit MAO, a minimum of two weeks should be allowed before an SSRI is started after MAOI treatment. This enables sufficient new MAO to be synthesised. The time period may be shorter for moclobemide. For the reverse situation, that is starting an MAOI after stopping an SSRI, a two-week period is necessary to allow washout of citalopram, fluvoxamine, paroxetine and sertraline, but a five-week washout is required after stopping fluoxetine, because of the long half-life of its metabolite norfluoxetine.

Initially there were reports of neurotoxicity when fluoxetine was combined with lithium, but a lithium augmentation trial revealed neurotoxicity to be no more frequent with the combination of lithium and fluoxetine than with the combination of lithium and lofepramine (Katona *et al*, 1995). SSRIs do not potentiate the sedative effects of alcohol. There have been a few reports of fluoxetine being associated with hypoglycaemia in patients taking insulin or oral hypoglycaemic drugs.

Efficacy of SSRIs

Double-blind placebo-controlled trials have shown unequivocally that SSRIs are more effective than placebo. Debate continues about the relative efficacies of SSRIs and TCAs.

Table 4.2 Half-lives of SSRIs at therapeutic dose ranges

Drug	Half-life (hours) (Approximate unless a range is shown)
Citalopram	33
Metabolites (less active)	
Fluoxetine	48–96
Norfluoxetine	168–360
Fluvoxamine	22
11 metabolites largely inactive	
Paroxetine	21
M2 metabolite	<24
Sertraline	26
Desmethylsertraline	48–96

A meta-analysis of 63 randomised controlled trials of an SSRI versus a TCA (or related drug such as a tetracyclic) found, overall, that there was no difference between the two antidepressant types (Song *et al*, 1993). For those studies in which standard deviations were given it was possible to pool the Hamilton scores to estimate a difference in efficacy. For the 10 studies using the 17-item Hamilton scale a statistically significant, but clinically small difference in favour of the TCAs was shown. This did not appear in the six studies included in the 21-item Hamilton pooled comparison.

Anderson & Tomenson (1994) identified 90 reports of double-blind randomised controlled trials of SSRIs in depressed patients. They considered only 55 of these studies to be methodologically sound; these included 2325 patients who took an SSRI and 2305 patients on a TCA. In the main analysis both classes of drugs were superior to placebo and there was no difference in efficacy between the TCAs and SSRIs. However, subgroup analysis revealed some small differences. Studies restricted to in-patients showed a margin in favour of TCAs but the effect size was small, and disappeared when studies with paroxetine were removed from the analysis. TCAs were also marginally more effective than SSRIs in the group of studies with high initial Hamilton Scores. (Studies were classified into high and low depression scores based on a median split of initial Hamilton scores.) The effect size was also small and was mainly accounted for by the result for fluoxetine. Serotonergic TCAs (amitriptyline and clomipramine) were more effective than the SSRIs, which were marginally more effective than noradrenergic TCAs (imipramine and other TCAs), but the effect sizes for these differences were very small.

Most of the studies of SSRI efficacy have been limited to adults aged between 18 and 65. Boyer & Feighner (1991) have reviewed studies of elderly patients. They concluded that, as with younger patients, the SSRIs and TCAs are equally efficacious, although there is evidence for SSRIs being less efficacious on measures of sleep disturbance, but the SSRI side-effect profile may be more favourable for the elderly.

Individual SSRIs

Citalopram

Citalopram is a substituted phthalane derivative with a tertiary amino group in the side chain (see Fig. 4.4). It is the most serotonin-selective of the SSRIs and TCAs (see Fig. 4.2) but this does not mean that it is the most potent inhibitor of serotonin reuptake. It differs from other SSRIs in having a shorter time to reach peak plasma levels of around 2–4 hours. Citalopram is a weak inhibitor of the cytochrome P450 isoenzyme 2D6 and does not inhibit P450 1A2; on present evidence it appears to have a moderate effect in raising plasma TCA levels, by up to 40–50% (summarised by Baumann & Larsen, 1995). The starting dose of 20 mg daily may be increased to 40 mg but doses of 60 mg per day do not appear to confer any additional advantage (Montgomery & Johnson, 1995).

Fluoxetine

Fluoxetine has the biggest market share of the SSRIs in both the UK and the USA. Its structure is shown in Fig. 4.4. Both fluoxetine and its metabolite norfluoxetine have a long half-life and they both inhibit liver cytochrome P450 2D6 and other P450 isoenzymes (see Table 4.3). The oral dose is directly related to side-effects and non-linearly to plasma levels, but not to clinical response. For example, Wernicke *et al* (1987) found that fluoxetine 20 mg and 40 mg daily were superior to placebo, but fluoxetine 60 mg daily was not. Nausea, emergent anxiety and insomnia are among the most common side-effects and are more prevalent at higher doses (60 mg) than the recommended dose of 20 mg daily. A few reports have described the initiation of intense suicidal thoughts or the exacerbation of existing suicidal ideation. In the largest series, all six of the patients had been previously treated with MAOIs and all had reduced the dose of an antidepressant in the weeks prior to starting fluoxetine (Teicher *et al*, 1990). A subsequent meta-analysis showed that this phenomenon occurred just as frequently with TCAs (Beasley *et al*, 1991).

Fluoxetine is also available in syrup form so treatment can be initiated at much lower doses than the recommended 20 mg daily, for example, a starting dose of 5 mg daily can be used for patients who are particularly liable to suffer side-effects.

Fluvoxamine

Fluvoxamine is a monocyclic structure (see Fig. 4.4). The most common ADRs are nausea, vomiting, agitation, insomnia and somnolence. Nausea is less common if fluvoxamine is given at night. Gastro-intestinal side-effects diminish after the first two weeks (Stimmel *et al*,1991). The starting dose is 100 mg at night and the recommended dose is between 100 and 200 mg per day.

Unlike fluoxetine, paroxetine and sertraline, fluvoxamine has little effect on cytochrome P450 2D6 (Preskorn & Magnus, 1994; Nemeroff *et al*,1996) but it is a potent inhibitor of cytochrome P450 1A2 (Brosen *et al*, 1993), which is little affected by other SSRIs. A three-fold rise in plasma theophyllin levels was found following administration of fluvoxamine (Committee on Safety of Medicines, 1994; see Table 4.3); the CSM recommends avoiding the use of the two drugs together or, alternatively, halving the theophyllin dose together with monitoring plasma theophyllin levels.

Paroxetine

Paroxetine is chemically distinct from other SSRIs in its having a piperidine ring (the ring with -N-; see Fig. 4.4). The most common side-effects are nausea, anxiety, agitation and tremor. In its serotonin uptake inhibition it is second in potency only to sertraline (Hyttel, 1994). There is a wide

Table 4.3 SSRIs, P450 isoenzymes, and potential drug interactions

Enzyme system inhibited	Genetic polymorphism	SSRI[1]	Potential drug interaction	TCA interaction mechanism
1A2	Possible	Fluvoxamine (Paroxetine)	Theophyllin Caffeine Tertiary amine TCAs Haloperidol Clozapine Propranolol	N-demethylation
2C	For 2C19: 3–5% Caucasian 8% African 18% Japanese	Fluoxetine Fluvoxamine Sertraline	Tolbutamide Tertiary amine TCAs Diazepam Phenytoin	N-demethylation
2D6	5–10% of Caucasian population	(Citalopram) Fluoxetine (Fluvoxamine) Paroxetine Sertraline	Analgesics Flecainide Propafenone Quinidine Beta blockers Tertiary & secondary amine TCAs Trazodone Antipsychotic drugs including clozapine Antitussives	Ring hydroxylation
3A3 3A4	Absent Absent	Fluoxetine Fluvoxamine Sertraline	Nifedipine Terfenadine Astemizole Alprazolam Midazolam Triazolam Carbamazepine Tertiary amine TCAs Cyclosporin Ketoconazole	N-demethylation

1. Brackets indicate weak inhibition.
(Sources: Popli & Baldessarini, 1995; Nemeroff *et al*, 1996; Taylor & Lader, 1996.)

interindividual variability in plasma levels for a given dose of paroxetine (Kaye *et al*, 1989). Of the SSRIs, paroxetine is the most potent inhibitor of cytochrome P450 2D6 *in vitro* (Crewe *et al*, 1992) but it does not appear to have any significant effect on other isoenzymes (Table 4.3). However, because of its comparatively short half-life (Table 4.2) inhibition of cytochrome P450 2D6 is reversed within a week of stopping paroxetine, compared with one to two weeks for discontinuation of sertraline and up to five weeks for fluoxetine. The usual daily dose is 20 mg and this may be increased to a maximum recommended dose of 50 mg per day.

Sertraline

Sertraline is a naphthalenamine, with a two-ringed amine complex (see Fig. 4.4). In respect of serotonin uptake inhibition, it is the most potent of the SSRIs (Hyttel, 1994) and in serotonin selectivity it is second only to citalopram (Fig. 4.2). Like other SSRIs it is relatively slowly absorbed from the gastro-intestinal tract, reaching peak plasma levels after four to eight hours. With a half-life of approximately 26 hours, daily doses achieve a steady-state after one week. Sertraline inhibits cytochrome P450 2D6, but not as potently as fluoxetine, norfluoxetine or paroxetine. It also inhibits the P450 2C enzyme (see Table 4.3). This may explain the interaction with tolbutamide, and a 16% reduction in tolbutamide clearance occurs in conjunction with sertraline administration.

Sertraline (like fluoxetine and paroxetine) is highly protein-bound and these SSRIs may displace other protein-bound drugs such as warfarin from their binding sites. Warfarin is also metabolised by cytochrome P450 2C. The manufacturers report a small but statistically significant increase in prothrombin time when sertraline is co-administered with warfarin. Sertraline clearance is also reduced during co-administration with cimetidine. Sertraline and paroxetine were stimulants as measured by critical flicker frequency while fluoxetine and fluvoxamine were no different from placebo. Citalopram was not included (Hindmarsh, 1995). Sertraline has a similar prevalence of ADRs to fluoxetine (Aguglia *et al*, 1993).

The manufacturers recommend a starting dose of 50 mg daily and the usual maintenance dose is also 50 mg daily. The dose may be increased over several weeks to a maximum of 200 mg daily but the manufacturers recommend that doses of 150 mg or more per day should not be used for periods exceeding eight weeks.

ADRs of SSRIs

Gastro-intestinal effects

Nausea, the most common SSRI side-effect, is usually transient and dose related. It may be most common with fluvoxamine (36%), compared with imipramine (20%) and placebo (16%) (Feighner *et al*, 1989) since other SSRIs have had lower rates in similar comparative studies (Rouillon *et al*, 1992). Loss of appetite represents a milder form of this phenomenon, and diarrhoea sometimes occurs. Gastro-intestinal distress may occasionally be severe, possibly accompanied by vomiting. Weight loss of a few pounds may occur with fluoxetine and fluvoxamine but is less likely with citalopram, paroxetine or sertraline. This side-effect is sometimes welcomed by those depressed patients who complain of gaining weight during TCA therapy.

Central nervous system effects

Nervousness, emergent anxiety and agitation have been reported with all SSRIs. They usually occur early in treatment and generally subside. Over time the SSRIs are as effective as TCAs in reducing anxiety. Associated with initial nervousness may be racing thoughts, insomnia, headache and tremor. Headache has been reported in 20–30% of patients taking SSRIs but in these studies there was a similar prevalence with placebo (Feighner *et al*, 1989). For studies with fluoxetine there was a 5% drug–placebo difference in the prevalence of headache but this figure did not reach significance (Preskorn, 1995). Although there may be insomnia, SSRIs occasionally produce sedation. This is more pronounced with paroxetine, with which a prevalence of up to 50% has been reported, and least with fluoxetine (8–11%). Seizures may occur, particularly in overdose.

Apart from tremor, extrapyramidal features including akathisia, dystonia and, rarely, an oro-lingual dyskinesia have been reported. Adding an SSRI to patients already taking antipsychotic drugs may result in a worsening of extrapyramidal effects. There is a wealth of evidence (Arya, 1994) that brain-stem serotonergic neurones have a tonic inhibitory influence on dopamine function and in this respect play a role in the acetylcholine–dopamine balance (see page 440). In keeping with this hypothesis serotonergic receptor blockade by methysergide relieves extrapyramidal signs. Extrapyramidal effects also occur with TCAs, but it is unknown whether they are more common with the SSRIs.

The serotonin syndrome

Among patients taking L-tryptophan in the 1960s, there were reports of drowsiness, nystagmus, hyperreflexia, ankle clonus and clumsiness in a few subjects. Similar neurological features as well as excessive sweating and an agitated delirium were noted in patients taking MAOIs with L-tryptophan and an MAOI–TCA combination, even in the absence of an elevation in blood pressure. Animal studies suggested that serotonin may be responsible. Thus rats given the combination of tranylcypromine and L-tryptophan developed hyperactivity (Grahame-Smith, 1971). Tetrabenazine, which inhibits the uptake and storage of serotonin and other amines by intraneuronal vesicles, greatly increases the speed of onset and development of this hyperactivity, while pretreatment with a decarboxylase inhibitor which blocks the synthesis of serotonin from its precursor 5-hydroxytryptophan prevents the development of the syndrome.

Sternbach (1991) reviewed reports of 38 patients said to have the 'serotonin syndrome'. In 16 the syndrome was due to a combination of an MAOI with L-tryptophan (with or without lithium), 14 patients had been treated with fluoxetine and an MAOI, five with fluoxetine and L-tryptophan, and there were three miscellaneous cases. Among those who took lithium the blood levels were within normal limits. The main clinical features were restlessness (45%), confusion (42%), myoclonus (34%), hyperreflexia (29%), diaphoresis (26%), shivering (26%), tremor (26%), hypomania (21%), diarrhoea (16%) and incoordination (13%). The delineation of the syndrome is unclear and it may be mild in some cases but severe in others, and there may be overlap with the neuroleptic malignant syndrome.

Usually the syndrome resolves within 24 hours once the offending drugs are withdrawn. Supportive measures include cooling for hyperthermia, anticonvulsants for seizures and, if required, artificial ventilation for respiratory insufficiency. If supportive measures are ineffective, serotonin receptor blockade by methysergide or propranolol (which blocks certain 5-HT receptors as well as beta-adrenergic ones) should be considered, although there are no controlled studies of these drugs.

Sexual dysfunction

Adverse effects on sexual function are probably a direct consequence of serotonin agonism, but are often only reported at a later stage when the depression has improved. For men the placebo-adjusted incidence of abnormal ejaculation and orgasm is as follows: paroxetine 13%, sertraline 13%, venlafaxine 12% and nefazodone 1%. For paroxetine the placebo-adjusted rates of other sexual dysfunctions, such as erectile impotence was 10%, and libido was decreased in 3%. SSRI-associated sexual dysfunction in women was under 2% (Preskorn, 1995). Because of its low incidence of sexual problems and different mechanism of action, nefazodone (and by implication trazodone) may be considered in those who develop SSRI-associated sexual dysfunction.

Cardiovascular effects

The only consistent cardiovascular effect of the SSRIs has been a minor degree of slowing of the pulse rate. While TCAs slow cardiac conduction via a quinidine-like effect on the His–Purkinje system, this is not the SSRI mechanism (Fisch, 1985). Thus SSRIs are much safer in overdose than TCAs and are usually preferred in those with cardiovascular disease. Since SSRIs do not block adrenergic receptors, postural hypotension does not occur.

Anticholinergic effects

Although SSRIs do not have anticholinergic side-effects, dry mouth, blurred vision and constipation have been reported. The mechanisms probably involve noradrenergic innervation of the salivary glands, and serotonergic innervation of the pupil and gut. Urinary retention has not been reported.

Monoamine oxidase inhibitors

The enzyme monoamine oxidase (MAO) inactivates the amine neurotransmitters serotonin, noradrenaline and dopamine. The observation that iproniazid is a monoamine oxidase inhibitor (MAOI) was an important contribution to the amine hypothesis of depression. However, a single dose of phenelzine will give 80% MAO inhibition in a few hours, but the antidepressant effect takes weeks to develop. As with TCAs, the initial explanation for MAOI action of a deficiency of synaptic monoamines was followed by a later theory of down-regulation of post-synaptic receptors, which takes a few weeks to develop and is thought to be associated with recovery (see page 112).

The MAOI clorgyline was found to discriminate between two forms of the enzyme, MAO-A and MAO-B, which led to studies of the distributions and specificities of the two forms. Both MAO-A and MAO-B are found in the cerebral cortex (approximately 45% MAO-A, 55% MAO-B), intestine (75% MAO-A, 25% MAO-B), liver, stomach and kidney. MAO-A is selectively located in the adrenergic and serotonergic nerve endings in the CNS and peripheral sympathetic system, while platelets contain only MAO-B. Serotonin and noradrenaline are broken down almost exclusively by MAO-A but adrenaline, dopamine and tyramine are catabolised by both MAO-A and MAO-B. Clinical studies indicate that while MAO-A inhibitors such as clorgyline have antidepressant activity, MAO-B inhibitors may not, although deprenyl (later relabelled selegiline), an MAO-B inhibitor, may have antidepressant effect if given in sufficient dose (Mann *et al*, 1989).

The chemical structures of phenelzine and tranylcypromine are similar to dextroamphetamine (Fig. 4.5) which has a catecholamine-releasing effect on nerve endings. Thus in addition to inhibiting MAO, the amine-releasing properties of MAOIs may also contribute to their therapeutic and stimulant effects. A third possible mechanism of action, resembling that of TCAs and SSRIs, is inhibition of amine reuptake. This is particularly important for tranylcypromine.

MAOIs may be classified in three ways: (i) selectivity for MAO-A or MAO-B; (ii) hydrazides (-C-N-N configuration, see Fig. 4.5) or non-hydrazides. Non-hydrazides such as tranylcypromine were thought to be less toxic to the liver, but may have a greater risk of hypertensive reactions; (iii) whether the inhibition of MAO is reversible or irreversible. Moclobemide is a reversible inhibitor.

Pharmacokinetics

Absorption and first-pass metabolism

All the MAOIs are rapidly absorbed. Peak plasma levels occur within 1–3 hours when the risk of postural hypotension is greatest. Steady-state plasma levels of phenelzine increase over the first 6–8 weeks of treatment suggesting that the drug inhibits its own metabolism.

Metabolism

As noted previously MAOIs are structurally similar to the catecholamines and amphetamine and up to 20% of tranylcypromine may be converted to amphetamine. Phenelzine is converted to beta-phenylethylamine and phenylacetic acid. Metabolites may be responsible for some of the stimulant effects that occur with MAOIs as well as their potential for abuse and dependence. Irreversible MAOIs like phenelzine are consumed by their mechanism of action, that is irreversibly binding to MAO and deactivating it, and they have short half-lives ranging from 2 to 4 hours. Although moclobemide is a reversible MAOI it also has a short half-life of two hours. The plasma levels of these drugs show considerable variability. There is no clear relationship between plasma levels and MAO inhibition and plasma drug monitoring is of no value.

ADRs of the MAOIs

Daytime drowsiness and dizziness due to postural hypotension are common at the start of treatment. Anticholinergic ADRs such as blurred vision, dry

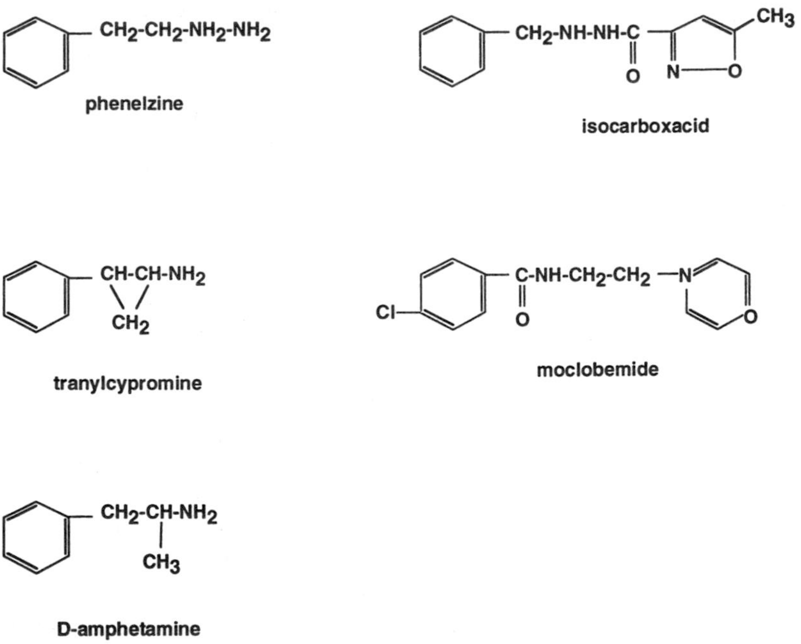

Fig. 4.5 Chemical structure of some MAOIs and D-amphetamine.

mouth and constipation also occur but less commonly than with the TCAs. Hepatocellular jaundice is a rare complication as are peripheral neuropathy and bone marrow suppression.

Cardiovascular ADRs

MAOIs can both lower and raise blood pressure. The hypotensive effect of MAOIs is common when treatment is started and may limit the dose taken because tolerance sometimes does not develop. Both supine and erect blood pressures are lowered so the postural component is less than with the TCAs.

A rarer ADR is the hypertensive crisis or 'cheese reaction' explained as follows: (i) The breakdown of monoamines such as tyramine in the gut, liver and blood is blocked by MAOIs, therefore in the presence of an MAOI there is enhanced absorption of tyramine from the intestine, and reduced catabolism elsewhere; (ii) certain foods (see Box 4.1) are rich in tyramine. Indirectly acting sympathomimetic agents such as tyramine and ephedrine release stored catecholamines from the neuronal vesicles; (iii) because of inhibition of neuronal MAO located in the mitochondria, the vesicles in the neurones will have accumulated large amounts of noradrenaline. Indirectly acting amines release these large quantities of noradrenaline from the vesicle stores into the synapse stimulating post-ganglionic sympathetic adrenergic neurones and so causing the hypertension; (iv) an MAOI itself might function as an indirect sympathomimetic agent. This might explain why hypertension can sometimes occur during MAOI treatment in the absence of a dietary insult.

Hypertensive reactions have varying degrees of severity. They usually have an abrupt onset from within minutes to up to three hours after the ingestion of an inappropriate food or medication. They frequently start with an occipital pounding headache which radiates, or with palpitations, nausea or vomiting. Apprehension, chills, sweating, restlessness, photophobia, neck stiffness, dilated pupils and a rise in blood pressure may occur. Typically during such a reaction systolic blood pressure may range from 150 to 220 mmHg and diastolic blood pressure from 100 to 130 mmHg. The headache will lessen in severity after an hour but a dull ache may persist. There may be persistent hypertension, alteration of consciousness, hyperpyrexia, convulsions and cerebral haemorrhage. The fatality rate has been estimated as 1 in every 8000 hypertensive reactions, or more generally as one per 100 000 patients treated with tranylcypromine (Davidson, 1992).

Treatment is with an alpha-adrenoceptor blocking agent such as phenoxybenzamine or phentolamine. Most emergency boxes should contain these drugs but if they are not available, chlorpromazine, with its powerful alpha-adrenergic blocking activity can be used. Parenterally, chlorpromazine is licensed only for intramuscular use and should not be given intravenously.

Drug interactions and food restrictions

MAOIs interact with a variety of drugs and foodstuffs (reviewed by Bernstein, 1995*b*). When MAOIs are dispensed, the pharmacist provides the patient with an information card which lists foods and medicines to be avoided. Patients should carry this card at all times and show it to any doctor or dentist who treats them. The two most serious reactions are hypertensive crises and the serotonin syndrome. Hypertensive reactions may occur with stimulants (e.g. dexamphetamine, methylphenidate and pemoline), diet pills (fenfluramine and diethylpropion), other sympathomimetics (ephedrine and adrenergic-based bronchodilators used in asthma), and over-the-counter cold cures, nose-drops, nasal decongestants and cough syrups (containing phentermine, phenylephrine and phenylpropanolamine). Patients with asthma preferably should not take an MAOI, but if they do, only steroid-based inhalers should be used.

A MAOI may interact with another MAOI producing hypertension, and severe reactions have been reported with the phenelzine–tranylcypromine combination. L-dopa may result in CNS stimulation as well as hypertension. Both hypotension and hypertension can occur with TCAs. Guanethidine initially releases noradrenaline from nerve endings; thus MAOI-treated patients who are given guanethidine may experience a hypertensive reaction followed by severe hypotension and the same may occur with clonidine. Hypotension has been reported with phenothiazines presumably through the mechanism of alpha-adrenergic blockade. A similar mechanism may explain the hypotension which occurs with an MAOI and spinal anaesthesia.

The serotonin syndrome may be severe and fatalities have been reported. This may occur with opiates, particularly pethidine (both CNS excitatory and depressant effects may occur, leading to coma and death), but may also happen with any of the SSRIs, clomipramine, imipramine and sumatriptan. The effects of antidiabetic agents such as insulin, metformin and the sulphonylureas may be enhanced and there is a small risk of hypoglycaemia. The effect of anticonvulsants may be antagonised. There may be increased effects with alcohol, benzodiazepines, barbiturates, and chloral hydrate resulting in excessive sedation.

Although emergency surgery with a general anaesthetic can be safely accomplished if a patient is on an MAOI, there are several potential interactions. Halothane and enflurane may result in muscle stiffness and hyperpyrexia, and as MAOIs decrease plasma pseudocholinesterase activity there may be prolonged muscle relaxation and muscle paralysis with muscle relaxants such as suxamethonium and d-tubocurarine. Anaesthetists may prefer to delay elective surgery to permit a one- to two-week drug washout.

Dietary restrictions while taking MAOIs

Tyramine-rich foods (Box 4.1) should be avoided while the patient is on an MAOI and for two weeks after the drugs have been stopped (Bernstein, 1995*b*).

This list is somewhat more extensive than that in the BNF, which similarly advises patients to eat fresh foods. Foods that could be stale or 'going off' should be avoided and this is especially important with meat, fish, poultry or offal. The BNF also advises patients to avoid game. Despite this extensive list, serious hypertensive crises among those taking MAOIs are rare although milder hypertensive reactions are more common. The risk of harm is small in comparison with the risk of suicide associated with depressive episodes.

Individual MAOIs

Phenelzine

This was the MAOI used in the Medical Research Council (1965) study of depression which found phenelzine to be no more effective than placebo. Since then it has been suggested that higher doses are needed to achieve an antidepressant effect. It may be more useful in atypical depression and as an anxiolytic, particularly for phobic anxiety (Tyrer *et al*, 1973). Although tolerance does not develop, when the drug is stopped the original anxiety symptoms may reappear. A dose of 30–90 mg per day is used.

Isocarboxazid

In a placebo-controlled trial of 130 anxious depressed patients isocarboxazid was more effective than placebo. This particularly applied to patients with major depression and those with atypical depression showing reversed vegetative symptoms, such as weight gain and excessive sleep (Davidson *et al*, 1988). The usual dose is 20–50 mg per day.

Tranylcypromine

This is a non-hydrazine which some suggest may increase the risk of a 'cheese' reaction. Some regard it as the most potent antidepressant of the MAOIs and it also inhibits neuronal amine reuptake as well as having amine-releasing properties like amphetamine. The usual dose is 10–30 mg per day.

Selegiline

This selective MAOI inhibits MAO-B. In the UK it is licensed only for use in Parkinsonism because it reduces the catabolism of dopamine. It may be used alone or with a lower dose of L-dopa than would otherwise be required. Its efficacy in depression was shown by Mann *et al* (1989).

Recent case reports (reviewed by Livingston, 1995) have brought into question the safety of the newer selective MAOIs, particularly selegiline, in combination with other drugs. Life-threatening paroxysmal hypertension has been induced by noradrenaline, a condition known as pseudo-phaeochromocytoma. Medications known to cause this include those

Box 4.1. Foods to be avoided while taking an MAOI drug

Cheeses (particularly mature cheese).
Broad (sava) bean pods (green beans may be eaten).
Alcohol, especially chianti, vermouth, wines, draught beer.
Sausages, pepperoni, salami, liver, spam, canned ham.
Pickled herring, sardines, anchovies.
Any non-fresh or fermented meat, fish or protein product.
Yeast extract (e.g. Marmite), brewers' yeast, meat extracts
    (e.g. Bovril).
Sauerkraut, banana peel.

affecting both the catecholamine and indoleamine systems, for example terbutaline, phenylephrine, fluoxetine and TCAs. In addition, Bernstein (1995*b*) recommends avoiding the use of SSRIs with the reversible MAOI moclobemide. Symptoms include paroxysmal hypertension, vaso-constricton, confusion, abdominal pain and sweating. Livingston (1995) concluded that even for the selective MAOIs patients need to moderate their dietary consumption of amine-rich foodstuffs such as matured cheese and yeast extract, and be advised about other drug preparations.

Reversible MAOI

Moclobemide

Moclobemide is a reversible inhibitor of MAO-A; the chemical structure is shown in Fig. 4.5. Reversible inhibition permits any excess tyramine to displace the drug from its binding site on the enzyme and so enables intestinal mucosa MAO to catabolise tyramine, making a hypertensive reaction about 10 times less likely compared with tranylcypromine. Because of the reversible inhibition and short half-life, the drug should be prescribed twice daily and its effects decline rapidly once the drug is stopped. This contrasts with the irreversible MAO inhibition of traditional MAOIs because once the enzyme is irreversibly inhibited, it may take several weeks to regenerate new enzyme.

Large trials have shown moclobemide to be as effective as TCAs, with a similarly delayed onset of action (7–21 days; Baumhackl *et al*, 1989; Versiani *et al*, 1989). In many studies the TCA doses were not increased to recommended maximums and fewer than expected patients in the TCA groups responded (*Drug and Therapeutics Bulletin*, 1994). Among the elderly one study found it to be less efficacious than nortriptyline, but anticholinergic and orthostatic side-effects were less common (Nair *et al*, 1995). The main side-effects are insomnia and nausea occurring in about 10% of patients. The incidence of postural hypotension is low, about 1%, which is much less than with traditional MAOIs. Moclobemide has no appreciable effect on body weight and lacks cardiotoxic effects or the stimulant effect of older MAOIs.

Studies of 2300 patients taking moclobemide without dietary restrictions reported no tyramine-related hypertensive reaction (*Drug and Therapeutics Bulletin*, 1994). Patients should avoid eating large amounts of tyramine-rich foods, for example, more than 50 g of strong ripe cheese. The risk of a cheese reaction can be minimised by taking moclobemide a sufficient period after meals when any ingested tyramine would have been absorbed. There are no reports of interaction between alcohol and therapeutic doses of moclobemide.

Cimetidine blocks moclobemide metabolism and so reduces the dose requirement of moclobemide by 50%. In therapeutic doses combinations of moclobemide with a tricyclic appear safe but combinations with an SSRI are probably best avoided (Amrein *et al*, 1992; *Drug and Therapeutics Bulletin*, 1994; Bernstein, 1995*b*). In patients who took overdoses, of 13 patients who took moclobemide alone, 12 required no treatment, but there were five fatalities when the moclobemide was taken together with an overdose of clomipramine or citalopram (Neuvonen *et al*, 1993). As moclobemide is short-acting, interactions can be avoided if moclobemide is stopped 24 hours before another drug is given. The recommended starting dose is 150 mg b.d. with a maximum daily dose of 600 mg.

Other substances used in the treatment of depression

Antipsychotic drugs used as antidepressants

Antipsychotic drugs may also be effective antidepressants (reviewed by Robertson & Trimble, 1982; Willner, 1995). Early placebo and TCA comparator trials had shown that chlorpromazine, thioridazine and oral flupenthixol are all effective antidepressants. However the risk of extrapyramidal effects may be greater during a depressive episode and they are not used as a first-line treatment.

Thioridazine is sometimes used in combination with an antidepressant for the management of insomnia, anxiety and agitation, particularly in the early weeks of treatment. In contrast to the benzodiazepines it is not addictive. Some patients with ideas of reference may benefit from a small dose of an antipsychotic drug. Chlorpromazine may be used in severe agitated or psychotic depression (see page 196).

Lithium

In spite of its proven value in mania, and as a prophylactic agent (see chapter 2), there are little data on its acute antidepressant effects. A placebo-controlled trial showed it to be as effective as imipramine, but antidepressant effects did not appear until the third week (Worral *et al*, 1979). In the USA, the Food and Drug Administration does not recognise it as an antidepressant. Its main use in acute treatment of depression is in augmentation (see page 208).

Treatment of a depressive episode

Depressive episodes are common. Their treatment is probably the most frequent single intervention made by general adult psychiatrists, and it is also among the more common interventions made by general practitioners. The initial psychiatric interview will establish whether the patient's disorder satisfies diagnostic criteria for a depressive episode, while the degree of the patient's distress will usually determine whether or not antidepressant treatment should be instituted. For a depressive episode the indication for antidepressant treatment is clear, but for cyclothymia, dysthymia and other persistent mood disorders the indications for treatment are less certain. The presenting depressive symptoms should always be carefully listed at the initial diagnostic assessment as monitoring these symptoms will provide the best guide to progress, or lack of it.

The three treatment modalities are antidepressant drugs, ECT (chapter 5) and cognitive–behavioural therapy (chapter 6). Patient preference, the severity of the depression, the presence of melancholic features, suicidal ideation, the availability of cognitive–behavioural therapy and other factors will determine which treatment is selected. Although data are not available, most patients with depressive episodes presenting to psychiatric clinics are treated with medication.

Non-compliance and reluctance to take antidepressants

The psychiatrist's task is to ensure that patients who agree to take an antidepressant receive an *efficacious* drug, in *sufficient dose* and for an *adequate duration* of time. This might seem obvious, but it is often surprisingly difficult to implement. Many factors may interfere with the administration of a course of antidepressants, and it is essential to seek out information in the follow-up interviews concerning the patient's degree of compliance.

Illness factors which contribute to non-compliance with antidepressants include: lack of motivation, feelings of hopelessness, and a mild degree of cognitive impairment leading to forgetfulness. Drug factors include side-effects and the delay in antidepressant effect. Patient factors include a distaste for taking any medication, and misinformation, for example, the belief that it is addictive or that taking an antidepressant might lead to a change of personality. Life events may also contribute. Depressive episodes, whether or not accompanied by recent life events, appear to respond equally well to antidepressants, but patients who have experienced a recent life event may find this approach difficult to understand. They may question how a tablet can help in a social crisis, feel such an approach is inappropriate, and refuse to take medication.

The management of non-compliance requires careful consideration and it is usually possible to help patients through this impasse. The initial assessment interview establishes a relationship and this should be of a quality such that the patient is able to trust the doctor's advice concerning treatment. Eliciting the possible reasons for non compliance or reluctance to take medication, which may include other factors than those described above, is essential. Excessive pressure on the patient to take medication may prove counter-productive, so that a patient may drop out of treatment altogether. On occasion severely suicidal patients will need a compulsory hospital admission. In general it is best to continue to offer reviews in the clinic as patients who initially refuse medication may later change their minds. Sometimes at an appropriate moment it is helpful to point out that the natural history may be lengthy. For example Braftos & Haug (1968) state that the average duration of an untreated depressive episode is about eight months. The prospect of relief of symptoms in 3–6 weeks may lead some patients to reconsider an earlier decision not to take an antidepressant.

Prescribing

Medication is part of an overall management plan and most patients appreciate a supportive relationship and education about their psychiatric disorder while taking a course of antidepressants. It is helpful to explain at the outset that some guesswork is involved in prescribing and that changes in both the dosage and the drug may be necessary. Patients should be advised to telephone the clinic if they experience unwanted side effects, as dealing with such problems speedily may diminish the risks of defaulting from treatment. An essential component of the treatment programme is the communication of important items of information about antidepressant drugs. Though verbal information may be reinforced by drug leaflets these cannot be relied on alone because depressed patients may not be motivated to read the leaflets, or be able to concentrate well enough to take in their contents.

Information for patients

Doctors should convey the following information to patients and, if appropriate, to their relatives or carers as well.

(1) All antidepressants have side-effects. The patient should know the common side-effects of the drug prescribed. Judgement is required to assess the amount of detail that should be conveyed. This is good practice and is also part of the right to information in the Patients' Charter. From December 1998 European Community legislation will require that patients are provided with detailed written information about dispensed drugs.

(2) Improvement in mood and other symptoms may be noticed only after one to three weeks and may not be maximal until two months or more. Patients may be reassured to hear that some symptoms such as poor sleep and depressed mood may improve relatively early, although other symptoms such as lack of interest and pessimistic thoughts may take longer to disappear.

(3) Emotional lability is common during improvement and may be very distressing. Patients should be told that during recovery 'bad days' may occur and on these occasions they may feel as depressed as ever. This distress may incline a patient to stop treatment. It is helpful to explain that these days gradually become less frequent and eventually disappear.

(4) Side-effects commonly diminish after a few days, but if they persist, a lower dose or an alternative antidepressant may be used. There is no need for patients to soldier on in the face of severe side-effects.

(5) Stopping antidepressants at any time may precipitate a relapse. This is most likely to occur soon after the relief of symptoms. Even well-informed individuals may want to stop their antidepressants once the depression has resolved. Although life events are important in precipitating depression, in their search for a cause patients often blame an event which has occurred in the past and is unlikely to recur, but at the same time they fail to appreciate their individual susceptibility to depression. Most patients need to be specifically counselled not to stop their antidepressants prematurely and some may require this advice to be repeated.

(6) The names of the drug which resulted in improvement as well as the names of those drugs which could not be tolerated should be noted by the patient. A drug which has proved to be beneficial in one episode is likely to be helpful during future episodes. The patient may encounter other doctors in the future and previous records may not always be available.

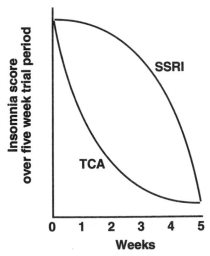

Fig. 4.6 Representation of improvement in insomnia scores.

Factors influencing the choice of an antidepressant

A variety of factors may influence antidepressant drug choice. These include side-effects, certain clinical features, and comorbid medical disorders.

Many patients with depression will respond to a TCA or an SSRI; the BNF (1996) states these drugs should be used in preference to the older MAOIs because of the MAOIs' dietary restrictions and risks of interactions with other medications. For patients in primary care the majority will probably respond to the first antidepressant they receive, but in secondary care there is a higher proportion of resistant cases. As both TCAs and SSRIs are probably equally effective in depression, the decision will depend more on the side-effect profile of each drug and which drug best meets the patient's particular needs. It is better to become thoroughly acquainted with a few drugs in each class than to use a bewildering array of different drugs on an occasional basis.

The dose of TCAs needs to be titrated gradually upwards, with anticholinergic and sedative side-effects sometimes being a limiting factor. Most patients can be started on 50–75 mg of a TCA such as amitriptyline, dothiepin or doxepin with increments over the course of a few weeks to the full therapeutic dose. For patients who are overly affected by side-effects, starting doses can be very low, for example amitriptyline or doxepin 10 mg daily with small weekly increments, at least until the patient's concern over side-effects has diminished. MAOIs should also be gradually titrated up. Some SSRIs are prescribed in their full therapeutic dose from the start.

Sedation and weight gain

Sleep disorder is a cardinal feature of depression and if insomnia is a distressing symptom, a tricyclic taken at night will provide rapid relief of initial insomnia, interrupted sleep and early waking. Although an SSRI will help insomnia once the depression has resolved, during the first weeks of treatment a tricyclic has a definite advantage as shown in Fig. 4.6. Sedative tricyclics include amitriptyline, dothiepin and doxepin. Trimipramine is probably the most sedative TCA. Trazodone, which is not a tricyclic, is also strongly sedative.

Daytime drowsiness particularly in the mornings is sometimes associated with the use of high doses of TCAs at night. In these cases dose reduction, or giving divided doses during the day may be helpful. Alternatively the patient can be switched to an SSRI.

Some patients express a fear of weight gain and most TCAs can cause weight gain. In these cases an SSRI may be helpful, as fluvoxamine and fluoxetine may cause weight loss, while citalopram, paroxetine and sertraline are neutral in this respect.

Anxiety, obsessions and atypical depression

The presence of obsessional symptoms or comorbid obsessional disorder may favour a serotonergic TCA such as clomipramine or an SSRI. The use of irreversible MAOIs in the treatment of atypical depression, anxiety depression, agoraphobia with depression or social phobia has become less common. Panic disorder responds to both TCAs and SSRIs.

Psychotic depression

Making the distinction between psychotic and non-psychotic depression has implications for treatment because psychotic depression usually responds poorly to an antidepressant drug as a single treatment. Psychotic depression may be overlooked and should be suspected in any case of severe or resistant depression, and among the elderly. Charney & Nelson (1981) found that in unipolar depression with delusions only 22% of patients responded to a TCA alone, compared with 80% of the patients with non-delusional depression. However, 82% of the delusional depressives responded to ECT. An antipsychotic drug alone gave a response rate of 31% while a combination of an antipsychotic with a TCA gave a 68% response rate.

A meta-analysis of treatment response in psychotic depression used "effect size" for comparison. Effect size is the improvement in depression rating score divided by the standard deviation of the initial severity level. Parker *et al* (1992) found that the effect size was highest for ECT at 2.3 (based on 21 studies), while a combination of an antipsychotic and a TCA had an effect size of 1.6 (based on 12 studies) and a TCA alone had an effect size of 1.2 (28 studies). There was a tendency for bilateral ECT to be superior to unilateral ECT in this meta-analysis.

Most cases of psychotic depression will require in-patient treatment. If a patient is not eating or drinking sufficient fluids or is suicidal, ECT is likely to be the first line of treatment. Otherwise an antidepressant may be combined with an antipsychotic drug. Price *et al* (1983) reported that some patients with psychotic depression who were already taking a combination of chlorpromazine with a TCA responded well to lithium augmentation.

Antidepressants and suicide

The newer antidepressants including the SSRIs, taken in overdose, are less toxic than the older tricyclics (Henry *et al*, 1995), but the importance of this can be overstated. Some authors had gone so far as to say that SSRIs should be the antidepressant of first choice because of their safety in overdose, but more recent studies have shown that prescribing of newer antidepressants is not associated with lower suicide rates.

The largest study (Isacsson *et al*, 1994*a*) examined 3400 patients who committed suicide in Sweden. At autopsy, toxicological screening was done for all antidepressants, while at a national level, the type, number and dose of prescribed antidepressants were obtained from the National Corporation of Pharmacies. Antidepressants were detected in only 585 (17% of the total) of the 3400 cases of which 190 (6% of the total) had toxic concentrations. Thus 94% of suicides did not have toxic antidepressant concentrations. Although the study was done before SSRIs were widely prescribed in Sweden, it shows that the newer antidepressants mianserin and moclobemide had significantly higher standardised mortality ratios (SMRs) for suicide (2.0 and 1.8 respectively) while lofepramine had a significantly lower SMR of 0.14. In a second study in the UK based on data from the General Practice Research Database (Jick *et al*, 1995), 172 598 patients received 1 198 303 prescriptions and there were 143 suicides. Table 4.4 (column 2) shows the adjusted relative risk of suicide for each antidepressant; these were raised only for fluoxetine and mianserin. It also shows (column 1) (from Henry *et al*, 1995) how the various antidepressants compare in relation to risk of fatal poisoning. The difference is due to the fact that fatal antidepressant poisoning constitutes only a small proportion of completed suicides, and patients kill themselves by a variety of other means.

There are several possible biases that could explain these results. Suicidal features at initial assessment might favour the prescription of a newer, non-toxic antidepressant so that patients are non-randomly allocated to different antidepressant types. Those at high risk might then subsequently kill themselves by other means such as a paracetamol overdose or by hanging. Alternatively, some of the new antidepressants might be less effective in preventing suicide. Available studies cannot distinguish between these possibilities.

The problem is compounded by high levels of comorbidity, which might increase suicide risk. Isometsa *et al* (1994) found that among 71 Finnish cases of suicide with a diagnosis of major depression, only 11 had no

Table 4.4 Antidepressants by deaths from fatal poisoning and all causes of suicide

Antidepressant	Fatal poisonings per million defined daily doses[1] (95% CI)	Adjusted relative risk for all causes of suicide[2] (95% CI)
Lofepramine	0.08 (0.03–0.11)	0.5 (0.2–1.6)
Amitryptiline	1.64 (1.46–1.74)	0.7 (0.4–1.2)
Imipramine	1.47 (1.2–1.74)	0.7 (0.3–1.7)
Clomipramine	0.38 (0.25–0.54)	0.8 (0.4–1.8)
Dothiepin	1.54 (1.42–1.63)	1.0 (reference drug)
Doxepin	1.40 (0.98–1.88)	1.0 (0.3–3.7)
Trazodone	0.6 (0.21–0.99)	1.2 (0.4–4.0)
Flupenthixol	Not available	1.5 (0.7–3.0)
Mianserin	0.2 (0.22–0.35)	1.6 (0.7–3.3)
Fluoxetine	0.02 (0–0.07)	3.8 (1.7–8.6)

1. Henry *et al*, 1995.
2. Jick *et al*, 1995.

comorbidity. The remainder (85%) were affected by physical illness, substance misuse, personality disorder and anxiety disorder. Of these 71 suicides with major depression, 44 (67%) had received no antidepressant treatment. Isacsson *et al* (1994*b*) suggested that the major problem in treating suicidal patients is inadequate or no antidepressant therapy rather than the use of any particular antidepressant type. Suicide prevention entails more than choosing a particular drug and may involve hospital admission, the use of ECT, and other measures (see chapter 11).

Comorbid medical disorders

Because of their more favourable side-effect profile the SSRIs are the preferred drug for depression comorbid with some medical disorders. In cardiovascular disease the SSRIs and mianserin are relatively non-cardiotoxic. In patients with glaucoma or prostatism, in whom anti-cholinergic side-effects must be avoided, SSRIs are the treatment of choice. In cases of epilepsy with depression it is thought that the SSRIs are less epileptogenic than the TCAs. In hepatic and renal disease, with impairment of drug clearance, tricyclics have an advantage because their plasma levels can be monitored and so toxic accumulations may be avoided. Of the few studies comparing different antidepressants in medical disorders, most have been in the area of cardiovascular disease.

Driving

Patients frequently ask whether antidepressants will affect their driving. Depression itself, particularly in the presence of impaired concentration or retardation, is more likely to impair psychomotor performance than antidepressant drugs and there have been only a few studies which separate out the effects of the depression from those caused by drugs. The topic has been reviewed by Edwards (1995*a*) and Freeman & O'Hanlon (1995). The latter authors reported four studies which showed that treatment with imipramine improved psychomotor performance and memory in conjunction with depressive symptoms, whereas those whose depressive symptoms failed to respond to the antidepressant continued to show impaired psychomotor performance.

Among healthy volunteers who take a tricyclic, performance is impaired initially but tolerance for the drug soon develops so that by the seventh day there is no difference from placebo. Tolerance for these effects has been observed for clomipramine, dothiepin, doxepin, mianserin and maprotiline. SSRIs cause less initial sedation and impairment than TCAs on tests of critical flicker fusion, choice reaction time, memory and simulated car tracking (Edwards, 1995*b*). Older drivers may be at greater risk from TCAs. In road trials in specially instrumented cars driven around closed circuits, single doses of antidepressants such as mianserin, trazodone, amitriptyline and dothiepin may increase the stopping distance of a car travelling at 70 m.p.h. by up to 10 feet.

Affective disorder may contribute to road traffic accidents; patients with depression concentrate poorly, those with mania may drive recklessly or at great speed and patients sometimes commit suicide in fatal accidents. The overall contribution of antidepressant drugs to road traffic accidents is probably small and the adverse effect of alcohol is greater than that of all other drugs combined. Everest *et al* (1989) analysed the body fluids from subjects in 1273 fatal road traffic accidents and found the following substance prevalence: alcohol 35%, cannabis 2.4%, benzodiazepines 1.6%, anticonvulsants 1.0%, phenothiazines 0.3%, hypnotics 0.3%, antidepressants 0.2%, decongestants 0.2% and other drugs 0.2%.

For most patients with depression, driving can continue but if patients report feeling impaired in respect of driving (whether due to depression or medication), they should not drive. Among the elderly there should be increased caution while taking antidepressants. Periods of greater risk are when first starting antidepressants, and after a dose increase, although sedative effects wear off. Patients should be cautioned about driving long distances or at speed while taking antidepressants.

The responsibility for determining fitness to drive rests with the driving and vehicle licensing authority (DVLA). All drivers have the responsibility to notify the DVLA of a relevant medical condition or any change in it. In most instances of depression drivers of group 1 vehicles (private cars and motor cycles) are permitted to continue to drive even if taking antidepressants, and only a small minority whose driving is likely to be affected need to notify the DVLA. However for drivers of group 2 vehicles (lorries, buses and taxis) who have a serious acute mental illness it is obligatory for the individual to inform the DVLA. The doctor should advise patients to do this and record in the case notes that this advice has been given. It should be noted that section 4 of the Road Traffic Act 1988 states, "A person who when driving a motor vehicle on a road or other public place is unfit to drive through drink or drugs is guilty of an offence".

Long-term treatment of depression

Terminology

Figure 4.7 shows the natural history of a depressive episode with response to treatment shown by the dotted line. Remission refers to alleviation of symptoms during the natural history of the episode while recovery implies that the natural history of the particular episode is past. Relapse means a recrudescence of symptoms during the episode; recurrence refers to a different episode. Figure 4.7 illustrates the three different phases of treatment: acute, continuation and maintenance.

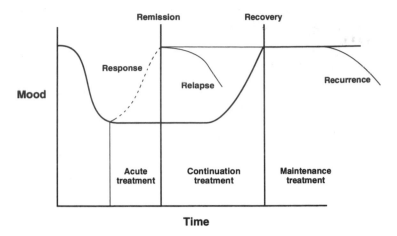

Fig. 4.7 Terms used to describe phases of treatment

Continuation therapy after an acute episode

Continuation drug therapy reduces the risk of relapse after remission; thus the relapse rate on placebo was 50% compared with 22% on a tricyclic over a two- to eight-month period (Kupfer & Frank, 1992). It is not known whether drug treatment shortens the episode or whether it only serves to relieve the symptoms until the episode has completed its natural course. Withdrawal of antidepressants in the six months following remission is more likely to be associated with relapse if there are residual depressive symptoms (Mindham *et al*, 1973; Faravelli *et al*, 1986). Individuals who are free of significant symptoms or who have returned to their usual level of inter-episode functioning, both for at least four months, have a lower rate of relapse when their continuation therapy is withdrawn than those who have not reached these levels (Prien & Kupfer, 1986; Frank *et al*, 1990). Other variables which increase the risk of relapse when antidepressants are withdrawn are: a history of previous episodes of depressive illness, poor social support and the presence of continuing social difficulties, such as unemployment or disharmony in interpersonal relationships (Prien, 1992).

The World Health Organization consensus statement (WHO, 1989) is for antidepressant medication to be continued for at least six months after remission, and then discontinued gradually, and the patient should be seen subsequently to check their mental state. A joint consensus statement from the Royal Colleges of Psychiatrists and General Practitioners also stated that the continuation phase should last from four to six months. Drugs should be continued near to the dose at which clinical response was achieved unless side-effects make this unacceptable; there is no reason for a steep reduction in dose with longer-term treatment (Paykel & Priest,

1992). Continuation treatment also reduces the relapse rate after ECT. Thus, prescribing a tricyclic after ECT was associated with a relapse rate of 20% compared with 50% with placebo.

Maintenance treatment (prophylaxis)

The decision to recommend prophylactic treatment depends on the risk of recurrence, the degree of disruption during an episode of depression, the risk of suicide associated with previous episodes and the patient's attitude to long-term treatment. Although there is a risk of recurrence after a first episode, in most cases an attempt is made to withdraw patients from their antidepressants. An exception may be made for illnesses that have been resistant to treatment.

From the available studies (reviewed by Angst, 1992) the only known predictors of a recurrent course are an early age of onset, a greater number of previous episodes, and bipolarity. Angst has shown that the time period between episodes tends to decrease with each successive episode, reaching a plateau after four to five bouts. This time period drops from three years following a first episode to 18 months after the third episode (Angst *et al*, 1973; see also page 40).

The WHO (1989) consensus statement recommends that maintenance treatment should be considered if a patient has had more than one severe episode of depressive illness, but especially if there have been several episodes in the previous five years. The antidepressant the patient is known to have responded to in the acute episode should also be used for maintenance. The Royal Colleges of Psychiatrists and General Practitioners have similar guidelines. The US Department of Health Care Policy and Research clinical practice guidelines recommend maintenance treatment for individuals who have had three or more episodes. The guidelines also recommend maintenance medication for individuals with two episodes who have one or more of the following characteristics: a family history of bipolar or recurrent depression; early onset of the first episode (before age 20); both episodes occurring in the previous three years, with sudden onset and being severe or life-threatening (Agency for Health Care Policy and Research, 1993). These guidelines have in common the recom-mendation for maintenance treatment after two or three depressive episodes. Particular patient characterisitcs, for example intervals of many years between episodes, may lead to modification of the recommendation. It is the task of the psychiatrist to discuss longer-term treatment issues and advise the patient once the recurrent nature of the disorder is apparent.

Efficacy of drug prophylaxis

There are few controlled trials of long-term maintenance treatment (in contrast to the large amount of data available for acute episodes)

(Montgomery & Montgomery, 1992). In part, this is due to the practical difficulty of conducting long-term studies, but there is also the ethical problem of how long a patient can be kept on placebo in a research trial. One of the longest studies of unipolar depression is that of Frank *et al* (1990) who reported the three-year survival figures for being free of recurrence as: imipramine with interpersonal psychotherapy 60%, imipramine alone 46%, interpersonal psychotherapy alone 31%, placebo 9% (see also chapter 6). After the three-year trial a small number of patients were randomised to receive imipramine or placebo and over a further two years imipramine appeared to prevent recurrence. Prien (1992) pooled data from four studies on imipramine and found that over a two-year period 78% of patients on placebo relapsed compared with 48% of those taking imipramine. Among the elderly, Jacoby & Lunn (1993) reported that dothiepin reduced the risk of relapse over a two-year period by a factor of 2.5 in comparison with placebo.

The SSRIs are also effective in long-term prophylaxis. Montgomery *et al* (1988) treated 220 patients with fluoxetine 40 mg over a one-year period and found that 57% of those on placebo had recurrences compared with 26% on fluoxetine. Franchini *et al* (1994) compared fluvoxamine to lithium in a two-year maintenance study following recovery from an episode of major depression, and found significantly more patients relapsed on lithium (eight (25%) of 32) compared with fluvoxamine (four (13%) of 32). A double-blind study of sertraline extending over 44 weeks showed 46% relapsed on placebo compared with 13% on sertraline (Doogan & Caillard, 1992). Claghorn (1991) reported on a one-year study of prophylactic paroxetine (10–50 mg daily) compared with imipramine (65–275 mg daily) and placebo, and the corresponding relapse rates were paroxetine 14%, imipramine 12% and placebo 23%.

Lithium may be the treatment of choice if there is a risk of mania as all antidepressants are capable of precipitating a manic episode. Lithium by itself has also been shown to have prophylactic effects in unipolar depression in some studies (Coppen *et al*, 1971) but the practice of adding lithium to an antidepressant for the purpose of prophylaxis in unipolar depression has not been shown to confer any additional benefit (Prien *et al*, 1984). The combination may be useful in a few bipolar patients who are at risk for both manic and depressive episodes if lithium alone has failed to prevent the depression.

Post (1993) has reported a "discontinuation-induced refractoriness" in respect of lithium; the term applies to patients who have been well maintained on long-term lithium therapy who relapse when the lithium is withdrawn and then fail to respond when lithium is reinstituted. The prevalence of this condition and whether it applies to other maintainance treatments are unknown.

Carbamazepine may also be helpful in prophylaxis. For example Stuppaeck *et al* (1994) treated 15 patients with recurrent unipolar depression with melancholia (four of whom had previously failed with lithium) with carbamazepine 600 mg daily. Over the next five years the number of episodes per year fell significantly from a pretreatment rate of 1.9 to 0.8; five patients had no further episodes.

The selection of which prophylactic drug to use will depend on the characteristics of the depression and a patient's ability to tolerate side-effects. In general the drug which has proved most useful during the acute phase and can be easily tolerated is also used in the long term. Most authorities now advocate using the drug in the same dose as was used to induce the remission, that is, "the dose to keep is the same as the dose to treat"; for example, Frank *et al* (1990) used imipramine 200 mg both in the acute phase and long term. Some authorities suggest a lower maintenance dosage, such as imipramine 50–100 mg, which may be better tolerated over the long term with fewer side-effects. Bridges (1992) argues against this and suggests that an excessive preoccupation with side-effects results in many patients taking doses that are too low and consequently suffering unnecessary depressive relapses. No prophylactic trial extends beyond five years yet many patients take antidepressants for 10 or more years and there are few guidelines as to how long prophylactic treatment should last. Prien (1992) suggests that after three to four years the issue of further treatment should be discussed with the patient to consider whether drug withdrawal should be undertaken.

Withdrawing antidepressants

Patients should be symptom-free for a minimum of four to six months before antidepressant withdrawal is attempted. With TCAs the time period over which to taper will depend on the dose, but TCAs should not be stopped abruptly. The usual period is one to two months, but this may be extended for patients who are on high doses. With SSRIs, when only one tablet a day is taken it is possible to stop abruptly because the long half-lives will ensure a phase of gradual clearing of the drug. Another option is to take the SSRI drug on alternate days for a period. The patient's mood needs to be observed carefully during drug withdrawal, both during out-patient visits and by family members. If depression returns, the antidepressant regime will need to be reinstated in full dosage and a further attempt to withdraw should be delayed for 6–12 months.

Treatment-resistant depression

There is no agreed definition of treatment-resistant depression (TRD). It is important to distinguish between treatment-resistant and treatment-intolerant patients in whom side-effects have prevented an adequate trial of pharmacotherapy. In research trials treatment resistance is usually defined by a failure to respond to a specified dose of an antidepressant for a specified period of time. For example, de Montigny *et al* (1981) provided a definition of TRD as "failure to respond to imipramine 150 mg daily or equivalent after three weeks". Most would regard this duration of treatment as too brief, and the dose too low. Thase & Rush (1995) describe a staging of the degree of resistance according to the amount of previous exposure to antidepressant treatments (Box 4.2). A favourable response to a treatment is usually defined as a 50% reduction in the patient's baseline depression rating scale score.

Prevalence and aetiology

The definition of TRD determines its prevalence. Nierenberg & Amsterdam (1990) estimated there were a total of 750 000 cases of TRD in the USA. A survey of Canadian psychiatrists reported that approximately 12% of their depressed patients had TRD (Chamowitz, 1991).

In their study of 55 subjects with two or more years of depression, Scott (1991) reported two predictors of chronicity. These were a greater time interval between the onset of symptoms and presentation to a clinician, together with neuroticism on the Eysenck Personality Questionnaire, and these findings replicated earlier observations by Keller (1986). Keller also noted that protracted recovery from depression was associated with secondary depression (depression secondary to some other psychiatric disorder such as anorexia nervosa or schizophrenia), a long previous episode, low family income, and older age.

A more recent Australian study found patients with TRD, as compared with those with treatment-responsive depression, were more likely to: be older, have longer episodes of depression, have a later age of onset for their first episode, and be more severely depressed. In terms of their phenomenology, 18% of the patients with TRD in this series had a major

---

Box 4.2 Staging of treatment-resistant depression (after Thase & Rush, 1995)

Stage   Previous treatment

0   Has not had a single adequate trial of medication

         Failure to respond to:
1   an adequate trial of one medication
2   an adequate trial of two medications with different profiles
3   stage 2 plus one augmentation strategy
4   stage 2 plus two augmentation strategies
5   stage 4 plus ECT

depressive episode (DSM–III–R criteria), 28% had melancholia, and 43% had psychotic depression (Wilhelm *et al*, 1994). The association of a comorbid personality disorder also increases the likelihood of treatment resistance (Black *et al*, 1988).

There is a significant prevalence of undetected physical illness as well as known medical disability among those with TRD. Depression may be a presenting feature of thyroid disease, carcinoma (particularly carcinoma of the pancreas), Huntingdon's disease, Parkinson's disease and other organic disorders. In a lithium augmentation trial of TCA-resistant depression, four (12%) of 34 patients had an undiagnosed physical disease which was unrecognised at the time of recruitment into the trial and only came to light later (Stein & Bernadt, 1993). MRI studies in TRD have recently demonstrated the presence of subcortical white matter hyperintense regions which suggest areas of cortical hypoperfusion (Coffee *et al*, 1990; Wilhelm *et al*, 1994). In the latter study, the number and severity of the hyperintense regions were correlated with a worse response to somatic treatment.

Management of TRD

The first step is to reconsider the diagnosis. It is important to confirm that the patient at some stage satisfied diagnostic criteria for a depressive episode since a partial response to treatment might mean that some key depressive symptoms such as sleep disturbance are alleviated. Does the patient have an undiagnosed medical illness? Physical investigations such as a full blood count, thyroid function and chest X-ray may be indicated. Are covert psychological factors operative? Psychological issues which have not been elicited during the original history-taking may emerge later, for example undisclosed sexual abuse, an oppressive marital relationship or work difficulties.

The patient's drug compliance must be assessed. This can be done on the basis of the history from the patient as well as an informant who might have kept a check on the patient's drug supply. The presence of side-effects and a blood antidepressant level are useful pointers. Admission to hospital may be considered in the more severe cases and this will assist in the assessment of drug compliance. Further information may be sought about possible alcohol abuse, personality disorder and undisclosed individual problems.

Further treatment strategies include high-dose monotherapy, switching to another antidepressant, augmentation strategies, ECT, and, very rarely, psychosurgery (see page 234).

High-dosage monotherapy

A recent study of patients with TRD showed that only 60% had received TCA treatment equivalent to 150 mg or more daily of imipramine or amitriptyline for three to four weeks. The 40% who received lower doses were younger, had more personality problems and less often had melancholia (Wilhelm *et al*, 1994). In most cases the failure to raise doses to higher levels was due to intolerance of side-effects. Numerous authors have advocated the use of high doses of TCAs; for example Quitkin (1985) suggested the use of imipramine 300 mg, or phenelzine 90 mg daily before a patient is designated as having TRD.

High doses of TCAs over longer periods are probably even more effective. Thus Greenhouse *et al* (1987) found that by five weeks only 25% of patients taking imipramine 150–300 mg responded, but by 17 weeks 75% had responded. This study suggests that if sufficient time is given, increases in dosage may be effective. Plasma drug levels should be monitored closely, as well as the ECG in which a prolonged QT_c is an important sign of toxicity. Although those who advocate TCAs in high dosage claim that this is safe, a survey of Canadian psychiatrists found that most doctors were reluctant to prescribe such high doses; thus 71% used doses of TCAs between 100 and 200 mg, only 7.7% gave doses above 200 mg daily and less than 1% ventured to prescribe doses of 300 mg or more daily (Chamowitz, 1991).

Switching to another antidepressant

When an antidepressant has been given an adequate trial and shown not to be working, switching to another antidepressant drug is often helpful. Switching antidepressants is one of the most common manoeuvres made in the clinic but its empirical basis is relatively weak. There are no studies of whether it is best to adopt a switching or an augmentation strategy in cases of TRD and guesswork is required. One suggestion is that among patients with a partial response to an antidepressant, augmentation should be tried, but if there has been little or no response, switching may be better. Increased vigilance is needed soon after the switch is made. Stopping the first antidepressant may exacerbate the depression because the first drug may have had a partial antidepressant effect. Starting the new drug exposes the patient to a different range of side-effects which the patient may not be able to tolerate. Most depressed patients will not be able to endure a drug-free washout period and so at the time of the switch there is also the risk of a toxic interaction between the two antidepressants. With a TCA for TCA substitution the new drug should be substituted for the old one gradually over a period of weeks, but when a mono-dose SSRI is being introduced it is started in full dosage.

A switch between different TCAs was a commonly used manoeuvre before the advent of the SSRIs. Controlled studies showed that this change was helpful only in around 10–30% of cases (Charney *et al*, 1986). The theory underlying this strategy was that some TCAs had a predominantly noradrenergic effect and others a serotonergic effect, and that switching from a predominantly noradrenergic drug such as imipramine or desipramine to a serotonergic drug such as amitriptyline or clomipramine (or vice versa) might help. The move sometimes worked, but its theoretical basis was never verified. As Nystrom & Halstrom (1987) point out, the critical factor may have been the use of any different antidepressant in the second trial period. For a few patients who cannot tolerate TCA anticholinergic side-effects a switch from a tertiary amine (such as amitriptyline) to a secondary amine such as desipramine or nortriptyline which has less severe anticholinergic side-effects may be helpful. If this is done, each week 50 mg of desipramine is substituted for 50 mg of amitriptyline, but the total TCA dosage is kept constant until the switch is complete.

Most authorities now advocate that the TCAs and SSRIs should be used in sequential mono-drug therapy. The majority of depressed patients will respond to one or other of the two classes of antidepressant. Early double-blind cross-over studies showed that 60–65% of patients who failed to respond to an SSRI responded to a TCA and similar percentages responded when switched from a TCA to an SSRI. Unfortunately, some of these studies were conducted with zimelidine, the SSRI which had to be withdrawn. More recently Beasley *et al* (1990) in a well-controlled double-blind trial showed that higher than usual doses of fluoxetine (mean 70 mg daily) led to a successful outcome in 51–62% of TCA-resistant subjects, and the drop-out rate for this regime was 18%, similar to that found when fluoxetine is used as the initial antidepressant. Patients who cannot tolerate a TCA may also benefit from switching to an SSRI and 80% of the TCA-intolerant subjects in the study of Beasley *et al* (1990) were able to tolerate fluoxetine.

Thase & Rush (1995) summarise studies of switching to another antidepressant in cases of TCA-resistant depression. Ten studies of switching to the older MAOIs showed a 40–70% response rate, and response rates of 40–60% are shown for trazodone, fluvoxamine and paroxetine. Fluvoxamine and fluoxetine have been the most studied drugs. It should be noted that for individual drugs the studies are few and that most of them have small patient numbers. For the few available studies on in-patients (presumably having more severe depressions), switching is less often successful.

By contrast to the relatively large database for TCA non-responders there are few data concerning SSRI non-responders. Bernstein (1995) argues that these patients should be switched to a TCA rather than another SSRI because all the SSRIs have a similar, selective action. There is only one controlled trial of switching from an SSRI to a TCA. Peselow *et al* (1989) treated 40 patients with paroxetine 20–50 mg daily and 15 subjects failed to respond. Of these 15 patients, 11 (73%) responded to six weeks of imipramine 150–300 mg daily. Switching from an SSRI to a TCA runs the risk of TCA toxicity, particularly in the case of switching from fluoxetine and paroxetine, and therefore the TCA should be introduced gradually.

Augmentation strategies

In general, an attempt is made to restrict prescribing to a single antidepressant. However a patient's failure to respond to adequate doses of different classes of antidepressant drugs, as described above, will on occasion warrant adding a second medication to the existing antidepressant drug. Lithium, triiodothyronine, an antipsychotic drug, and a second antidepressant such as an MAOI, a TCA or an SSRI have all been used.

Lithium augmentation

According to Thase & Rush (1995) lithium augmentation is the best-studied out-patient treatment strategy for TRD. The technique was first introduced by de Montigny *et al* (1981) who demonstrated a rapid resolution of symptoms in eight TCA-resistant subjects. There have been a number of open studies, but few randomised double-blind controlled reports. Stein & Bernadt (1993) found that of 34 TCA-resistant subjects, 44% responded to lithium 750 mg, while lithium 250 mg was no better than placebo (16% and 22% responding respectively). Katona *et al* (1995) first treated a large group of depressed patients ($n = 144$) with either lofepramine or fluoxetine; 62 patients were non-responders and they entered into the second phase of the study in which lithium and placebo augmentation were compared. Excluding those with low blood lithium levels, 15 (52%) of 29 subjects on lithium responded versus eight (25%) of 32 patients on placebo.

Price *et al* (1986) studied the effect of lithium augmentation in 84 depressed patients and the response to lithium was variable, with 31% of patients showing a good response, 25% a partial response, and the remainder showing no response. Dinan & Barry (1989) found that lithium augmentation was as effective as ECT in TCA-resistant depression; 10 of 15 (67%) lithium-treated patients responded and 11 of 15 (73%) of those given ECT responded. Improvement occurred earlier with lithium augmentation than with ECT.

The mechanism underlying lithium augmentation is uncertain and two contrasting theories have been proposed. The first is that lithium enhances serotonergic transmission and the second is that there is no augmentation, rather that lithium itself acts as an antidepressant, that patients who respond to the lithium–tricyclic combination represent those patients who might have responded to lithium alone (Worral *et al*, 1979). Thase *et al* (1989) observed recovery at two different rates among patients who respond to lithium augmentation. A few patients improve in the first two weeks which suggests an acute synergistic effect, and a second group of subjects improve after 6–8 weeks, which raises the possibility of a more slowly emerging direct antidepressant effect.

Lithium augmentation therapy requires close monitoring; symptoms of lithium toxicity may occur at normal serum lithium levels. Tremor and nausea are more frequent, as lithium and antidepressants may cause each independently. A trial should continue for at least eight weeks because there are a few late responders. In the face of non-response or severe side-effects, lithium augmentation should be stopped. Some elderly patients cannot tolerate lithium in the usual dose range, yet still derive therapeutic benefit, and in these cases lithium augmentation in lower than usual doses may be helpful (Kushnir, 1986).

Thyroid augmentation

Prange *et al* (1969) added triiodothyronine (T_3) to imipramine and noted a diminished latency of onset of action of imipramine. A controlled study by Goodwin *et al* (1982) in 12 patients previously unresponsive to amitriptyline or imipramine showed that the addition of T_3 in doses of 25 or 50 µg daily gave a statistically significant improvement in depression scores in nine subjects and this occurred within the first three days. Joffe & Singer (1990) found a significantly better response for T_3 (nine (53%) of 17) compared with thyroxine (four (19%) of 21) among TCA-resistant patients. In a later study, Joffe *et al* (1993) randomly assigned 50 TCA-resistant out-patients to either lithium, T_3 or placebo; 53% of the lithium group, 50% of the T_3 group and 19% of the placebo group responded. Targum *et al* (1984) found that thyroid augmentation was more useful in a small subgroup of patients who had an exaggerated thyrotropin response to thyrotropin-releasing hormone, although this finding has not been confirmed by others. Thyroxine is used to treat lithium-induced hypothyroidism. The rationale for preferring T_3 to thyroxine in augmentation is not clearly established. In their review, Thase & Rush (1995) summarise data from 10 studies and suggest that between 25 and 60% of TCA-resistant subjects will respond to augmentation with 25–50 µg T_3 daily. Side effects are infrequent; if the patient starts to lose weight, the dose of T_3 should be decreased.

L-tryptophan

This amino acid, a precursor of serotonin, was previously used as an adjunct to treatment with an MAOI or, less commonly, a tricyclic (usually clomipramine). Because it is mildly sedative it was also taken in a chocolate powder form in milk as a nightcap.

In April 1990, oral tryptophan preparations were withdrawn following reports of an eosinophilia–myalgia syndrome (EMS). This potentially fatal multi-system disorder is characterised by eosinophilia (more than 2000 eosinophils per mm³), severe myalgia, arthralgia, oedema and a rash together with lung and CNS involvement. EMS might have been due to an impurity in the L-tryptophan. The CSM (1994) recommends it should only be prescribed (i) by hospital specialists, (ii) for patients who have severe depressive illness of more than two year's duration, (iii) after adequate trials of standard drug treatments have failed, (iv) as an adjunct to other medication, and (v) it should not be given with an SSRI. Patients on tryptophan require regular eosinophil counts and surveillance for features of EMS, and prescribing is monitored by the product licence holder.

A combination of a TCA and an MAOI

This augmentation strategy was used more frequently in the past for cases of TRD. If the two drugs are not started together, the order to be followed must be an MAOI added to a TCA, as a hypertensive reaction is likely if the reverse order is used.

Phenelzine is the MAOI most commonly added to a TCA such as amitriptyline or trimipramine. Pare *et al* (1982) present evidence that the risk of a hypertensive reaction is reduced for patients taking combined antidepressants (MAOI and TCA) compared with MAOI monotherapy, and suggest that the tricyclic mechanism of action prevents the uptake of a secondary amine such as tyramine into the presynaptic neurone, and so stops tyramine from having a pressor effect. However, combinations of MAOIs with clomipramine, imipramine and all five SSRIs must be avoided because of the risk of the serotonin syndrome; there have been reports of fatalities with these combinations. There is no study showing that the combination of a TCA and an MAOI is more effective than either used separately.

Combining a TCA and an SSRI

The effect of combining an SSRI with a TCA has been reviewed by Taylor (1995). TCA levels are usually increased and there is an increased risk of toxicity; for example, paroxetine and sertraline raised desipramine levels by 400 and 250% respectively (see Taylor, 1995). If the combination is used, plasma TCA levels should be monitored.

There are two reports suggesting therapeutic synergism and that both drugs are required for beneficial effects. Weilburg *et al* (1989) added fluoxetine to the medication of 30 depressed out-patients who had failed to respond to a variety of other antidepressants (mainly TCAs) and 26 (86%) responded. It appeared that the combination of drugs was important because eight patients relapsed when the TCA was withdrawn so that they remained on fluoxetine alone. Seth *et al* (1992) reported that eight patients who had been resistant to both nortriptyline and ECT improved when fluoxetine was added to their nortriptyline. No adverse effects to the combination were reported in this study, but Cowen & Power (1993) reported increased anxiety and agitation for patients on this combined regime.

ECT

The indications for ECT as an inital treatment for depression are discussed in chapter 5. ECT may also work when a course of drug therapy has failed:

response rates of 50–70% are consistently seen (reviewed by Thase & Rush, 1995). For patients with severe depression, for example those with psychotic depression, it may be best to administer ECT after a first course of antidepressant drugs has failed rather than trying a second course of medication.

Bilateral ECT may be more efficacious than unilateral ECT. The number of ECTs may be increased, depending on whether some improvement is shown. However after a successful course of ECT, TRD patients have a high risk of relapse. There is anecdotal evidence that patients with TRD who do not respond to ECT may be more responsive to antidepressant drugs after the ECT than they were before (Thase & Rush, 1995). Shapira *et al* (1988) studied 12 patients, eight of whom were resistant to ECT and four who showed a partial response. In the two months following ECT all 12 patients responded to medication (clomipramine in seven patients, maprotiline in one patient, lithium alone in four patients). Changes in receptor sensitivity induced by ECT may explain the subsequent response to medication.

There are few studies of ECT-resistant depression. Sackheim *et al* (1990) investigated a group of depressed patients who were resistant to ECT. They found that those who had been previously resistant to very large doses of TCAs (300–400 mg daily) prior to the ECT were also resistant to ECT, but those who had shown a partial response to these high doses sometimes responded to ECT.

Psychosurgery

This infrequently used treatment, for long-standing, disabling TRD is discussed in chapter 5.

Conclusion

Associated with major biological, psychological and sociological advances in our knowledge of depression there is now available a diversity of antidepressant treatments which allows a far better matching of a therapeutic regime to a patient's needs than ever before. It is the responsibility of psychiatrists to ensure that their education keeps pace with developments in related disciplines.

Acknowledgements

My thanks to Dr John Cookson, Dr Alan Lee, Dr Hamish McAllister-Williams and Professor N. Ferrier for helpful comments on earlier drafts of this chapter.

References

Agency for Health Care Policy and Research (1993) Depression guideline panel. *Depression in Primary Care: Volume 1. Treatment of Major Depression. Clinical Practice Guidelines.* Rockville, MD: US Department of Health Care Policy and Research.

Aguglia, E., Casacchia, M., Cassano, G., *et al* (1993) Double-blind study of the efficacy and safety of sertraline versus fluoxetine in major depression. *International Clinical Psychopharmacology*, **8**, 197–202.

Amrein, R., Guntert, T. W., Dingemanse, J., *et al* (1992) Interactions of moclobemide with concomitantly administered medication: evidence from pharmacological and clinic studies. *Psychopharmacology*, **106**, S24–S31.

Anderson, I. & Tomenson, B. (1994) The efficacy of selective serotonin re-uptake inhibitors in depression: a meta-analysis of studies against tricyclic antidepressants. *Journal of Psychopharmacology*, **8**, 238–249.

Angst, J. (1992) How recurrent and predictable is depressive illness? In *Long-term Treatment of Depression* (eds S. Montgomery & F. Rouillon). Chichester: Wiley.

——, Baastrup, P. C., Grof, P., *et al* (1973) The course of monopolar depression and bipolar psychoses. *Psychiatrica Neurologie et Neurochirugie (Amersterdam)*, **76**, 489–500

APA Task Force (1985) Tricyclic antidepressant – blood level measurements and clinical outcome: an APA Task Force report. *American Journal of Psychiatry*, **142**, 155–162.

Arya, D. (1994) Extrapyramidal symptoms with selective serotonin reuptake inhibitors. *British Journal of Psychiatry*, **165**, 728–733

Asberg, M., Cronholm, B., Sjoqviost, F., *et al* (1971) Relationships between plasma level and therapeutic effect of nortriptyline. *British Medical Journal*, **3**, 331–334.

Baldwin, D. & Johnson, F. (1995) Tolerability and safety of citalopram. *Reviews in Contemporary Pharmocotherapy*, **6**, 315–325.

Baumann, P. & Larsen, F. (1995) The pharmacokinetics of citalopram. *Reviews in Contemporary Pharmacotherapy*, **6**, 287–295.

Baumhackl, U., Biziere, K., Fischbach, R., *et al* (1989) Efficacy and tolerability of moclobemide compared with imipramine in depressive disorder (DSM–III): an Austrian double-blind multicentre study. *British Journal of Psychiatry*, **155** (suppl. 6), 78–83.

Beasley, C., Sayler, M., Cunningham, G., *et al* (1990) Fluoxetine in tricyclic refractory major depressive disorder. *Journal of Affective Disorders*, **20**, 193–200.

——, Dornsief, B. E., Bosomworth, J. C. (1991) Fluoxetine and suicidality. *British Medical Journal*, **303**, 685–692.

Benet, L., Kroetz, D. & Sheiner, L. (1996) Pharmacokinetics. The dynamics of drug absorption distribution and elimination. In *The Pharmacological Basis of Therapeutics* (9th edn) (eds L. Goodman & A. Gilman). New York: McGraw Hill.

Bernstein, J. G. (1995*a*) Tricyclic, heterocyclic and serotonin selective antidepressants. In *Drug Therapy in Psychiatry* (3rd edn). St Louis, MO: Mosby.

—— (1995*b*) Monoamine oxidase inhibitors. In *Drug Therapy in Psychiatry* (3rd eds). St Louis, MO: Mosby.

Black, D., Bell, S., Hulbert, J., *et al* (1988) The importance of personality disorders in major depression: a controlled study. *Journal of Affective Disorders*, **14**, 115–122.

Bloch, R. G., Dooneief, A. S., Buckberg, A. S., *et al* (1954) The clinical effects of isoniazid and iproniazid in the treatment of pulmonary tuberculosis. *Annals of Internal Medicine*, **40**, 881–900.

BNF (1996) *British National Formulary No. 31 (March 1996)*. London: British Medical Association and the Royal Pharmaceutical Society of Great Britain.

Boston Collaborative Drug Surveillance Program (1972) Adverse reactions to tricyclic antidepressant drugs: Report from Boston Collaborative Drug Surveillance Program. *Lancet*, *i*, 529–531.

Boyer, W. & Feighner, J. (1991) The efficacy of selective serotonin inhibitors in depression. In *Selective Serotonin Re-Uptake Inhibitors* (eds J. Feighner & W. Boyer). Chichester: Wiley.

Braftos, O. & Haug, J. O. (1968) The course of manic depressive psychosis: a follow up of 215 patients. *Acta Psychiatrica Scandinavica*, **44**, 89–112.

Bridges, P. (1992) Resistant depression and psychosurgery. In *Handbook of Affective Disorders* (ed. E. S. Paykel), pp. 437–452. Edinburgh: Churchill Livingstone.

Brosen, K., Skjelbo, E., Rasmussen, B., *et al* (1993) Fluvoxamine is a potent inhibitor of cytochrome P450-1A2. *Biochemical Pharmacology*, **45**, 1211–1214.

Cade, J. F. J. (1949) Lithium salts in the treatment of psychiatric excitement. *Medical Journal of Australia*, **36**, 359–352

—— (1970) The story of lithium. In *Discoveries in Biological Psychiatry* (eds F. Ayd & B. Blackwell). Philadelphia, PA: J. B. Lippincott.

Chamowitz, L. (1991) Treatment resistant depression: a survey of the prescribing habits of Canadian psychiatrists. *Canadian Journal of Psychiatry*, **36**, 353–356.

Charney, D. S. & Nelson, J. C. (1981) Delusional and non delusional unipolar depression: further evidence for distinct subtypes. *American Journal of Psychiatry*, **138**, 328–333.

——, Price, L. H. & Henninger, D. R. (1986) Desipramine–yohimbine combination treatment of refractory depression. *Archives of General Psychiatry*, **43**, 1153–1161.

Claghorn, J. (1991) Paroxetine: long term efficacy and tolerability. *Biological Psychiatry*, **29** (suppl. 115), 205S.

Coffee, C. E., Figiel, G. S., Djang, W. T., *et al* (1990) Subcortical hyperintensity on magnetic resonance imaging: a comparison of normal and depressed elderly subjects. *American Journal of Psychiatry*, **147**, 187–189.

Committee on Safety of Medicines (1994*a*) Fluvoxamine increases plasma theophylline levels. *Current Problems in Pharmacovigilance*, **20**, 12.

—— (1994*b*) L-tryptophan (OPTIMAX): Limited availability for resistant depression. *Current Problems in Pharmacovigilance*, **20**, 2.

Cookson, J. (1993) Side-effects of antidepressants. *British Journal of Psychiatry*, **163** (suppl. 20), 20–24.

Coppen, A., Noguera, R., Bailey, J., *et al* (1971) Prophylactic lithium in affective disorder. *Lancet*, *ii*, 326–329.

Cowen, P. J. & Power, A. C. (1993) Combination treatment of depression. *British Journal of Psychiatry*, **162**, 266–267.

Crewe, H., Lennard, M., Tucker, G., *et al* (1992) The effect of selective serotonin re-uptake inhibitors on cytochrome P450-2D6 (CYP2D6) activity in human liver microsomes. *British Journal of Clinical Pharmacology*, **34**, 262–265.

Davidson, J. (1992) Monoamine oxidase inhibitors. In *Handbook of Affective Disorders* (ed. E. S. Paykel). Edinburgh: Churchill Livingstone.

——, Giller, E., Zistook, S., *et al* (1988) An efficacy study of isocarboxacid and placebo in depression, and its relationship to depressive nosology. *Archives of General Psychiatry*, **45**, 120–127.

Davis, J. M. & Glassman, A. H. (1989) Antidepressant drugs. In *Comprehensive Textbook of Psychiatry* (eds H. Kaplan & B. Sadock). Baltimore, MD: Williams & Wilkins.

de Montigny, C., Grunberg, F., Mayer, A., *et al* (1981) Lithium induces rapid relief of depression in tricyclic antidepressant drug non-responders. *British Journal of Psychiatry*, **138**, 252–256.

Dinan, T. G. & Barry, S. (1989) A comparison of electroconvulsive therapy with a combined lithium and tricyclic combination among depressed tricyclic nonresponders. *Acta Psychiatrica Scandinavica*, **80**, 97–100.

Doogan, D. & Caillard, V. (1992) Sertraline and the prevention of depression. *British Journal of Psychiatry*, **160**, 217–222.

Drug and Therapeutics Bulletin (1994) Moclobemide for depression. *Drugs and Therapeutics Bulletin*, **32**, 6–7.

Edwards, J. G. (1995*a*) Depression, antidepressants and accidents. *British Medical Journal*, **311**, 887–888.

—— (1995*b*) Drug choice in depression. Selective serotonin reuptake inhibitors or tricyclic antidepressants. *CNS Drugs*, **4**, 141–159.

El-Fakahany, E. & Richelson, E. (1983) Antagonism by antidepressants of muscarinic acetylcholine receptors of human brain. *British Journal of Pharmacology*, **78**, 97–102.

Everest, J., Tunbridge, R. & Widdop, B. (1989) *The Incidence of Drugs in Road Accident Fatalities*. (TRRL research report 202.) Cowthorne: Transport Research Laboratory.

Faravelli, C., Ambonetti, A., Pallanti, S., *et al* (1986) Depressive relapses and incomplete recovery from index episode. *American Journal of Psychiatry*, **143**, 888–891.

Feighner, J., Boyer, W., Meredith, C., *et al* (1989) A placebo-controlled inpatient comparison of fluvoxamine maleate and imipramine in major depression. *International Clinical Psychopharmacology*, **4**, 239–244.

Fisch, C. (1985) Effect of fluoxetine on the electrocardiogram. *Journal of Clinical Psychiatry*, **46**, 42–44.

Franchini, L., Gasperini, M. & Smeraldi, E. (1994) A 24-month follow up study of unipolar subjects: a comparison between lithium and fluvoxamine. *Journal of Affective Disorders*, **32**, 225–231.

Frank, E., Kupfer, D., Perel, J., *et al* (1990) Three-year outcomes for maintenance therapies in recurrent depression. *Archives of General Psychiatry*, **47**, 1093–1099.

Freeman, H. & O'Hanlon, J. (1995) Acute and subacute effects of antidepressants on performance. *Journal of Drug Development and Clinical Practice*, **7**, 7–20.

Garvey, M. & Tollefson, G. (1987) Occurrence of myoclonus in patients treated with tricyclic antidepressants. *Archives of General Psychiatry*, **44**, 269–272.

Goodwin, F., Prange, A., Post, R., *et al* (1982) The augmentation of antidepressant effects by L-triiodothyronine in tricyclic non-responders. *American Journal of Psychiatry*, **139**, 34–38.

Grahame-Smith, D. (1971) Studies *in vivo* on the relationship between brain tryptophan, brain 5-HT synthesis and hyperactivity in rats treated with a monoamine oxidase inhibitor and L-tryptophan. *Journal of Neurochemistry*, **18**, 1053–1066.

Greenhouse, J. B., Kupfer, D. J., Frank, E., *et al* (1987) Analysis of time to stabilization in the treatment of depression. Biological and clinical correlates. *Journal of Affective Disorders*, **15**, 259–266.

Guengerich, F. (1992) Human cytochrome P-450 enzymes. *Life Sciences*, **50**, 1471–1478.

Harris, B., Young, J. & Hughes, B. (1986) Comparative effects of seven antidepressant regimes on appetite, weight and carbohydrate preference. *British Journal of Psychiatry*, **148**, 590–592.

Harrison-Read, P. & Tyrer, P. (1995) The application of drug treatment in psychiatric practice. In *Seminars in Clinical Psychopharmacology* (ed. D. King), pp. 59–102. London: Gaskell.

Henry, J., Alexander, C. & Sener, E. (1995) Relative mortality from overdose of antidepressants. *British Medical Journal*, **310**, 221–224.

Hindmarsh, I. (1995) The behavioural toxicity of the selective serotonin reuptake inhibitors. *International Clinical Psychopharmacology*, **9** (Suppl. 4), 13–17.

Hyttel, J. (1994) Pharmacological characterization of selective serotonin reuptake inhibitors (SSRIs). *International Clinical Psychopharmacology*, **9** (suppl.), 19–26.

Inman, W. (1988) Blood disorders and suicide in patients taking mianserin or amitriptyline. *Lancet*, *ii*, 90–92.

Isacsson, G., Holmgren, P., Wasserman, D., *et al* (1994*a*) Use of antidepressants among people committing suicide in Sweden. *British Medical Journal*, **308**, 506–509.

——, ——, ——, *et al* (1994*b*) Suicide and the use of antidepressants. *British Medical Journal*, **308**, 916.

Isometsa, E., Henriksson, M., Aro, H., *et al* (1994) Suicide in major depression. *American Journal of Psychiatry*, **151**, 530–536.

Jacoby, R. & Lunn, D. (1993) How long should the elderly take antidepressants? A double-blind placebo-controlled study of continuation/prophylaxis therapy with dothiepin. *British Journal of Psychiatry*, **162**, 175–182.

Jick, S., Dean, A. & Jick, H. (1995) Antidepressants and suicide. *British Medical Journal*, **310**, 215–218.

Joffe, R. & Singer, W. (1990) A comparison of triiodothyronine and thyroxin in the potentiation of tricyclic antidepressants. *Psychiatry Research*, **32**, 241–251.

——, ——, Levitt, A. J., *et al* (1993) A placebo-controlled comparison of lithium and triiodothyronine augmentation of tricyclic antidepressants in unipolar refractory depression. *Archives of General Psychiatry*, **50**, 387–393.

Karch, F. & Lasagna, L. (1975) Adverse drug reactions. *Journal of the American Medical Association*, **234**, 1236–1241.

Katona, C., Abou-Saleh, M., Harrison, D., *et al* (1995) Placebo-controlled trial of lithium augmentation of fluoxetine and lofepramine. *British Journal of Psychiatry*, **166**, 80–86.

Kaye, C., Haddock, R., Langley, P., *et al* (1989) A review of the metabolism and pharmacokinetics of paroxetine in man. *Acta Psychiatrica Scandinavica*, **80**, 60–75.

Kowalski, A., Stanley, R., Dennerstin, I., *et al* (1985) The sexual side-effects of antidepressant medication: a double blind comparison of two antidepressants in a non-psychiatric population. *British Journal of Psychiatry*, **147**, 413–418.

Keller, M. B., Klerman, G. L., Lavori, P. W., *et al* (1986) The persistent risk of chronicity in recurrent episodes of non bipolar depression: a prospective follow up study. *American Journal of Psychiatry*, **143**, 24–28.

Kuhn, R. (1958) The treatment of depressive states with G-22355 (imipramine hydrochloride). *American Journal of Psychiatry*, 111, 459–464.

Kupfer, D. & Frank, E. (1992) The minimum length of treatment for recovery. In *Long-Term Treatment of Depression* (eds S. Montgomery & F. Rouillon). Chichester: Wiley.

Kushnir, S. L. (1986) Lithium antidepressant combination in the treatment of depressed physically ill geriatric patients. *American Journal of Psychiatry*, 143, 378–379.

Leonard, B. (1987) A comparison of the pharmacological properties of the novel tricyclic antidepressant lofepramine with its major metabolite, desipramine: a review. *International Clinical Psychopharmacology*, 2, 281–297.

Livingston, M. (1995) Interactions with selective MAOIs. *Lancet*, 345, 533–534.

Mann, J., Aarons, S., Wilner, P., *et al* (1989) A controlled study of the antidepressant efficacy and side-effects of (−)-deprenyl: a selective monoamine oxidase inhibitor. *Archives of General Psychiatry*, 46, 45–50.

Marneros, A. & Philipp, M. (1979) A double-blind trial with amitriptyline and lofepramine in the treatment of endogenous depression. *International Pharmacopsychiatry*, 14, 300–304.

Meader-Woodruff, J., Akil, M., Wisner-Carlson, R., *et al* (1988) Behavioural and cognitive toxicity related to elevated plasma tricyclic antidepressant levels. *Journal of Clinical Psychopharmacology*, 8, 28–32.

Medical Research Council (1965) Clinical trial of the treatment of depressive illness. *British Medical Journal*, 1, 881–886.

Mindham, R. H. S., Howland, C. & Shepherd, M. (1973) An evaluation of continuation therapy with tricyclic antidepressants in depressive illness. *Psychological Medicine*, 3, 5–17.

Montgomery, S., Dufour, H., Brion, S., *et al* (1988) The prophylactic efficacy of fluoxetine in unipolar depression. *British Journal of Psychiatry*, 153 (suppl. 3), 69–76.

—— & Montgomery, D. (1992) Prophylactic treatment in recurrent unipolar depression. In *Long-term Treatment of Depression* (eds S. Montgomery & F. Rouillon). Chichester: Wiley.

—— & Johnson, F. (1995) Citalopram in the treatment of depression. *Reviews in Contemporary Pharmacotherapy*, 6, 297–306.

Morris, J. B. & Beck, A. T. (1974) The efficacy of antidepressant drugs. *Archives of General Psychiatry*, 30, 667–674.

Nair, N., Amin, M., Holm, P., *et al* (1995) Moclobemide and nortriptyline in elderly depressed patients. A randomised, multicentre trial against placebo. *Journal of Affective Disorders*, 33, 1–9.

Nemeroff, C., De Vane, L. & Pollock, B. (1996) Newer antidepressants and the cytochrome P450 system. *American Journal of Psychiatry*, 153, 311–320.

Neuvonen, P., Pohjola-Sintonen, S., Jacke, U., *et al* (1993) Five fatal cases of serotonin syndrome after moclobemide–citalopram or moclobemide–clomipramine overdoses. *Lancet*, 342, 1419.

Nierenberg, A. A. & Amsterdam, J. D. (1990) Treatment resistant depression. Definition and treatment approaches. *Journal of Clinical Psychiatry*, 51 (suppl. 6), 39–47.

Nystrom, C. & Hallstrom, T. (1987) Comparison between a serotonin and a noradrenaline reuptake blocker in the treatment of depressed outpatients. *Acta Psychiatrica Scandinavica*, 75, 377–382.

Pare, C., Kline, N., Hallstrom, C., *et al* (1982) Will amitriptyline prevent the "cheese" reaction of monoamine oxidase inhibitors? *Lancet, ii,* 183–186.

Parker, G., Roy, K., Hadzi-Pavlovic, D., *et al* (1992) Psychotic (delusional depression): a meta-analysis of physical treatments. *Journal of Affective Disorders,* **24,** 17–24.

Paykel, E. & Priest, R. (1992) Recognition and management of depression in general practice: consensus statement. *British Medical Journal,* **305,** 1198–1202.

Peselow, E. D., Filippi, A. M., Goodnick, P., *et al* (1989) The short-and long-term efficacy of paroxetine HCl: B. Data from a double-blind crossover study and from a year-long trial vs. imipramine and placebo. *Psychopharmacology Bulletin,* **25,** 272–276.

Petit, J., Spiker, D., Ruwitch, J., *et al* (1977) Tricyclic antidepressant plasma levels and adverse effects after overdosage. *Clinical Pharmacology and Therapeutics,* **21,** 47–51.

Pete, T., Tienari, P. & Jaskari, M. (1977) A comparison of the cardiac effects of mianserin and amitriptyline in man. *Pharmacopsychiatry,* **10,** 309–312.

Popli, A. & Baldessarini, R. (1995) Interactions of serotonin reuptake inhibitors with tricyclic antidepressants. *Archives of General Psychiatry,* **52,** 784–785.

Post, R. (1993) Issues in the long-term management of bipolar affective illness. *Psychiatric Annals,* **23,** 86–92.

Prange, A. J., Wilson, I. C., Robon, A. M., *et al* (1969) Enhancement of imipramine antidepressant activity by thyroid hormone. *American Journal of Psychiatry,* **126,** 457–469.

Preskorn, S. (1993) Pharmacokinetics of antidepressants: why and how they are relevant to treatment. *Journal of Clinical Psychiatry,* **54** (suppl.), 14–34.

—— (1995) Comparison of the tolerability of bupropion, fluoxetine, imipramine, nefazodone, paroxetine, sertraline and venlafaxine. *Journal of Clinical Psychiatry,* **56** (suppl. 6), 12–21.

—— & Fast, G. (1991) Therapeutic drug monitoring for antidepressants: efficacy, safety, and cost-effectiveness. *Journal of Clinical Psychiatry,* **52** (suppl. 6), 22–33.

—— & Magnus, R. (1994) Inhibition of hepatic P-450 isoenzymes by selective serotonin reuptake inhibitors: in vitro and in vivo findings and their implications for patient care. *Psychopharmacology Bulletin,* **30,** 251–259.

Price, L. H., Conwell, Y. & Nelson, J. C. (1983) Lithium augmentation of combined neuroleptic–tricyclic treatment in delusional depression. *American Journal of Psychiatry,* **140,** 318–322.

——, Charney, D. S. & Henniger, G. R. (1986) Variability of response to lithium augmentation in refractory depression. *American Journal of Psychiatry,* **143,** 1387–1392.

Prien, R. F. (1992) Maintenance treatment. In *Handbook of Affective Disorders* (ed. E. S. Paykel), pp. 419–435. London: Churchill Livingstone.

——, ——, Mansky, P. A., *et al* (1984) Drug therapy in the prevention of recurrences in unipolar and bipolar affective disorders. Report of the NIMH Collaborative Study Group. *Archives of General Psychiatry,* **41,** 1096–1104.

—— & —— (1986) Continuation drug therapy for major depressive episodes: how long should it be maintained? *American Journal of Psychiatry,* **143,** 18–23.

Quitkin, F. (1985) The importance of dosing in prescribing antidepressants. *British Journal of Psychiatry,* **247,** 593–597.

Richelson, E. (1983) Are receptor studies useful in clinical practice? *Journal of Clinical Psychiatry*, **44**, 4–9.

Robertson, M. M. & Trimble, M. R. (1982) Major tranquillizers used as antidepressants. A review. *Journal of Affective Disorders*, **4**, 173–193.

Roose, F., Glassman, A., Firis, S., *et al* (1981) Comparison of imipramine and nortriptyline-induced orthostatic hypertension: a meaningful difference. *Journal of Clinical Psychopharmacology*, **1**, 316–319.

Rouillon, F., Lejoyeux, M., Filteau, M., *et al* (1992) Unwanted effects of long-term treatment. In *Long-Term Treatment of Depression* (eds S. Montgomery & F. Rouillon). Chichester: Wiley.

Sackheim, H., Prudic, J., Devanand, D., *et al* (1990) The impact of medication resistance and continuation pharmacotherapy on relapse following response to electroconvulsive therapy in major depression. *Journal of Clinical Psychopharmacology*, **10**, 96–104.

Schapira, B., Kindler, S. & Lerer, B. (1988) Medication outcome in ECT resistant depression. *Convulsive Therapy*, **4** (suppl. 3), 192–198.

Schmidt, L., Grohmann, R., Müller-Oerlinghausen, B., *et al* (1986) Adverse drug reactions to first- and second-generation antidepressants. A critical evaluation of drug surveillance data. *British Journal of Psychiatry*, **148**, 38–43.

Scott, J. (1991) Epidemiology, demography and definition of chronic depression. *International Clinical Psychopharmacology*, **6** (suppl.), 1–12.

Seth, R., Jennings, A. L., Bindham, J., *et al* (1992) Combination treatment with noradrenalin and serotonergic reuptake inhibitors in resistant depression. *British Journal of Psychiatry*, **161**, 562–565.

Song, F., Freemantle, N., Sheldon, T., *et al* (1993) Selective serotonin reuptake inhibitors: meta-analysis of efficacy and acceptability. *British Medical Journal*, **306**, 683–687.

Stein, G. & Bernadt, M. (1993) Lithium augmentation therapy in tricyclic-resistant depression. A controlled trial using lithium in low and normal doses. *British Journal of Psychiatry*, **162**, 634–640.

Sternbach, H. (1991) The serotonin syndrome. *American Journal of Psychiatry*, **148**, 705–713.

Stimmel, G., Skowron, D. & Chameides, W. (1991) Focus on fluvoxamine: a serotonin reuptake inhibitor for major depression and obsessive–compulsive disorder. *Hospital Formulary*, **26**, 635–643.

Stuppaeck, C. H., Barnes, C., Schwitzer, J., *et al* (1994) Carbamazepine in the prophylaxis of major depression. A five year follow up. *Journal of Clinical Psychiatry*, **55**, 146–150.

Targum, S. D., Greenberg, R. D., Harmon, R. L., *et al* (1984) Thyroid hormone and the TRH stimulation test in refractory depression. *Journal of Clinical Psychiatry*, **45**, 345–346.

Taylor, D. (1995) Selective serotonin reuptake inhibitors and tricyclic antidepressants in combination. Interaction and therapeutic uses. *British Journal of Psychiatry*, **167**, 575–580.

—— & Lader, M. (1996) Cytochromes and psychotropic drug interactions. *British Journal of Psychiatry*, **168**, 529–532.

Teicher, M., Glod, C. & Cole, J. (1990) Emergence of intense suicidal preoccupation during fluoxetine treatment. *American Journal of Psychiatry*, **147**, 207–210.

Thase, M. E. & Rush, A. J. (1995) Treatment resistant depression. In *Psychopharmacology: The Fourth Generation of Progress* (eds F. Bloom & D. Kupfer), pp. 1081–1097. New York: Raven Press.

Thase, M., Kupfer, D., Frank, E., *et al* (1989) Treatment of imipramine-resistant recurrent depression. II: An open clinical trial of lithium augmentation. *Journal of Clinical Psychiatry*, **50**, 413–417.

Tyrer, P., Candy, J. & Kelly, D. (1973) A study of the clinical effects of phenelzine and placebo in the treatment of phobic anxiety. *Psychopharmacologia*, **32**, 237–254.

Versiani, M., Oggero, U., Alterwain, P., *et al* (1989) A double-blind comparative trial of moclobemide versus imipramine and placebo in major depressive episodes. *British Journal of Psychiatry*, **155** (suppl. 6), 72–77.

Warner, M., Peabody, C., Whiteford, H., *et al* (1987) Trazodone and priapism. *Journal of Clinical Psychiatry*, **50**, 256–261.

Warrington, S., Padgham, C. & Lader, M. (1989) The cardiovascular effects of antidepressants. *Psychological Medicine, Monograph Supplement 16*. Cambridge: Cambridge University Press.

Weilburg, J. B., Rosenbaum, J. F., Biederman, J., *et al* (1989) Fluoxetine added to non-MAOI antidepressants converts nonresponders to responders: a preliminary report. *Journal of Clinical Psychiatry*, **50**, 447–449.

Weller, R. & Preskorn, S. (1984) Psychotropic drugs and alcohol: pharmacokinetic and pharmacodynamic interactions. *Psychosomatics*, **25**, 301–309.

Wernicke, J., Dunlop, S., Dornseif, B., *et al* (1987) Fixed-dose fluoxetine therapy for depression. *Psychopharmacology Bulletin*, **23**, 164–168.

WHO (1989) Pharmacotherapy of depressive disorders. A consensus statement. *Journal of Affective Disorders*, **17**, 197–198.

Wilde, M., Plosker, G. & Benfield, P. (1993) Fluvoxamine. An updated review of its pharmacology and therapeutic use in depressive illness. *Drugs*, **46**, 895–924.

Wilhelm, K., Mitchell, P., Sengoz, A., *et al* (1994) Treatment resistant depression. Outcome of a series of patients. *Australian and New Zealand Journal of Psychiatry*, **28**, 23–33.

Willner, P. (1995) Dopaminergic mechanism in depression and in mania. In *Psychopharmacology: The Fourth Generation of Progress*. (eds F. Bloom & D. Kupfer), pp. 921–931. New York: Raven Press.

Worral, E., Moody, J., Peet, M., *et al* (1979) Controlled studies of the acute antidepressant effects of lithium. *British Journal of Psychiatry*, **35**, 255–262.

Young, R., Alexopoulis, G., Sharmoian, C., *et al* (1987) Plasma 10-hydroxy nortriptyline and renal function in elderly depressives. *Biological Psychiatry*, **22**, 1283–1287.

5 Electroconvulsive therapy and other treatments

Alistair G. Hay & Morris Bernadt

---

*Indications • Contraindications • Side-effects • Efficacy of ECT •
Mode of action • Clinical administration of ECT • Consent •
Psychosurgery*

Electroconvulsive therapy (ECT) is widely used in modern day psychiatry. Properly applied it is rapidly acting and effective, particularly in severe depressions, but it remains a controversial treatment still arousing some fear in the public.

Convulsive therapy was introduced into psychiatry through the mistaken belief that schizophrenia was an opposite to epilepsy, and observations that in patients with both schizophrenia and epilepsy a convulsion produced a temporary improvement of the psychotic symptoms. It was also thought that epilepsy was less common in schizophrenia, a view that is probably also erroneous. In the early 1930s, Meduna, a Hungarian psychiatrist, first started to induce fits with camphor and cardiazol. Of the first 26 patients with schizophrenia treated by Meduna, 10 recovered, three improved and 13 were unchanged. In 1937 Ugo Cerletti and Lucio Bini, two Italian psychiatrists, applied an electroconvulsive stimulus to animals in an attempt to alleviate temporal lobe epilepsy by producing sclerosis of Ammonn's horn. From this experiment they speculated that electricity could be used as a simple, safe agent with which to induce fits in humans. The following year they carried out the first successful electroconvulsion in man. Their first patient was found wandering in a fugue, almost mute and needed 11 ECTs to be cured. In the early days ECT was conducted without anaesthesia and was quite a hazardous procedure, often resulting in vertebral fractures and occasionally fat embolism. With the introduction of short acting anaesthetic induction agents and muscle relaxants, ECT is no longer a crude procedure but a well recognised, safe and acceptable treatment for the modern-day psychiatrist.

All psychiatrists using ECT should be familiar with what the procedure involves, the indications and potential pitfalls of treatment and should have a clear idea about the practical issues concerning the clinical administration of ECT. The guidelines of *The ECT Handbook* (Royal College of Psychiatrists' Special Committee on ECT, 1995) must be followed if ECT is used.

Indications

Electroconvulsive therapy is most commonly prescribed in the treatment of depressive illness although its use extends to the treatment of both mania and schizophrenia.

Depression

ECT is widely and effectively used as an integral part of the treatment for depressive disorders. Patients at the more severe end of the spectrum of depressive disorders who exhibit more psychotic or endogenous symptoms are more likely to respond to ECT (Table 5.1).

ECT, in comparison with other treatments available for depression, provides rapid relief from the more serious immediate life threatening symptoms of depressive illness. It is particularly indicated in cases of severe psychomotor retardation in which there may be immediate concerns about the patient's physical well being, for example, if fluid intake is poor. It may also be used on an emergency basis when there is an acute risk of harm to the individual or to others due to the patient acting on psychotic delusions or hallucinations. The indications for ECT in depression are given in Box 5.1.

Mania

Prior to the introduction of neuroleptic drugs and lithium, ECT was widely used in the treatment of mania, but once these drugs became established ECT was little used, although in recent years there has been some renewed interest. In cases of severe manic illness for example, where there is severe exhaustion or manic stupor, ECT has the advantage of producing a rapid response without having the risks associated with the side-effects of the very high doses of neuroleptic medication patients otherwise require.

Black *et al* (1987) in a retrospective study involving 438 patients found that a greater number, 78%, improved with ECT compared with 62% receiving adequate doses of lithium, 52% on inadequate doses of the

Table 5.1 Predictors of response to ECT

Good response	Poor response
Depressive delusions	Hypochondriacal symptoms
Psychomotor retardation	Histrionic features
Premorbid personality problems	
Biological symptoms	Fluctuating course
Previous response to ECT	Poor previous response to ECT
(in similar illness)	(in previous illness)

Box 5.1 Indications for ECT in depression

Severe depression where poor fluid intake is potentially life
    threatening
Depressive stupor
Depression with strong suicidal features
Psychotic depression
Puerperal psychosis (depressive)
Failure to respond to oral antidepressants
Intolerance of oral antidepressants due to side-effects
Previous response to ECT

---

drug and 37% who received neither. In a prospective study comparing
ECT with lithium, Small *et al* (1988) showed that ECT produced a more
rapid response than lithium, although relapse rates were similar for the
two groups. It was suggested that appropriate treatment might be ECT in
the early acute stages of the illness followed by maintenance lithium (i.e.
the same treatment as given to the ECT group in the study). ECT can also
be useful for patients with mania whose psychotic symptoms remain in
spite of adequate pharmacotherapy.

Schizophrenia

Concerns about the side-effects of high dose neuroleptic drugs have led
to ECT being reconsidered as a treatment for the acute symptoms of
schizophrenia. Most studies have included patients already taking
neuroleptic medication. One early study (May 1968) showed ECT to be
less beneficial than phenothiazines but better than a general ward
programme or analytic psychotherapy.

However ECT in combination with neuroleptics will produce a more
rapid improvement in the psychotic and depressive symptoms of acute
schizophrenia than drug treatment alone (Taylor & Fleminger, 1980;
Abraham & Kulhara, 1987). This suggests that ECT has a useful and effective
place in the management of schizophrenia although it is not commonly
used. In particular it is effective in individuals with delusions of passivity,
delusional mood and delusions of a persecutory nature especially if there
are associated depressive features. Predictors of good response to ECT
include short duration of illness, few premorbid schizoid personality traits
and the presence of perplexity (Dodwell & Goldberg, 1989).

Similarly ECT is useful in the treatment of schizoaffective disorder in
particular if depressive symptoms predominate. ECT had also been
recommended for the treatment of acute catatonic symptoms associated
with both schizophrenia and affective disorders.

Chronic schizophrenia

ECT has no place in the management of symptoms of withdrawal, apathy and social incongruence that are associated with the defect state of chronic schizophrenia. It may be used to treat intercurrent acute depressive episodes which occur within the context of chronic schizophrenia.

Puerperal psychosis

ECT is strongly indicated and highly effective in the management of puerperal psychosis especially when affective symptoms predominate. It allows for a rapid improvement in psychotic symptoms in a situation in which there is a need to have the mother fit to care for her baby in as short a time as possible.

Maintenance ECT

A review of the literature (Munroe, 1991) finds a lack of reliable data looking at the indications for and efficacy of maintenance ECT. The American Psychiatric Association (1990) has suggested that maintenance ECT may be indicated for patients with recurring illness which has been acutely responsive to ECT or for whom maintenance pharmacotherapy is ineffective or intolerable due to side-effects. Maintenance ECT should be considered in the treatment of illnesses which relapse frequently or where relapse occurs early following a course of treatment. It may also be useful in patients whose compliance with drug treatment is unreliable or who are at high risk of suicide by overdose.

Little is known about the practical details concerning the administration of maintenance treatment. Questions such as how frequently treatment should be administered and for how long treatment should be continued remain largely unanswered. It is probably best to start maintenance ECT at a frequency sufficient to prevent depressive symptoms recurring while avoiding side-effects from it. As maintenance treatment progresses the psychiatrist should watch for any evidence of the patient relapsing and increase the frequency of ECT to counteract this. On the other hand, especially in elderly patients, the psychiatrist should watch for signs of confusion from too frequent treatments. Cognitive function, including memory, should be regularly monitored for evidence of any deterioration suggestive of overtreatment. If side-effects are detected the frequency of treatment should be reduced.

ECT in other disorders

ECT has been suggested as a treatment for a number of other non-psychiatric disorders. Generally there are few adequate studies to support these claims and much of the evidence is based on isolated case reports.

Some reports have demonstrated ECT to be of benefit in Parkinson's disease including relief of the "on–off" phenomenon (Andersen *et al*, 1987) and as a maintenance therapy in refractory cases (Zervas & Fink, 1991). ECT may also have a role in the management of the neuroleptic malignant syndrome in combination with conventional drug and supportive treatment (Schefter & Schuman, 1992).

There is no evidence to suggest that ECT is of benefit in the treatment of any other psychiatric disorder. It has no therapeutic use in the control of violent or aggressive patients, and should not be prescribed as a last resort measure, without any clear indication, when other treatments have failed.

Contraindications

There are no absolute contraindications to ECT (Box 5.2). All patients should be individually assessed and the benefits of ECT weighed against its potential hazards. General anaesthesia and the ECT itself produce a number of physiological changes affecting primarily the heart, the blood vessels and the brain. The cardiovascular changes accompanying the procedure can be quite profound. There is an initial tachycardia accompanying the induction of anaesthesia. Administration of the ECT produces a bradycardia followed by a tachycardia both of which can lead to marked swings in blood pressure and cardiac output (Perrin, 1961). These may be accompanied by various arrhythmias and ECG changes consistent with myocardial ischaemia. The routine use of an antimuscarinic agent e.g. atropine or glycopyrrolate (which does not cross the blood–brain barrier) to reduce secretions and prevent the vagally mediated bradyarrythmias and occasional extra systoles is no longer recommended in every case. The ECT induced seizure results in a marked increase in regional cerebral blood flow and an increase in permeability of the blood–brain barrier (Bolwig, 1988).

As a consequence of these physiological changes patients who have pre-existing cardiovascular or cerebral diseases are more prone to develop complications following ECT (Alexopoulos, 1984). Potential problems in such patients can be reduced by appropriate medical management prior to ECT.

The management of these patients during ECT should include such measures that are required to minimise the swings in blood pressure and heart rate that occur during the treatment and will involve close liaison with both the anaesthetist and any other medical specialists involved as well as ECG monitoring during the procedure. Short acting beta blockers (Esmolol), nifedipine and labatolol have been used to combat the hypertension that occurs with ECT. Careful blood pressure control is required in certain rare instances such as retinal detachment, raised intracranial pressure due to a tumour and in phaeochromocytoma. In the case of tumours dexamethazone has been used to decrease intracranial pressure before ECT.

In the event of complications occurring during ECT it is essential that there are sufficient staff present who are adequately trained in cardiopulmonary resuscitation and that the appropriate first line equipment is immediately at hand and in good working order (for review see Abrams, 1991).

In all patients it is advisable to discuss as early as possible potential complicating factors including current drug treatment with the anaesthetist before giving the ECT. It may be worth considering other types of treatment such as antidepressant drugs, or if necessary postponing ECT until a patient's physical condition improves. In certain situations the urgent need for treatment outweighs the risks and the psychiatrist should proceed with caution.

It is good practice to involve a patient's relatives in making a decision about whether to proceed with ECT. The psychiatrist should explain to the family about the risks of ECT as well as the necessity and benefits of treatment. All decisions, as well as the rationale behind them, should be clearly documented in the medical notes.

Special populations

ECT is often helpful in the elderly because many elderly depressives cannot tolerate antidepressants. It is important to note that seizure threshold

---

Box 5.2 Relative contraindications of ECT

Within three months of myocardial infarction
Congestive cardiac failure
Ischaemic heart disease
Poorly controlled hypertension
Cardiac pacemaker *in situ* (induced currents can cause arrhythmias)
Aortic aneurysm
History of cerebral aneurysm/cerebral haemorrhage
Raised intracranial pressure, e.g. space occupying lesion
Poorly controlled epilepsy
Recent cerebral trauma
Active cerebral infection
Respiratory impairment, e.g. from chest infection, asthma, etc.
Difficulties in tolerating anaesthesia, e.g. previous or family history of malignant hyperpyrexia
Relevant orthopaedic problems, e.g. cervical spondylosis

rises with age, and therefore higher stimulus intensities are required. Anaesthetic risks, the presence of an increased prevalence of cardiovascular disorder, and the increased use of a variety of other medications are additional risks among the elderly.

ECT is safe and effective among adolescents with acute psychotic disorders particularly catatonia, depression, mania and schizophrenia, but there is limited experience and a general reluctance to use ECT in this age group. ECT is safe in pregnancy, the risks being associated only with anaesthesia. It is important to ensure good muscular relaxation as the movement of the abdominal muscles in later pregnancy may be a risk.

Side-effects

The mortality rate associated with ECT is relatively low (one per 22 000 treatments). Anaesthetic factors are the commonest cause of death (Hesche & Roeder, 1976). Most of these deaths occur as a result of a fatal arrhythmia or myocardial infarction. This can be reduced by careful pre-treatment assessment notifying the anaesthetist about potential complicating factors at an early stage. Patients should receive ECT in a designated setting which includes a separate recovery area allowing for close monitoring of the patient, and resuscitation equipment should be readily at hand. Doctors involved in administering of ECT must be familiar with basic resuscitation techniques.

The mortality from giving ECT is similar to that from a minor surgical procedure although the repeated administration of ECT adds to its risks. On the other hand, ECT is given to patients suffering from disorders which in their own right carry a certain mortality. This factor should be remembered when weighing up the risks and benefits of treatment. Over a three year period Avery & Winokur (1976) showed the mortality from ECT was significantly lower than treatment with low dose antidepressants or psychotherapy.

Serious side-effects include myocardial infarction, status epilepticus, aspiration pneumonia and pulmonary embolus. These are all relatively rare and the risk of their occurring is reduced by good medical and nursing management before, during and after each treatment. Crushed vertebrae and other fractures, although common in the past, should not happen now that neuromuscular relaxants are given.

Minor side-effects are common and experienced by up to 80% of patients receiving ECT (Freeman *et al*, 1980). They include a short lived confusional state, nausea, vomiting, headache, muscle pains and memory impairment. The majority of these are related to post-anaesthetic and post-ictal factors, and settle within hours of treatment. Of these effects memory impairment is longer lasting and more controversial, and is discussed below.

There is no doubt that ECT affects short-term memory. Almost all patients report some difficulty in recalling events that occurred immediately before and after a treatment with ECT. The memory disturbance can last for up to three months after the last treatment. Autobiographical memory (the recall of personal events) is more likely to be disrupted than other types of long-term memory. For many patients the amnesia provides relief from painful recollections of their illness and how it affected them. The memory disturbance is directly related to the number of treatments a patient has received and is less with unilateral non-dominant electrode placement (D'Elia & Raotma, 1975; Hesche *et al*, 1978; Squire, 1986). However, these patients may require more treatments (Abrams *et al*, 1983; Sackeim *et al*, 1987) which adds to their memory loss. Patients with depression also complain of memory loss, but depressive memory loss appears to be associated with impairment of the acquisition of new information whereas ECT causes transient disruption of the retention of new information.

ECT and brain damage

Of more concern is the question of whether ECT causes long-term irreversible brain damage. It has been claimed that ECT leads to brain damage due to neuronal loss (Freidberg, 1977). There is little evidence for this view and many of the changes that have been found at postmortem can be attributed to the changes in pulse and blood pressure associated with unmodified treatment or prolonged generalised seizures. A review of the evidence (Weiner, 1984) failed to substantiate claims that ECT itself can cause gross structural brain damage. A more recent prospective study (Scott *et al*, 1991*b*) using NMR scans failed to detect any parenchymal loss following ECT while an isolated postmortem report (University of Louisville, 1985) of a woman who had received more than one thousand treatments did not show gross morphological changes.

The absence of gross structural damage does not rule out the possibility that ECT may result in long-term deficits in brain functioning. Such changes may become apparent as subtle deficits in cognitive function that are difficult to detect and even more difficult to separate from other confounding factors, such as simple forgetting, the effects of depression, current medications, or alcohol intake. Available evidence suggests that there is no difference in long-term memory for events occurring after ECT between treated and untreated groups (Johnstone *et al*, 1980; Weeks *et al*, 1980) for patients who received average courses of ECT. Testing for long-term retrograde amnesia is more unreliable. If there is any effect it is likely to be rare (Squire & Chace, 1975). The evidence against ECT causing permanent brain damage is supported by studies on patients who have received longer courses of treatment which fail to show any cognitive impairment over pre-ECT assessments (Devanand *et al*, 1991; Scott *et al*, 1991*b*; Hay & Scott, 1994).

Efficacy of ECT

The UK Medical Research Council trial (1965) showed a significantly greater improvement in patients with depression receiving ECT compared with the other treatments (71% improved with ECT, 52% with imipramine, 30% with phenelzine and 39% with placebo). A large controlled study in America found a 76% response rate with ECT compared to 45% with placebo (Greenblatt *et al*, 1964).

The treatment package of ECT involves a number of interventions, apart from the induction of a seizure, any of which might influence recovery. These include the therapeutic milieu of the clinical setting (usually in-patient), the administration of an anaesthetic, the short term induction of unconsciousness, the passage of electricity through the brain, and the production of a grand mal seizure. Evidence that it is the seizure itself rather than the passage of electricity through the brain which results in clinical improvement was first demonstrated by Ottoson (1960) who also found the degree of memory loss to be proportional to the amount of electricity used. Further support for the argument that the seizure is the key factor comes from evidence that intravenous lignocaine will reduce seizure length and result in prolonged recovery (Cronholm & Ottoson, 1960) and that intravenous flurothyl is equally efficacious when substituted as the convulsant agent (Laurell, 1970).

In an attempt to separate these issues in a clinical setting the effects of real ECT have been compared with those of sham ECT. Sham ECT involves exactly the same procedure as real ECT except that once the patient is unconscious no electrical stimulation is applied. These studies have shown that bilateral ECT is significantly superior compared to sham treatment (Freeman *et al*, 1978; Johnstone *et al*, 1980; West, 1981; Brandon *et al*, 1984). In two of the studies (Johnstone *et al*, 1980; West, 1981) when patients were followed up after treatment the differences between the control and treated groups disappeared at one and three months respectively. Both studies noted that patients with more severe delusional depression tended to respond better to treatment. In the studies by Freeman *et al* (1978) and West (1981) substitution of real ECT for sham resulted in a rapid improvement in the patient's condition. Another study (Gregory *et al*, 1985) found that patients receiving bilateral ECT treatment responded significantly better than those receiving unilateral treatment who in turn responded better than those receiving sham treatment. Patients receiving bilateral treatment required fewer treatments than those receiving unilateral ECT. Although most studies show real ECT is superior to sham ECT, Lambourn & Gill (1978) failed to detect any differences between unilateral ECT and sham ECT, although both groups improved over the study period.

Mode of action

Details of the precise neurophysiological changes that underly the therapeutic affect remain unclear (see review by Fink, 1990; also Cooper *et al*, 1995).

Investigation into monoamine receptor changes following ECT have revealed an increase in $5HT_2$ receptors (Green, 1988). Neuroendocrine investigations have focused on the effects of ECT on a number of substrates including prolactin, ACTH, cortisol, TSH, GH and various posterior pituitary peptides (Aperia *et al*, 1985; Scott, 1989; Kronfol *et al*, 1991). Most of these rise following ECT although the therapeutic implications of the changes are unclear. Of note is the rise in prolactin following ECT, which is blocked by the serotonin antagonist methysergide suggesting a major role for this neurotransmitter system (Papakostas *et al*, 1988), although its inter-relationship with other transmitter systems and relevance to therapeutic effects is unknown. At present there are no physiological measures or tests which are more reliable than clinical judgement in predicting which patients will respond to ECT (Cooper *et al*, 1990).

Clinical administration of ECT

Hospitals in which ECT is administered should have facilities that meet the requirements recommended by the Royal College of Psychiatrists (1995). These include having a designated ECT suite comprising a minimum of three rooms, a quiet waiting area, the treatment room and an adequately equipped recovery room.

A consultant psychiatrist should have direct responsibility for the ECT suite and should take an active role in the running of the clinic. This should include having responsibility for the junior doctors' ECT rota, making sure that adequate training is given to junior staff and that they have adequate supervision while performing their clinical duties. If possible junior staff should have the opportunity to follow individual patients through a course of ECT. A senior anaesthetist should be responsible for supervising anaesthetic matters and should liaise closely with the psychiatrists. The hospital should ensure that there are adequate numbers of nursing staff attached to the ECT suite and that these nurses have received appropriate training. A senior experienced nurse should be designated with overall responsibility for the day to day running of the ECT suite.

Pre-treatment preparation

Before receiving ECT it is the responsibility of the psychiatrist and the nursing staff to ensure that the patients are adequately prepared.

The psychiatrist should take a full history (including recent drug use) and carry out a full clinical examination looking for factors which might interfere with the ECT process (Lock, 1994) or compromise patients from the anaesthetic point of view. It is important to ask about psychotropic medication the patient is taking as it may have significant cardiovascular side-effects which could increase the likelihood of a fatal arrhythmia during anaesthesia. If possible the psychiatrist should stop such treatment before ECT although in clinical practice this may not be feasible. Some drugs alter the seizure threshold. Benzodiazepines and anticonvulsant drugs increase the seizure threshold making it harder to electrically induce seizures while other drugs e.g. SSRIs, tricyclic antidepressants and neuroleptics reduce the seizure threshold. In particular there are reports of SSRIs being associated with status seizures.

A full list of factors known to affect seizure threshold can be seen in Table 5.2. Details of relevant information should be recorded on a standard ECT prescription form which the anaesthetist can see at a glance. This

Table 5.2 Factors which alter seizure threshold (T) and duration (D). From Weiner *et al* (1991), by permission of W. B Saunders Co.

Lower threshold/longer duration	Higher threshold/shorter duration
Gender – female (T)	Gender – male (T)
Young (T, D)	Elderly (T, D)
Multiple seizures over the last few minutes (D)	Multiple seizures over the last few weeks (T, D)
Unilateral ECT (d'Elia et al, 1975)	Unilateral ECT (other types) (T, D)
	Bilateral ECT (T)
Low initial seizure threshold (D)	High initial seizure threshold (D)
Moderate supra threshold stimulus (D)	Maximal supra threshold stimulus (D)
Hyperventilation (low Pco_2) (D)	Hypoventilation (High Pco_2) (D)
Hyperoxygenation (D)	Hypooxygenation (D)
Muscle relaxation (D)	General anaesthesia (T, D) (particularly propofol and methohexitone > 1.2 mg/kg) (except for ketamine)
Adenosine antagonists (?T, D) (Caffeine, theophylline etc.)	
Stimulants (?T, D)	Anticonvulsants (T, D)
Reserpine (T)	
Adrenaline (?T)	Benzodiazepines (T, D)
Sedative/hypnotic withdrawal (?T, D)	L-tryptophan (D)
Sensory stimulation (T)	Lignocaine (T, D)
	Beta-blockers (centrally acting) (D)
	Clonidine (?D)
	Opioids (?T)

form should include information about the patient's age, physical health, relevant past history, drug treatments and details of past and present ECT treatments. It is the responsibility of the psychiatrist to review the medication of all patients about to receive ECT and to make certain that the anaesthetist is aware of any aspect of the patient's physical state, drug treatment and so forth that could be potentially hazardous during ECT. If necessary the psychiatrist should liaise directly with the anaesthetist at an early stage to discuss any areas of concern. Consent should be obtained (see page 233).

The psychiatric nursing staff have a continuing role in support, explanation and reassurance in the time leading up to ECT. They should also supervise standard pre-anaesthetic procedures, for example, fasting, emptying of the bladder and bowels and checking that the treatment has been prescribed properly and consent given. A psychiatric nurse should accompany the patient throughout the treatment.

The practical administration of ECT

All psychiatrists who are involved in the clinical administration of ECT should have adequate training in the practical aspects of delivery. An official video teaching pack from the Royal College of Psychiatrists' Special Committee on ECT should be used.

Details on stimulus dosing, seizure thresholds and duration, placement of electrodes and the features of modern ECT machines can be found in Lock (1994), Cooper *et al* (1995), Robertson & Fergusson (1996), and *The ECT Handbook* (Royal College of Psychiatrists, 1995).

Debate about the relative merits of unilateral and bilateral electrode placement continues (Abrams, 1986). While there is good evidence that right unilateral ECT produces fewer cognitive side-effects compared with bilateral treatment it seems that more treatments are required. Bilateral ECT gives a more rapid clinical improvement but produces more cognitive side-effects. It would seem reasonable therefore to use unilateral treatment for the elderly, and others who may be more sensitive to the cognitive side-effects and for those who have responded well in the past to unilateral ECT. Bilateral treatment, however, is the most widely used treatment in the UK.

It is best to commence treatment at a relatively lower setting and restimulate the patient if necessary titrating the dose of electricity up over the first two to three treatments. There is considerable individual variation in seizure threshold and this also tends to rise by about 70% during a course of treatment and so a higher charge may be required for later treatments. Accurate placement of the electrodes is necessary to ensure that sufficient current passes through the brain. A large part of the charge administered is required to overcome the resistance of the soft tissues, bone and CSF that separate the electrodes from the brain. It is helpful to slightly moisten the hair at the site and immediately adjacent to the site of electrode placement to reduce the electrical resistance. The ECT stimulus should only be administered once the muscle fasciculation caused by the depolarising effects of the muscle relaxant have worn off. Seizure length should be recorded either from the beginning or the end of the stimulus although the latter is a more representative measure. The length of the convulsion is not reliably related to the therapeutic efficacy of treatment. In a clinical setting the ultimate test about whether ECT is working is the observed clinical state of the patient. If the patient is improving the seizures duration is probably irrelevant. In older patients, and those further on in a course of ECT, shorter seizures may still result in a good clinical response.

If seizure duration is in doubt EEG monitoring will yield more accurate information (Christensen & Koldbaek, 1982). ECT causes a generalised central seizure that spreads through the cerebral cortex and ends with a post-ictal electrical silence that lasts up to 90 seconds. Post-ictal suppression is then followed by high voltage delta waves and theta waves and then a return to the pre-seizure EEG in 20–30 minutes. The EEG may take some months to return to normal after a course of ECT. Unfortunately monitoring is usually impractical because most hospitals lack the necessary equipment. A more accessible but less accurate method is the Hamilton "cuff method" which involves pumping a blood pressure cuff to beyond the systolic blood pressure prior to the administration of any muscle relaxant. Twitching in the forearm distal to the cuff indicates seizure activity. However, it should be remembered that seizure activity detectable using an EEG can occur without any obvious peripheral motor manifestations. Three types of inadequate seizure may occur: failed seizure (no seizure or a seizure lasting less than 15 seconds), a seizure of insufficient duration (15 - 25 seconds) or a prolonged seizure. It is always best to confirm with other staff present that seizure activity has not occurred or has been too brief. Faults due to the equipment or inadvertently using the wrong setting or poor connections should be quickly ruled out. Before applying a second stimulus the anaesthetist should be asked to ventilate the patient with 100% oxygen, which not only prevents hypoxia, but also lowers seizure threshold. A second stimulus at approximately 25–100% of the original charge (American Psychiatric Association, 1990) is then applied but if no further fit occurs treatment should be abandoned for that session. A few patients may consistently fail to have adequate seizures and as a consquence no clinical improvement occurs. In these instances it is important to confirm that seizures have actually occurred, either by the cuff method or by EEG monitoring if this is available. Lateral skull x-rays may help determine the thinnest part of the skull and electrode placement over these areas may lessen electrical resistance of the bone. Seizure threshold may also be reduced by asking the anaesthetist to hyperventilate the patient, or by administering neuroleptics, caffeine, or theophyleine (Coffey *et al*, 1990; Swartz *et al*, 1991).

An appropriate length of time for defining a prolonged seizure is more than one minute, although no clear guidelines exist. Studies based on EEG monitoring suggest that the prevalence of prolonged seizures is lower than reported and that they are often wrongly attributed to prolonged apnoea (Weiner *et al*, 1980). In these circumstances the setting on the ECT machine should be reduced for future treatments. Occasionally a patient will have a prolonged seizure that has to be terminated pharmacologically using intravenous diazepam. The length of time a seizure should be permitted to continue without intervening is also not clearly defined but it seems reasonable to consider terminating seizures that have lasted more than two minutes. Before continuing the course of ECT the clinician should look for factors that could be acting to prolong seizure activity such as other drugs, and make appropriate changes. The machine setting should also be reduced. It is essential that the psychiatrist records details of seizure activity and recommendations for future ECT treatments in the ECT record.

Consent

The psychiatrist has a responsibility to ensure that if possible patients have given their explicit written consent to the procedure (Royal College of Psychiatrists, 1995). The psychiatrist needs to explain why ECT has been selected as a treatment, the procedure and its side-effects, that a general anaesthetic is used, and the likely consequences of not having the ECT. The language used as well as the amount of detail should be tailored according to the needs and sophistication of the patient, but it should be as clear and simple as possible.The psychiatrist should explain the nature of the procedure, including the risks involved clearly and simply. In the UK this involves giving an explanation to a level "based on what a reasonable member of the medical profession would give to the patient in a particular set of circumstances to enable him to make a decision" (Sideaway, 1985). Consent should be clearly documented on a typed consent form which should be filed in the patient's notes. Patients may withdraw their consent at any time during the course of treatment. It is a sad reminder that in one study (Freeman & Kendell, 1980) only one fifth of the patients who had received ECT felt they had been given an adequate explanation. It is good practice to offer patients a written information sheet about the treatment. It is also sensible to fully inform the relatives of the decision to treat and explaining the potential side-effects.

The ability of a patient to give informed consent as outlined above is not always possible. Some very severely depressed, often psychotic or mute patients whose thought processes, reasoning and judgement are impaired are not able to give informed consent. In practice this is a clinical decision that the psychiatrist must make. If a patient seems unable to give consent or refuses treatment in the face of severe or life threatening illness then the psychiatrist should use the relevant section in the Mental Health Act and then seek a second opinion of an independent colleague, through the Mental Health Commission in England, Wales and Northern Ireland and the Mental Welfare Commission in Scotland (see Cooper *et al* (1995) for details).

In cases of dire emergency, for example if poor fluid intake becomes life threatening, ECT may be given without consent under the "duty to care principle", but after doing this the relevant Mental Health Commission must be contacted and a second opinion arranged.

Psychosurgery

History

Trepanation, the boring of holes through the skull, began between four and five thousand years ago in Europe and North Africa and its use spread to Siberia, Asia, Tahiti and New Zealand and in South America to Peru and Bolivia. It was used to treat a variety of pathological conditions (Swayze, 1995). The modern era of psychosurgery was started by the Portuguese neurologist, Egas Moniz, who had already made a name for himself in developing cerebral angiography. In 1935 he and his neurosurgical colleague, Almeida Lima, attended the Second International Neurological Congress in London where Fulton and Jacobson of Yale University reported the effects of ablating the frontal lobe association areas in two chimpanzees, Becky and Lucy. In a learned task involving which of two cups contained food the chimpanzees displayed emotional upset including one chimpanzee having a violent temper if she forgot where the food was. After the operation the chimpanzees made similar errors but without any evidence of emotional response. At the end of the lecture, Moniz stood up and asked whether the operation might be used to help disturbed psychiatric patients. Later that year Moniz and Lima injected alcohol as a sclerosing agent into a patient's frontal lobe white matter through bilateral trephine openings in the skull. They later developed a special instrument called a leucotome which had a retractable wire loop used to crush discrete cores of white matter in the frontal lobes. They reported effects of this procedure on nearly 100 patients, and those with depression, anxiety and obsessional neurosis did better than those with schizophrenia. In the absence of any other effective treatment at the time it was thought to be a great advance and in 1949 Moniz received the Nobel Prize for Medicine.

In 1936 Freeman, a neurologist, and Watts, a neurosurgeon, modified Moniz's procedure by using a lateral approach. Thus incisions and burr holes were made behind the canthus of the eye destroying white matter in a coronal plane. This closed procedure became known as the "standard leucotomy of Freeman and Watts". It soon became the standard operation in Europe and North America and many thousands of patients were operated on. By the mid 1940s severe side-effects were reported. Many patients became apathetic, lethargic, placid and lacking in any emotional spontaneity and 10% subsequently developed epilepsy. Postmortem studies of these early leucotomy cases showed that the lesion sometimes increased in size in the years following surgery. The outcome was particularly poor in cases of schizophrenia and 40% of those operated on remained in hospital. With the advent of chlorpromazine the operation fell into disrepute and its use in schizophrenia eventually ceased.

Modern techniques

Psychosurgery is still practiced today, but on a much smaller scale and only in three centres in the world, Boston, Stockholm and London (Bridges, 1994). All the present day operations have in common the interruption of tracts between the frontal cortex and the limbic system. The advent of stereotactic surgery, combined with the new imaging techniques such as CT and MRI has helped to make the modern operations more accurate. The three operations in use today are described below.

Stereotactic subcaudate tractotomy (SST)

This is the main operation practiced in the UK. The target site is the lower medial quadrant of the frontal lobe and the lesion is made beneath the head of the caudate nucleus, severing connections between the supra-orbital part of the frontal lobe and the limbic system. The term tractotomy was introduced to avoid the unhappy associations of the earlier terms leucotomy and lobotomy (Bridges, 1992). Using a stereotactic technique, radioactive yttrium 90 rods, each about 7mm long, are inserted in two rows. These decay with a half life of 68 hours to zirconium which is a stable isotope and the lethal radiation extends no more than 2mm from the rods, allowing areas of destruction in the brain to be strictly delimited. This is a much safer and more accurate method than using the earlier leucotomies.

Capsulotomy

This operation is used in Sweden mainly for depression, severe anxiety and obsessive–compulsive disorders. Capsulotomy entails interruption of the anterior limb of the internal capsule bilaterally thus disconnecting the limbic system from the frontal lobes. Heated electrodes, radioactive implants, or beams focused from an external gamma radiation source are used to make the lesions.

Cingulotomy

The cingulum is a bundle of association fibres which run from the orbital frontal cortex around the corpus callosum terminating in the cortex of the temporal lobe and also connecting with the hippocampal gyrus. Cingulotomy is most commonly performed in the USA. Two bilateral burr holes are made and electrodes are passed through them; with the help of MRI and a stereotactic frame the electrodes are accurately placed in the cingulum bundles. The lesion is made by heating the tips of the electrodes to 80–85°C for 100 seconds. The incidence of side-effects is low but a second operation may be required 6–12 months later if the first operation is ineffective. It is used mainly in the treatment of anxiety, obsessive–compulsive disorder, depression, and pain.

Post operative course

The operations appear to be safe with a negligible mortality. Patients get out of bed on the second day and are mobile on the third day. With SST, confusion develops in around 10% of those over 50 years of age and MRI scans have shown this is the result of cerebral oedema. Haemorrhage and significantly adverse effects on personality are rare but 1–2% may develop fits. Rehabilitation is important in the first few months because there is a gradual improvement over a period of several weeks, sometimes lasting for 3–6 months or more. Post operative tests of cognitive function usually show an improvement because of the symptom relief, for example the poor concentration associated with depression.

Indications and frequency of use

The operation is only considered for serious, incapacitating, and persistent treatment-resistant non-schizophrenic illnesses. These include both unipolar and bipolar depression, anxiety states, phobic anxiety, obsessive–compulsive disorders, as well as persistent suicidal behaviour and self-mutilation. Contraindications include the presence of even mild dementing processes which can now be detected on pre-operative CT scans, other cerebral lesions, schizophrenia (but not schizo-affective disorder), adverse premorbid personality traits, and the presence of addictions.

Before embarking on psychosurgery treatment resistance must be confirmed. In the London unit (Bridges, 1994) this entails: two full courses of ECT separated by several months; a trial of a high dose of a tricyclic, such as amitriptyline up to 400mg daily; lithium augmentation for two months; a trial of a MAOI such as phenelzine 90mg daily if this can be tolerated. For obsessive–compulsive disorder an adequate trial of behaviour therapy would have failed. Treatment resistance usually develops over a period of years and establishing the degree of treatment resistance described above will take more time. In the UK the operation is declining in frequency, thus in 1979 there were 70 operations but by 1989 there were only 23 operations and of those referred to one centre only 22% were operated on (Bridges, 1992). Thus while psychosurgery remains an option for treating severe and resistant disorders it is very rarely used today.

Outcome

As might be expected there are no double-blind placebo-controlled trials for psychosurgery, but there are several reports comparing patients before and after the operation. Strom Olson & Carlyle (1971) reported on a series of 150 cases with mixed diagnoses and found that 56% of those with depression, 50% of the obsessionals and 41% of those with anxiety did well. None of the nine schizophrenic patients did well. Modest but longlasting personality change was found in only 2.4% of the subjects but minor changes were detected in a further 11%. There was also some reduction in the number of suicide attempts. Goktepe (1975) found in the pre-operative review period that 33 out of 78 patients had made suicidal attempts compared to only five in the post-operative period, although over the longer term 3% committed suicide. This figure should be placed in the context of a long-term suicide risk of 15% for depressive illnesses. Poynton *et al* (1988) examined a small series of nine patients with bipolar disorder refractory to other treatments. He reported a greater reduction in severity of the mania than for depression and stated there had been some amelioration of the mood swings.

Mindus (1988) reported on the result of 300 cases of capsulotomy and found 70% improvement in cases of obsessive–compulsive disorder, generalised anxiety disorder and severe phobic conditions. Ballantine *et al* (1990) reported on 198 patients who had a cingulotomy in Boston and some nine years later found that 66% of those with depression did well but the 4% with personality disorders and the 6% with schizophrenia "improved less predictably". In this series a late suicide rate of 9% was noted. In a second report from the Boston group Martuza *et al* (1990) reported that 25% of those with obsessive–compulsive disorder treated with cingulotomy were functionally improved and well, and another 31% showed some improvement.

Although a multi-centred double-blind control trial would be desirable it would be difficult to undertake as there is no adequate control group. The Royal College of Psychiatrists (1977) made an attempt to devise a trial where some of the patients referred for psychosurgery received the operation and others were to be placed on a waiting list to serve as controls for a period of one year, but the project floundered partly for lack of funding but also on the issue of consent. Thus patients with severe intractable psychiatric disorders whose hopes had been raised that they might be cured, would be unlikely to give their consent to be placed in a control group, and have to wait for a year before receiving any treatment (Bridges, 1992).

The Mental Health Act

In the UK, Section 57 of the Mental Health Act 1983 was introduced to supervise psychosurgery and applies to "any surgical operation for destroying brain tissue or for destroying the function of brain tissue as well as such forms of treatment as may be specified for the purpose of this section by regulations made by the Secretary of State", the latter applying at the present time only to surgical implantation of hormones. Section 57 requires both the consent of the patient *and* a second opinion, and the second opinion doctor should certify that the treatment has a likelihood of alleviating or preventing deterioration. Section 57 requires a doctor (who is not responsible for the patient's care), and two other persons (neither being doctors, one a nurse and the other not a nurse or a doctor) appointed by the Mental Health Act Commission to have "certified in writing that the patient is capable of understanding the nature, purpose and likely effects of the treatment in question and has consented to it".

References

Abrams, R. (1986) Is unilateral electroconvulsive therapy really the treatment of choice in endogenous depression? *Annals of the New York Academy of Sciences*, **462**, 50–54.
—— (1991) Electroconvulsive therapy in the medically compromised patient. *Psychiatric Clinics of North America*, **14**, 871–885.
——, Taylor, M. A., Faber, R., *et al* (1983) Bilateral versus unilateral electroconvulsive therapy: efficacy in melancholia. *American Journal of Psychiatry*, **140**, 450–463.
Abraham, K. R. & Kulhara, P. (1987) The efficacy of electroconvulsive therapy in the treatment of schizophrenia: a comparative study. *British Journal of Psychiatry*, **151**, 152–155.
Alexopoulos, G. S., Shamoian, C. J., Lucas, J., *et al* (1984) Medical problems of geriatric psychiatric patients and younger controls during electroconvulsive therapy. *Journal of the American Psychiatric Society*, **32**, 651–654.
American Psychiatric Association Task Force on Electroconvulsive Therapy (1990) *The Practice of Electroconvulsive Therapy: Recommendations for Treatment, Training and Privileging*. Washington, DC: American Psychiatric Association.

Andersen, K., Balldin, J., Gottfries, C. G., *et al* (1987) A double blind evaluation of electroconvulsive therapy in Parkinson's disease with "on–off" phenomena. *Acta Neurologica Scandinavica*, **76**, 191–199.

Aperia, B., Bergman, H., Ecklebrekston, K., *et al* (1985) Effects of electroconvulsive therapy on neurophysiological functioning and circulating levels of ACTH, cortisol, prolactin and TSH in patients with major depressive illness. *Acta Psychiatrica Scandinavica*, **72**, 536–541.

Avery, D. & Winokur, G. (1976) Mortality in depressed patients treated with electroconvulsive therapy and antidepressants. *Archives of General Psychiatry*, **33**, 1029–1037.

Ballantine, H. T. Jr., Bouckoms, A. J., Thomas, E. K., *et al* (1987) Treatment of psychiatric illness by stereotactic cingulotomy. *Biological Psychiatry*, **22**, 807–819.

Black, D. W., Winokur G. & Nasrallah, A. (1986) ECT in unipolar and bipolar disorders: a naturalistic evaluation of 460 patients. *Convulsive Therapy*, **2**, 231–237.

——, —— & —— (1987) Treatment of mania: A naturalistic study of electroconvulsive therapy versus lithium in the treatment of 438 patients. *Journal of Clinical Psychiatry*, **48**, 132–139.

Bolwig, T. G., Hertz, M. M., Paulson, O. B., *et al* (1977) The permeability of the blood–brain barrier during electrically induced seizures in man. *European Journal of Clinical Investigation*, **7**, 87–93.

Brandon, S., Cowley, P., McDonald, C., *et al* (1984) Electroconvulsive therapy: results in depressive illness from the Leicestershire trial. *British Medical Journal*, **288**, 22–25.

Bridges, P. K. (1992) Resistant depression and psychosurgery. In *Handbook of Affective Disorders* (ed. E. S. Paykel), pp. 437–452. Edinburgh: Churchill Livingstone.

——, Bartlett, J. R., Hale, A. S., *et al* (1994) Psychosurgery: stereotactic subcaudate tractotomy, an indispensable treatment. *British Journal of Psychiatry*, **165**, 599–611.

Coffey, C. E., Figiel, G. S., Weiner, R. D., *et al* (1990) Caffeine augmentation of ECT. *American Journal of Psychiatry*, **147**, 579–585.

Cooper, S. J., Scott, A. I. F. & Whalley, L. J. (1990) A neuroendocrine view of ECT. *British Journal of Psychiatry*, **157**, 740–743.

——, Kelly, C. B. & McClelland, R. J. (1995) Affective disorders: 3. Electroconvulsive therapy. In *Seminars in Clinical Psychopharmacology* (ed. D. King), pp. 224–258. London: Gaskell.

Christensen, P. & Koldbaeck, I. B. (1982) EEG monitored ECT. *British Journal of Psychiatry*, **141**, 19–23.

Cronholm, B. & Ottoson, J. O. (1960) Experimental studies of the therapeutic action of ECT in endogenous depression. *Acta Psychiatrica Scandinavica*, **Suppl. 145**, 69–101.

D'Elia, G. & Raotma, H. (1975) Is unilateral ECT less effective than bilateral ECT. *British Journal of Psychiatry*, **126**, 83–89.

Devanand, D. P., Verma, A. K., Tirumalasetti, F., *et al* (1991) Absence of cognitive impairment after more than 100 lifetime ECT treatments. *American Journal of Psychiatry*, **148**, 929–932.

Dodwell, D. & Goldberg, D. (1989) A study of factors associated with response to electroconvulsive therapy in patients with schizophrenic symptoms. *British Journal of Psychiatry*, **154**, 635–639.

Fink, M. (1990) How does convulsive therapy work. *Neuropsychopharmacology*, **3**, 73–82.

Freeman, C. P. L., Basson J. V. & Crighton, A. (1978) Double blind controlled trial of electroconvulsive therapy (ECT) and simulated ECT in depressive illness. *Lancet*, *i*, 738–740.

—— & Kendell, R. E. (1980) ECT: patients' experiences and attitudes. *British Journal of Psychiatry*, **137**, 17–25.

——, Weeks, D. & Kendall, R. E. (1980) ECT: patients who complain. *British Journal of Psychiatry*, **137**, 8–16.

Freidberg, J. (1977) Shock treatment, brain damage and memory loss; a neurological perspective. *American Journal of Psychiatry*, **134**, 1010–1014.

Goktepe, E. O.,Young, L. B. & Bridges, P. K. (1975) A further review of the results of stereotactic subcaudate tractotomy. *British Journal of Psychiatry*, **126**, 270–280.

Green, A. R. (1988) The mechanism of action of antidepressant treatments: basic aspects. *Pharmacopsychiatry*, **21**, 3–5.

Gregory, S., Shawcross, C. R. & Gill, D. (1985) The Nottingham ECT study. A double blind comparison of bilateral, unilateral and simulated ECT in depressive illness. *British Journal of Psychiatry*, **146**, 520–554.

Hay, A. G. & Scott, A. I. F. (1994) ECT and brain damage (letter). *British Journal of Psychiatry*, **165**, 120–121.

Hesche, J. & Roeder, E. (1976) Electroconvulsive therapy in Denmark. *British Journal of Psychiatry*, **128**, 241–245.

——, ——, Theilgaard, A. (1978) Unilateral and bilateral ECT. *Acta Psychiatrica Scandinavica*, **Suppl. 275**.

Johnstone, E. C., Deakin, J. F W., Lawler, P., *et al* (1980) The Northwick Park electroconvulsive therapy trial. *Lancet*, *ii*, 1317–1320.

Kronfol, Z., Hamden-Allen, G., Goel, K., *et al* (1991) Effects of single and repeated electroconvulsive therapy sessions on plasma ACTH, prolactin, growth hormone and cortisol concentrations. *Psychoneuroendocrinology*, **16**, 345–352.

Laurell, B. (1970) Comparison of electric and flurothyl convulsive. *Acta Psychiatrica Scandinavica*, **Suppl. 145**, 22–35.

Lambourn, J. & Gill, D. (1978) A controlled comparison of simulated and real ECT. *British Journal of Psychiatry*, **133**, 514–519.

Lock, T. (1994) Advances in the practice of electroconvulsive therapy. *Advances in Psychiatric Treatment*, **1**, 47–56.

Martuza, R. L., Chiocca, E. A., Jenike, M. A., *et al* (1990) Stereotactic radiofrequency thermal cingulotomy for obsessive–compulsive disorder. *Neuropsychiatric Practice and Opinion*, **2**, 331–336.

May, P. R. A. (1968) *Treatment of Schizophrenia*. New York: Science House.

Medical Research Council Clinical Psychiatry Committee (1965) Clinical trial of the treatment of depressive illness. *British Medical Journal*, *i*, 881–886.

Mindus, P. (1988) *Capsulotomy, a Psychosurgical Intervention Considered in Cases of Anxiety Disorders Unresponsive to Conventional Therapy*. Pp. 151–167. National Board of Health and Welfare, Drug Information Committee, Sweden.

Munroe, R. R. (1991) Maintenance electroconvulsive therapy. *Psychiatric Clinics of North America*, **14**, 947–960.

Ottoson, J. D. (1960) Experimental studies on the mode of action of electroconvulsive therapy. *Acta Psychiatrica Scandinavica*, **Suppl. 145**, 35.

Papakostas, Y., Markianos, M. & Stefanis, C. (1988) Methysergide reduces the prolactin response to ECT. *Biological Psychiatry*, **24**, 465–468.

Perrin, G. M. (1961) Cardiovascular aspects of electric shock therapy. *Acta Psychiatrica Scandinavica*, **Suppl. 152**.

Poynton, A., Bridges, P. K. & Bartlett, J. R. (1988) Resistant bipolar affective disorder treated by stereotactic subcaudate tractotomy. *British Journal of Psychiatry*, **152**, 354–358.

Robertson, C. & Fergusson, G. (1996) Electroconvulsive therapy machines. *Advances in Psychiatric Treatment*, **2**, 24–31.

Royal College of Psychiatrists (1977) Research Committee evaluation of the surgical treatment of functional mental illness: proposal for a prospective controlled trial. In *Neurosurgical Treatment in Psychiatry, Pain and Epilepsy*. (eds W. H. Sweet, S. Obrador & J. G. Martin-Rodriguez). Baltimore: University Park Press.

Royal College of Psychiatrists' Special Committee on ECT (1995) *The ECT Handbook*. Council Report CR 39. London: RCPsych.

Sackeim, H. A., Decina, P., Kanzler, M., *et al* (1987) Effects of the electrode placement on the efficacy of titrated low dose ECT. *American Journal of Psychiatry*, **144**, 1449–1455.

——, Devenand, D. P. & Prudic, J. (1991) Stimulus intensity, seizure threshold and seizure duration: impact of the efficacy and safety of electroconvulsive therapy. *Psychiatric Clinics of North America*, **14**, 803–843.

Schefter, W. A. & Schuman, R. D. (1992) Treatment choice in neuroleptic malignant syndrome. *Convulsive Therapy*, **8**, 267–279.

Scott, A. I. F. (1989) Which depressed patients will respond to electroconvulsive therapy? The search for biological predictors of recovery. *British Journal of Psychiatry*, **154**, 8–17.

Scott, A. I. F., Weeks, D. & MacDonald, C. (1991*a*) Continuation electroconvulsive therapy. Preliminary guidelines and an illustrative case report. *British Journal of Psychiatry*, **159**, 867–870.

——, Turnbull, L. W., Blane, A., *et al* (1991*b*) Electroconvulsive therapy and brain damage. *Lancet*, **338**, 264.

Selected Staff, University of Louisville School of Medicine (1985) 1250 Electroconvulsive treatments without evidence of brain injury. *British Journal of Psychiatry*, **147**, 203–204.

Sideaway v. Board of Governors of Bethlam Royal Hospital and The Maudsley (1985) 2WLR 480; (1985) 1 All E.R. 643 HLL.

Small, J. G., Milstein, V., Klapper, M. H., *et al* (1988) Electroconvulsive therapy in the treatment of manic episodes. *Annals of the New York Academy of Sciences*, **462**, 37–49.

Squire, L. R. (1986) Memory functions as affected by electroconvulsive therapy. *Annals of the New York Academy of Sciences*, **462**, 307.

—— & Chace, P. (1975) Memory functions six and nine months after electroconvulsive therapy. *Archives of General Psychiatry*, **32**, 1557–1564.

Strom-Olsen, R. & Carlisle, S. (1971) Bifrontal stereotactic tractotomy. *British Journal of Psychiatry*, **118**, 141–154.

Swartz, C. M. & Lewis, R. K. (1991) Theophylline reversal of electroconvulsive therapy (ECT) seizure inhibition. *Psychosomatics*, **32**, 47–51.

Swayze, V. W. (1995) Frontal leucotomy and related surgical procedures in the era before antipsychotics (1935–1954): an historical overview. *American Journal of Psychiatry*, **152**, 505–515.

Taylor, P. J. & Fleminger, J. J. (1980) ECT for schizophrenia. *Lancet*, *i*, 1380–1382.

Wiener, R. D., Volow, M. R., Gianturco *et al* (1980) Seizures terminable and interminable with ECT. *American Journal of Psychiatry*, **137**, 1416–1418.

Weeks, D., Freeman, C. P. L. & Kendell, R. E. (1980) ECT III: Enduring cognitive deficits. *British Journal of Psychiatry*, **137**, 26–37.

Weiner, R. D. (1984) Does electroconvulsive therapy cause brain damage? *Behaviourial Science*, **7**, 1–53.

——, Coffey, C. E. & Krystal, A. D. (1991) The monitoring and management of electrically induced seizures. *Psychiatric Clinics of North America*, **14**, 845–869.

West, E. D. (1981) Electric convulsion therapy in depression: a double blind controlled trial. *British Medical Journal*, **282**, 355–357.

Zervas, I. M. & Fink, M. (1991) ECT for refractory Parkinson's disease. *Convulsive Therapy*, **7**, 222–223.

6 Psychological treatment of depression

Stirling Moorey

Individual therapy ● Group therapy ● Marital and family therapy ● Principles of psychological management ● Psychotherapy research in depression ● Conclusions

---

Psychosocial intervention, in its broadest sense, is a vital component in the management of all types of depression, from mild depressive reactions to psychotic episodes. Even if ECT or pharmacological therapy is the main treatment, the way in which the clinician assesses, engages the patient, gives information about the illness and its treatment, and provides support contributes significantly to successful outcome. In addition to this basic level of supportive work, many patients will benefit from more structured forms of psychotherapy. This chapter will consider the various psychological therapies available for individual, group, family and marital treatment of depression. Some general principles of psychological management for the depressed patient will be described. The final section will review studies of the effectiveness of various therapies.

Antidepressants and psychotherapy

Antidepressant medication is the main line of treatment for most depression seen by psychiatrists but it is not a panacea. In a recent multicentre trial appropriately conservative criteria for recovery revealed that only 57% of depressed patients could be said to have recovered after antidepressant therapy plus clinical management (Elkin *et al,* 1989). Side-effects of drugs may prevent adequate dosage, while compliance is rarely complete. The value of maintenance antidepressants to prevent relapse is now recognised; relapse rates rise when medication is discontinued. Relapse on a placebo following active treatment can be as high as 89% over three years (Glen *et al,* 1984). Psychological treatments can seem more attractive to many patients. They offer no physical side-effects, and hold the promise of perhaps deeper and more lasting change than can be obtained with drug therapy. In patients whose physical state contraindicates drug treatment, psychological therapy may be the only treatment option.

Some concern has been expressed in the past about combining antidepressant medication with psychotherapy. Taking an antidepressant might for instance lead patients to attribute gains to this and not the therapy, and thus reduce the extent to which they internalise the effects of therapy. Klerman & Schechter (1985) reviewed the ways in which the two treatments might interact. There is evidence to suggest that the two modalities may complement each other in the short term (Weissman *et al*, 1979; Blackburn *et al*, 1981) and follow-up studies do not suggest that there is any negative long-term effect of combined treatments (Blackburn *et al*, 1986; Simons *et al*, 1986).

Individual therapy

Most descriptive and research work has been done using individual therapy with depressed patients. There are two broad approaches to therapy with depressed patients. Firstly, there are therapies which aim to relieve depressive symptoms, such as cognitive, behavioural and interpersonal therapies. These problem-oriented therapies are used during the depressive phase itself with or without accompanying antidepressants. In addition to relieving distress they also attempt to reduce vulnerability to relapse. The second approach is associated with therapies such as psychoanalysis. Here the primary aim is not symptom relief, but resolution of conflict and modification of deeper personality structures. Treatments based on psychoanalytic theory are usually applied after the patient has recovered from the depressive episode.

Cognitive therapy

Cognitive therapy (CT) is the most widely known and most thoroughly evaluated psychological treatment for depression. The therapy is firmly based on Beck's cognitive model of depression (Beck *et al*, 1979). This states that depression is characterised by a negative bias in information processing. There is a depressive cognitive triad: a negative view of the self, the world and the future. Depressed patients believe themselves to be inadequate and worthless, their surroundings seem bleak and uninteresting and the future seems hopeless. Interpretations of current events and predictions about future events are distorted. Beck identifies particular biases in information processing, called cognitive distortions or thinking errors (See Box 6.1). These often take the form of faulty inferences. One of the commonest thinking errors is 'overgeneralisation', where a single negative event is seen as the beginning of a never-ending pattern of defeats. For example, a depressed person may forget to buy some items at the supermarket, concludes from this that his memory is beginning to fail, and becomes convinced that he is facing an inexorable decline into senility.

The depressed person's distorted view of the world shows itself in the form of frequent negative automatic thoughts. These are spontaneous, plausible thoughts and images associated with unpleasant emotions, which enter the mind unbidden. When viewed logically they appear to be exaggerated and unrealistic. For instance, if criticised for a small mistake at work a depressed patient might have the following negative automatic thoughts:

Negative view of self – 'I'm stupid, this job's beyond me. I never get anything right.'

Negative view of world – 'nobody likes me here, I just don't fit in.'

Negative view of future – 'what's the point? It's useless even trying. They'll give me the sack soon.'

Other symptoms of depression are derived from this cognitive bias: behavioural symptoms such as social withdrawal and low activity levels; loss of motivation and interest; cognitive deficits such as poor concentration. Cognitive factors are not the cause of depression, but mediate between various factors such as biological and environmental

---

Box 6.1 Examples of information processing errors in depression (from Blackburn & Davidson, 1990)

Situation: my boss laughed at two typing errors I had made in a draft.

Selective abstraction: the patient selects one aspect of a situation and interprets the whole situation on the basis of this one detail.

Interpretations: he dismissed two hours' hard typing with derision.

Arbitrary inference: the patient reaches a conclusion without enough evidence to support that conclusion or even in the face of contrary evidence.

Interpretations: he thinks I am a poor typist.

Overgeneralisation: the patient draws a general conclusion on the basis of one aspect of a situation which has been arbitrarily selected from a whole context.

Interpretations: nobody appreciates me.

Magnification and minimisation: the patient exaggerates the negative aspect of a situation and minimises the positive aspect.

Interpretations: what is wrong with me? I make nothing but mistakes.

Personalisation: the patient relates to himself external events when there is no basis for making such a connection.

Interpretations: no wonder he looks so harassed all the time. He cannot even rely on me to type his work correctly.

stressors and depressive symptoms. Depressed mood is associated with more depressive thinking which distorts reality in a negative way and produces more depression. Because the future looks so hopeless patients give up trying to solve their problems and no longer engage in rewarding activities, which further depresses their mood. Cognitive therapy is aimed at breaking into these vicious circles of negative thinking, depressed mood and maladaptive behaviour.

The final component of the model relates to cognitive vulnerability factors. Beck suggests that idiosyncratic beliefs or rules make the person susceptible to depressive reactions to critical events, usually involving loss. These underlying assumptions are derived from experiences in childhood and later life. They often have the form of imperatives such as 'I must always be nice to people,' or conditional statements such as 'I can only be happy if I'm a success at everything I do'.

> A woman presenting with depression had experienced her parents divorce at the age of six. She believed she was responsible for the break up of the marriage, and developed the assumption that she had to make the perfect marriage to make up for it. Whenever she got into a relationship this assumption was activated and she put so much effort into the affair that her partner backed off. She ended up rejected and depressed, feeling her negative beliefs about herself were correct.

Like many assumptions this one remained latent until activated by a critical event (the relationship) when its true maladaptive nature became apparent. It also illustrates the rigid, global and idiosyncratic characteristics of these silent rules.

Beck's cognitive theory is a tripartite one; consisting of cognitive structures (assumptions) which when activated bias cognitive processing (cognitive distortions) and produce depressive cognitions (automatic thoughts).

Characteristics of cognitive therapy

Cognitive therapy is a form of problem-solving. As such, the emphasis is on teaching the patient to identify problems and learn strategies for coping with and resolving them. The therapist is therefore more active and directive than in traditional psychotherapy, and the relationship is a collaborative partnership in problem-solving. The focus is on how maladaptive thinking is maintaining current problems, less than the origins of these problems. From the first session patients are told that the therapy is time-limited and that it will involve learning and practising self-help skills which the patient will be able to continue when therapy ends. In addressing the problems patients are encouraged to view thoughts and beliefs as hypotheses which can be examined and tested. In challenging these maladaptive beliefs the therapist uses questioning and guided discovery, rather than confrontation. Box 6.2 summarises some of the techniques used in cognitive therapy which are described in more detail below.

Behavioural techniques in cognitive therapy

In the treatment of depression behavioural assignments are important in the early stages since they often lead to a rapid improvement in mood. The tasks are set up as experiments for testing negative beliefs and

---

Box 6.2 Cognitive therapy techniques

Behavioural techniques

Activity scheduling – patients structure time to distract themselves from negative thoughts and to encourage pleasurable and rewarding activities.

Graded task assignment – large or complex tasks are divided into smaller achievable ones to give graded success experiences.

Mastery and pleasure ratings – patients rate activities for mastery and pleasure on 10-point scale. Tasks scoring high are scheduled more frequently over coming weeks.

Behavioural experiments – homework tasks are assigned to test negative beliefs.

Cognitive techniques

Identifying negative automatic thoughts – patients learn to monitor negative thoughts associated with exacerbations of depressed mood, and to link external event, thought and affect.

Challenging negative automatic thoughts – patients keep a mood diary and replace negative thoughts with more realistic alternatives. Various methods of challenging thoughts exist:
– labelling distortions
– reality testing
– search for alternatives
– decatastrophising.

Preventative strategies

Challenging assumptions – underlying assumptions are challenged using a cost benefit analysis followed by logical disputation and experimental behaviour change.

Relapse prevention – risk factors for future relapses are identified and strategies for coping reviewed before the end of therapy.

---

predictions. For instance, a depressed patient believed his family would be better off without him because he was useless and a burden to them. The therapist was aware that his relatives were very supportive, so he encouraged the patient to test the belief by asking them if they did indeed feel they would be better off if he were dead. The response was a very moving, open display of affection from his grown-up children which they had not been able to show before. This convinced him that he was valued and needed and led to a marked improvement in his mood.

Activities which give a sense of pleasure or achievement are particularly useful in raising the depressed person's mood. The therapist establishes what activities the patient used to find rewarding and then helps him or her to plan these on a daily basis. A daily activity schedule is used to log what is actually done and the degree of pleasure or achievement recorded for each activity. This gives information about which tasks are most rewarding.

Sometimes tasks need to be broken down into small manageable steps so that they are achievable - many depressed people have very high expectations of themselves even when they are ill, and they set themselves up for failure. For instance, if a patient has a problem with concentration, a graded task programme would involve reading for increasing time spans, reading materials of increasing complexity and gradually increasing the amount of time spent on work related activities. Success at a homework task helps to build self-esteem.

In grading tasks care must be given to ensuring the task is not too difficult for the depressed patient. However, even if the patient is unable to carry out the assignment it is not considered a failure, but gives valuable information about the patient's negative thoughts.

A woman who had some difficulty deciding which problems she wanted to tackle in therapy was asked to write down three problems as homework and to fill out the assessment questionnaires. She came back feeling despairing that the therapy could not help her, because she had such difficulty in doing the homework. This gave information about the degree of her problems with concentration and decision-making; the therapist used her catastrophic reaction (based on the thought 'If I can't do this homework it means the therapy can't help me') to show her how she was overgeneralising from the failure on one task to conclude that she would never get anything out of cognitive therapy.

Strategies for changing cognition

Cognitive interventions are aimed at helping patients to identify and change the cognitive processes which are at the centre of their depression. This can be seen as a three step process:

Step 1. Teaching the model.   In the early stages of therapy the patient is introduced to the cognitive model of emotion, and the problems conceptualised using this framework. The patient is shown how his or her problems are part of the depressive syndrome, and the central role of negative thinking in depression is illustrated. The link between events, cognitions and emotion is described and the patient encouraged to look at how this fits in with their own experiences. For instance, the patient may be asked to recall a day during the week when the depression was more severe, then asked what events might have triggered this exacerbation. The negative interpretation made of the situation will then demonstrate how negative thinking increases depressed mood. If the patient became more depressed after a friend did not return a phone call, a link might be found between this trigger and negative thoughts such as; 'She's not interested in me; if I was worth anything people would want to be with me; I must be boring'. The material from behavioural assignments is often used to illustrate the model, for example when thinking about a task the patient may say 'I won't be able to do it' or 'there's no point in trying'. The link between these negative thoughts and depressed mood and lack of motivation can then be demonstrated. A booklet outlining the model and form of therapy is often given at the first session (*Coping with Depression*; Beck & Greenberg, 1974) to reinforce the discussion within the session. There is evidence to suggest that patients who respond positively to the cognitive model are more likely to benefit from therapy (Fennell & Teasdale, 1987).

Step 2. Identifying negative automatic thoughts.   Once the patient understands the basic concepts involved, the next step is to identify their repetitive automatic thoughts. Initially the therapist elicits negative automatic thoughts in the session, and then the patient records instances of these as homework. A daily form monitoring upsetting events, associated emotions and intervening thoughts can be used to structure this exercise. No matter how pervasive the mood disorder there is usually a fluctuation with everyday events, and noticing this change is a step towards gaining control over the mood. Labelling the type of distortions in thinking can be helpful at this stage (Box 6.1). Most patients, if they are given clear instructions about how to monitor thoughts with examples, can catch their thoughts with a little practice. If they have difficulty, their thoughts about the monitoring itself can be examined. This may reveal negative thoughts about the therapist despising them if they reveal themselves, fear of exposing themselves to the painful cognitions, or hopeless thoughts about the whole exercise being pointless. Once these cognitions are identified they can be challenged with the usual cognitive techniques.

Step 3. Challenging negative automatic thoughts.   As the behavioural work helps to lift the patient's mood and he or she becomes familiar with automatic thoughts, the therapy moves into a more cognitive mode. From session one the therapist has used cognitive techniques to question the reality of the patient's negative thinking. Now the patient learns to do this for himself, recording the automatic thoughts as they occur and challenging them with rational responses. The aim is not to think positively, but to subject thoughts and beliefs to reality testing, and thus overcome the depressive bias. This is known as cognitive restructuring. Several techniques are commonly used to challenge automatic thoughts. Patients can be taught to ask these as questions:

(i) *What's the evidence?*   This is one of the core cognitive techniques. It could be argued that the whole of cognitive therapy is getting the patient to stop accepting thoughts at face value and instead to always ask the question, 'What's my evidence?'. A simple way of doing this is to draw a line down the centre of a piece of paper and list on one side the evidence for and on the other side the evidence against a particular belief.

If you were a depressed psychiatrist you might have the following automatic thought: 'I'm incompetent, I can't do my job properly.'
Evidence for:
– I keep putting off writing that court report.
– I can't concentrate when talking to my patients.
– My colleagues seem to look down on me.
– I've taken weeks off work lately, and I'm letting people down.
Evidence against:
– I know I'm depressed at the moment, and my concentration and motivation are badly affected by that.
– Until six months ago I never had any problems with my work.
– I know I'm not the only person to procrastinate.
– I've no evidence that my colleagues really look down on me, I'm just making assumptions. In fact I know they value me for my contributions because they have told me so in the past.
– Taking time off work is not a sign of incompetence.
– No one has ever criticised my work or complained about my efficiency.
With practice this questioning of evidence becomes automatic, and gradually challenges the ingrained negative bias in the patient's thinking.

(ii) W*hat alternative views are there?*   Alternative interpretations of an event are considered. The depressed person usually chooses the most negative interpretation of an event and automatically assumes this is correct. The therapist teaches the patient to generate alternatives. At first these are also quite negative, but as more and more alternatives are asked for by the therapist the patient is forced to think of more positive ones. This starts to break up the depressive bias in interpretations. After practising in the session the patient is able to question their immediate response to situations in the outside world. For instance, if a friend passes the patient in the street, rather than automatically thinking 'He's deliberately ignoring me', the patient starts to consider other explanations such as 'He's busy and he probably didn't notice me'. The likelihood of these various explanations being correct can then be assessed, and a less biased judgement made about the situation.

(iii) *What are the advantages and disadvantages of this way of thinking?* Even if a negative thought is accurate it is not necessarily helpful. Looking at the usefulness of a belief or thought can help to change it. In this exercise the patient can list the advantages and disadvantages of the negative belief or thought.

Ruminations about real life problems such as unemployment, loss, or even impending death may be accurate reflections of reality, but in depression they rarely lead to effective problem-solving or emotional working through. In fact they have the disadvantage of making the person feel worse, preventing them from engaging in life, and even alienating them from loved ones. Once patients see these disadvantages they are often able to reduce the frequency of these thoughts themselves, or to use distraction techniques.

(iv) *If my interpretation is correct, are things as catastrophic as they seem?* – patients who are anxious and depressed often catastrophise, but rarely think beyond the catastrophe. Facing up to the worst fear often reveals that it is not as terrible as it seems, or that the person has the resources to cope with it. For example, a depressed student convinced he will fail his exam can explore what would be so terrible if he did. He may never have even thought about the fact that he would be able to retake it again without any bad effect on his career.

Preventative strategies

These are aimed at changing the underlying assumptions about the world which make people vulnerable to psychological problems. The same cognitive change techniques which were applied to thoughts can be used with assumptions. Evidence for and against the reasonableness of these assumptions is sought, the advantages and disadvantages of the assumption explored and its origins plotted. Finally a more flexible, less punitive rule is developed and behavioural assignments set so the patient can experiment with acting differently. The final sessions of therapy usually involve some preparation for the future with the discussion of relapse prevention strategies.

Case illustration:

A patient had a very negative relationship with her mother, who had been critical and rejecting throughout her childhood. A typical painful memory was of her mother refusing to give her a goodnight kiss. The one way she did get acceptance was through achievement, and the patient developed the rule that she must do things perfectly or she would be rejected. A specific example of this rule applied in her relationship with her partner: she believed completely that if she was not a perfect partner, giving no cause for criticism, her lover would eventually leave her. The reality and usefulness of this assumption was challenged in the session. Then the patient showed her partner the beliefs she had written down. She was astonished to find that her partner did not agree with her at all, and in fact had a more flexible rule that no one was perfect, and it was healthy to have the occasional row about the irritating things the other person did. As a result her belief in this diminished greatly, and with help from the therapist she began to gradually give up her perfectionistic view of relationships.

Other cognitive and behavioural approaches

Behavioural models of depression are based on learning theory. Depression is seen to be a behavioural deficit (e.g. social withdrawal) resulting from a reduction in rewarding experiences or an increase in aversive experiences. The depressive's environment itself may be unrewarding or the person may lack the skills necessary for obtaining reinforcement (Lewinsohn *et al*, 1976). In treatment emphasis is placed on functional assessment of each case, monitoring of mood and behaviour, increasing pleasant activities and graded tasks. Other behavioural approaches emphasise social interaction and propose social skills training as a treatment (McLean & Hakstian, 1979). Cognitive therapy has been enhanced by the addition of behavioural techniques. Similarly most behavioural theories of depression now contain a cognitive component (Lewinsohn *et al*, 1985).

Interpersonal therapy

Interpersonal therapy (IPT) is a treatment which was developed by Weissman and Klerman in the New Haven-Boston Collaborative Depression Project. It is a brief (12–16 weeks) weekly treatment originally devised for out-patient, non-psychotic, unipolar depressives, which focuses on improving the patient's interpersonal functioning.

Theoretical framework

IPT is based on the assumption that psychosocial and interpersonal factors are of major significance in the development and maintenance of depression, and possibly contribute to vulnerability to further episodes. Its fundamental view of the person derives from Adolf Meyer's psychobiological approach which emphasised the interpersonal and psychosocial context of psychiatric disorder (Meyer, 1957). More specifically, Sullivan's *Interpersonal Psychiatry* (1953) and Bowlby's *Attachment Theory* (1981) have been influential (see page 589). Two main areas of empirical evidence support the contention that problems with social roles are important in depression. Firstly, there is strong evidence that interpersonal relations are impaired in depression. Weissman & Paykel (1974) found that a group of depressed women had more impairment in social functioning, particularly with husbands and children, than a control group of non-depressed neighbours. On recovery marital relationships often remained problematic. Research also shows that depressives behave in a way that elicits negative responses from others (Coyne, 1976). Although these findings may be a result rather than a cause of the depression, their role in maintenance and relapse may still be significant. High expressed emotion in the form of hostile criticism from a family member is a strong predictor of relapse (Hooley *et al*, 1986). The second source of empirical support for the interpersonal theory is research on social stresses and social support. A close confiding relationship with a spouse is a buffer against depression (Brown & Harris, 1978) (see also page 129).

Role impairments in depression. IPT sees all roles, in the nuclear and extended family, work, friendship and community, as having a potential buffering effect. Any disruption of these roles may lead to depression. This psychosocial contribution will interact with the effects of biological factors to produce the final common pathway to depression. Four main problem areas are defined, and become the focus of treatment: grief; interpersonal disputes; role transitions and interpersonal deficits.

Clinical application of interpersonal therapy

This section will give a brief description of the techniques used in IPT. A manual describing the therapy in detail has been published (Klerman *et al*, 1984). Like cognitive therapy IPT is a here-and-now therapy. Current relationships, rather than childhood experiences are the focus of attention. The therapeutic techniques are eclectic, incorporating reassurance, clarification of emotional states, improvement of communication and reality testing of perceptions and performance. These methods are used to achieve two main goals: the alleviation of depressive symptoms, and the development of strategies for dealing with the interpersonal problems associated with the depressive episode.

Managing the depressive state

This phase is supportive and educational. Patients are educated about the nature of depression. The therapist reviews all the patient's symptoms and describes how they are all part of a syndrome of depression which is a well recognised and treatable condition. Information is then given about the prevalence of the condition. Hopelessness may be directly addressed by informing the patient that their belief that they will never recover is part of the depressive syndrome just like symptoms of weight loss or sleep disturbance. Symptom management is another component of this phase and is similar in many ways to the behavioural techniques used in cognitive therapy. Situations which exacerbate the depression are identified and strategies devised to avoid them or reduce their impact. For instance, if the patient feels worse when alone, measures for increasing social contact can be explored; or if the patient is overwhelmed at work they may be helped to reduce their expectations and plan essential tasks. Antidepressant medication may be considered in this symptom reduction phase.

Targeting interpersonal problem areas

Once there has been some reduction in depressive symptoms the therapist adopts a more interpersonal focus. The initial assessment will show which of the four interpersonal problem areas are affected, and one or two of these will be dealt with in therapy. If an unresolved grief reaction is part of the problem the therapist will help the patient to mourn by expressing feelings about the lost person, particularly suppressed anger, reconstruct more realistically the relationship and finally go on to re-establish interests and new relationships. This latter stage may involve the prescription of quite specific tasks such as joining social organisations. Dealing with role transitions involves a similar approach to handling the loss, plus developing a more positive attitude to the new role. Interpersonal role disputes most frequently occur with the spouse. During treatment the patient is helped to identify the dispute, to make choices about a plan of action, and then encouraged to modify maladaptive patterns of communication. IPT works individually with the patient to either change the patient's or spouse's behaviour, or to change the patient's attitude to the problem. Finally, interpersonal deficits may contribute to depression. Social isolation, lack of social skills, or low self-esteem may all be present. IPT reviews past relationship problems and adopts problem-solving and role play to develop social skills. The therapeutic relationship is also used as a vehicle for demonstrating and working with the interpersonal problems in the session.

Psychodynamic therapy

The individual therapies described above were designed specifically to treat the depressive syndrome. They focus on problems and symptoms. In contrast to this, therapies derived from psychoanalysis are not primarily concerned with changing symptoms. They seek to bring about a more radical change of personality or resolution of unconscious conflicts. Depression is merely a manifestation of an underlying disturbance, and recovery from depression does not mean that the true underlying disturbance has been modified. A distinction should be made between psychoanalysis, which is a highly specialised form of psychotherapy carried out 3–5 times weekly for years, where the therapist adopts a deliberately impersonal passive stance; and psychoanalytically-oriented therapies which may be shorter, once weekly and involve a more active therapist. While individual psychoanalysis provides many insights and hypotheses about depression, there is no place for it as a treatment in the NHS, but it may have an important educational role, for example, in the training of psychotherapists.

Psychodynamic theories

Psychoanalysts have produced a wealth of theoretical writing on the subject of depression, with relatively little practical advice on technique and virtually no research on the effectiveness of their methods. Freud (1917) was the first to point out the similarities of depressive reactions to grief reactions. He suggested that the depressed patient has high dependency needs for a parental figure, with consequent ambivalent feelings (love mixed with anger and frustration because of the dependency). In depression the loss of a real or imagined object results in an introjection of the lost object (i.e. an internal unconscious representation of the lost person as an attempt to avoid the real loss). The anger towards this object then becomes unleashed on the ego itself resulting in depression. Freud believed the depressive's self-reproaches were not really anger at the self, but an indirect attack on the lost loved object. Subsequent psychoanalytic theories have used similar themes: loss, internal objects, dependence and ambivalence, and anger directed at the self (see page 129). The work of Klein (1935) and Bowlby (1981) have been particularly influential in this field.

In summary, psychoanalytic theories all propose a 'narcissistic injury' at an early stage of the child's development (at an age where the child is just beginning to relate to others as whole beings rather than part objects). This injury is a failure of the parents, usually the mother, to sustain the child's physical and emotional needs at this key stage. It may be due to separation, loss, abandonment or lack of affective response from the mother. At this age the child still finds it difficult to form a representation of a real parent who is a mixture of love and weakness. There is a bipolar view of the mother as either all good or all bad. The child rages against the 'bad mother'.

In an attempt to regain the lost object the child introjects it but the angry feelings mean that there is an ambivalent attitude to the internal representation of the mother, with sadistic fantasies. The mother is not seen as a separate entity now but has become a part of the child itself, and there is a regressive dependency on this internal figure. The child feels guilt over the hostile impulses to the mother and the superego may lead to self-punishing behaviour. As the child grows up it becomes overly dependent on significant others. A real or symbolic loss causes reactivation of the unresolved conflict over dependency and hatred and the aggressive impulses are directed at the self and experienced as depression. Psychoanalytic theory supposes that psychotic depression results from a disruption of earlier child-mother bonds than neurotic depression.

Treatment

Psychoanalytically oriented treatment of depression uses the relationship between the patient and therapist as the major vehicle for change. The way the patient relates to what Arieti refers to as the 'dominant other' influences the way he or she relates to the therapist. As treatment progresses the patient becomes dependent on the therapist recapitulating the relationship with the lost object. Treatment involves interpreting the links between the patient-therapist relationship and early childhood relationships. The progress of therapy often involves helping the patient to see how this dependence and attachment extends to various ongoing relationships, and to uncover the underlying ambivalence and anger. The patient works through these feelings to a point where he can establish a view of himself as his own person.

Psychoanalytic therapy involves challenging the patient's defences, and requires commitment and concentration from the patient. Orthodox analytic techniques such as the use of the couch and the therapist's impersonal style may actually be counterproductive with the depressed patient, and so psychodynamic therapy with severely depressed patients is very specialised work. Arieti & Bemporad (1978) describe a modified form of psychoanalysis for severely depressed patients. Psychodynamic concepts may, however, be useful in understanding the behaviour of severely depressed patients even if the therapy is not used. Jackson (1991) describes how these ideas can be applied to patients with psychotic depression.

Even in less severe forms of depression long-term psychoanalytic psychotherapy is not cost effective. Other forms of psychological and physical treatment can produce more rapid recovery. Psychotherapy is best used to help selected patients explore their vulnerability to depression and change relationship patterns. In the NHS this will mean either group therapy (see below) or brief psychotherapy. Ryle (1991) describes the application of a form of integrated brief psychotherapy (cognitive analytic therapy) in depression.

Group therapy

One of the themes running through much depression research is the relevance of interpersonal factors to vulnerability and maintenance of depression. There is therefore a rationale for using group therapy in depression, but surprisingly little research on outcome. This is possibly because group work often makes heterogeneous selections of patients rather than homogeneous ones.

Group cognitive and behavioural therapies

Cognitive and behavioural therapies (CBT) can be applied in groups. They have the advantage that more patients can be treated in the same time than with individual therapy. Most CBT groups are structured and educational in nature, paying little attention to group dynamics. A good example of this psycho-educational model is Lewinsohn's *Coping with Depression Course* (Lewinsohn *et al*, 1984). This approach is probably appropriate for straightforward depressed out-patients, but may be less easy to apply to chronic or personality disordered groups. Eidelson (1985) described a group cognitive therapy which made use of the group format to challenge dysfunctional interpersonal beliefs such as 'I can't give anything to others,' 'no one understands what I'm going through,' and 'I can't relate to other people'. Some studies have found group treatment to be effective but less powerful than individual CT (Rush & Watkins, 1981; Wierzbicki & Bartlett, 1987), while others have shown that the two modes of presentation are equally effective (Scott & Stradling 1990).

Cognitive and behavioural groups are probably indicated for less depressed patients in primary care or community settings. Skills-based groups e.g. social skills and assertiveness training can be used as an adjunct to other treatments. The indication for these treatments will depend upon the problems identified at assessment. Many depressed people have longstanding difficulties with assertiveness, and tend to suppress their own wishes and try excessively to accommodate and please others. This may predispose them to depression, and assertiveness training can help to make them less vulnerable to depression in the future.

Psychodynamic and interpersonal groups

Two main approaches to group work are the psychodynamic group which applies psychoanalytic principles to the group setting, and the interpersonal approach pioneered by Yalom (1985) which emphasises 'here and now' experiences. Stein (1985), writing from a psychodynamic perspective, believes group therapy can be particularly helpful in depression. In a group, the member's relationship with the therapist can provide valuable interpersonal learning. The therapist's realistic, supportive and tolerant attitude replaces the patient's harsh self-criticism, and allows the members to gradually treat themselves in a more accepting way (in analytic terms the members internalise the therapist's more tolerant superego which replaces the depressive's punitive superego). The group also allows patients to express guilt and hostile feelings in a supportive atmosphere. He suggests that the group helps patients to identify and deal with their regressive conflicts 'more quickly, realistically and effectively than in individual therapy'. The effectiveness of this type of group work in actively depressed patients has not been evaluated. The eclectic, interpersonal form of group therapy is often used with hospital in-patients. Ward groups are frequently led by inexperienced therapists, with little supervision. Group psychotherapy with in-patients demands quite specialist skills and modifications of techniques used with out-patients (Yalom, 1983). Because the depressed in-patient may show psychomotor retardation their capacity to engage in group work is limited. In-patient groups need to be less challenging, less demanding and more focused than out-patient groups.

Group therapy has more to offer after the resolution of the acute depressive phase. Recovered depressives can explore and change interpersonal patterns which predispose to depression. Groups can also function as vehicles for support in chronic cases. For instance, several studies have demonstrated decreased hospitalisation and improved social functioning in manic depressive patients on lithium maintenance treatment (Davenport *et al*, 1977; Volkmar *et al*, 1981).

Marital and family therapy

As with group therapy, marital and family therapy describes a mode of delivery rather than a model of therapy. Cognitive, behavioural and psychodynamic forms of therapy all exist. These approaches have in common the idea that the interactional patterns in the family contribute to depression and can be used as a vehicle for change.

Behavioural marital therapy

This is a well developed and researched method of treatment for marital dysfunction (see Schmaling *et al*, 1989). The evidence mentioned above linking marital difficulties to depression has led to the application of the therapy to couples in which one partner is depressed. To date the research has been limited to depressed wives. Behavioural marital therapy (BMT) is a social learning approach which uses techniques such as teaching positive interchanges between partners, communication skills and problem-solving. In the last decade cognitive techniques have been introduced into the package.

Two studies have compared CT with BMT. Jacobson *et al,* (1991) compared individual CT, BMT, and CT plus BMT in depressed married women. In couples with no initial marital distress CT was more effective in alleviating depression. In those with marital distress the two treatments were equally effective, but BMT improved relationships more than CT. O'Leary & Beach (1990) compared the two treatments and a waiting list control in couples with marital problems and a depressed wife. Both treatments improved depression, but only BMT improved marital satisfaction. These two studies suggest that a therapy like CT, with its emphasis on changing individual thinking, does not have a strong effect on marital difficulties. Further research is needed, but these studies suggest that depressed patients with poor marriages might be most effectively treated with behavioural marital therapy.

Systems theory in marital and family therapy

Outside the cognitive–behavioural field, family and marital therapy has been strongly influenced by systems theory. Mood disturbance is seen as arising in the context of a family system. Interactional patterns may include complementary role fits between the dependent depressive partner and a controlling caring partner. Byng-Hall & Whiffen (1982) see depression as a result of problems in distance regulation in the family: 'depressive disorder is ...only one element in the web of emotional bonds which have been broken, are breaking or are threatening to break. The techniques for dealing with affective disorder cannot then be isolated from those which aim at resolving the conflicts in the regulation of the distances between family members'.

Gotlib & Colby (1987) presented an interpersonal systems approach to the conceptualisation of depression and outlined strategies for change. Their model combines both cognitive and systems theory, the latter adding techniques such as reframing and altering family boundaries. Haas *et al* (1988) reported results of an in-patient family intervention for depressed patients. Six family sessions focused on the identification of stressors, and stressful family interactions and the development of strategies for dealing with these. In-patient family intervention was more effective than standard hospital treatment, but this applied only to women.

Weber *et al* (1988) have developed a form of systems family therapy for manic depressives. They report a 70% reduction in relapse rates after an average of 6.6 family sessions, and suggest that this effect is not explained by changes in prescribing of psychotropic medication (Retzer *et al,* 1991).

Systems based therapies for depression need further investigation. In particular, it would be interesting if these approaches have any advantages over simpler problem-based family interventions, such as those described by Falloon (1988) for schizophrenia.

Principles of psychological management

Two major themes run through the psychological literature on depression and its treatment. One is the cognitive-behavioural axis, with substantial evidence that the depressed patients show behavioural deficits and cognitive abnormalities. The second is the interpersonal axis. Critical losses of important relationships or current relationship difficulties are closely related to depression. These two lines of research and the treatment associated with them should inform the psychiatrist's clinical management of the depressed patient.

Therapeutic relationship

The doctor–patient relationship is important in the management of all psychiatric disorders. In depression the doctor needs to achieve a balance between under- and over-involvement with the patient. Too distant a stance will fail to engage the patient and confirm the depressive's view that he is isolated and not understood. Over-involvement can lead the psychiatrist to 'buy into' the depressive's negative world view, and see the situation as hopeless and overwhelming. A warm, friendly, supportive and empathic manner is necessary, but this needs to be balanced with objectivity and professionalism. The patient's negative bias may influence the therapeutic relationship. He or she may think, 'He's not interested in me, I'm boring.' These automatic thoughts about the therapist can be checked out periodically, and corrected with appropriate information.

Psychodynamic theory can inform the clinician of transference phenomena which might interfere with the supportive relationship. The depressive's ambivalence towards important relationships means that the psychiatrist is likely to be perceived as both hostile and punishing, as well as being nurturing at various times in the relationship. The negative thoughts described above illustrate a transference in which the therapist is seen as critical. When a good rapport exists the therapist may be idealised and a dependent transference may develop. This, and the depressive's sensitivity to loss, means that cancellations of appointments, holidays etc. may be particularly difficult for the patient to tolerate. The psychiatrist should also be aware of how his or her own feelings to the patient may be part of the depressive's interpersonal pathology. These counter-transference feelings occur when the therapist is drawn into a reciprocal role, playing unconsciously a real or fantasised relationship from the patient's childhood (e.g. the role of a critical parent). Strong feelings of anger, wanting to punish or get rid of the patient, as well as positive urges to look after or rescue the patient are indications of possible countertransference reactions. If these occur the clinician should discuss the patient with a colleague or obtain supervision.

Information gathering

The process of taking the history and assessing mental state can be therapeutic in its own right. To be able to tell your story and to have someone empathically listen is helpful. This can challenge beliefs such as 'I'm the only person like this,' and 'no one can understand me'. Defining problems and drawing up problem lists helps to diminish the idea that depression is overwhelming, and starts to engender hope. Giving the patient a diagnostic formulation helps to give meaning to their experience, and helps to encourage trust.

Education

The depressive's negative bias can lead to misinterpretation of the symptoms of depression. Lack of motivation and loss of energy are seen as signs of weakness, failure or laziness. Education about the nature of depression can dispel these self-criticisms:

(1) depression is a syndrome with characteristic symptoms
(2) depression is associated with negative views of the self, experience and the future
(3) depression is treatable.

Similarly education about the side-effects of medication prevents misattribution of symptoms and improves compliance (see chapter 4). Many patients expect antidepressants to work immediately, and if they are not told otherwise become disillusioned and may give up taking the drugs before they can take effect. The treatment plan should be explained to the patient and the rationale for any intervention given.

Fatigue, poor concentration and a negative bias may all contribute to difficulties in decision-making and impairment of work performance. It is therefore wise to advise patients not to make any major life decisions and to delay large difficult tasks until the depression has lifted.

It is vital to check the patient's understanding of information given. In severe depression impairment of concentration may reduce the amount that is taken in, and even in less severe cases misunderstandings can occur.

Interviews with significant others

Partners, friends and relatives can not only give information about the patient and his or her relationships, but can also be directly involved in treatment. Education about the nature of depression can be helpful for them too. If the relationship is good the partner can be used as a co-therapist. If the relationship is poor, some simple work on communication combined with education about the nature of depression may be helpful. In assessing relationship problems think of the IPT problem areas:

(1) grief
(2) role disputes
(3) role transitions
(4) interpersonal deficits.

Guidance and environmental change

Sometimes guidance and advice is necessary. A good assessment may indicate activities which can be discouraged (e.g. a depressed patient visiting a friend who overloads her with her own problems), or those which can be encouraged. Behavioural techniques of self-monitoring, activity scheduling and graded task assignment (see above) can easily be incorporated into the psychiatric interview. Patients can also be taught simple problem-solving skills.

In the long run larger environmental changes may be indicated such as moving house, changing job, divorce, or medical retirement. Sometimes it may be clear that environmental stresses are maintaining the depression, and the psychiatrist can contribute by helping to remove them.

> A patient presented one month after a cot death with severe depression and suicidal thoughts. She reported that she was unable to go into the room where the baby had died. Despite classical biological features of depression she refused antidepressant medication and confided little in her community psychiatric nurse. She insisted that the only thing that would help her would be for the council to arrange a move to another flat. The psychiatrist wrote a letter strongly supporting such a move and once the patient had moved she felt considerably improved.

The following case of a depressed police officer in a stressful job demonstrates the therapeutic role of medical retirement.

> A 47-year-old Flying Squad officer worked in a very stressful job which involved waiting in banks which were thought to be the target of robberies. His teenage daughter had become delinquent because he was away for considerable periods of time, quite unpredictably, as part of his job. He presented with a classical depressive syndrome but once he had been off sick for a month he felt quite unable to return to his previous work. The psychiatrist offered to support retirement on medical grounds, and once this had been arranged his depression cleared completely, indicating that the underlying cause had been great fear associated with his stressful job, and the destructive effect it had on his family's life.

Both the above examples describe social interventions which are not really psychotherapy but may nevertheless have psychotherapeutic effects.

The psychiatrist can and should intervene on the patient's behalf whenever this is appropriate to diminish the external stresses on the patient.

Referral for specific psychological therapies

In considering referral for more specialised psychological treatment it is useful to distinguish between treatments that are designed to reduce symptoms of depression (such as CT) and treatments whose main aim is to treat other aspects of the person (more traditional therapies such as psychoanalysis). If the depression is a single episode arising in someone with a previously good adjustment to life, i.e. stable relationships and good work record, psychological therapy is not indicated. If conventional treatment is proving unsuccessful (e.g. only partial response to medication or recurrent depression) or if there are recurrent episodes of depression, a treatment aimed at the symptoms of depression and relapse prevention may be a useful adjunct. CT would seem to be the treatment of choice in this case.

More traditional forms of psychotherapy are indicated when there are other personal problems co-existing with the depression i.e. vulnerability factors. Current problems within the family are indications for marital or family therapy. Wider ranging relationship difficulties, particularly if associated with a disturbed early life (e.g. parental loss or family disruption in childhood), would make one consider individual or group psychodynamic therapy. This type of therapy, in contrast to CT, may well be more effective once the symptoms of depression have lifted. Table 6.3 summarises some of these clinical referral criteria. Unfortunately, the limiting factor is often the availability of psychological treatment. While CT is becoming more available from clinical psychologist and nurse behaviour therapists, IPT remains a research therapy. In many districts the length of individual psychodynamic therapy means that only a very small proportion of NHS patients can receive it, but group psychotherapy may be more easily accessible.

Psychotherapy research in depression

It is only relatively recently that psychological interventions in depression have become a legitimate focus for research. The conventional wisdom has often held that depressive illness is too severe to respond to psychotherapy while less severe depressions will be self-limiting and are best left alone. Research until the 1970s consistently found pharmacotherapy superior to psychotherapy (Morris & Beck, 1974). The first outcome study to demonstrate that a psychological treatment was as effective as antidepressants was that of Rush *et al* (1977). Since then numerous trials have shown cognitive, behavioural and other therapies

Table 6.3 Referral for psychological treatment

Problem	Therapy
Recurrent depression Depression not responsive to antidepressants Residual depression after severe depressive illness	CBT, individual or group
Current relationship problems	Marital therapy
Unresolved grief Maladaptive relationship patterns	IPT
Insight	Psychodynamic therapy
Chronic illness	Support group

to be effective in depression. Part of the problem with earlier studies was a result of methodological inadequacies. Over the last decade depression research has led the way in developing a more sophisticated methodology for psychotherapy research. Studies have attempted to overcome problems by addressing the following methodological issues:

(1) Adequate sample sizes
(2) reliable, operationally defined criteria for depression (RDC or DSM criteria)
(3) operationally defined treatments (often based on manuals)
(4) ensuring adequate and consistent training, experience and supervision of therapists
(5) objective outcome measures with demonstrated reliability and validity.

In considering the various approaches to the treatment of depression it is important to assess the extent to which trials have adhered to these methodological principles.

Cognitive therapy

Cognitive behaviour therapy (CBT) has been compared with no-treatment and waiting list controls in several studies. Overall the results show a significant advantage of therapy over no treatment (Miller & Berman, 1983). Of more interest to the psychiatrist is a comparison between CT and antidepressant medication. There have been several studies comparing Beck's CT with tricyclic antidepressants (Table 6.4). These studies took out-patient depressives who met criteria for unipolar major depression. Three studies allowed the prescribing doctors to choose the dosage best suited to the individual patient (Blackburn *et al*, 1981; Rush & Watkins 1981; Teasdale *et al*, 1984) while another measured antidepressant blood levels to ensure adequate dosage (Murphy *et al*, 1984). All of these trials found CT to be at least as effective as tricyclic medication. Blackburn *et al* (1981) looked at both out-patient and general practice depressives in Edinburgh. In general practice CT proved more effective than drugs. In the hospital group a combination of CT and drugs was more effective than either alone. A problem with all of these studies is the small sample size. There are rarely more than 20 patients per group, and while this is sufficiently large to show differences if the clinical effect is large it may not show up relatively small differences. But taken as a whole the effect cannot be ignored. None of these studies found CT to be less effective than drug treatment.

Four studies show reduced relapse rates in patients treated with CT compared with antidepressant medication (Kovacs *et al*, 1981; Beck *et al*, 1985; Blackburn *et al*, 1986; Simons *et al*, 1986). In these studies the antidepressant was not given as a maintenance treatment, though the studies were 'naturalistic' and allowed for further treatment over the one or two year follow-up. (See Shaw (1989) for a summary of the evidence of the effect of CT on relapse.)

Some results are now available for the effectiveness of CT with depressed in-patients. De Jong *et al* (1986) found that a treatment combining cognitive and behavioural components did better than a cognitive restructuring only treatment or an attention control.

Miller *et al* (1989) reported that both CT and social skills training produced more reduction in symptoms and greater percentages of responders at the end of treatment than standard in-patient treatment. Bowers *et al* (1990) compared nortriptyline, relaxation plus nortriptyline or CT plus nortriptyline over 12 sessions. At discharge the two psychological treatment groups reported fewer depressive symptoms and fewer subjects were judged depressed at discharge in the CT group. These studies give preliminary evidence that adding cognitive-behavioural treatments to the standard ward regime may improve the treatment of in-patient depression.

Interpersonal therapy

There have been fewer outcome studies of IPT than CT. Two major studies exist. In the first (Klerman *et al*, 1974; Weissman *et al*, 1974), depressed women who had responded to a 4–6 week treatment with amitriptyline were randomly allocated to maintenance treatment with amitriptyline, placebo or no medication, and then either received once monthly low contact or weekly IPT. Antidepressant medication reduced relapse rate and prevented symptom return, but had no impact on social functioning. Psychotherapy had little effect on symptoms, but had a significant effect

Table 6.4   Cognitive therapy and antidepressant therapy

Study	Outcome
Rush *et al*, 1977 ($n = 41$)	CT > imipramine
Beck *et al*, 1979 ($n = 26$)	CT = CT + amitriptyline
Blackburn *et al*, 1981 ($n = 64$)	Hospital out-patients: CT + TCA > CT = TCA General practice: CT = CT + TCA > TCA
Rush & Watkins, 1981 ($n = 38$)	Individual CT = individual CT + TCA > group CT
Murphy *et al*, 1984 ($n = 70$)	CT = nortriptyline = CT + nortriptyline = CT + placebo
Teasdale *et al*, 1984 ($n = 34$)	CT + treatment as usual > treatment as usual

CT: Cognitive therapy; TCA, tricyclic antidepressant.

on social functioning. In the second study DiMascio *et al* (1979) found that drugs and IPT both had effects on symptoms and the combination produced the greatest improvement. Results from the National Institute of Mental Health Study (see below) suggest that it may be applicable for severe as well as mild to moderate out-patient depression.

The National Institute of Mental Health Collaborative Study

The promising results of trials using CT and IPT encouraged the United States National Institute of Mental Health (NIMH) to set up a multicentre project to compare these two treatments with pharmacotherapy. This is the largest and most carefully designed trial to date. Patients were treated at Pittsburgh, Washington DC and Oklahoma. Two hundred and fifty patients who met Research Diagnostic Criteria for major depressive disorder and also had a score of 14 or more on the Hamilton Rating Scale for Depression (HRSD) were randomly assigned to four treatments:

(1) cognitive behaviour therapy (CBT)
(2) interpersonal therapy (IPT)
(3) imipramine plus clinical management (IMI-CM)
(4) placebo plus clinical management (PLA-CM).

The two psychotherapies were based on manuals and controlled for quality. Each session was 50 minutes. The clinical management consisted of minimal supportive therapy sessions of 20–30 minutes duration. Eleven patients dropped out before the first treatment session leaving 239 patients who received up to 20 sessions of therapy over 16 weeks.

Patients in all treatments showed a significant reduction in symptoms over the course of treatment. There were no significant differences between therapies, although there was a consistent ordering of treatments with the active drug doing best, placebo worst and the two psycho-therapies coming somewhere in between. A *post hoc* analysis was then carried out for subgroups of severe and mild depression. There were no significant differences for the less severely depressed group. For the more severe group there was some evidence for the specific effectiveness of imipramine and to a lesser extent IPT.

The use of the Beck Depression Inventory in this study permits a comparison of the proportionate change with other studies. In five other studies where CBT alone or TCA alone were compared (Rush *et al*, 1977; McLean & Hakstian, 1979; Blackburn *et al*, 1981; Murphy *et al*, 1984; Teasdale *et al*, 1984) the mean proportionate change for CBT was 0.72 and for TCA 0.63. In the NIMH study the change for CBT was 0.62, for TCA 0.76 and for IPT 0.70. The percentage of patients in the non-clinical range for depression after therapy was also less than in other trials. There is a possibility that the CT in this study was less effective than in others, although the reasons for this are not clear.

Psychodynamic therapy

Evidence for the effectiveness of psychodynamic therapy in depression is scant. Until recently psychoanalysts eschewed objective or symptom based measurement of their work and randomised trials of psychoanalysis have not been conducted. As Cawley (1983) points out, the aim of psychoanalysis is to expand the patient's 'comprehension, acceptance, control and self-fulfilment', which is very difficult to assess objectively. It can also be argued that because the therapy is very private and personal to the therapist, by pooling the data in a randomised trial essential components of an individual therapy would be lost to sight. Because of these reservations on the part of dynamic psychotherapists most of the studies that exist were carried out by behaviourally oriented researchers. Questions therefore can be raised about the quality of therapy given, whether the length of treatment is sufficient to give psychodynamic therapy a fair chance, and the length of follow-up.

Sloane *et al* (1975) compared behaviour therapy and psychodynamic therapy in neurotic out-patients, some of whom were depressed. Both treatments did equally well. McLean & Hakstian (1979) found behaviour therapy, tricyclics and relaxation to be superior treatments to insight oriented therapy, but Bellack *et al* (1981) found no difference between social skills training, amitryptiline, placebo and insight oriented therapy in a group of depressed patients. Shapiro & Firth (1987) compared a cognitive-behavioural (prescriptive) therapy and an interpersonal/ psychodynamic (exploratory) approach. Exploratory and prescriptive therapy were equally effective regardless of the order they were given, but the generalisability of this study is questionable because the subjects were all mildly depressed businessmen and not psychiatric patients.

Conclusions

A variety of psychological therapies for depression are now available, and there is a growing research literature to support their efficacy. Cognitive and behavioural treatments are the most extensively researched and there is some evidence to suggest they may be slightly more effective than other forms of therapy overall (Dobson, 1989). Questions remain about which of these therapies, if any, have long-term effects on vulnerability to depression. Some of the clinical insights from therapies demonstrated to be effective in depression can be used in the psychological management of depression even if formal psychotherapy is not being undertaken.

References

Arieti, S. & Bemporad, J. (1978) *Severe and Mild Depression*. New York: Basic Books.
Beck, A. T. & Greenberg, R. L. (1974) *Coping with Depression*. New York: Institute for Rational Living.
——, Rush, A. J., Shaw, B. F., *et al* (1979) *Cognitive Therapy of Depression*. New York: Guilford Press.
——, Hollon, S. D., Young, J. E., *et al* (1985) Treatment of depression with cognitive therapy and amitriptyline. *Archives of General Psychiatry*, **42**, 142–148.
Bellack, A. S., Hersen, M. & Harmondsworth, J. (1981) Social skills training compared with pharmocotherapy and psychotherapy for depression. *Behaviour Research and Therapy*, **21**, 101–107.
Blackburn, I. M., Bishop, S., Glen, A. I. M., *et al* (1981) The efficacy of cognitive therapy in depression: a treatment trial using cognitive therapy and pharmacotherapy each alone and in combination. *British Journal of Psychiatry*, **139**, 181–189.
——, Eunson, K. M. & Bishop, S. (1986) A two year naturalistic follow up of depressed patients treated with cognitive therapy, pharmacotherapy and a combination of both. *Journal of Affective Disorders*, **10**, 67–75.
Bowers, W. A. (1990) Treatment of depressed in-patients: cognitive therapy plus medication, relaxation plus medication, and medication alone. *British Journal of Psychiatry*, **156**, 73–78.
Bowlby, J. (1981) *Attachment and Loss* (Vols I, II & III). London: Penguin.
Brown, G. W. & Harris, T. (1978) *Social Origins of Depression: A Study of Psychiatric Disorder in Women*. New York: Free Press.

Byng-Hall, J. J. & Whiffen, R. (1982) Family and marital therapy. In *Handbook of Affective Disorders* (ed. E. S. Paykel). Edinburgh: Churchill Livingstone.

Cawley, R. H. (1983) The principles of treatment and therapeutic evaluation. In *Handbook of Psychopathology 1: General Psychopathology* (eds M. Shepherd & O. L. Zangwill). Cambridge: Cambridge University Press.

Coyne, J. C. (1976) Depression and the response of others. *Journal of Abnormal Psychology*, **85**, 186–193.

Davenport, Y. B., Ebert, M. H., Adland, M. L., *et al* (1977) Couples group therapy as an adjunct to lithium maintenance of the manic patient. *American Journal of Orthopsychiatry*, **47**,495–502.

de Jong, R., Treiber, R. & Henrich, G. (1986) Effectiveness of two psychological treatments for in-patients with severe and chronic depression. *Cognitive Therapy and Research*, **10**, 645–663.

DiMascio, A., Weissman, M. M., Prusoff, B. A., *et al* (1979) Differential symptom reduction by drugs and psychotherapy in acute depression. *Archives of General Psychiatry*, **36**, 1450–1456.

Dobson, K. (1989) A meta analysis of the efficacy of cognitive therapy for depression. *Journal of Consulting and Clinical Psychology*, **57**, 414–419.

Eidelson, J. I. (1985) Cognitive group therapy for depression. "Why and what". *International Journal of Mental Health*, **13**, 54–66.

Elkin, I., Shea, M. T., Watkins, J. T., *et al* (1989) National Institute of Mental Health treatment of depression collaborative research program. *Archives of General Psychiatry*, **46**, 971–982.

Falloon, I. R. M. (1988) Behavioural family therapy. In *Family Therapy in Britain* (eds E. Street & W. Dryden). Buckingham: OUP.

Fennel, M. J. V. & Teasdale, J. D. (1987) Cognitive therapy for depression: individual differences and the process of change. *Cognitive Therapy and Research*, **11**, 253–271.

Freud, S. (1917) *Mourning and Melancholia. Collected Papers 4*. London: The Hogarth Press.

Glen, A., Johnson, A. & Shepherd, M. (1984) Continuation therapy with lithium and amitriptyline in unipolar illness: a randomised double-blind controlled trial. *Psychological Medicine* **14**, 37–50.

Gotlib, A. H. & Colby, C. A. (1987) *Treatment of Depression: An Interpersonal Systems Approach*. New York: Pergamon.

Haas, G. L., Glick, I. D., Clarkin, J. F., *et al* (1988) In-patient family intervention: A randomised clinical trial. II. Results at hospital discharge. *Archives of General Psychiatry*, **45**, 217–224.

Hooley, J. M., Orley, J. & Teasdale, J. D. (1986) Levels of expressed emotion and relapse in depressed patients. *British Journal of Psychiatry*, **148**, 642–647.

Jackson, M. (1991) Psychotic disorders. In *Textbook of Psychotherapy in Psychiatric Practice* (ed. J. Holmes) Edinburgh: Churchill Livingstone.

Jacobson, N. S., Dobson, K., Fruzzetti, A. E., *et al* (1991) Marital therapy as a treatment for depression. *Journal of Consulting and Clinical Psychiatry*, **59**, 547–557.

Klein, M. (1935) A contribution to the psychogenesis of manic depressive states. In *The Selected Melanie Klein* (1986, ed. J. Mitchell). London: Penguin.

Klerman, G. L., DiMascio, A., Weissman, M. M.,*et al* (1974) Treatment of depression by drugs and psychotherapy. *American Journal of Psychiatry*, **131**, 186–191.

——, Weissman, M. M., Rounsaville, B. J., *et al* (1984) *Interpersonal Therapy of Depression.* New York: Basic Books Inc.

—— & Schechter, G. (1985) Drugs and psychotherapy. In *Handbook of Affective Disorders* (ed. E. S. Paykel). Edinburgh: Churchill Livingstone.

Kovacs, M., Rush, A. J., Beck, A. T., *et al* (1981) Depressed out-patients treated with cognitive therapy or pharmacotherapy: a one year follow up. *Archives of General Psychiatry*, **38**, 33–39.

Lewinsohn, P. M., Biglan, T. & Zeiss, A. (1976) Behavioral treatment of depression. In *Behavioral Management of Anxiety, Depression and Pain* (ed. P. Davidson). New York: Brunner/Mazel.

——, Antonuccio, D., Steinmetz, J., *et al* (1984) *The Coping with Depression Course: A Psychoeducational Intervention for Unipolar Depression.* Eugene OR: Castalia.

——, Hoberman, H. M., Teri, L., *et al* (1985) An integrative theory of depression. In *Theoretical Issues in Behavior Therapy* (eds S. Reich & R. Bootzin). New York: Academic Press.

McLean, P. & Hakstian, A. R. (1979) Clinical depression: comparative efficacy of out-patient treatments. *Journal of Consulting and Clinical Psychology*, **47**, 818–836.

Meyer, A. (1957) *Psychobiology: A Science of Man.* Springfield: Charles C. Thomas.

Miller, I. V., Norman, W. H. & Keitner, G. I. (1989) Cognitive-behavioural treatment of depressed in-patients: six and twelve month follow up. *American Journal of Psychiatry*, **146**, 1274–1279.

Miller, R. C. & Berman, J. S. (1983) The efficacy of cognitive behaviour therapies: a qualitative review of the research evidence. *Psychological Bulletin*, **94**, 39–53.

Morris, J. B. & Beck, A. T. (1974) The efficacy of antidepressant drugs: a review of research (1958 to 1972). *Archives of General Psychiatry*, **30**, 667–674.

Murphy, G. E., Simons, A. D., Wetzel, R. D., *et al* (1984) Cognitive therapy and pharmacotherapy: singly and together in the treatment of depression. *Archives of General Psychiatry*, **41**, 33–41.

O'Leary, K. D. & Beach, S. R. H. (1990) Marital therapy: a viable treatment for depression and marital discord. *American Journal of Psychiatry*, **147**, 183–186.

Retzer, A., Simon, F. B., Weber, G., *et al* (1991) A follow up study of manic depressive and schizoaffective psychoses after systemic family therapy. *Family Process*, **30**, 139–153.

Rush, A. J., Beck, A. T., Kovacs, M., *et al* (1977) Comparative efficacy of cognitive therapy and pharmacotherapy in the treatment of depressed out-patients. *Cognitive Therapy and Research*, **1**, 17–37.

Rush, A. J. & Watkins, J. T. (1981) Group versus individual cognitive therapy: a pilot study. *Cognitive Therapy and Research*, **5**, 95–103.

Ryle, A. (1991) Depression. In *Textbook of Psychotherapy in Psychiatric Practice* (ed. J. Holmes). Edinburgh: Churchill Livingstone.

Schmaling, K. B., Fruzzetti, A. E. & Jacobson, N. (1989) Marital therapy. In *Cognitive Behaviour Therapy for Psychiatric Problems: A Practical Guide* (eds K. Hawton, P. M. Salkovskis, J. Kirk & D. M. Clark). Oxford: Oxford Medical Publications.

Scott, M. J. & Stradling, S. G. (1990) Group cognitive therapy for depression produces clinically significant reliable change in community-based settings. *Behavioural Psychotherapy*, **18**, 1–19.

Shapiro, D. A. & Firth, J. (1987) Prescriptive v. exploratory psychotherapy: outcomes of the Sheffield psychotherapy project. *British Journal of Psychiatry*, **151**, 790–799.

Shaw, B.F. (1989) Cognitive behaviour therapies for major depression: current status with an emphasis on prophylaxis. *Psychiatric Journal of the University of Ottowa* **14**, 403–408.

Simons, A. D., Murphy, G. E., Levine, J. L., *et al* (1986) Cognitive therapy and pharmacotherapy for depression: sustained improvement over one year. *Archives of General Psychiatry*, **43**, 43–49.

Sloane, R. B., Staples, F. R., Cristol, A. H., *et al* (1975) Psychotherapy versus behaviour therapy. Cambridge: Harvard University Press.

Stein, A. (1985) Group therapy. In *Handbook of Affective Disorders* (ed. E. S. Paykel). Edinburgh: Churchill Livingstone.

Sullivan, H. S. (1953) *The Interpersonal Theory of Psychiatry.* New York: W. W. Norton.

Teasdale, J. D., Fennell, M. J. V., Hibbert, G. A., *et al* (1984) Cognitive therapy for major depressive disorder in primary care. *British Journal of Psychiatry*, **144**, 400–406.

Volkmar, F. R., Bacon, S., Shakir, S. A., *et al* (1981) Group therapy in the management of manic depressive illness. *American Journal of Psychotherapy*, **35**, 226–234.

Weber, G., Simon, F. B., Stierlin, H., *et al* (1988) Therapy for families manifesting manic-depressive behaviour. *Family Process*, **27**, 33–49.

Weissman, M. M., Klerman, G. L., Paykel, E. S., *et al* (1974) Treatment effects on the psychosocial adjustment of depressed patients. *Archives of General Psychiatry*, **30**, 771–778.

—— & Paykel, E. S. (1974) *The Depressed Woman: A Study of Social Relationships.* Chicago: University of Chicago Press.

——, Prusoff, B. A., DiMascio, A., *et al* (1979) The efficacy of drugs and psychotherapy in the treatment of acute depressive episodes. *American Journal of Psychiatry*, **136**, 555–558.

Wierzbicki, M., & Bartlett, T. S. (1987) The efficacy of group and individual cognitive therapy for mild depression. *Cognitive Therapy and Research*, **11**, 337–342.

Yalom, I. D. (1983) *In-patient Group Psychotherapy.* New York: Basic Books.

—— (1985) *The Theory and Practice of Group Psychotherapy* (3rd edn). New York: Basic Books.

7 Schizophrenia – the clinical picture

Peter F. Liddle

*The origins of the concept ● The phenomena of schizophrenia ●
Disorders of thought, affect and volition ● Cognitive impairment in
schizophrenia ● Neurological signs ● Subtypes and syndromes of
schizophrenia ● Course and prognosis of schizophrenia ● Standardised
assessment and diagnosis ● The boundaries of schizophrenia*

Schizophrenia is a psychotic illness that undermines fundamental aspects
of the personality. It erodes the ability to initiate and organise self-directed
mental activity, and to recognise oneself as the source of such activity.
It can produce a diverse array of disturbances within the domains of
thought, perception, affect and volition. Typically, the illness follows a
course in which acute episodes of hallucinations, delusions, and florid
disorganisation of thought, are superimposed upon more persistent and
subtle disorders in the initiation and organisation of thought and
behaviour. These persistent disorders can produce profound disruption
of occupational activities and social relationships. However, the severity
of the persisting disorder varies greatly between cases.

The origins of the concept

The concept of schizophrenia emerged from 19th century attempts to
describe the psychotic illnesses of young and middle adult life. At the
beginning of that century, the English psychiatrist Haslam (1809)
recognised a state of insanity unaccompanied by furious or depressing
passions. In 1860, the French psychiatrist Morel (1860) described a
condition, which he named *demence precoce*, that had its onset in late
adolescence with odd behaviour and self-neglect, leading to a
deterioration in mental function. However, the major developments that
led to the concept of schizophrenia occurred in Germany in the four
decades which extended from Griesinger's (1861) formulation of the
concept of a unitary psychosis, including both affective psychoses and
the condition we now call schizophrenia, to Kraepelin's recognition that
these two conditions should be separated on the grounds of their tendency
to differ in time course.

The seminal figure of these four decades was Kahlbaum. He described three chronic psychotic conditions: catatonia, hebephrenia and dementia paranoides. He is best known for his description of catatonia (Kahlbaum, 1874), a condition dominated by disturbances of voluntary motor activity. Kahlbaum emphasised the importance of evaluating not only the current symptoms but also the course of an illness. Catatonia runs a course which includes atonic or stuporous periods of under-activity, and periods of excitement and over-activity. In some instances it progresses to a demented state. Kahlbaum also emphasised the association between affective symptoms and catatonic motor symptoms. This provided an empirical basis for the notion which we will develop later, that there are pathophysiological processes common to affective psychosis and schizophrenia. Kahlbaum's colleague Hecker (1871), recorded the classic description of hebephrenia, a condition beginning in young adult life with silly behaviour, inappropriate affect, disordered form of thought and fragmentary delusions. Dementia paranoides is characterised by delusions in a setting of deteriorating personality.

Kahlbaum's seminal ideas came to fruition at the turn of the century, when Emil Kraepelin (1896) separated manic-depressive psychosis, in which there is virtually normal mental function between episodes, from the chronic psychoses, hebephrenia, catatonia and dementia paranoides, which tend to produce persisting disability. He amalgamated these three chronic psychoses to form a single illness which he named dementia praecox in recognition of its tendency to begin in early adult life and its propensity to lead to a state of mental enfeeblement. In a later essay (Kraepelin, 1920) which reflected a distillation of his views on psychopathology, he described the essential feature of the illness as:

> "that destruction of conscious volition...which is manifest as loss of energy and drive, in disjointed volitional behaviour. This rudderless state leads to impulsive instinctual activity: there is no planned reflection which suppresses impulses as they arise or directs them into proper channels".

Although Kraepelin regarded impaired volition and loss of unity of mental processes as cardinal features of the illness, he also emphasised the prevalence of auditory hallucinations, especially in the acute phase.

The illness was renamed schizophrenia by Eugen Bleuler in 1911. He wished to discard the name dementia praecox because he recognised that many cases did not show progressive deterioration. Also in at least some cases, the illness began in mid-adult life. He regarded fragmentation of psychic functions as the hallmark of the illness, and chose the name schizophrenia to denote this fragmentation of mental activity. He specified a number of fundamental symptoms including affective flattening, looseness of associations, ambivalence and autism, which he considered were present in every case. He gave special weight to looseness of associations:

> "Of the thousands of associative threads which guide our thinking, this disease seems to interrupt, quite haphazardly, sometimes such single threads, sometimes a whole group, and sometimes even large segments of them. In this way thinking becomes illogical and often bizarre" (Bleuler, 1911, p. 14).

He considered that many of the other symptoms arose from looseness of associations. Bleuler regarded hallucinations and delusions as accessory symptoms:

> "Besides these specific permanent or fundamental symptoms we can find a host of other more accessory manifestations such as delusions, hallucinations or catatonic symptoms. The fundamental symptoms are characteristic of schizophrenia, while the accessory symptoms may also appear in other types of illness" (Bleuler, 1911).

Thus, in the evolution of the concept of schizophrenia, the emphasis was initially on fragmentation of mental functions and enduring deficits. Delusions and hallucinations were recognised as concomitant of the disorder, but were considered to be a transient though potentially recurring feature of the illness. However, as attempts were made to improve the reliability of diagnosis, delusions and hallucinations, especially those identified as first rank symptoms by Schneider (see below), assumed greater importance, and the emphasis shifted from the enduring deficits to the acute phases of the illness during which delusions and hallucinations are usually prominent. This shift in emphasis was reinforced in the second half of the 20th century by the development of pharmacological treatments which were relatively successful in alleviating the symptoms of the acute phase. However, these treatments do not cure the illness; the chronic deficits present a persisting challenge.

Case illustration:

> Schizophrenia is a very diverse illness and no single case can encapsulate all of its features. Nonetheless, many of the features are illustrated by the case of Alan. His father, a watch-maker, was a solitary and anxious man. Alan's mother suffered from schizophrenia herself, and eventually committed suicide when Alan was 34. He had a younger sister who was mentally well, and married when in her twenties. As a child Alan had only a small number of friends. He was intelligent and passed examinations in four subjects at O-level, but by that time his teachers had noted that his school performance was deteriorating. He left school at 16. He obtained

a series of jobs, the longest lasting for about eight months. At the time of his first admission to a psychiatric hospital he was a laboratory technician. He never had a girl friend.

At age 19 he suffered his first episode of schizophrenia. He began to develop delusions of reference and to hear hallucinatory voices commenting on his actions. By the time he was admitted to hospital he had disordered form of thought, blunted affect and poverty of speech. His IQ at that time was 113. The hallucinations and delusions gradually resolved during treatment with trifluoperazine and fluphenazine decanoate, but his blunted affect and poverty of speech persisted.

He was discharged from hospital after one year, but in the following 12 years was admitted to hospital a further 11 times, for periods ranging from two to 18 months. Throughout this time, hallucinations tended to recur whenever the dose of his antipsychotic medication was decreased. At age 33, he was admitted to hospital after a conflict with his father and remained an in-patient for the following six years.

During this long period in hospital it was extremely difficult to engage him in realistic constructive activities. He spent most of each day sitting in an arm chair. He virtually never initiated conversation, His verbal responses were slow and rarely comprised more than a few words. However, he maintained an interest in science and obtained scientific books by mail order, in spite of lacking any means of paying for them. Although his concentration and immediate recall were within the normal range, he was incapable of pursuing his interests. Much of the time, several of his science books lay unread on the floor beside the chair in which he sat blank and inactive.

Inquiry about his emotions sometimes led to confused and contradictory responses, though he usually denied having any emotions at all. He established a relatively close relationship with one of his doctors. When the doctor told him that he would be leaving the hospital in a few months time, Alan was unexpectedly aroused from his usual torpor. He decided that it was time he left hospital. He planned that he would write to Lord Cadbury to ask for money. His logic was that he needed money and Lord Cadbury had plenty of money, so surely Lord Cadbury would give him some. He thought a bank manager would want to see his birth certificate, so he left the hospital and walked several miles home to get it. Unfortunately the house was locked and he returned empty handed. While the reversal of his prior inactivity was striking, he appeared to lack a common sense grasp of daily affairs and tended to dissipate his energies in a futile manner.

It was possible to arrange for his discharge from hospital to sheltered accommodation in a staffed hostel. Six months later, he had returned to a state of somewhat impoverished speech and affect, but he was still perceptibly more animated than during his long period in hospital.

The phenomena of schizophrenia

The Schneiderian first rank symptoms

In his attempt to define of set of symptoms which might provide a reliable basis for the diagnosis of schizophrenia, Kurt Schneider identified a group of experiences (Box 7.1), which have become known as first rank symptoms. Schneider did not give explicit definitions of the first rank symptoms, and clinicians have subsequently employed various definitions that differ in detail. Mellor (1970) formulated a set of strict definitions and reported that 72% of schizophrenic patients exhibited at least one such symptom. The following descriptions of first rank symptoms are based on Mellor's definitions, though where possible, illustrations from Schneider's account (trans. 1959) are given.

Voices commenting: the patient hears a voice describing his/her actions as they occur. The actions are often quite mundane, but in some instances a special significance might be suspected. Schneider (p. 97) describes a schizophrenic woman who heard a voice say whenever she wanted to eat: "Now she is eating, here she is munching again".

Voices discussing or arguing: the patient experiences hallucinations of voices which discuss him, or argue about him, referring to him in the third person. Schneider (p. 97) refers to a schizophrenic patient who experienced auditory hallucinations night and day "like a dialogue, one voice always arguing against the other".

Audible thoughts (Gedankenlautwerden; Echo de la pensee): the experience of hearing one's own thoughts aloud. The thoughts might be heard either simultaneously with the act of thinking, or after a very brief delay. One of Schneider's patients reported: "I hear my own thoughts. I can hear them when everything is quiet". Another complained: "When I try to think, my head gets full of noise; it's as if my own brain were in an uproar with my thoughts" (p. 97).

Thought insertion: the experience of thoughts which are not one's own being inserted into one's mind. It is not merely a matter of being influenced to think a particular thought; the essence of the symptom includes the experience that the thought is not one's own. "A skilled shirtmaker knew how large the collars should be but when she proceeded to make them there were times when she could not calculate at all. This was not ordinary forgetting, she had to think thoughts she did not want to think, evil thoughts. She attributed all this to being hypnotised by a priest" (Schneider, p. 101).

Thought withdrawal: the experience that thoughts are removed by an alien influence. Schneider (p. 100) gives as an example: "A schizophrenic man stated that his thoughts were 'taken from me years ago by the parish council'. They had constantly robbed him of all his thoughts". The experience that one's thinking has stopped, leaving a state in which all

---

Box 7.1 Schneider's first rank symptoms

Voices commenting
Voices arguing or discussing
Audible thoughts
Thought broadcast
Thought withdrawal
Thought insertion
Made will
Made acts
Made affect
Somatic passivity
Delusional perception.

---

thought is absent (thought blocking) is less specific to schizophrenia and is not regarded as a first rank symptom.

Thought broadcasting: the experience that one's thoughts are broadcast so that others might share them. Schneider (p. 101) describes a female patient who was so convinced that the doctor knew exactly what she was thinking that she suggested that she would stop talking and he could just listen. The belief that others can read one's thoughts is not in itself a first rank symptom; the essential feature is the experience that one's thoughts are available to others.

Made will: the patient is impelled by an impulse to act which is experienced as arising from an alien source. The impulse is usually so strong that it is acted upon. The execution of the action itself is not experienced as alien. Mellor (p. 17) gives as an example the account of a patient who had emptied a urine bottle over the dinner trolley. "The sudden impulse came over me that I must do it. It was not my feeling; it came into me from the X-ray department." Schneider (p. 119) describes a patient who was unable to respond to suggestions because "thousands and thousands of wills act against me".

Made acts: the patient experiences his actions as being executed by an external influence, such that he is a passive observer of his own actions. Mellor (p. 17) reports a patient who described his fingers moving to pick up objects, "but I don't control them... I sit there watching them move, and they are quite independent, what they do is nothing to do with me. I am just a puppet... I am just a puppet who is manipulated by cosmic strings."

Made affects: affects are experienced as imposed by an alien influence. A young woman described by Mellor (p. 17) complained "I cry, tears roll down my cheeks and I look unhappy, but inside I have a cold anger because they are using me in this way, and it is not me who is unhappy, but they are projecting unhappiness into my brain".

Somatic passivity: the experience of alien influence over bodily functions; Mellor (p. 18) specifies that there are two essential components: a somatic experience which is usually, but are not always hallucinatory, combined with a delusional belief in alien origin of that experience. The experience is most commonly one of visceral function. He gives the example of a young man who experienced "X-rays entering the back of my neck, where the skin tingles and feels warm; they pass down the back in a hot tingling strip about six inches wide to the waist. Then they disappear into the pelvis which feels numb and cold and solid like a block of ice. They stop me from getting an erection."

Schneider was less strict, and allowed that the symptom might entail either a somatic hallucination or belief in strange influences acting on the body. Schneider also points out that the content is frequently sexual in nature. He gives as an illustration a woman who described "a sort of intercourse as if a man was really there. He was not there of course... but it was as if a man was with me...that is what I felt." In this case, the patient reports a somatic hallucination, but her explanation does not have the conviction of a delusion.

Delusional perception: the attribution of abnormal significance, usually with self-reference, to a genuine perception without any understandable rational or emotional justification. Delusional perception is sometimes preceded by a delusional atmosphere, a sense of oddness or strangeness. Mellor (p. 18) describes a young Irishman at breakfast with a fellow lodger who felt a sense of unease as if something frightening was about to happen. When the lodger pushed the salt cellar towards him he perceived the event and understood his companion's intentions correctly, but suddenly knew he must return home to greet the Pope who was visiting Ireland to see his family and reward them "because Our Lord is going to be born again of one of the women... and because of this they are all born with their private parts back to front."

Schneider (p. 113) emphasised that there is sometimes a substantial delay, which might be hours or even years, between the perception and the development of a delusional belief in its significance. He gives as an example a girl employed in domestic service who 'later on' decided that an earlier visitor to the house was the disguised son of the household who intended to test her out and marry her.

Schneider was careful to emphasise that schizophrenia involves not merely first rank symptoms but also more widespread changes in mental function. "A psychotic phenomenon is not like a defective stone in an otherwise perfect mosaic" (p. 95).

First rank symptoms are not unique to schizophrenia; they are reported in approximately 10–15% of patients with manic–depressive psychosis and in patients with overt organic brain conditions. However, clinicians have differed in their interpretation of Schneider's concepts, and there has been no adequate study which has established the prevalence of

Olfactory hallucinations occur, as do other olfactory disorders including disturbances of the affective connotations of smells. Sometimes patients become convinced that they are giving off an unpleasant odour. Somatic hallucinations are common and are often associated with delusional interpretations. A man who experienced a strange sensation in his bowels was convinced that a snake had entered through his anus. Another described the experience of being cut with a knife by his parents. While this statement might well have been understood as an expression of his tense relationship with his parents, he was adamant that the experience was real, not merely a metaphor.

Although visual hallucinations are usually regarded as evidence suggesting an overtly organic psychosis, such hallucinations are not uncommon in schizophrenia, especially in cases with severe persistent illness. Sometimes the patients experience them as personal, intended only for themselves, yet they believe in their reality. A patient described the appearance of King George V and Queen Mary regularly at the ward entrance. Both were dressed in full coronation regalia. When asked why others could not see them she replied "because they have come to see me" (Mellor, personal communication).

Rarely, visual hallucinations occur at the onset of an acute episode of illness as a feature of a dream-like (oneiroid) state in which the patient is detached from reality. In this altered state of consciousness, complex vivid visual hallucinations sometimes occur, as may visual illusions in which perceptions of real stimuli are distorted. Objects can be surrounded by an aura; have either an unnatural intensity of colour or be muted and grey; be changed in shape, reduced in size (micropsia) or enlarged (macropsia). Patients might have an unrealistic experience of having encountered the present situation before (deja vu). These specific distortions of reality are not characteristic of schizophrenia, and unless they are accompanied by other clinical features more typical of schizophrenia, some other organic disorder of the brain should be suspected.

Delusions

Virtually all schizophrenic patients suffer from delusions at some time in their illness, and a wide variety of types of delusions can occur. Especially characteristic of schizophrenia are delusional beliefs that appear to defy logic, either because they arise suddenly and without any foundation based on preceding mental processes, or because they refer to fantastic events or circumstances which could not possibly occur. For example, a young woman suddenly knew, with total conviction, that she was a cat. It was not possible to elicit any mental precursor to this notion. Such a belief arising suddenly from unaccountable origins is called a primary or autochthonous delusion. While the non-understandability of a primary delusion is a feature typical of schizophrenia, the difficulty of determining whether or not such a delusion might be accounted for by antecedent mental processes presents a practical problem.

Also characteristic of schizophrenia are the delusions of alien control of thought, action, will, affect and somatic function which express the disordered experience of autonomy lying at the heart of many of the Schneiderian first rank symptoms described previously. These phenomena are delusions in that they entail beliefs based on a faulty evaluation of reality, but they involve disturbance in more than just the process of evaluating reality. They reflect disorder of the mental process that creates awareness of oneself as the source of one's own thoughts, feelings and actions. Although Schneider's primary purpose in identifying the first rank symptoms was to assemble a group of phenomena of special use for making diagnosis, the fact that the experience of alien control is common to the majority of the first rank symptoms suggests that a disturbed experience of self is a cardinal feature of schizophrenic psychopathology.

Schneider also drew attention to the phenomenon of delusional mood. This is a scarcely tangible experience that something strange or unusual is happening. It can occur for a period of hours or days before the emergence of more clearcut delusional beliefs. In Mellor's account (described above) of the Irishman who had the delusional perception when his companion pushed the salt cellar towards him there was evidence of a preceding delusional mood, a sense of unease as if something frightening was about to happen. Sometimes the delusional mood encompasses a sense of exaltation. A young woman woke one morning with a feeling of cosmic strangeness and power as if she could ride a bicycle (which she had never previously done). She then stabbed herself in the abdomen with a bread-knife, but after her recovery could give no explanation of why she had done this.

Schizophrenic patients sometimes exhibit delusional memories. These are accounts of fictitious events or circumstances which the patient is convinced they had experienced in the past. For example, a young man was convinced that several years previously he had had an operation in which his abdominal organs had been removed. He held tenaciously to this belief in spite of absence of any surgical scar.

Delusions of persecution and of reference have little diagnostic specificity but are common in schizophrenia. In the IPSS (WHO, 1973) ideas of reference were reported in 70% of cases and suspiciousness in 66% of cases. Patients commonly report that television programmes make special reference to them. Delusions of grandiose identity or grandiose ability also occur in schizophrenia, though they are more typical of mania. Unlike mania in which grandiose thinking is associated with elated mood, grandiose delusions in schizophrenia are usually not congruent with mood. Similarly, nihilistic delusions, which entail a belief that a part or all of one's own body is non-functioning or even absent, and are characteristic of depressive psychosis, can occur as mood-incongruent delusions in schizophrenia. For example, a middle-aged man suffering from schizophrenia stated that his head was absent, but apart from accompanying agitation, his mental state betrayed no underlying feelings or thoughts that might account for this nihilistic delusion.

Delusions can be either fragmentary or part of a system of linked, relatively self-consistent delusions. The man who claimed his head was absent also reported that there was blood all over his face, and showed no awareness of the contradiction implied by these statements. Another patient repeatedly referred to the fact that an axe had split his head but could give no explanation of how this had happened or what consequences it had produced. By contrast, a middle-aged woman, who had been experiencing auditory hallucinations and thought insertion for several months prior to a real burglary at her home, subsequently developed a relatively self-consistent persecutory delusional system based on the premise that the intelligence services were keeping her under surveillance and placing pressure on her by transmitting messages to her. Such organised delusional systems are most frequently encountered in female patients with the onset of illness in middle-age.

In acute episodes, patients often act in accordance with their delusions, but in the more chronic phase of the illness, it is common to encounter double orientation, in which there is a dissociation of affect and behaviour from the implications of the delusion. A man who maintained he was the Duke of Hamilton, and from time to time referred casually to a family member named Liz (Queen Elizabeth II), accepted without question the rather lowly accommodation and lack of privacy afforded by the hospital ward in which he lived. Although the dissociation between belief, affect and behaviour during the stable phase of his illness was typical of schizophrenia, during acute exacerbations of his illness his grandiosity was accompanied by irritability and hyperactivity. At these times his clinical state resembled mania, demonstrating an overlap between schizophrenia and affective psychosis.

Disorders of thought, affect and volition

Disorders of the form and flow of thought

Form of thought

In spite of many attempts to define and classify disorders of form of thought, since Bleuler introduced the apt term 'loosening of associations' more than 80 years ago, these disorders remain perhaps the most enigmatic of all schizophrenic phenomena. One of the problems lies in the variety of manifestations of disordered form of thought, and it is difficult to tease out the essential elements. There are at least three distinguishable classes

Box 7.2 Disorders of the form and flow of thought (synonyms or variants in brackets)

Unstable goal
Tangentiality – responses that are off the point.
Derailment – inappropriate shift to a loosely related or unrelated idea during flow of speech. (asyndetic thought).
Distractability – shift to an irrelevant idea triggered by an external stimulus.
Perseveration – unwarranted intrusion of a previously expressed word or idea.

Idiosyncratic thought and language
Idiosyncratic word use – normal words used in an inappropriate context (word approximations, metonyms) or non-words (neologisms).
Idiosyncratic ideas – unusual ideas that appear to reflect peculiar, personal concepts, or ideas expressed in an unusual manner that impedes comprehension.
Idiosyncratic logic – reasoning that does not follow normal rules of logic (autistic logic).
Incoherence[1] – incomprehensible speech, apparently reflecting absent or idiosyncratic connections between words (word salad).

Weakening of goal
Empty speech – utterances lacking an identifiable goal composed mainly of vacuous phrases of the type normally used merely to maintain flow of speech (poverty of content of speech).
Generalisation – speech lacks specificity and conveys little information because of over-generalisation.
Unelaborated ideas – ideas lack normal development; speech contains few adjectives, adverbs or modifying clauses.

Disorders of flow
Poverty of speech – decreased amount of speech; brief replies, lack of spontaneous speech.
Pressure of speech – excessive rate of speech.
Blocking – transient interruptions of speech during which the subject experiences absence of thought.

1. Incoherence apparently involves both unstable goal and idiosyncrasy.

of formal thought disorder in schizophrenia, each of which tend to occur at particular phases of the illness.

First, there are phenomena such as tangentiality, derailment, perseveration, and distractability which appear to reflect instability of the goal in thinking (see Box 7.2 for definitions of the various phenomena). The classification of perseveration, which involves the arbitrary intrusion of a previous idea into the present stream of thought, as an instance of instability of goal is debatable, but is justified by the observation that it often occurs with the other manifestations of unstable goal. This class of disorders is most prominent during acute exacerbations of the illness.

Second, there are idiosyncrasies of thought and language, including use of words, ideas and logic. The idiosyncrasies of logic do not usually involve a failure of strict, syllogistic logic. Rather, they appear to reflect unusual lines of thought which, at least in some instances, appear to reflect a private logic and ignore the common knowledge of the world guiding normal thinking. For example the woman who was asked why only she could see King George and Queen Mary at the doorway and replied "because they have come to see me" (see above), appears to be following an internally consistent line of thought but ignores common knowledge of the world. In the past, clinicians might have described this as autistic logic, but it is best to avoid the term 'autistic' because the thinking is not identical to that characteristic of childhood autism. Idiosyncrasies of thought and language can occur at any phase of the illness. They are sometimes prominent among the residual symptoms that persist after the resolution of the acute phase of illness. They also occur relatively frequently in some first degree relatives, suggesting they might be a marker for a schizophrenic trait.

Third, there are disorders which appear to reflect weakening of the goal of thinking, such as empty speech, uninformative generalisations, and lack of elaboration of ideas. Empty speech is characterised by utterances beginning without any identifiable goal and is dominated by vacuous phrases, of the type which are used from time to time in normal speech to maintain flow (e.g. 'you know'). The patients do not seem to be sure of what they are saying, thinking or perceiving. Empty speech is similar in concept to poverty of content of speech defined by Andreasen (1982), but unfortunately, ratings of poverty of content according to Andreasen's definition tend to correlate with ratings of derailment, which reflects instability rather than weakening of goal. Weakened goal is occasionally encountered during acute episodes, but is more common among patients with chronic illness.

There are also some disorders that appear to reflect the coincidence of two different classes of phenomena. For example, the combination of an unstable goal with idiosyncratic use of language generates incoherence, and in extreme cases, word salad (verbigeration).

Of these three classes of formal thought disorder, idiosyncrasy of thought and language is perhaps the most specific to schizophrenia, although instances occur occasionally in manic speech. In contrast, instability of goal is commonly encountered in mania. Weakening of goal is not a feature of mania, but can be a prominent feature of speech in a variety of chronic brain disorders other than schizophrenia. The coexistence of all three types of thought disorder is very rarely encountered in any condition other than schizophrenia. It should, however, be noted that occasional instances of all three classes of formal thought disorder occur in the speech of normal individuals; it is the frequency of occurrence and degree of disorder that distinguishes the thoughts of schizophrenic patients.

Flow of thought

There are also a variety of disorders of the flow of thought. During acute phases, the flow of thought can be accelerated, generating pressure of speech. When this is combined with unstable goal, the pattern of speech closely resembles that seen in mania. During any phase of the illness, but especially in chronic illness, there may be an impoverishment or slowing of thought leading to poverty of speech, which is manifest as a lack of spontaneous speech and brevity of replies. Slowing of thought also occurs in depression; but poverty of speech tends to be more persistent in schizophrenia. It is probable that there is only a partial overlap between the mechanism of poverty of speech in the two conditions. Poverty of speech, which refers to the flow of speech averaged over periods of several minutes or more, differs from the phenomenon of blocking, which is manifest as brief interruptions of speech during which the patient has the experience of having no thoughts at all. It is possible that this phenomenon is closely related to the experience of thought withdrawal, but lacks the delusional attribution of alien influence.

Positive and negative thought disorder

The various disorders of form and flow of thought might be grouped into two major divisions: positive thought disorder comprising unstable goal, idiosyncrasy, and pressure of speech; and negative thought disorder comprising weakening of goal and poverty of speech. Such a dichotomy is consistent with the overlap in the nature of unstable goal and idiosyncrasy in that both involve a tendency to make connections between words or ideas on the basis of incidental features. However, it scarcely does justice to the variety and temporal course of thought disorders in schizophrenia.

Assessment

The clinical assessment of thought disorder is difficult because the expression of these disorders depends on the extent to which the patient is given the opportunity to exhibit spontaneity and to direct the flow of conversation. Thought disorder can be more overt when the patient faces an intellectually challenging task, or when explaining delusional beliefs.

There are several useful rating scales for thought disorder, but none are completely satisfactory. Andreasen (1979) devised a scale for disorders of thought, language and communication (TLC) providing definitions of 23 items that can be rated with reasonable reliability in a clinical interview. However, the TLC scale is not sensitive to the relatively subtle idiosyncratic uses of language that are perhaps most characteristic of schizophrenia. Holzman *et al* (1986) have constructed the Thought Disorder Index (TDI) which is much more sensitive to these subtle idiosyncrasies of schizophrenic thought. However, the procedure devised by Holzman *et al* for assigning TDI scores involves assessment of thinking during the completion of both the Rorschach Test and the verbal subtests of the Wechsler Adult Intelligence Scale (WAIS), making it too cumbersome for use in the setting of a clinical interview.

Clinical illustration:

A 48-year-old female patient who suffered from a sustained florid illness reported having a telephone in her head. When she was asked what she heard on the telephone, she replied: "Well, it's like meeting people and I (pause) have a jug of hot tea and relax therapy, relaxation, and I can speak to the sinus arrhythmia doctor." Her reply begins in a slightly tangential manner, and then becomes derailed. At times she has difficulty in finding words. The term sinus arrhythmia doctor appears to be an idiosyncratic use of words to describe a psychologist or psychiatrist. At another point in the interview, in an attempt to delineate suspected ideas of reference, the interviewer asked: "Has there been anything about you on the TV?" She replied: "There's been the union jack and the hospital fire alarm and plastic surgery." Interviewer: "Did those things have anything to do with you?" Patient: "The Boer war". These replies illustrate marked tangentiality and derailment.

When asked about a scene depicting a boat tied to a tree, a patient with persisting stable symptoms replied: "I'd like to get in the boat, put in on the canal and row it away, 'cos there's a waistline there. The tree here is er.. somebody.. a man or a woman will come there... they'll sit down because that's there.. they'll feel uneasy and they'll take it and burn it." His reason for wanting to get in the boat reveals both idiosyncratic logic and idiosyncratic use of the word waistline. The subsequent sentence exhibits derailment. When asked whether he meant that they would burn the boat he said: "Yes, only for a person in the mind... you put that up there so it's a Van Gogh, you know, Christ knows. What the hell is the boat doing there, you know you give five million quid for it, he'd change his mind." The reply begins tangentially and becomes derailed. As a result of the derailment, it is unclear to whom the pronoun 'he' refers. 'Only for a person in the mind' is an idiosyncratically expressed idea whose meaning is difficult to discern.

The idiosyncrasy of thought and language can be quite subtle. When asked about his daily activities, a 37-year-old man with only slight evidence of residual schizophrenic symptoms replied: "I look at walls and windows and that bothers my life." In poetry, such a sentence might be accepted as legitimate. Indeed, his reply might be regarded as a poignant description of the impoverishment of life faced by many schizophrenic patients. However, when idiosyncrasy in everyday speech impedes communication substantially, it indicates pathological thought.

Poverty of speech and lack of elaboration are illustrated in the following response by a chronic patient to an invitation to describe a picture which depicted an active dockside scene in bright sunshine: "Reminds me of some...um...er...sun...er...clouds and sun...(long pause)...that's all."

Disorders of affect

Although disorders of thinking and perception are the most distinctive features of schizophrenia, disorders of affect are also a major component of the condition. Affect can be blunted, incongruous, unstable, irritable, depressed or elevated.

Blunted affect

Blunted affect has long been regarded as a cardinal feature of chronic schizophrenia, but it is also prevalent in acute schizophrenia. For example, in the IPSS it was reported in 66% of cases of acute schizophrenia (WHO, 1973). It is manifest as a failure to express feelings either verbally or non-verbally even when talking about issues which would normally be expected to engage the emotions. Expressive gestures are rare, and there is little animation in facial expression and in vocal inflection.

In some cases, objective evidence of affective blunting is accompanied by subjective awareness of loss of the ability to experience emotion. More commonly, the patient is unaware of having blunted emotions. However, friends and relatives often find the difficulty in establishing emotional contact with the patient a source of frustration and distress.

Incongruous affect

The expression of affect can be markedly inconsistent with the circumstances. A schizophrenic patient might laugh in a hollow and meaningless way for no understandable reason. However, this degree of incongruity of affect is not common. A shallow, fatuous affect similar to that arising from damage to the frontal lobes of the brain is more common.

Depression

Depression can occur during different phases of schizophrenia. Dysphoric mood is very common in the prodromal phases preceding a psychotic episode. Overt depression is often present during acute psychotic episodes. Knights & Hirsch (1981) found an extensive range of depressive features in 65% of a sample of acute schizophrenic patients. In general, this overt depression shows some evidence of diminution as the psychotic episode itself resolves, but it is also common to find depression persisting or becoming apparent in the months following an acute episode. Finally, depression may occur in the chronic stable phase of the illness. Cross-sectional examination reveals depression in 15–25% of chronic cases.

In both the acute and stable phases of the illness, depressed mood is usually part of a syndrome of depression similar to that occurring in primary depressive illness. In particular, the depressed mood is likely to be accompanied by anhedonia and negative cognitions such as low self-esteem, pessimism, hopelessness, and suicidal ideation. Suicide itself is not rare, though in some instances, suicide in schizophrenia occurs when there is no significant evidence of depression, suggesting that factors such as delusional ideation, hallucinatory voices, idiosyncratic judgement, and reduced impulse control can play a part. Biological features of depression such as disturbance of sleep and appetite also occur in association with depressed mood.

The observation that depression is a feature of virtually all phases of schizophrenia has prompted various proposals regarding the relationship between depression and schizophrenia. Some of the evidence suggests that a liability to depression is simply one aspect of the diathesis to schizophrenia. However, it appears that there is also a more intimate relationship between psychotic episodes in schizophrenia and depression. The observation that depression tends to resolve as psychotic symptoms respond to treatment with antipsychotic medication (Donlon *et al*, 1976) raises the possibility that the neuropharmacological processes associated with acute episodes of schizophrenia produce both psychotic symptoms and depression. By contrast, there is also evidence that antipsychotic medication can have a depressive effect in addition to inducing Parkinsonian symptoms (Rifkin *et al*, 1975). While at first sight this is inconsistent with the proposal that depression can be an intrinsic part of the pathological process of an acute schizophrenic episode, it is possible that the depressive component of an acute episode actually reflects a compensatory neuronal response. The psychological response to the implications of having schizophrenia might also be a factor in the pathogenesis of depression.

Anhedonia

Anhedonia, which is a loss of the ability to experience pleasure, can be a feature of depression in schizophrenia. It also occurs independently of depression, especially in the chronic phase of the illness, when it tends to be associated with flattened affect, poverty of thought and decreased volition. If it is part of a depressive syndrome it often comprises loss of ability to experience satisfaction in achievement and also loss of consummatory pleasure. When associated with flattened affect, anhedonia usually entails loss of the pleasures of the hunt rather than of the feast.

Disorders of volition

In schizophrenia, volition can be either weakened or disjointed.

Weakened volition

Weakened volition is manifest as a lack of spontaneous motor activity often accompanied by a lack of spontaneity in speech and affect. The patient is inclined to sit inertly in an armchair, or to remain in bed throughout much of the day.

Case illustration:

A 63-year-old woman, who had lived alone in a flat provided by the local authority after her discharge from mental hospital several years previously, lay in bed throughout the day, despite attempts by the community nurse, occupational therapist and doctor to engage her in activity. Left to her own devices, she would eat only confectionery bought for her by a friend. Her flat became increasingly squalid and her physical health was at risk. She was re-admitted to hospital compulsorily, and after treatment for a month, showed some marginal improvement in her level of activity. However, her cooperation was limited by resentment concerning her compulsory admission. After discharge, she returned to her former state.

Disjointed volition

The patient can be overactive in an ill-directed manner. There is a reduced ability to withstand impulses to act.

Case illustration:

An intelligent and artistic young woman who had been unable to re-establish either stable social relationships or regular occupation after her psychotic symptoms abated, lived alone in a poorly furnished rented room. One day she felt cold, so she gathered together a pile of paper and lit a fire on the carpet beside her bed. Fortunately, she managed to extinguish it before serious damage was done, but the carpet was ruined. She was quite capable of appreciating the consequences of acts such as lighting a fire. It appeared that she had been unable to suppress the impulse to act in spite of her ability to appreciate the likely consequences.

Catatonia

Catatonia is a disturbance of voluntary motor activity, and so overlaps with the disorders of volition described above. Catatonia is reflected in abnormalities of the form of motor activity and in the amount of activity, with either under-activity or over-activity.

At times, an apparently normal motor act is arrested in mid-flight. For example, a patient might become frozen in the act of reaching out for the door handle to open a door, and stand with his arm extended for many minutes. Catatonic phenomena described in the early years of this century were often more dramatic in character. Patients were more commonly reported to exhibit *flexibilitas cereus* (waxy flexibility), a condition in which the patient adopts a posture which can be adjusted by an examiner as if the patient is a passively deformable wax model. Catatonic under-activity can be manifest as an apparently stuporous state in which consciousness is usually maintained.

A catatonic act can appear to reflect abnormal compliance with or resistance to cues for action, resulting in a movement or posture that is inappropriate in the circumstances. For example, the patient might mimic a movement made by the examiner (echopraxia). At times it as if the patient is continually changing his mind about whether or not to execute a socially appropriate action such as shaking hands on meeting, and alternates between extending and withdrawing his hand. Such ambivalence when exhibited in the sphere of motor actions is known as ambitendence. Catatonic acts can also be negativistic, such as withdrawing the hand when interviewers appropriately proffer their hand.

Case illustration:

> The wife of a 42-year-old man who had a 14 year history of schizophrenia summoned an ambulance to their house because her husband had collapsed. The ambulancemen found him inert on the floor, mute but with his eyes open. In an attempt to establish his level of consciousness, they first rubbed the skin over his sternum and then twisted a handful of the trapezius muscle above his scapula. He did not respond. Several days later in hospital, when he had resumed a normal level of activity he reported being fully aware of the ambulancemen's attempts to elicit a response and was angry at the way they had treated him. He could not account for his failure to respond.

Catatonic over-activity takes the form of apparently pointless activity that is usually repetitive, such as walking rapidly round and round a table for a period of an half an hour or more. In at least some cases, an abrupt switch from a state of under-activity to over-activity can occur.

Violent behaviour

Violent behaviour is usually the product of an interaction between individuals and their surroundings. The type and frequency of violent behaviour by schizophrenic patients is strongly dependent on social circumstances, and any attempt to describe such violence as if it were purely a manifestation of schizophrenia would be misleading. Occasionally, schizophrenic patients perpetrate serious violence against others. Violence against self, such as self-mutilation or suicide, is more common. Minor physical violence against people or property, and verbal aggression is very common.

There are several aspects of the mental disturbances in schizophrenia that can contribute to violence. Delusional misinterpretations might generate fear or anger. Hallucinatory voices sometimes instruct the patient to carry out a violent act. Irritability might arise as a consequence of persistent, intrusive and unpleasant psychotic experiences, or possibly, as a direct consequence of the disease process on the level of cerebral arousal. Disturbance of volition might diminish control over impulses that are recognised to be inappropriate. Lack of judgement might result in a faulty evaluation of the consequences of an act or of its ethical implications.

Aggression can be directed against members of the patient's family, against mental health professionals, and occasionally against members of the general public. The families of patients living at home, or nursing staff caring for patients in hospital, are commonly the target of verbal aggression and minor physical violence. Serious violence driven by delusions or hallucinations, although much rarer, sometimes has a fatal outcome. Again, family and professionals are at greatest risk. Even matricide, an extremely rare crime, can occur in schizophrenia. Therefore careful assessment of the risk of violence is an important aspect of the assessment of acutely disturbed patients. This assessment will take account of any past history of violence, the current level of arousal and irritability, the content of delusions and hallucinations, and degree of insight. Preparing in advance for the possibility of violence is an important aspect of a domiciliary visit. Pharmaceutical aspects of treating violent behaviour are described in chapter 9 and the psychosocial aspects of management in chapter 10.

Case illustration:

> A patient who was in general considerate and gentle towards
> others, developed grandiose and persecutory delusions, and

became irritable and aggressive. The police were summoned, and when a policeman appeared at his front door, the patient shot him with a bolt from a cross-bow. After conviction in court, he was detained in a secure unit for treatment under the Mental Health Act. The episode of acute disturbance settled and the patient was eventually transferred to an unlocked ward. He once again resumed his characteristic gentle and considerate manner in most matters, but continued to maintain that the policeman deserved to be shot and he had been right to do so. In light of this evidence of limited insight and lack of judgement, he was very closely supervised following discharge to a group home under a Home Office restriction order. After he had been living in the group home for about a year, the community nurse noted that he was again becoming agitated. When the community nurse returned a few days later, the patient was suspicious and angry. An urgent psychiatric assessment confirmed that he was harbouring the delusional belief that the community nurse was part of a conspiracy against him. He was compelled to return to hospital immediately under the terms of the restriction order. The manager of the group home subsequently found a partially assembled cross-bow in the patient's room.

Cognitive impairment in schizophrenia

Patients with schizophrenia often perform poorly in formal tests of cognitive function, although the patterns of impaired performance vary between cases. Executive functions, associated with the frontal lobes, memory functions associated with both frontal and temporal lobes, and various aspects of attention, are especially prone to impairment, but virtually all aspects of cognitive function have been reported to show impairment in at least some patients. Examination of twins discordant for schizophrenia reveals that the schizophrenic twin usually exhibits a lower level of performance in tests than the unaffected twin, even though the affected twin's performance might be within the normal range (Goldberg *et al*, 1992). This suggests that even in cases where there is no marked cognitive impairment, the illness inhibits the realisation of potential cognitive ability.

The failure in executive functions is illustrated by the deficit in performance in word-generation tasks in which the patient is asked to generate as many words as possible in a given category in a specified time. Some patients with schizophrenia, like patients with Alzheimer's disease, tend to produce few words. However, unlike the situation in Alzheimer's disease, if the patient is asked to perform the same task on numerous occasions, many different words are generated, indicating that the store of words is intact. Instead the problem lies in employing strategies to obtain access to the store. Ability to change strategies in response to changing task demands is another aspect of executive function commonly impaired in schizophrenia. This can be demonstrated by tasks such as the Wisconsin Card-Sorting Test, in which the subject is required to discover the rule governing the sorting of cards according to specific features, and when given feedback indicating that the rule has been changed, to discover the new rule. Patients with schizophrenia, like individuals with frontal lobe lesions, tend to make incorrect perseverative responses.

Although virtually all aspects of memory function can be impaired, in the verbal domain it is typical to find a disproportionate impairment of recall compared with recognition. At least in cases which are not too chronic, the deficit in recall can be overcome by preparing the patients with strategies for organising the material to be recalled (Calev *et al*, 1983) which suggests that even here much of the deficit lies in the domain of developing strategies for the task.

Among the attentional impairments observed in schizophrenia are impairment of selective attention, and of the ability to sustain attention. Selective attention involves the ability to attend to a specific aspect of a situation in the face of competition from other features that tend to intrude. The Stroop Task, in which the subject is presented with colour names printed in ink which is not congruent with the colour name, and required to name the colour of the ink, tests selective attention and also ability to select response. Patients with schizophrenia, especially those suffering disorganisation of thought, exhibit evidence of decreased ability to suppress the influence of the irrelevant colour name. The ability to sustain attention (vigilance) is commonly assessed using the continuous performance test (CPT). In this test, the subject is presented with a long series of varying stimuli, including irrelevant stimuli and designated target stimuli, and is required to respond whenever a target stimulus appears. Patients with schizophrenia, and also a substantial number of their first degree relatives, perform poorly.

The observed impairment of performance in a variety of language tasks in schizophrenia supports the hypothesis that there is disordered activity in the left hemisphere. However, functions such as the recognition of facial expression, normally regarded as a predominantly right hemisphere activity, can also be impaired.

While the evidence of a multiplicity of different patterns of cognitive impairment in schizophrenia indicates it is unlikely that a single cognitive defect accounts for all the manifestations of the condition, impairment of working memory, which lies within the overlap of the domains of executive function, attention and memory, possibly plays a cardinal part in the illness. Working memory is the mental system responsible for the temporary storage and manipulation of information essential for complex cognitive tasks such as comprehension of language, learning and reasoning (Baddeley, 1992). There appear to be three major components of this system: a central executive whose tasks include the allocation of attentional resources, a visuo-spatial sketch pad which manipulates visual images, and a phonological loop which stores and rehearses speech-based information. The neuronal substrate of working memory is association cortex, especially prefrontal cortex. The neurotransmitter dopamine plays an important part in modulating the activity of working memory.

Chronic schizophrenic patients, especially those with persistent disorders of the form and flow of thought and speech, tend to have more marked cognitive impairments than acute cases. In the time when patients with persistent illness usually remained in hospital, approximately one-fifth of those who became long-term in-patients suffered from age disorientation. In many cases the patient reported an age within a few years of that on admission to hospital, in spite of a duration of hospital stay of 20 years or more. This phenomenon was associated with a severe, global impairment of intellect (Liddle & Crow, 1984). In spite of this evidence suggesting the progression of cognitive impairment in a small proportion of cases, the majority of the evidence suggests that there is no consistent tendency towards an inexorable deterioration in cognitive function with time in most patients with schizophrenia. One of the few longitudinal studies of cognitive function in schizophrenia found that the mean WAIS score in a group of 42 patients actually increased by six points between the initial assessment approximately 12 years after the onset of illness and the follow-up assessment eight years later (Klonoff *et al*, 1970). Neuropsychological dysfunction is further discussed on page 352.

Neurological signs

Abnormal involuntary movements

Several decades before the development of antipsychotic medication, Farran-Ridge (1926) described a range of abnormal involuntary movements, which he attributed to basal ganglion disorder, in schizophrenic patients. The movements include tics, twitches and grimaces. After the introduction of anti-dopaminergic antipsychotic medication in the mid 1950s, abnormal involuntary movements became more prevalent, although the onset of abnormal movements related to treatment usually only starts after prolonged treatment. Hence, these medication-related dyskinetic movements are called tardive dyskinesia. The movements can be exacerbated by withdrawal of antipsychotic medication, and often persist long after cessation of treatment.

Dyskinetic movements in schizophrenia fall into two distinguishable groups: orofacial dyskinesia, and trunk and limb dyskinesia. While the former are more characteristic of drug induced dyskinesia, it is probable that aspects of the disease process itself contribute to both types of dyskinesia. In particular, core negative symptoms such as poverty of speech and flat affect are associated with both types of dyskinesia. However, the two types of dyskinesia differ in their relationship to ageing. The prevalence of trunk and limb dyskinesia is virtually independent of age, while orofacial dyskinesia is rare in young patients and increases rapidly in late middle-age. This increase in prevalence occurs about a decade earlier in patients with marked negative symptoms in comparison with those without negative symptoms, suggesting the pathological process underlying negative symptoms interacts with age-related neuronal degeneration in a way that hastens the onset of orofacial dyskinesia (Liddle *et al*, 1993*a*).

Cortical signs

Both dyspraxia and agnosia are common, at least among chronic schizophrenic patients. Typically, patients are clumsy or hesitant in performing motor sequences, or have impairments of integration of sensory information such as dysgraphaesthesia or impaired two point discrimination. These neurological signs have limited localising power, but are probably indicative of impaired function of the association cortex. They are related to core negative symptoms and to a lesser extent, to disorganisation of mental activity (Liddle *et al*, 1993*b*).

Abnormal eye movements

Saccadic intrusions in smooth pursuit eye movements have been reported in 50–85% of patients and 40–50% of first degree relatives (Holtzman *et al*, 1988). The familial pattern prompted Holtzman and colleagues to propose the existence of a heritable neurological characteristic (a latent trait) which may be manifest as either schizophrenia or as an abnormality of smooth pursuit or both disorders. Since eye movements are governed by the cortical frontal eyefields and by brainstem nuclei, the relevant deficit in patients with schizophrenia might in principle be at either or both of these two sites. A large body of evidence favours involvement of the frontal eyefields (Levin, 1980).

In addition to saccadic intrusions in smooth pursuit, other abnormalities of eye movement occur. For example, some patients fail to suppress an automatic saccade towards a stimulus in the periphery when instructed to perform a saccadic movement away from the side of the stimulus (an antisaccade).

Insight

While some impairment of insight is implicit in the classification of schizophrenia as a psychotic illness, the degree to which unrealistic thinking interferes with the patient's understanding of the nature of the illness is variable, both over the course of the illness in an individual case and between cases. At its most severe, impaired insight might lead patients to deny that they are suffering from an illness at all. It is difficult to engage them in any therapeutic programme. At less severe levels, patients may accept that they have an illness, but deny that it is a mental illness. More commonly, the patients accept, at least implicitly, that they have a mental illness, but have unrealistic ideas that diminish their ability to evaluate issues regarding treatment, or to comprehend the impact of the illness on their lives. Assessment of the level of insight is especially important where there is a risk of dangerous behaviour.

Case illustration:

> A 22-year-old man who had suffered a schizophrenic episode one year previously, developed a delusional belief that he belonged to the Knights Templar, and had to defend the temple against enemies. He assembled a collection of weapons including guns and swords. His parents informed his general practitioner, but the man maintained he was not ill and was unwilling to accept medical assessment. When a social worker and psychiatrist came to his house to assess him with a view to compulsory admission to hospital under the Mental Health Act, he threatened them with a shotgun. The police were called and in the ensuing gun battle, the patient and two police officers were injured. The patient was admitted to hospital under section two of the 1983 Mental Health Act, and treated with haloperidol. In the following weeks, he accepted that he required treatment with antipsychotic medication in hospital. However, he continued to believe that he was besieged by enemies. In particular, he regarded his parents as enemies, possibly because of their attempts to seek medical help for him. Thus, despite an increase in the level of his insight during treatment, he developed only a partial appreciation of the nature of his condition and remained potentially dangerous.

Subtypes and syndromes of schizophrenia

The classical subtypes

The classical subdivision partitions schizophrenia into hebephrenic, paranoid, catatonic and simple subtypes, reflecting the fact that the disease has its origins in Kraepelin's amalgamation of hebephrenia, catatonia and dementia paranoides into a single disease entity, to which Diem (1903) had added dementia simplex.

In practice, it is difficult to allocate patients within this classical subdivision because many patients show features of more than one subtype in the course of their illness. The most successful of the various attempts to define discrete subtypes of schizophrenia have been those that collapsed the classical subdivision into paranoid and non-paranoid types. Provided that the criteria for paranoid schizophrenia emphasise not only the presence of systematised delusions and hallucinations, but also the absence of formal thought disorder and affective deterioration, paranoid schizophrenia is distinguished by having a relatively good outcome.

Dimensions of psychopathology

The limited success of attempts to divide schizophrenia into discrete sub-types vindicates Kraepelin's proposal that hebephrenia, catatonia and dementia paranoides might best be regarded as different manifestations of a single disease. However, it is clear that the clinical manifestations are heterogeneous which suggests that several distinguishable but related psychopathological processes can occur within schizophrenia. In recent years, accumulating evidence concerning the nature of the associated brain disorder has pointed towards the existence of several distinguishable underlying neuropathological processes. This has led to the proposal that schizophrenia is a disease in which there are a number of dimensions of psychopathology, reflecting distinct but related neuropathological processes, that might or might not occur together in a single case.

The type 1/type 2 dichotomy

The first model that linked dimensions of psychopathology to neuropathology was proposed by Crow (1980). He suggested there were two independent dimensions which he designated type 1 and type 2. Type 1 schizophrenia was characterised by positive symptoms which tend to be acute. Positive symptoms entail the presence of an abnormal mental process, and include delusions, hallucinations and formal thought disorder. Crow proposed that type 1 schizophrenia reflected a biochemical imbalance, such as dopaminergic hyperactivity. Type 2 schizophrenia was characterised by negative symptoms which tend to be chronic. Negative symptoms reflect the absence of a mental function present in normal individuals, and include poverty of speech and blunted affect. Crow proposed that type 2 schizophrenia arose from a structural abnormality of the brain.

As predicted by Crow's hypothesis, a great deal of evidence indicates that negative symptoms are more strongly associated with various indices of brain abnormality than are positive symptoms. However, the structural abnormalities revealed by X-ray computed tomography and magnetic resonance imaging are not associated exclusively with negative symptoms. Also the efficacy of atypical antipsychotic drugs such as clozapine in treating persistent negative symptoms in at least some cases, implies that a biochemical imbalance plays some role in the genesis of these symptoms.

While the type 1/ type 2 proposal now appears to be an oversimplification of the relationship between symptoms, chronicity, and neuropathology, it was perhaps the first credible attempt to link the symptoms of schizophrenia with underlying neuropathology in a way that accounted for the occurrence of episodes of acute disturbance superimposed upon a background of enduring deficits. In particular, it provided a major stimulus to investigation of the enduring deficits.

Three syndromes of characteristic schizophrenic symptoms

Most of the studies that have performed a detailed analysis of the pattern of correlations between schizophrenic symptoms reveal at least three distinguishable groups of symptoms. In studies limited to patients with persistent, stable symptoms (e.g. Liddle, 1987), three groups of symptoms emerge: psychomotor poverty (the core negative symptoms – poverty of speech, blunted affect; decreased spontaneous movement); disorganisation (disorders of the form of thought, inappropriate affect); and reality distortion (the core positive symptoms – delusions, hallucinations). Many other studies have reported a similar segregation of schizophrenic symptoms, even in groups of patients which were more heterogeneous with regard to chronicity of symptoms (e.g. Arndt *et al*, 1991; Frith, 1992; Peralta *et al*, 1992).

In many ways these three syndromes resemble the three principal psychotic illnesses which Kraepelin amalgamated to form dementia praecox. Reality distortion comprises symptoms which were a feature of dementia paranoides; disorganisation is similar to hebephrenia; and psychomotor poverty, which reflects diminished spontaneous activity, resembles the hypoactive phase of catatonia. It is important to emphasise that the syndromes can coexist within an individual patient reflecting distinguishable dimensions of psychopathology within a single illness.

Each of the three syndromes is associated with a distinct pattern of impairment in neuropsychological tests, suggesting three different patterns of underlying brain function. The evidence suggests that psychomotor poverty, disorganisation, and reality distortion are associated with impairment of the supervisory mental functions responsible for initiation, selection, and monitoring of self-generated mental activity, respectively. A study of regional cerebral blood flow (rCBF) using positron emission tomography confirmed that each syndrome is associated with a particular pattern of cerebral activity (Liddle *et al*, 1992). For each syndrome, the associated pattern of rCBF embraces anatomically connected regions of association cortex, and related sub-cortical nuclei. In each instance the cerebral regions involved include those areas of cortex implicated in the corresponding supervisory mental function in normal individuals. Thus, the evidence suggests that there are several distinct patterns of brain malfunction in schizophrenia. The details of these patterns require confirmation, but it is reasonable to expect that as the patterns of neural malfunction are delineated more clearly, new light will be thrown on the common factors that link them and ultimately lead to the identification of the essential characteristics of schizophrenia in neurological terms.

Five dimensions of psychopathology in schizophrenia

The three characteristic schizophrenic syndromes which emerge from exploration of the relationships between persistent symptoms do not embrace the entire gamut of symptoms occurring in schizophrenia. In particular, there are two additional syndromes which are usually transient: depression, characterised by low mood and depressive cognitions such as low self-esteem and pessimism; and psychomotor excitation, characterised by motor over-activity and excited labile affect, which appears to be the polar opposite of psychomotor poverty and resembles the excited phase of catatonia.

A factor analysis of the symptoms assessed using the positive and negative syndrome scale (PANSS; Kay, 1991), which covers the symptoms of schizophrenia in a comprehensive manner, revealed a complex pattern with five main factors: core negative symptoms (including social withdrawal, lack of spontaneity and flow of conversation, blunted affect, motor retardation); core positive symptoms (delusions and hallucinations); excitement (including excitement, poor impulse control, tension, hostility); depressive symptoms (including anxiety, guilt feelings, depression, somatic concern); cognitive disorders (including difficulty in abstract thinking, disorientation and conceptual disorganisation).

The group of cognitive disorders resembles the disorganisation syndrome. Unfortunately, PANSS ratings do not provide a clear delineation of the disorganisation syndrome because several negative symptom items

---

Box 7.3 Dimensions of psychopathology in schizophrenia

Reality distortion – delusions, hallucinations
Disorganisation – (positive) formal thought disorder, inappropriate affect, disjointed volition
Psychomotor poverty – poverty of speech, flat affect, motor under-activity
Psychomotor excitation – pressure of speech, irritability, motor over-activity
Depression – depressed mood, pessimism/hopelessness, low self-esteem/guilt, anhedonia
Non-specific psychopathology – attentional impairment, disorientation, anxiety, sleep disturbance, somatic complaints

of the PANSS are defined in a manner which includes features of the disorganisation syndrome. In particular, the blunted affect item includes inappropriate affect. With this relatively minor caveat, Kay's factor analysis confirmed that virtually the entire gamut of schizophrenic symptoms can be accounted for by five principal dimensions of psychopathology.

Box 7.3 presents the five principal dimensions of schizophrenic pathology in a way which reflects the consistent patterns of relationships between symptoms identified by recent factor analytic studies. If psychomotor poverty and psychomotor excitation are regarded as lying at opposite poles of a bipolar continuum, it would perhaps be more correct to say that there are four independent dimensions, one of which is bipolar. These dimensions apparently reflect five major pathological processes that generate five distinguishable syndromes. Although these five syndromes are distinguishable in that they can occur separately, evidence of more than one syndrome is detectable in the majority of patients. The probability of observing a particular combination of syndromes depends on the phase of illness, suggesting that there are various shared features linking these distinguishable syndromes. Overall, the symptoms of schizophrenia appear to form a constellation of symptoms all of which are related, but some of the relationships are closer than others, with the symptoms clustering into five major groups.

The course and prognosis of schizophrenia

Although Kraepelin distinguished dementia praecox from affective psychosis largely on the basis of the time course, with dementia praecox typically beginning in adolescence and persisting throughout adult life, the course of the illness now known as schizophrenia shows substantial variability. There is variability in the mode of onset; in the degree of persistence of symptoms through the mid-stage of the illness; and in the long-term outcome.

The onset

At one extreme, the onset can be insidious, with subtle evidence of abnormality beginning in childhood, or even in infancy. In some cases, a patient's mother declares that even in the first year of life the patient differed from his siblings in responsiveness. At school, one of several different patterns of behaviour might emerge: in some cases, the child is shy and socially awkward; in others cases, hostile and disruptive in class. During adolescence these patterns develop further. The shy, awkward child becomes introspective and socially isolated. The more disruptive child might as an adolescent become quite erratic in behaviour. In either case, the developing young adult finds it difficult to form stable intimate relationships, or establish a consistent work record. Sooner or later, perhaps while still at school, a decline in performance becomes noticeable. In unfavourable circumstances, there might be a drift into a vagrant lifestyle with marked neglect of personal hygiene. In most cases, the illness eventually declares itself with delusions and hallucinations.

At the other extreme, the onset can be quite abrupt. Over the course of a few weeks, the patient becomes unsettled. He might experience dysphoric mood or irritability and a puzzled sense that something odd is happening. He often appears preoccupied. In some instances, obsessional thoughts intrude. Concentration deteriorates and sleep is disturbed. From this unsettled state, delusions or hallucinations emerge and behaviour is likely to become disruptive, even aggressive. There is a rapid deterioration in occupational performance and social activity. Such an onset often follows a stressful experience.

In less extreme instances, the onset of florid symptoms occurs after a prodromal phase lasting many months, which begins with a subtle alteration of behaviour and may progress through a phase of preoccupation and social withdrawal before agitation becomes prominent and overt psychosis appears. Not uncommonly, onset occurs during the first year of a university or college course. The young person might be living away from home for the first time and as pressures build up, perhaps as first-year examinations approach, the breakdown occurs.

The distribution of age of onset of overt symptoms is one of the most characteristic features of schizophrenia. In men, the frequency of onset rises rapidly through adolescence to a peak at about age 22, followed by a steady decrease so that onset after 40 is rare. In women, the frequency of onset rises through adolescence, but the peak is later, the distribution is somewhat broader, and an appreciable risk of onset persists into middle age.

Outcome of the first episode

In a study from New York of the course of illness in a large cohort of patients satisfying Research Diagnostic Criteria for schizophrenia or schizoaffective disorder of predominantly schizophrenic type, Lieberman *et al* (1993) found that 83% of the schizophrenic cases achieved a remission within the first year, though in 14% remission was only partial. The mean time to achieve remission was 42 weeks, although the median time was only 10 weeks.

The medium-term evolution of the illness

In a minority of cases, there is complete recovery after the first episode. A systematic five-year follow-up study of a comprehensive, representative cohort of patients from a defined catchment area in Buckinghamshire, a relatively affluent rural English county, 16% of cases had had only one episode and showed no residual impairment (Watt *et al*, 1983). The patients had been selected according to Present State Examination diagnostic criteria which places emphasis on the presence of Schneiderian first rank symptoms, but do not demand persistence of symptoms.

A synthesis of findings from the major longitudinal studies (Bleuler, 1974; Huber *et al*, 1975; Ciompi & Muller, 1976; Watt *et al*, 1983) indicates that 20–30% of cases run an episodic course with relatively minor disability intervening between episodes. Even in such relatively good outcome cases, it is common to find that the patient experiences brief periods of mild dysphoric symptoms and attentional difficulties several times a year. Some of these episodes of mild disturbance prove to be the prodromal phase of florid psychotic relapse.

In the middle range of severity of illness are cases in which an appreciable degree of disability persists between episodes of florid symptoms. Between episodes the patient typically exhibits abnormal sensitivity to stress, and some oddities of behaviour or lack of initiative, but is able to sustain relationships and perform an occupation, although at a lower level than might otherwise have been expected. The middle range also includes patients who have persisting delusions or hallucinations which interfere minimally with daily life so that occupational and social activities suffer only mild disruption. Some patients who initially exhibit an illness of medium severity, appear to suffer a stepwise deterioration after successive episodes. The rate of remission in later episodes is lower than in first episodes.

Box 7.4 Prognostic factors

Factors indicating poor prognosis
  Poor premorbid adjustment
  Insidious onset
  Onset in adolescence
  Marked cognitive impairment
  Enlargement of cerebral ventricles

Factors indicating good prognosis
  Evidence of schizoaffective features
  (a) Marked mood disturbance at onset
  (b) Family history of affective illness

Outcome is better in females than in males.
Outcome is better in less developed countries.

(Adapted from WHO, 1973).

Towards the severe end of the spectrum of illness, about 20–25% of cases achieve at best partial remission of symptoms and suffer from substantial persisting disability. The most severe 5–10% of cases suffer from persistent symptoms and behavioural disorder that seriously disrupts all aspects of life.

Persistent symptoms and the defect state

The features most likely to persist are psychomotor symptoms such as apathy, flat affect and poverty of speech, and signs of disorganised mental activity, such as formal thought disorder and disjointed volition. Delusions and hallucinations tend to be intrinsically more episodic, and furthermore, usually respond to treatment with conventional dopamine blocking antipsychotic medication. Nonetheless, they persist in 15–20% of cases despite such treatment. The use of atypical antipsychotic drugs such as clozapine, which can alleviate not only hallucinations and delusions but also disorganisation and psychomotor poverty symptoms, produces substantial improvement in about 40% of hitherto treatment-resistant patients.

In a small proportion of the patients at the severe end of the spectrum, the clinical picture is dominated by persistent active psychotic symptoms and chaotic or aggressive behaviour. In a larger number, the dominating feature is a defect state characterised by negative symptoms (psychomotor poverty) and a disintegration of occupational and social behaviour. Sociable greetings and polite conversation disappear, table manners deteriorate and basic hygiene is neglected. In such cases, there is often overt cognitive impairment.

In the era when a large number of schizophrenic patients lived as long-stay residents of large institutions which afforded them little opportunity to take responsibility for their own lives, many developed a severe defect state. Bleuler (1918) described in graphic terms the way in which patients "sit about the institutions to which they are confined with expressionless faces, hunched-up, the image of indifference". As might be expected, it appears that depriving individuals, whose illness diminishes their ability to initiate mental activity, of the opportunity to exercise what remains of their capacity for initiative, exacerbates the intrinsic problems. It is likely that interaction between intrinsic cognitive impairment and lack of stimulation in the institutional environment plays an important part in the age-disorientation which occurs in a minority of long-stay schizophrenic patients.

Long-term outcome

In contrast to the implication of Kraepelin's original choice of the name dementia praecox, there is a tendency for schizophrenia to resolve eventually in many cases, though the time-scale of improvement can be several decades. The pooled data from the major studies that have followed patients for more than 20 years (Bleuler, 1974; Huber *et al*, 1975; Ciompi & Muller, 1976; Harding *et al*,1987) shows that 57% of 1117 schizophrenic patients followed up over a mean of 27 years showed either recovery or significant improvement. Improvement was not confined only to those with mild illness. For example, Harding *et al* (1987) studied 118 patients satisfying DSM–III criteria for schizophrenia who had been representative of the most impaired third of the Vermont State Hospital in-patient population prior to a programme of active rehabilitation in the mid 1950s. They were re-settled in the community and three decades later, 68% were judged to have either recovered or improved significantly.

In patients who have not yet recovered after several decades, acute exacerbations are less common than in earlier years. A minority suffer chronic delusions or hallucinations. A larger number exhibit a defect state which can range in severity from mild apathy, flattened affect and social withdrawal, to a severely disabling impoverishment or dis-organisation of mental activity combined with serious self-neglect and asociality. Some patients exhibit a state which Huber (1966) called the non-characteristic defect state, dominated by subjective awareness of psychological deficits, such as attentional impairment and anergia, and somatic sensations (coenaesthesia).

Factors predicting outcome

There are no reliable guidelines for predicting outcome in an individual case. However, there are constitutional factors and also features of the onset of illness that indicate an increased likelihood of better outcome. Female gender, good pre-morbid social adjustment and a family history of affective disorder are associated with better outcome. Abrupt onset associated with major precipitants, onset at a later age, and the presence of marked mood disturbance at onset, are indicators of a relatively good prognosis (Box 7.4).

Among neurobiological features, extent of structural abnormality of the brain is perhaps the feature most consistently observed to be associated with poor outcome, though some studies have not confirmed this association. In his review of X-ray CT studies of ventricular size in schizophrenia, Lewis (1990) reported that five of the nine studies which addressed the issue found a significant relationship between increased ventricular size and poorer response to treatment. It should be noted that ventricular enlargement tends to be present from the beginning of the illness, and hence can be regarded as predictive of outcome, rather than a consequence of poor outcome.

Once the illness is established, certain clinical features are predictive of poor occupational and social outcome. In particular, symptoms of psychomotor poverty or disorganisation, and evidence of overt cognitive impairment, are associated with poor occupational and social adjustment. On the other hand, patients who report the use of coping strategies to minimize their symptoms tend to have a better outcome. While this might merely be an indicator that better insight reflects less severe illness that has a better outcome, it raises the possibility that a style of therapy that fosters coping strategies might enhance prognosis.

Case illustration:

> An 32-year-old architect had maintained his professional role despite three admissions to hospital with acute episodes of illness dominated by hallucinations and delusions of reference. He lived with his parents and found an active social life too stressful. He developed the ability to recognise the prodromal signs of impending relapse. For example, he would become aware of increasing preoccupation with car number plates, and recognised that this was a precursor to the delusional belief that the numbers contained a significant message concerned with espionage. When he became aware of the intensifying preoccupation he sought additional medication and organised his life to minimise the demands upon him.

Standardised assessment and diagnosis

The issue of reliable, valid assessment of symptoms and diagnosis remains vexed. As we have seen, the fragmentation of mental activity emphasised by Kraepelin and Bleuler appears to lie at the heart of the illness, yet is difficult to assess. On the other hand the first rank symptoms identified by Schneider can be defined with reasonable precision, but are only loosely correlated with the disruption of the patient's life.

The US–UK diagnostic project (Cooper *et al*, 1972) demonstrated substantial discrepancies between diagnostic practices in the United States where a relatively broad concept of schizophrenia had evolved from a tradition influenced by Bleuler; and the UK, where the prevailing concept of schizophrenia placed more emphasis on Schneiderian first rank symptoms. The IPSS (WHO, 1973), demonstrated that consistency across cultures was possible using semi-standardised criteria leaning heavily on Schneiderian symptoms. However, this consistency in diagnosis is achieved at the expense of excluding cases who suffer sustained fragmentation of mental activity without delusions or hallucinations.

Symptom assessment

The approach to symptom assessment adopted by the IPSS is embodied in the Present State Examination (PSE). The PSE is a semi-standardised clinical interview in which a set of standard questions, augmented by additional questions as required to clarify the nature of the patient's symptoms, is used to detect the presence and determine the severity of designated symptoms which are defined carefully in a glossary. The IPSS employed a modified 360 item version of the eighth edition.

The ninth edition (Wing *et al*, 1974), which has proved to be a very successful and practical instrument for the assessment of psychotic illnesses, includes 140 symptom items, each scored 0, 1 or 2. The text includes a glossary of the definitions of each of the 140 symptoms and the interviewer's task is to decide whether the subjects' responses fit with the definition given in the glossary. In general, a score of 2 denotes greater severity than a score of 1, but for some of the psychotic items, a score of 2 denotes a qualitatively different phenomenon. For example, for item 57 (thought echo or commentary), the experience of hearing one's thoughts echoed is scored 1, whereas the experience of alien thoughts related to one's own thoughts is scored 2.

In order to condense the amount of information contained in the full set of 140 symptom scores, the symptoms are grouped into 38 syndromes, defined on the basis of clinical judgement, in a way that brings symptoms of similar character commonly occurring within a single illness together, while keeping symptoms with different diagnostic implications apart. For example, Schneiderian first rank symptoms, including both the delusional and hallucinatory phenomena, are grouped together to form the nuclear syndrome, while grandiose and religious delusions are grouped together in a separate syndrome. Some syndromes, such as the nuclear syndrome, have strong diagnostic significance alone. The diagnostic implication of others, such as the grandiose and religious delusions syndrome, depends on the presence or absence of other syndromes. Yet other syndromes, such as non-specific psychosis, include a miscellaneous collection of items and have little diagnostic specificity. Syndrome scores can also be assigned from clinical case-notes, making it possible to assemble a comparable, though less reliable, data set covering a period of time different from the one month examined in the PSE interview.The full version of the PSE measures both neurotic and psychotic disorders. A shorter, screening version focuses principally on neurotic disorder.

In the tenth edition of the PSE there are 299 symptom items, mostly scored on a scale ranging from 0–4 reflecting increasing degrees of severity. The greater range allows greater sensitivity, but it is more difficult to achieve inter-rater reliability. Teasing out a sufficiently detailed description of the patient's experience to rate severity on a five point scale for a substantial number of the 299 items would be extremely demanding of a patient's attention and cooperation. For many purposes, only a sub-set of items would be assessed. Although subjected to detailed evaluation since the mid-1980s, the tenth edition has not yet been widely used.

The PSE does not lend itself easily to sensitive measurement of change in overall severity of illness. The Brief Psychiatric Rating Scale (BPRS), constructed by Overall & Gorham (1962), allows the scoring of each of 16 items commonly occurring in psychotic illnesses on a seven-point ordered scale, and is potentially suitable to measure change in severity of individual symptoms and of overall severity of illness. It was used in the majority of pharmacological treatment trials in the three decades after its introduction. However, some items embrace a variety of different phenomena, while some particular classes of phenomena are scattered over several different items. For example, delusions contribute to the scores for several different items, making it difficult to quantify overall severity of delusions.

The Manchester Symptom Scale developed by Krawieka *et al* (1977) allows the scoring of eight phenomena common in chronic schizophrenia according to a five-point ordered scale. Concise definitions of the phenomena and descriptions of each level of severity are provided for each item. Its brevity makes it a very suitable scale for assessing severely disabled chronic patients. However, the limited range of phenomena measured restricts its utility for assessing other patient groups.

In the 1980s several scales were developed which emphasised the observable deficits of speech, affect and behaviour in schizophrenia. For example, the Scale for the Assessment of Negative Symptoms (SANS) (Andreasen, 1982) comprises five sub-scales concerned with affective flattening, alogia, avolition, anhedonia and attentional impairment. There are 25 individual items, each scored in the range 0–5. It is possible to score the observable behavioural items with acceptable reliability. This scale has been widely used in the exploration of the clinical and neurobiological correlates of negative symptoms of schizophrenia.

However, the grouping of items within subscales of SANS does not adequately reflect the relationships between the various aspects of the psychopathology of schizophrenia, so sub-scale scores have limited utility. In particular, in the original version, the affective flattening subscale included inappropriate affect, which would no longer be regarded as a negative symptom. Similarly, the inclusion of blocking in the alogia subscale is dubious. Furthermore, the assignment of scores for avolition and anhedonia in SANS are based on assessment of performance in aspects of everyday life, such as achievement at work or school and involvement in relationships. Clearly, many factors apart from avolition and anhedonia might interfere with performance in everyday life. Even more troublesome is the inclusion of attentional impairment as a negative symptom, because attentional impairments arise in association with a wide variety of schizophrenic symptoms, especially with disorders of the form of thought. Thus, while the items within SANS provide a comprehensive coverage of the negative syndrome, the inclusion of some phenomena that are more closely related to the disorganisation syndrome weakens the validity of sub-scale scores and of the total score. On the other hand, because the main limitation of SANS lies in the grouping of items, rather than in the definitions of the individual items themselves, by using SANS in conjunction with Andreasen's Scale for the Assessment of Positive Symptoms (SAPS), it is possible to obtain a comprehensive coverage of schizophrenic phenomena.

Shortly after the development of the SANS, Kay and colleagues drew on concepts embodied in both the BPRS and SANS to develop a scale for measuring a wide range of schizophrenic symptoms, the Positive and Negative Syndrome Scale (PANSS; Kay, 1991). It contains three subscales: positive symptoms (including delusions, hallucinations and positive formal thought disorder); negative symptoms (including lack of spontaneity, blunted affect) and general psychopathology. Although it was designed on the basis of a view of schizophrenic symptoms that afforded special importance to a positive-negative dichotomy, subsequent factor analysis of PANSS symptom scores revealed a more complex pattern of relationships between symptoms, consistent with the five-dimensional model of schizophrenic pathology. Unfortunately, some of the PANSS items embrace differing phenomena which are not closely related, and, as in the BPRS, delusional thinking is included in several different items in combination with non-delusional phenomena. Because the contamination occurs within items, it is intrinsically difficult to tease apart aspects of psychopathology which probably should be assessed separately. Nonetheless, PANSS provides an efficient comprehensive measure of schizophrenic psychopathology which is suitable for use in serial assessments of the severity of illness.

Unfortunately, there is no single symptom scale which combines the virtues of reliability, sensitivity to change in clinical state, and efficient coverage of the major phenomena of schizophrenia within a relatively small set of items defined and assembled in a manner that provides sub-scale scores reflecting current understanding of the relationships between symptoms. It is probably unreasonable to expect all of these qualities in one scale. The PSE provides rigorous assessment, but is cumbersome and relatively unsuitable for monitoring clinical change. SANS when combined with SAPS provides good coverage of schizophrenic phenomena but the original sub-scale composition differs from current understanding. PANSS offers the possibility of efficient measurement of overall severity of illness and a reasonably adequate estimation of severity of the five major syndromes that occur within schizophrenia, but there are some problems with item composition.

Standardised diagnosis

The success of the ninth edition of the PSE demonstrates that the presence or absence of symptoms can be assessed reliably, and offers the foundation for diagnosis. PSE scores from either the eighth, ninth or tenth editions can be entered into a computer algorithm, CATEGO (Wing *et al*, 1974), together with data from a brief questionnaire designed to elicit possible aetiological factors, to yield a diagnosis which is relatively free of subjective bias. CATEGO employs a hierarchical strategy, such that the presence of features of schizophrenia leads to the assignment to the class schizophrenia despite the presence of features typical of other conditions. As well as giving a diagnostic class, the programme gives an index of severity in its 'Index of Definition', which has eight levels based on the number, type and severity of individual symptoms. Level 5 is the threshold for regarding a subject as a psychiatric case. Level 8 represents patients with most severe pathology (generally psychotic in-patients) while levels 1 to 4 represent milder degrees of disturbance such as might be found in a community survey. Although CATEGO provides a diagnostic class and a measure of severity that are relatively objective, it takes relatively little account of the time-course of illness. Many clinicians have been reluctant to assign the diagnosis of schizophrenia without evidence of a relatively sustained disorder affecting personal adjustment.

The inclusion of aspects of the time course of illness and personal adjustment, in addition to symptoms, within a set of operational criteria for the diagnosis of schizophrenia, was proposed by Feighner *et al* (1972) from St Louis, Missouri. The Feighner criteria specifically demand that the illness be chronic, lasting for at least six months without return to premorbid social adjustment. This particular criterion, subsequently adopted in DSM–III, shifted the definition of schizophrenia nearer to Kraepelin's original concept of dementia praecox. Spitzer *et al* (1975) developed a set of Research Diagnostic Criteria which attempted to steer a middle path by formulating criteria that demanded an illness of at least two weeks duration, to exclude brief situational psychoses, yet avoid limiting the diagnosis to chronic cases only. With the rapidly accumulating evidence that schizophrenia is associated with long-lasting abnormality of the brain, there is a developing consensus that schizophrenia is characterised by at least subtle disturbances of mental function persisting over a substantial period of time. A definitive conclusion regarding time course is unlikely until the pathophysiology of the condition has been established.

The Diagnostic and Statistical Manual of the APA

The third edition of the DSM (DSM–III), published in 1980, attempted to apply relatively rigorous criteria to diagnosis while taking account of a variety of clinical features in addition to psychiatric symptoms. It did this in two ways. Firstly, it introduced a multi-axial description of illness. Axis 1 deals with clinical syndromes; axis 2, personality disorders; axis 3, physical disorders and conditions; axis 4, severity of psychological stressors; axis 5, highest level of adaptive function in the preceding year. Secondly, axis 1 diagnosis is based on operational criteria which demand not only the presence of a specified number of items from a list of symptoms or signs considered characteristic of the illness, but also criteria concerning features such as duration of the illness, age at onset and absence of clinical features sufficient to justify certain alternative diagnoses.

In DSM–III, the first criterion for an Axis 1 diagnosis of schizophrenia was the presence of one of several possible combinations of characteristic symptoms, with greatest diagnostic weight afforded to bizarre delusions and Schneiderian auditory hallucinations. The other criteria included age of onset before 45 years, but this requirement was dropped from the revised third edition (APA, 1987). In DSM–IV (APA, 1994), the list of characteristic symptoms was simplified. Although bizarre delusions and Schneiderian auditory hallucinations still carried the greatest weight, negative symptoms were given increased emphasis. The DSM–IV criteria are summarised in Box 7.5.

DSM–IV defines various types of schizophrenia, but acknowledges that the presentation frequently includes symptoms characteristic of more than one type, and adopts a hierarchical approach to assigning type. The catatonic type (295.20) is assigned whenever prominent catatonic symptoms are present, regardless of the presence of other symptoms. Disorganised type (295.10) is assigned to cases with prominent disorganised speech and behaviour and flat or inappropriate affect, unless catatonia is also present. Paranoid type (295.30) is assigned whenever there is preoccupation with delusions or frequent auditory hallucinations, but there are no prominent features of either catatonia or disorganisation. Undifferentiated type (295.90) is assigned when the case does not satisfy criteria for catatonic, disorganised or paranoid type, despite satisfying the criteria for schizophrenia. Residual type (295.60) is assigned when there has been at least one episode of schizophrenia, and the current picture is dominated by either negative symptoms, or by several attenuated positive symptoms.

The diagnosis schizophreniform disorder (295.40) is assigned to cases in which an episode (including prodromal, active and residual phases) lasts at least one month but less than six months. The diagnosis of schizophreniform disorder does not require impaired social or occupational function, although it may occur. The diagnosis delusional disorder is assigned to cases in which there are non-bizarre delusions lasting at least one month but without other characteristic schizophrenic symptoms. The diagnosis schizoaffective disorder is assigned when a mood episode and characteristic schizophrenic symptoms occur together, but are either preceded or followed by at least two weeks of delusions or hallucinations without prominent mood symptoms.

Box 7.5 Summary of DSM–IV criteria for schizophrenia (APA, 1994)

Characteristic symptoms
Either one or more of the following:
(1) bizarre delusions (clearly implausible and non-under-standable delusions, including delusions of control over mind or body)
(2) hallucinations in the form of voices commenting or conversing
Or two or more of the following:
(1) other delusions
(2) other hallucinations occurring in a clear sensorium
(3) disorganised speech
(4) grossly disorganised or catatonic behaviour
(5) negative symptoms (i.e. affective flattening, alogia, avolition)
The required characteristic symptoms must be present for a significant proportion of time throughout a one month period, or less if successfully treated. The period during which the required characteristic symptoms are present is referred to as the active phase. In addition, there might be prodromal or residual phases during which there are either negative symptoms alone, or at least two attenuated characteristic symptoms.
Social/occupational dysfunction
For a significant proportion of the time since the onset of disturbance, at least one major area of functioning such as work, interpersonal relations, or self-care is markedly below that achieved before the onset, or there has been failure to achieve the expected level of interpersonal, academic or occupational achievement in cases with onset during childhood or adolescence.
Six month duration
Continuous signs of disturbance for at least six months, including an active phase of at least one month (or less if successfully treated).
Exclusion of affective or schizoaffective psychosis
Any episodes of mood disorder accompanying the active phase of characteristic symptoms must be brief in relation to the total duration of active and residual symptoms.
Exclusion of toxic substances or a general medical condition
The disturbance is not due to the direct physiological effects of a substance (drug of abuse or medication) or a general medical condition.
Relationship to pervasive developmental disorder
If there is a history of pervasive developmental disorder such as autistic disorder, schizophrenia can only be diagnosed if prominent delusions or hallucinations are present for at least one month (or less if successfully treated).

Box 7.6 Summary of ICD–10 criteria for schizophrenia

Either one or more of the following specific symptoms:
(1) Thought echo, insertion, withdrawal or broadcast.
(2) Delusions of control of the body, thoughts, actions, or sensations; delusional perception.
(3) Hallucinatory voices commenting or discussing, or coming from a part of the body.
(4) Persistent delusional beliefs that are completely impossible.

Or two or more of the following specific symptoms or signs:
(5) Other persistent hallucinations, if either occurring daily for many weeks, or accompanied by evidence of delusional thinking or sustained overvalued ideas.
(6) Formal thought disorder (incoherent or irrelevant speech, neologisms).
(7) Catatonic behaviour (excitement, posturing, waxy flexibility, negativism, mutism, stupor).
(8) Apathy, paucity of speech, flat or inappropriate affect, usually resulting in social impairment (but not due to neuroleptic medication or depression).

Or (for a diagnosis of simple schizophrenia only):
A consistent change in behaviour manifest as loss of interest, aimlessness, idleness, a self-absorbed attitude and social withdrawal over a period of at least one year.

Duration of symptoms
Symptoms or signs must be clearly present for most of the time for at least one month (and at least one year for a diagnosis of simple schizophrenia).

Exclusion of affective psychosis
If there are extensive manic or depressive symptoms, the schizophrenic symptoms must antedate the mood disturbance.

Exclusion of overt brain disease
Schizophrenia should not be diagnosed in the presence of overt brain disease or during states of drug intoxication or withdrawal.

The International Classification of Diseases

The ICD–10, compiled by the World Health Organization (1993), offers guidelines for diagnosis which are summarised in Box 7.6. The ICD code for schizophrenia is F20.xy where x denotes subtype and y denotes course of illness. In making the diagnosis, Schneiderian first rank symptoms and persistent 'impossible' delusions are given special weight, but other persistent hallucinations, formal thought disorders, catatonic behaviour, and negative symptoms such as apathy, poverty of speech or blunted affect, can contribute to the diagnosis. Significant consistent change in personal behaviour manifest as loss of interest, aimlessness, self-absorbed attitude or social withdrawal are taken into account in the diagnosis of simple schizophrenia.

The guidelines specify that specific symptoms be clearly present most of the time during a period of a month or more, but acknowledge that prodromal symptoms often precede the onset of specific symptoms. In the case of simple schizophrenia, a duration of at least one year is required. A diagnosis of schizophrenia should not be made in the presence of extensive depressive or manic symptoms, unless it is clear that schizophrenic symptoms antedated the affective disturbance. When schizophrenic and affective symptoms develop together and are evenly balanced, a diagnosis of schizoaffective disorder should be made. Disorders presenting with clinical features resembling schizophrenia but arising from overt brain disease are classified as organic disorders, and those occurring during drug intoxication or withdrawal are classified as drug-induced disorders, not schizophrenia. Delusional disorders, in which the delusions are neither Schneiderian nor bizarre, nor accompanied by other characteristic schizophrenic features such as hallucinations, are also classified separately from schizophrenia.

The four classic subtypes, paranoid, hebephrenic, catatonic and simple schizophrenia are recognised, but in addition, the category undifferentiated schizophrenia is introduced to accommodate cases not conforming to the definitions of the sub-types, or with mixed features without a clear preponderance of the features of any one sub-type. In addition, there are categories for post-schizophrenic depression and residual schizophrenia for cases which previously exhibited features sufficient to satisfy criteria for schizophrenia, but the clinical picture is currently dominated by either depression or long-term negative symptoms.

The course of illness is classified into six types: continuous, episodic with progressive deficit, episodic with stable deficit, episodic remittent, incomplete remission or complete remission. While ICD–10 clearly recognises the possibility of complete remission, the demand that specific symptoms be present for most of the time for at least one month, defines a concept of schizophrenia which excludes brief, transient psychoses. Illnesses which meet the symptomatic requirements but have a duration of less than one month are diagnosed as acute schizophrenia-like psychotic disorders.

The retention of simple schizophrenia is perhaps the most controversial aspect of the ICD–10 concept of schizophrenia. Simple schizophrenia is defined as an uncommon disorder in which there is an insidious but progressive development of oddities of conduct, inability to meet the demands of society and decline in total performance. The characteristic negative features of residual schizophrenia develop without being preceded by any overt psychotic symptoms. The criteria include a marked loss of interest, idleness, and social withdrawal over a period of at least one year. With increasing social impoverishment, the patient may drift into vagrancy.

While it is clearly important to avoid overuse of this category by including individuals who should simply be regarded as eccentric, a strong case can be made for regarding simple schizophrenia as closely related to other schizophrenic illnesses. First, overt schizophrenia is often preceded by a prolonged prodromal phase which can resemble simple schizophrenia. Furthermore, at least some cases satisfying criteria for simple schizophrenia would fall within the spectrum of disorders which are genetically related to overt schizophrenia (see below). It is very likely that the cerebral abnormalities that predispose to overt schizophrenia can also produce the clinical picture described by the ICD–10 definition of simple schizophrenia.

The boundaries of schizophrenia

The schizophrenia spectrum

Family studies reveal that there is a range of disorders that have an increased prevalence among the relatives of schizophrenic patients. These disorders include affective psychosis, depression, alcohol misuse and schizotypal personality disorder. It is likely that a heritable cerebral abnormality that plays a part in schizophrenia can contribute to the development of any disorder in this spectrum.

Relationship between schizophrenia and affective psychosis

The observation that depression and excitation occur in schizophrenia, while conversely, features of the three characteristic schizophrenic syndromes, reality distortion, disorganisation and psychomotor poverty, can occur in affective psychosis, suggests that there are common elements in the pathophysiology of these two psychotic conditions. Furthermore, the evidence from family studies indicating at least a degree of familial relationship between schizophrenia and affective illness is consistent with the proposal that there is a continuum of psychotic illnesses, extending from affective psychosis, through schizoaffective disorder to schizophrenia.

Nonetheless, if we follow Kahlbaum and Kraepelin and examine the overall picture of the illness, there can be little doubt that it is useful to distinguish between schizophrenia and affective psychosis. Although similar clusters of symptoms can occur in the two conditions, there are differences in both the cross-sectional and the longitudinal picture. As emphasised by both Kraepelin and Eugen Bleuler, in schizophrenia there is a lack of unity in the mental processes. For example, the delusions and hallucinations are less readily understood on the basis of the prevailing mood. Longitudinally, the impoverishment and fragmentation of mental activity are prone to persist even when the transient mood disturbance has abated.

When an illness presents features characteristic of both disorders, a diagnosis of schizophrenia should be made if the periods of marked depression or elation are brief in comparison with the total duration of discernable illness, whereas a diagnosis of affective psychosis should be made if depression or elation are prominent throughout the period of discernable illness. In the majority of cases, it is possible to distinguish between schizophrenia and affective psychosis on this basis. In a minority, the distinction cannot be made, and a diagnosis of schizoaffective psychosis is appropriate.

Schizophrenia and other organic psychoses

Brain imaging studies reveal that the association cortex of temporal, frontal and parietal lobes, and the related sub-cortical nuclei, are all implicated in the pathophysiology of the schizophrenia. The symptoms that occur in schizophrenia are the symptoms associated with disorder of the neural systems linking these brain areas (for a review, see Liddle, 1993). Many different diseases affecting these neural systems can produce symptoms similar to those of schizophrenia. This raises the question of whether or not schizophrenia is a specific disease that should be distinguished from other organic psychoses exhibiting similar symptoms, and has led some clinicians to question the logic of excluding organic psychosis before making a diagnosis of schizophrenia.

While there is little doubt that schizophrenia is an organic psychosis, the observation that many cases exhibit a characteristic episode time course beginning in early adult life suggests that schizophrenia is a distinct disorder that should be distinguished from other organic psychoses with similar symptoms. (This issue is discussed further in the next section.) However, until the pathophysiology of the condition is delineated, the principal basis for distinguishing schizophrenia from other organic psychoses will remain the exclusion of those organic conditions whose aetiology or pathophysiology are known. From a practical point of view, in the clinical assessment of a patient presenting the symptomatic picture of schizophrenia, it is necessary to carry out investigations to identify any other organic psychosis which might have a specific treatment. These investigations should include screening tests for the known infectious, metabolic, endocrine and neoplastic diseases that can affect the central nervous system.

What is the essence of schizophrenia?

As details of the neural basis of schizophrenia have begun to emerge, it is pertinent to seek to define the essence of schizophrenia. Which of the various clinical features that we have considered is likely to be most relevant to the identification of the essence of the condition? The overlap between the symptoms of schizophrenia and those of affective psychosis and other organic psychoses indicates that the cross-sectional clinical picture alone is not adequate to define a discrete disease. In general, symptoms reflect the neural systems involved rather than the specific disease process. Course of illness appears more specific, but which features of the course are most relevant? A degree of persistence is probably an essential feature of the condition, though the evidence from the long-term follow-up studies provides very little evidence of a tendency to life-long deterioration in mental function implied by the word 'dementia' in Kraepelin's term dementia praecox. In contrast, the tendency for the disease to become manifest early in adult life, indicated by the word 'praecox', has been repeatedly confirmed.

The characteristic form of the distribution of age of onset in men, with its peak in early adult life, is one of the strongest reasons for proposing that schizophrenia in men is a single disease (or group of closely related diseases). In women, the somewhat broader distribution of age of onset indicates either that female gender can exert a moderating influence on onset, or alternatively, that schizophrenia in women embraces several different diseases, including the early onset condition seen in men, and also other conditions with later onset.

Overall, the data on age of onset supports the proposal that the majority of cases currently diagnosed as schizophrenia (including virtually all male cases and a substantial proportion of female cases) represent a single type of disease with a characteristic tendency to have onset in early adult life. This proposal is in accord with recent neurobiological evidence, reviewed in other chapters of this book, suggesting that the essential feature of schizophrenia is disordered connections between association cortical areas and related subcortical nuclei, arising during intra-uterine development and becoming manifest after the highest functions of association cortex come into action in adolescence. Although this hypothesis requires further confirmation, the concept of a subtle disruption of the development of connections between cerebral areas provides a neuroscientific description of schizophrenia that might account for the fragmentation of mental activity implied in the clinical descriptions provided by Emil Kraepelin and Eugen Bleuler nearly a century ago.

References

American Psychiatric Association (1980) *Diagnostic and Statistical Manual of Mental Disorders* (3rd edn) (DSM–III). Washington, DC: APA.

—— (1987) *Diagnostic and Statistical Manual of Mental Disorders* (3rd edn, revised) (DSM–III–R). Washington, DC: APA.

—— (1994) *Diagnostic and Statistical Manual of Mental Disorders* (4th edn) (DSM–IV). Washington, DC: APA.

Andreasen, N. C. (1979) Thought, language and communication disorders. I Clinical assessment, definition of terms, and evaluation of their reliability. *Archives of General Psychiatry*, **36**, 1315–1321.

—— (1982) Negative symptoms in schizophrenia: definition and reliability. *Archives of General Psychiatry*, **39**, 784–788.

Arndt, S., Alliger, R. J. & Andreasen, N. C. (1991) The distinction of positive and negative symptoms: The failure of a two-dimensional model. *British Journal of Psychiatry*, **158**, 317–322.

Baddeley, A. (1992) Working memory. *Science*, **255**, 556–559.

Bleuler, E. (1911) Dementia praecox or the group of schizophrenias. (Trans. by J. Zinkin, 1950). New York: International Universities Press.

Bleuler, M. (1974) The long-term course of the schizophrenic psychoses. *Psychological Medicine*, **4**, 244–254.

Calev, A., Venables, P. H. & Monk, A. F. (1983) Evidence for distinct verbal memory pathologies in severely and mildly disturbed schizophrenics. *Schizophrenia Bulletin*, **9**, 247–263.

Ciompi, L. & Muller, C. (1976) Lebensweg und Alter der Schizophrenen: Eine karamnertische Langzeitstudie bis ins Senium. Berlin: Springer Verlag.

Crow, T. J. (1980) The molecular pathology of schizophrenia. *British Medical Journal*, **280**, 1–9.

Cooper, J. E., Kendall, R. E., Gurland, B. J., *et al* (1972) *Psychiatric Diagnosis in London and New York*. London: Oxford University Press.

Diem, O. (1903) Die einfach demente Form der Dementia Praecox. *Archiv fur Psychiatrie und Nervenkrankheiten*, **37**, 81–87.

Donlon, P. T., Rada R. T. & Arora, K. K. (1976) Depression and the reintegration phase of acute schizophrenia. *American Journal of Psychiatry*, **133**, 1265–1268.

Farran-Ridge, C. (1926) Some symptoms referable to the basal ganglia occurring in dementia praecox and epidemic encephalitis. *Journal of Mental Science*, **72**, 513–523.

Feighner, J. P., Robins, E., Guze, S. B., *et al* (1972) Diagnostic criteria for use in psychiatric research. *Archives of General Psychiatry*, **32**, 343–347.

Frith, C. D. (1992) *The Cognitive Neuropsychology of Schizophrenia*. Hove: Lawrence Erlbaum.

Goldberg, T. E., Torrey, E. F., Gold, J. M., *et al* (1992) Learning and memory in monozygotic twins discordant for schizophrenia. *Psychological Medicine*, **23**, 71–85.

Griesinger, W. (1861) *Die Pathologie und Therapie der Psychischen Krankheiten*. Stuttgart: Krabbe.

Harding, C. M., Brooks, G. W., Ashikaga, T., *et al* (1987) The Vermont longitudinal study of persons with severe mental illness. *American Journal of Psychiatry*, **144**, 727–734.

Haslam, J. (1809) *Observations on Madness and Melancholy* (2nd edn). London: Hayden.

Hecker, E. (1871) Die hebephrenie. *Virchows archiv fur pathologische anatomie und physiologie und klinische medizin*, **52**, 394–429.

Holzman, P. S., Shenton, M. E. & Solloway, M. R. (1986) Quality of thought disorder in differential diagnosis. *Schizophrenia Bulletin*, **12**, 360–371.

——, Kringlen, E. & Matthysse, S. (1988) A single dominant gene can account for eye tracking dysfunctions and schizophrenia in offspring of discordant twins. *Archives of General Psychiatry*, **45**, 641–647.

Huber, G. (1966) Reine Defectsyndrome und Basisstadien endogener Psychosen. *Fortschrift fur Neurologie und Psychiatrie*, **34**, 409–426.

——, Gross, G. & Schuttler, R. (1975) A long term follow-up study of schizophrenia: psychiatric course of illness and prognosis. *Acta Psychiatrica Scandinavica*, **52**, 49–57.

Kahlbaum, K. L. (1874) *Die Katatonie oder das Spannungsirrescien*. Berlin: Hirschwald.

Kay, S. R. (1991) *Positive and Negative Syndromes in Schizophrenia*. New York: Brunner/Mazel.

Klonoff, H., Fibiger, C. H. & Hutton, G. H. (1970) Neuropsychological patterns in chronic schizophrenia. *Journal of Nervous and Mental Disease*, **150**, 291–300.

Knights, A. & Hirsch, S. R. (1981) Revealed depression and drug treatment for schizophrenia. *Archives of General Psychiatry*, **38**, 806–811.

Kraepelin, E. (1896) Dementia Praecox. In *The Clinical Roots of the Schizophrenia Concept* (1987) (Trans. J. Cutting & M. Shepherd from *Lehrbuch der Psychiatrie*, pp. 426–441. Leipzig: Barth), pp. 15–24. Cambridge: Cambridge University Press.

—— (1919) *Dementia Praecox and Paraphrenia* (Trans. R. M. Barclay, ed. G. M. Robertson). Edinburgh: Churchill Livingstone.

—— (1920) Die Erscheinungsformen des Irresciens. (Trans. by H. Marshall (1974) as Patterns of Mental Disorder, in *Themes and Variations in European Psychiatry* (eds S. R. Hirsch & M. Shepherd). Bristol: Wright

Krawieka, M., Goldberg, D. & Vaughan, M. (1977) A standard psychiatric assessment for rating chronic psychotic patients. *Acta Psychiatrica Scandinavica*, **55**, 299–308.

Lewis, S. W. (1990) Computerised tomography in schizophrenia 15 years on. *British Journal of Psychiatry*, **157**, 16–24.

Levin, S. (1980) Frontal lobe dysfunction in schizophrenia 1. Eye movement impairments. *Journal of Psychiatric Research*, **18**, 27–55.

Liddle, P. F. (1987) The symptoms of chronic schizophrenia: a re-examination of the positive–negative dichotomy. *British Journal of Psychiatry*, **151**, 145–151.

—— (1993) The psychomotor disorders: disorders of the supervisory mental processes. *Behavioural Neurology*, **6**, 5–14.

—— & Crow, T. J. (1984) Age disorientation in chronic schizophrenia is associated with global intellectual impairment. *British Journal of Psychiatry*, **144**, 193–199.

——, Friston, K. J., Frith, C. D., *et al* (1992) Patterns of cerebral blood flow in schizophrenia. *British Journal of Psychiatry*, **160**, 179–186.

——, Barnes T. R. E., Speller J., *et al* (1993a) Negative symptoms as a risk factor for tardive dyskinesia in schizophrenia. *British Journal of Psychiatry*, **163**, 776–780.

——, Haque, S., Morris D. L., *et al* (1993*b*) Dyspraxia and agnosia in schizophrenia. *Behavioural Neurology*, **6**, 49–54.

Lieberman, J. A., Jody, D., Geisler, S., *et al* (1993) Time course and biologic correlates of treatment response in first-episode schizophrenia. *Archives of General Psychiatry*, **50**, 369–376.

Mellor, C. S. (1970) First rank symptoms of schizophrenia. *British Journal of Psychiatry*, **117**, 15–23.

Morel, B. A. (1860) *Traite des Maladie Mentales*. Paris: Masson.

O'Grady, J. C. (1990) The prevalence and diagnostic significance of Schneiderian first rank symptoms in a random sample of acute psychiatric patients. *British Journal of Psychiatry*, **156**, 496–500.

Overall, J. E. & Gorham, D. R. (1962) The brief psychiatric rating scale. *Psychological Reports*, **10**, 799–812.

Peralta, V., deLeon, J. & Cuesta, M. J. (1992) Are there more than two syndromes in schizophrenia? A critique of the positive–negative dichotomy. *British Journal of Psychiatry*, **161**, 335–343.

Rifkin, A., Quitkin, K. & Klein, D. F. (1975) Akinesia: a poorly recognised drug-induced extrapyramidal behavioral disorder. *Archives of General Psychiatry*, **32**, 672–674.

Schneider, K. (1959) *Clinical Psychopathology*. (Trans. M. W. Hamilton). New York: Grune Stratton.

Spitzer, R. L., Endicott, J., Robins, E., *et al* (1975) Preliminary report on the reliability of research diagnostic criteria applied to case records. In *Predictability in Psychopharmacology* (eds A. Sudilovsky, S. Gershon, & B. Beer). New York: Raven Press.

Watt, D. C., Katz, K. & Shepherd, M. (1983) The natural history of schizophrenia: a 5-year prospective follow-up of a representative sample of schizophrenics by means of a standardized clinical and social assessment. *Psychological Medicine*, **13**, 663–670.

Wing, J. K., Cooper, J. E. & Sartorius, N. (1974) *The Measurement and Classification of Psychiatric Symptoms*. London: Cambridge University Press

World Health Organization (1973) *The International Pilot Study of Schizophrenia*. Geneva: WHO.

—— (1993) *The Tenth Revision of the International Classification of Diseases* (ICD–10). Geneva: WHO.

8 The aetiology of schizophrenia

Tom Fahy, Peter Woodruff & George Szmukler

Epidemiology • Genetics • Neurochemistry • Neuropathology of schizophrenia • Neuroimaging • Neuropsychology • Developmental factors • Social factors • Life events • Family factors

---

Elucidating the cause of schizophrenia presents a classic set of methodological challenges to researchers; perhaps more daunting than for any other disorder in medicine. The first problem is case definition. Researchers have developed several detailed sets of operational criteria, but in the absence of pathognomonic biological markers, the validity of these diagnostic criteria is unproven. There may be several types of schizophrenia, and the complexity and heterogeneity of the disorder is likely to reflect multiple and interacting aetiological and pathoplastic influences.

Epidemiological research addresses some of these concerns by studying the pattern of morbidity on a broad canvas, examining the interacting and confounding relationships between biological and social factors. We begin this chapter with a review of the epidemiology of schizophrenia, before examining in detail the robust evidence in support of the genetic contribution to aetiology. A large amount of circumstantial evidence points to neurochemical disturbance in schizophrenia, and although this area of research is bedevilled by methodological problems, this work has increased our understanding of neuroleptic drugs, leading to the most effective anti-psychotic treatment. Structural brain imaging provides direct evidence of brain abnormalities in schizophrenia. The importance of social and neuropsychological factors in the onset, phenomenology and course of schizophrenia is also reviewed, reflecting the increasing interest in non-pharmacological treatments.

Although the format of this chapter follows a traditional structure in placing the results of research under separate disciplinary headings, the most striking trend is towards interdisciplinary research, which combines perspectives and methods from different approaches, for example epidemiology and genetics, functional neuroimaging and neuropsychology. This combined approach holds the promise of greater success in unravelling the complexities of schizophrenia.

Epidemiology

Epidemiology is undergoing something of a renaissance in the area of schizophrenia research. This is in part due to improved methodology, particularly in terms of diagnostic uniformity which allows comparison across studies. What is perhaps more important, however, is the realisation that epidemiological findings can be integrated with data from other areas of schizophrenia research (phenomenology, psychology, genetics, neuroimaging) to provide clues to the aetiology of the condition. This section deals briefly with methodological problems in epidemiological research in schizophrenia; an overview of 'classic' epidemiological findings is provided; and finally some currently controversial areas of schizophrenia research are addressed.

Problems in schizophrenia epidemiology research

One of the problems of much early research in schizophrenia was a lack of diagnostic uniformity, which made comparison between studies almost impossible. For example, the diagnosis of schizophrenia was much more loosely applied in the US than the UK, leading to the quip that the easiest cure for the disease was a trans-Atlantic flight. Indeed, the US/UK diagnostic project (Cooper *et al*, 1972) investigated rates of schizophrenia and manic depression in the two countries using standardised criteria, and concluded that most of the previously reported difference in rates was due to variations in diagnostic practice. Lately, the advent of operationalised criteria for schizophrenia (e.g. Feighner criteria, RDC, DSM–IV) and standardised interviews (e.g. PSE, SADS, SAPS, SANS) have resulted in far more consistency in schizophrenia research in general. However, one difficulty with reliance on operationalised criteria is that, while showing good reliability, they are not necessarily valid, and their continued widespread use might result in the tacit acceptance that they are. Also, different sets of criteria emphasise different aspects of the illness (for example, two weeks duration in RDC versus six months in DSM–III–R; early onset of illness and family history of schizophrenia in Feighner's criteria), and this needs to be taken into account when conclusions are drawn.

The second major problem area in epidemiological investigations of schizophrenia is that of case-finding. Most studies have been based on hospital admissions, which are themselves subject to variations in service provision and admission policies. Reliance on admission statistics alone leads to bias from the inclusion of re-admissions. For example, more severely affected patients are more likely to be re-admitted, confounding work in such areas as gender differences, as males tend to have a more severe form of illness, resulting in an exaggerated male : female ratio in hospitalised samples. The inclusion of only first admissions is methodologically more sound, but biases still arise. For example, more severely affected patients are more likely to be admitted, as are those with a history of violence or disturbed behaviour.

Case registers, which record all first contacts with the psychiatric services for a specified area over a specified time-period, are a very useful resource, particularly for the determination of incidence rates for severe mental illness. However, while it might be anticipated that, in a country like England, most patients with a severe mental illness such as schizophrenia will eventually have contact with the psychiatric services, no such assumption can be made about countries with less well developed health services. There is an added problem in countries where a substantial proportion of psychiatric practice is in the private sector. Thus, thorough case-finding can be assured only by covering all caring agencies, or by doing population screens. An example of the former strategy was that employed by the World Health Organization Collaborative Study (Sartorius *et al*, 1986), which ascertained all psychiatric contacts with any caring agency in sites in ten countries. The five-centre Epidemiological Catchment Area Survey (ECA) in the US (see Keith *et al*, 1991) is an example of population screening. These studies require enormous financial and organisational input. Also, diagnostic issues remain troublesome. Thus, while the WHO study used the PSE administered by trained psychiatrists, the ECA resorted to lay interviewers using the Diagnostic Interview Schedule, which has been shown to be over-inclusive with respect to schizophrenia.

Prevalence and incidence

Prevalence and incidence studies of schizophrenia have been usefully reviewed by Eaton (1985; 1991). He found point prevalence rates ranging from 0.6 per 1000 in Ghana to 8.3 per 1000 in Ireland. Annual incidence rates showed less variation, with the lowest rate recorded in Salford, England (11 per 100 000), and the highest in Maryland, US (70 per 100 000). UK rates were uniformly lower than those in the US, reflecting the differences in diagnostic stringency. However rates did not differ by more than a factor of two.

The conclusion of many authors on reviewing incidence studies in schizophrenia is that the disease is fairly evenly distributed around the globe. Indeed, the WHO Collaborative Study (Sartorius *et al*, 1986), which specifically set out to ascertain incidence rates for schizophrenia in rural and urban settings, in developed and developing countries, concluded that "schizophrenic illnesses occur with comparable frequency in different populations". However, the reported annual incidence rates even for 'core' schizophrenia range from 7 per 100 000 in Aarhus, Denmark, to 14 per 100 000 in Nottingham, England, and the presentation and outcome of the illness differs between developed and developing countries. Furthermore, there are a number of areas which show much higher than expected rates of schizophrenia (extreme Northern Sweden, North-West Yugoslavia, Tamils in South India), while low rates have been found in Hutterites in the US (but not in Canada). Claims of high rates in Western Ireland have not been consistent, but of particular interest is a study of the prevalence of schizophrenia in 36 electoral divisions in rural Ireland which found a number of "high-prevalence pockets", implying "geographical variation in environmental or genetic factor(s) of aetiological relevance" (Youssef *et al*, 1991).

Geographical and social drift

An issue which is not addressed in the foregoing studies is the higher rates of schizophrenia in deprived inner-city areas. The pioneering study by Faris & Dunham (1939) in Chicago reported that prevalence rates for schizophrenia decreased in a zonal pattern from the city centre. Subsequently, Hare (1956), in Bristol, found higher rates of schizophrenia in areas where a high proportion of people were living alone. The clustering of patients with schizophrenia in deprived inner-city areas has been confirmed in more recent studies (e.g. Ineichen *et al*, 1984; Giggs & Cooper, 1987).

A related consideration is the reported excess of schizophrenic individuals in lower socioeconomic groups (for example, Redlich *et al*, 1953; Hollingshead & Redlich, 1954; Silverton & Mednick, 1984). Goldberg & Morrison (1963), in a widely cited study, claimed that although patients with schizophrenia were more likely than controls to be categorised as social class V, their fathers showed the same social class distribution as the general population.

Such data have led to a general conclusion that patients with schizophrenia 'drift' down the social stratum as a result of their illness or its prodrome, and that this also accounts for the high rates of schizophrenia in deprived inner city areas. More recently, however, there has been a renewal of interest in an alternative to the 'drift' hypothesis, namely that early environmental influences are of aetiological importance in schizophrenia. It is now widely accepted that at least some patients with schizophrenia have an illness consequent upon some subtle damage to the developing brain; such damage might be genetically or environmentally mediated (Jones & Murray, 1991). The 'environmental' factors which have attracted most attention have been obstetric complications (Lewis & Murray, 1987) and head injury or intrauterine infection. Such factors might be expected to be more common in deprived, overcrowded inner-city areas.

Support for this view comes from two sets of studies. First are studies suggesting that patients with schizophrenia are more likely than controls to have been born in cities. For example, in a Norwegian study, Astrup & Odegaard (1961) found higher rates of schizophrenia among those born in cities, and, while migrants generally showed lower rates, migrants from cities had higher rates than those from rural areas. Machon *et al* (1983) found that an excess of individuals who later manifested schizophrenia had been born in urban areas. In England and Wales, Takei *et al* (1992) found patients with schizophrenia to be significantly more likely than other psychiatric patients to have been born in cities, while Lewis *et al* (1992), using Swedish data, found that patients with schizophrenia were particularly likely to have been brought up in urban centres. Similarly, Castle *et al* (1993) found that, compared with non-psychotic controls, patients with schizophrenia were more likely to have been born into socially deprived households in inner London.

The second group of studies are those which challenge the conventional wisdom, based largely on the study of Goldberg & Morrison (1963; see above), that fathers of patients with schizophrenia have the same occupational distribution as the general population. For example, the work of Hollingshead & Redlich (1954) suggests that the fathers of schizophrenics were themselves from lower socioeconomic backgrounds, while Turner & Wagenfeld (1967) reported fathers of schizophrenics to be over-represented in the lower socioeconomic groups. In reviewing these studies, Kohn (1975) concluded that:

> "The weight of evidence lies against the drift hypothesis providing a sufficient explanation of the class-schizophrenia relationship. In all probability, lower class families produce a disproportionate number of patients with schizophrenia".

Immigration and ethnicity

Studies from a number of different countries have shown that immigrants tend to have a higher risk of schizophrenia than the general population of either their native or adopted country. For example, Odegaard (1932) showed Norwegian immigrants to Minnesota had higher rates than natives of Minnesota, while Malzberg & Lee (1956) found immigrants in New York to have higher rates than those born in New York. Harrison (1991) has recently reviewed studies of rates of schizophrenia in immigrants to the UK: Afro-Caribbean immigrants show rates of schizophrenia well above those of the indigenous population. Some authors have tried to explain these findings on methodological grounds. For example, most studies have been based on hospitalised samples, which might well show admission bias with regard to ethnic minorities. Help-seeking behaviour is also known to differ between different ethnic groups. Erroneous diagnosis by doctors who understand neither the culture nor the language of the immigrants has also been suggested. Littlewood & Lipsedge (1981) found that Afro-Caribbean immigrants to the UK more commonly had a short-lived illness characterised by paranoid and religious ideation, and suggested that in many cases the diagnosis of an acute psychotic reaction would be more appropriate.

Two sets of UK studies have tried to control for such biases. In Nottingham, Harrison *et al* (1988) performed a prospective study, using standardised PSE criteria, and found that both Caribbean-born and UK-born Afro-Caribbeans showed greatly elevated rates of schizophrenia. In a case register study in London, Castle *et al* (1991) showed a similar effect which was robust even when stringent diagnostic criteria were employed; a case-control study of the same cohort (Wessely *et al*, 1991) found that the risk of schizophrenia was greater in ethnic Afro-Caribbeans, irrespective of age, gender, or place of birth.

What is the explanation for such findings? There is no good evidence to support the contention that rates of schizophrenia in the Caribbean are particularly high, and selective migration of vulnerable individuals is unlikely. Migration itself is stressful, but it is not established that stress alone can cause schizophrenia, in any event, there is often a lag of many years between migration and onset of psychosis, and 'migration stress' cannot explain the high rates in UK-born (second generation) Afro-Caribbeans. It seems more plausible that at least part of the explanation lies in the fact that black people in the UK experience a range of social adversity, and that social adversity and schizophrenia go hand-in-glove. Indeed, controlling for socioeconomic status has been shown to account for much of the ethnic effect in schizophrenia (Boddington, 1992). A related explanation for the second generation effect is that mothers born in the Caribbean might not have been exposed to a number of viruses which are endemic in the UK, and exposure to such 'novel' viruses during pregnancy might result in damage to the developing brain of the foetus, leaving it vulnerable to later schizophrenia (see below).

Trends over time

Changes in the incidence of a disease over time can afford useful insights into the aetiology of the condition. It has been suggested that schizophrenia was virtually unknown before the industrial revolution and urbanisation. More recently, reports from a number of Western countries have suggested that there has been a decline in the treated incidence of schizophrenia in recent decades (see Der *et al*, 1990), but there are a number of potential biases that need to be taken into account in interpreting the results. Firstly, it is clear that the advent of operational definitions of schizophrenia may have altered clinicians' concept of the disease, possibly resulting in more reluctance in applying this label. However, Der *et al* (1990) found no reciprocal increase in the rate of other psychiatric disorders in their study, suggesting that the effect was not merely due to changes in diagnostic habit; a similar finding has been reported in a case register study in Oxfordshire (de Alarcon *et al*, 1990).

Secondly, it might be that changes in admission policies over the years could be a bias in those studies which have relied on first admission data. Certainly, there is a trend in most Western countries towards more community care for patients with mental disorders. However, two UK case register studies which included all first contacts with the psychiatric services in Aberdeenshire (Eagles *et al*, 1988) and Oxfordshire (de Alarcon *et al*, 1990), also found a decline in the incidence of schizophrenia. Such a decline could not have been a result of changes in numbers of psychiatric beds or of changing admission policies.

Season of birth

There is a substantial literature (reviewed by Bradbury & Miller, 1985) which shows that people with schizophrenia are more likely than the general population to be born in winter or early spring (the size of the effect is of the order of 5–10%). The excess of winter/spring births in schizophrenia suggests either that parents of schizophrenics have a conception pattern which differs from the normal population, or that it is due to some environmental agent which is aetiologically important in schizophrenia and which shows a seasonal variation in prevalence. The former hypothesis implies that siblings of schizophrenics would also show the season-of-birth effect, and this has not been convincingly demonstrated. The latter explanation implies that those schizophrenics born in winter/spring should have a lower familial loading for schizophrenia, compared with those born at other times; data on this issue are conflicting (for example, O'Callaghan *et al*, 1991a; Pulver *et al*, 1991). Some of the difficulty with the seasonality/family history dichotomy probably lies in too narrow a conception of genetic versus environmental influences in schizophrenia. Thus, it is quite plausible that in many individuals liability to the illness is determined by both genetic and environmental factors, and that a seasonal factor would act to 'produce' schizophrenia only in those individuals with some inherent (genetic) liability.

Viruses and schizophrenia

The winter–birth effect in schizophrenia could be due to some seasonal environmental agent, probably a neuropathogen, acting on the developing foetus and playing a critical role in the causation of the illness in some individuals. Attempts to find such a pathogen have focused mainly on the influenza viruses. Thus, Mednick *et al* (1988) in Finland, reported that individuals *in utero* (2nd trimester) during the 1957 influenza epidemic had a higher than expected risk of subsequent schizophrenia. Attempts to replicate this finding have not been conclusive. Kendell & Kemp (1989) in Scotland and Bowler & Torrey (1990) in the USA failed to do so. However, a re-analysis of Kendell & Kemp's data by Mednick *et al* (1990) suggested a significantly increased rate of subsequent schizophrenia in females, and O'Callaghan *et al* (1991*b*), using data from England and Wales, showed that foetuses in the fifth month of gestation during the epidemic had an 88% increased risk of later developing schizophrenia; again, the effect was confined to females. In a cohort study of children born in England, Scotland and Wales in the week 3–9 March 1958, Crow *et al* (1991) found no evidence that children of mothers who reported having had influenza during their pregnancies had any higher than expected risk of subsequent schizophrenia. Of course the cohort study has the most powerful design, but there are flaws which make it less than definitive: for example, reported rates of psychiatric illness were rather low, as were reported rates of influenza, suggesting a possible recollection bias in the mothers.

If there is indeed a 'schizophrenic effect' for the 1957 influenza epidemic, does influenza play a role in the aetiology of schizophrenia in individuals born at other times? Barr *et al* (1990) in Denmark, and Sham *et al* (1992) in England, studied the relationship between influenza and schizophrenia over a number of decades. Both studies found a correlation between rates of influenza at the time mothers were in the mid trimester of pregnancy, and rates of subsequent schizophrenic births. Sham and colleagues concluded that "maternal viral infection is an important cause of schizophrenia". While such a statement is compelling, blind acceptance would be premature before further confirmatory studies. It is also important to remember that any viral effect can account for only a small minority of patients with schizophrenia, and that most women who have a viral infection in pregnancy do not have children with any increased risk of schizophrenia.

Gender

The most robust finding regarding gender differences in schizophrenia is that females have a later onset of illness than males; the difference is usually of the order of five years (see Lewine, 1988). The effect is not due to differences in help-seeking behaviour between male and female patients with schizophrenia and their families, or differences in role-expectation (see Castle & Murray, 1991). Some data suggest that males are more prone to schizophrenia, but findings are inconclusive. What is clear, however, is that the age-at-onset distribution curves for males and females are very different. It is thus difficult to conceive of the male:female difference in age at onset being due entirely to factors which either precipitate the illness earlier in males (e.g. androgens), or serve to delay the onset in females (e.g. oestrogens, which are known to be dopamine antagonists). It has been argued that a more plausible explanation for gender differences in schizophrenia is that males and females are differentially prone to different aetiological subtypes of the illness (Castle & Murray, 1991; Murray *et al*, 1992). The subtype with most empirical support is an early 'dementia praecox' type associated with poor premorbid adjustment, low premorbid IQ, negative symptoms, poor outcome, and an excess of structural brain abnormalities; males are particularly prone to this subtype. The potential importance of sex differences in enhancing our understanding of aetiological factors in schizophrenia is now being recognised, and further research in this area is eagerly awaited.

Genetics

Family studies

The general design of family studies is to compare the incidence of a disorder in relatives of affected probands to the incidence in relatives of control probands (case–control study), or in the general population. Because schizophrenia has a variable age of onset, subjects who are included in a family study at a young age still have a chance of becoming ill in later life. To allow for this, and for different age distributions within families, family studies use a special type of incidence figure called the morbid risk (MR). This provides an estimate of the proportion of individuals who would eventually go on to develop the disorder if they were followed through the entire risk period.

Family studies of schizophrenia have repeatedly shown that the risk for schizophrenia in the close relatives of affected individuals exceeds the expected risk in the general population (1%) by 5 to 15 times (Kendler, 1988). Pooling data from several family studies, Gottesman & Shields (1982) calculated that the morbid risk for conservatively defined schizophrenia in second and first degree relatives of index cases was 3% and 10% respectively, and that this rose to 40% in those with two affected parents. The tendency for morbid risk figures to vary between studies is likely to reflect differences in the methods of selecting cases and collecting information, or the use of different diagnostic criteria. Thus, studies employing relatively broad definitions of schizophrenia will pick up more cases amongst relatives than those using narrow criteria. Likewise, more cases will be detected if psycho-pathology in relatives is determined by direct assessment (family study method) rather than by informant history (family history method) (Andreasen *et al*, 1977). Greater familial loading might also be observed if studies select index cases from specialised clinics (rather than from population samples) where the severity of illness may be greater, or where the disorder in a parent or sibling may have influenced the referral of the proband.

While the results of family studies of schizophrenia are certainly compatible with a genetic hypothesis of aetiology, familial clustering of cases could also result from common exposure to some 'schizophrenogenic' agent, such as a virus (Crow, 1983). Alternatively, psychosocial stressors may load in families as a result of cultural transmission (learnt behaviour) or because people tend to shape their own environments, partly as a result of genetic influences (Rutter *et al*, 1990). To disentangle the effects of genes and environment it is necessary to turn to the findings of twin and adoption studies.

Twin studies

Twin data can help differentiate between genetic and environmental influences. The most common strategy is to compare concordance rates between monozygotic (MZ) and same-sex dizygotic (DZ) twin pairs. Because monozygotic and dizygotic twins are assumed to share environmental factors to approximately the same extent, differences in concordance between the two types of twin are considered a reflection of genetic influences.

Concordance rates are described either as pairwise, which indicate the proportion of twin pairs in which both twins are ill, or as probandwise, which indicate the proportion of twin probands with an ill co-twin. Probandwise concordance tends to be higher than pairwise concordance because the same twin pair will be counted more than once if the co-twins are independently ascertained. For most studies, probandwise measures are more methodologically correct. Twin studies of schizophrenia reveal probandwise concordance rates ranging from 8% to 28% in same-sex DZ twins, and from 33% to 78% in MZ twins (Kendler, 1983). Pooling data from more recent studies, Gottesman & Shields (1982) calculated an overall probandwise concordance of 14% for same-sex DZ twins, in contrast to 40% for MZ twins. While these results provide convincing evidence of a genetic component in the aetiology of schizophrenia, lack of 100% concordance between MZ twins suggests that non-genetic factors must also operate. Thus, a measure of heritability is calculated. This provides a single estimate of the degree to which genetic factors (as opposed to environmental factors) contribute to the aetiology of the disorder. It is calculated from twin concordance data based on methods developed by Falconer (1965) and Smith (1974). One estimate of the heritability of schizophrenia (based on data from nine twin studies) indicates that approximately 68% of the variance in liability to disorder is due to (additive) genetic factors (Kendler, 1983).

The problems of twin studies have been well described (Gottesman & Shields, 1982; Rutter *et al*, 1990). Most criticism has been directed at the assumption that social and family environmental effects are similar for MZ and DZ twins. However, a number of studies suggest that MZ twins are exposed to a more similar environment than are DZ twins. In particular, they are more likely to be treated alike by their parents. This has led to suggestions that environmental similarities, and not genetic similarities, are the basis of higher levels of concordance in MZ twins. Against this, however, is evidence that parents may respond to, rather than create, similarities between twins (Scarr & Carter-Salzman, 1979).

Questions have also been raised about the applicability of twin data to non-twin populations (Tsuang & Farrone, 1990). Generalisations might not be appropriate if biological or psychosocial factors associated with twinning are of aetiological importance in schizophrenia. For example, it has been suggested that birth complications may have neurological sequelae which lead to schizophrenia in later life (Owen *et al*, 1988). As twins have a greater risk of pre- and perinatal complications than singletons, the role of these environmental factors may be exaggerated in twin studies. It has also been suggested that the unusual experience of being a twin might influence personality development in a way that creates greater susceptibility to psychiatric illness. If either of these hypotheses were true, twins would be expected to have higher rates of schizophrenia than the general population. However, existing data indicate that twins are no more likely than singletons to develop schizophrenia (Kringlen, 1967; Gottesman & Shields, 1982).

Finally, the interpretation of twin data might also be complicated by factors, such as the twin transfusion syndrome, which differentially affects MZ and DZ twins (Kendler, 1983). The twin transfusion syndrome occurs in about 15% of monochorionic (and therefore monozygotic) twins and is the result of blood being transferred from one twin to another via placental anastomoses. This can lead to marked disparity in foetal growth and intra-pair discrepancies in birth weight (MacGillivray *et al*, 1988). Because there is an association between schizophrenia and low birth weight (Lane & Albee, 1966; Woerner *et al*, 1971), it has been proposed that the twin transfusion syndrome might, in some cases, be responsible for discordance in MZ twins. This view is supported by reports that the schizophrenic twins of discordant MZ pairs are more likely to have been of low birth weight than their well co-twins (Gottesman & Shields, 1982). As the twin transfusion syndrome only occurs in MZ twins, its potential effect on twin studies will be to underestimate the role of genetic factors.

Adoption studies

Children who are adopted away at birth (adoptees) receive their genes from their biological parents but their rearing environment from their adoptive parents. This means that any similarities between the child and his biological family will be a consequence of having genes in common, whereas any resemblance between the child and his adoptive family will be the result of sharing the same family environment.

In adoptees' studies, the prevalence of the disorder in adopted offspring of affected parents is compared with the prevalence in control adoptees (i.e. the adopted offspring of unaffected parents). In the first adoption study of schizophrenia, Heston (1966) studied 47 adoptees born to schizophrenic mothers and 50 control adoptees. He reported rates of schizophrenia in the index group which were significantly higher (age-corrected rate of 16.4%) when compared with the control group, and which were comparable to rates predicted by family studies. Interestingly, he also reported that non-schizophrenic index adoptees were more likely than the control group to suffer from neurotic and sociopathic disorders. Subsequent adoptees' studies confirmed these findings (e.g. Rosenthal *et al*, 1971) but, along with Heston's study, have been criticised on various methodological grounds (Tienari *et al*, 1992). These issues have been largely addressed in a nationwide Finnish study which is still in progress (Tienari, 1992). Preliminary data on 124 index adoptees and 147 control adoptees indicate higher rates of schizophrenia in the index cases (7.3% *v.* 1.4%) (Tienari *et al*, 1987).

Other studies have used the adoptees' family method rather than the adoptees' study method. In other words, investigators first identified adoptees with schizophrenia and then assessed their biological and adoptive relatives for evidence of psychopathology. Using this design, Kety and his colleagues (1968) assessed the psychiatric status of the biological and adoptive parents of 33 schizophrenic adoptees and demonstrated significantly higher rates of schizophrenia and schizophrenia-related disorders in the biological relatives. In a later study, Wender *et al* (1968) compared rates of psychiatric illness in the biological and adoptive parents of 20 schizophrenic and 10 control adoptees. The biological relatives of the schizophrenic group were significantly more disturbed than either the adoptive or the control parent group. However, the adopting parents of schizophrenics showed slightly higher rates of psycho-pathology than the adopting parents of normals (Tienari, 1992). The same investigators (Wender *et al*, 1974) also examined the effect of a "schizophrenia rearing environment" by studying adoptees whose birth parents were not affected but whose adoptive parents were schizophrenic (cross-fostering study). Index adoptees did not differ from control adoptees, indicating that being reared by a schizophrenic parent is not sufficient to produce schizophrenia.

While adoption studies provide a powerful strategy for separating genetic and environmental influences, there are limitations to the method

(Rutter *et al*, 1990; Tienari, 1992). Firstly, an adoptee's environment before and during birth is provided by his biological, not his adoptive mother, and so a complete dichotomy of genetic and environmental influences is not possible. If schizophrenia in an adoptee is the result of some pre- or perinatal event this would be attributed, misleadingly, to genetic factors. A useful way of circumventing this problem is to study adopted half-siblings of schizophrenic fathers. For example, Kety *et al* (1975) diagnosed schizophrenia in 13% of the paternal half-siblings of schizophrenic adoptees, but in only 2% of control half-siblings. Taken with other adoption data, this favours a genetic rather than an obstetric aetiology.

Another factor which might complicate adoption studies is the tendency for adoption agencies to match, as closely as possible, biological and adoptive families (selective placement) (Bohman & Sigvardsson, 1980). A potential effect of selective placement is to make the adoptive and biological family environments more similar and thereby increase correlation for environmental effects which may be of aetiological importance. Thus, any deductions about genetic versus environmental causation will be confounded.

Mode of transmission

The genetic transmission of Mendelian disorders such as Huntington's disease (autosomal dominant), cystic fibrosis (autosomal recessive) or Duchenne's muscular dystrophy (X-linked recessive) is relatively easy to establish from family data. The transmission of other disorders may resemble classical Mendelian inheritance but deviate slightly. Thus, some individuals may possess the disease genotype but fail to manifest the disorder (reduced penetrance) whereas others may express the disorder in a modified form (variable expression). For some conditions, including schizophrenia, a genetic component is established but patterns of familial aggregation bear no resemblance to Mendelian inheritance. One reason might be that genetic susceptibility to these disorders is not conferred by single genes but rather by a small number of major genes (an oligogenic model), or by many genes of small and additive effect (polygenic model). Inheritance patterns might also be obscured by factors such as variable age of onset, reduced penetrance, non-genetic cases (phenocopies), genetic and aetiological heterogeneity, unclear phenotypic boundaries, and environmental influences.

In an effort to define the genetic transmission of these so-called 'complex genetic disorders', quantitative geneticists have put forward a number of hypothetical models. These mathematical models can be tested using morbid risk figures obtained from family studies (prevalence analysis) or information on the patterns of disease segregation within a defined set of families (segregation analysis).

Many of these models incorporate a liability-threshold construct (Falconer, 1965). 'Liability' is considered to be a continuously distributed variable in the general population which is determined both by genes and environmental factors (acting in a predominantly additive fashion) such that only those individuals whose liability exceeds a critical threshold develop the disorder (McGuffin *et al*, 1987). By specifying more than one threshold, models can be further extended to allow for different clinical forms of the disorder (Reich *et al*, 1975). Models which have been applied to schizophrenia include the generalised single locus model (GSL) in which genetic liability is endowed by a single major gene, and the multifactorial threshold model (MFT) in which liability is determined by many genes of small effect (polygenes) together with environmental factors. These models are not mutually exclusive and a 'mixed' model has also been proposed in which both major genes and polygenes operate.

Because the basic GSL model predicts mendelian segregation within families, investigators have modified the model when applying it to schizophrenia (Faraone & Tsuang, 1985). These refinements vary between studies but most allow for reduced penetrance and for the existence of sporadics (non-genetic cases). Although some studies have found the GSL model to be broadly compatible with schizophrenia family data, nearly all have observed an underprediction of MZ twin concordance (e.g. Elston & Campbell, 1970; Mathysse & Kidd, 1976). Others have been able to reject the model outright (for example, O'Rourke *et al*, 1982; McGue *et al*, 1985). Thus, the overall weight of evidence is against a single gene effect in which schizophrenia is viewed as a single homogeneous disorder (McGue & Gottesman, 1990). However, if schizophrenia is aetiologically heterogeneous, then the possibility of a single gene subtype still exists.

In contrast to the GSL model, the predictions of the MFT model appear to fit the observed patterns of familial aggregation of schizophrenia (Gottesman & Shields, 1967; McGue & Gottesman, 1990). Moreover, there are other data to support this model. For example, the risk of schizophrenia in relatives increases as a function of the number of affected individuals in the family. It also increases as a function of severity of illness in the proband. 'Mixed' models, which include both single major gene and polygenic effects have also been tested, but investigators have not been able to reject an MFT model in favour of a mixed model. This may be because there is not a single gene effect to be detected, or alternatively, it may reflect inadequate statistical power in these studies (McGue & Gottesman, 1990). It can be concluded that the genetic transmission of schizophrenia is still unclear and single gene effects, multifactorial transmission and aetiological heterogeneity remain contending possibilities.

Localising genetic defects

Once a genetic contribution to a disorder has been established, a natural progression is to try to localise a specific disease gene. If something is known about a gene product, then it may be possible to map the gene to its position on the chromosomes using molecular genetic techniques such as *in situ* hybridisation (Hindley, 1983) or somatic cell hybridisation (Puck & Kao, 1982). This process of localising genes on the basis of their protein products is sometimes referred to as 'forward genetics'. For some disorders, such as schizophrenia, we have no knowledge of specific gene products and, indeed, know hardly anything of the pathway leading from the disease gene to its clinical manifestation. In these circumstances, genetic linkage studies enable us to locate the disease gene, in the first instance, and then later define its protein product. This approach is known as 'reverse genetics'.

Genetic markers

Genetic linkage refers to the tendency for two genetic traits to be inherited together rather than independently. This will occur if the genetic loci for these traits are situated so close to each other on the chromosomes that recombination (crossing-over) during meiosis is unlikely. Genetic 'markers' correspond to gene loci of known chromosomal location. These are stable, easily detectable, polymorphic (exist in more than one form) traits which are inherited in a simple Mendelian manner. Alternate forms (polymorphisms) of the same genetic marker are called alleles. By demonstrating that a disorder is inherited along with a particular marker allele (i.e. the disease and marker are 'linked') it is possible to infer the position of a disease gene.

Early genetic markers included human leukocyte antigens, ABO blood types, red cell enzymes and certain protein polymorphisms (Owen & McGuffin, 1991). Taken together, these 'classic'" markers only provide information on a small fraction of the entire genome and so, a spectacular advance in the last decade has been the development of DNA markers (see Wetherall, 1992). These are sequences of DNA which are inherited in a Mendelian manner and which show considerable variation between individuals (i.e. are highly polymorphic). One type of marker is identified by means of enzymes (restriction endonucleases) which cleave DNA at specific (restriction) sites. A variation in DNA sequence may result in the creation or the elimination of one of these enzyme recognition sites and so DNA fragments of different lengths will be obtained. These are called restriction fragment length polymorphisms (RFLPs) and can be used as genetic markers to follow inherited variation in DNA sequences at different chromosomal locations.

Genetic linkage studies

The first step in a genetic linkage study is to collect families in which several members are affected with the disorder (multiplex families). Next, it is necessary to decide on a chromosomal region to study. A specific region might be indicated if it is known that particular genes (of known chromosomal location and for which markers are available) are likely to be involved in the pathological process of the disorder. These are known as 'candidate genes' and, for schizophrenia, might include those involved in monoamine pathways, such as the dopamine receptor genes or genes encoding enzymes like tyrosine hydroxylase. In the absence of candidate loci, the remaining strategy is to 'scan the genome' by systematically examining large numbers of anonymous DNA markers mapped to different chromosomes. This is how the gene responsible for Huntingdon's disease was localised to chromosome 4, and the gene for cystic fibrosis was mapped to chromosome 7.

Once a particular chromosomal region has been targeted, the next step is to trace the inheritance of genetic markers from this region through multiply affected families. If linkage is present, then one form (allele) of the marker will appear to be inherited along with the disorder. However, such co-segregation could also occur by chance and in order to ensure that this is not the case a statistical analysis is required. The most common approach is to perform a log of the likelihood ratio (LOD) score analysis. This initially involves calculating an odds ratio: the odds of the observed pattern of co-segregation (between marker and disease) occurring if the marker and the disorder are linked, over the odds of the same co-segregation occurring if the marker and the disorder are unlinked. The LOD score is this odds ratio expressed as a logarithm (see Ott, 1985). The interpretation of LOD scores is a complex issue, but traditionally, LOD scores of +3 or more have been taken to indicate a high chance of linkage (an odds ratio of 1000:1) whereas LOD scores below −2 exclude linkage.

Genetic linkage studies of schizophrenia

In the past decade, considerable effort has been expended on the search for the gene(s) which predispose to schizophrenia. Unfortunately, despite an impressive number of linkage studies, little progress has been made. Although systematic genome searches are in progress, data published so far have focused on chromosome 5, the sex chromosomes, and chromosomes 11.

Chromosome 5 became the centre of attention following a report from Canada in which an uncle and nephew were described, both suffering from schizophrenia, and both carrying an unbalanced translocation of chromosome 5 (Bassett *et al*, 1988). Shortly after, a paper was published claiming to have found linkage between schizophrenia and markers on the long arm of chromosome 5 (Sherrington *et al*, 1988). These findings were not replicated in subsequent studies (Kennedy *et al*, 1988; St. Clair *et al*, 1989; McGuffin *et al*, 1990), including a second study from Sherrington's group (Mankoo *et al*, 1991). Although the disparity between findings could be taken to indicate genetic heterogeneity (Lander, 1988), a recent meta-analysis suggests that the high LOD scores originally obtained by Sherrington *et al* (1988) were a chance occurrence and that there is no linkage (McGuffin *et al*, 1990).

The long arm of chromosome 11 (11q) became an obvious candidate region after the gene encoding the dopamine D_2 receptor was mapped to it (Grandy *et al*, 1989), and following three case reports of families in which translocations involving this region appeared to co-segregate with psychotic disorders (Smith *et al*, 1989; Holland & Godsen, 1990; St. Clair *et al*, 1990). Investigators have examined for linkage to the D2 receptor (Moises *et al*, 1991) and have completed a comprehensive study of the surrounding region (Gill *et al*, 1993). Data from these studies do not support linkage.

Although there is no evidence to indicate X-linked inheritance in schizophrenia, there are nonetheless reasons to suspect the involvement of sex chromosomes in its aetiology. Firstly, sex chromosomal anomalies are more common in psychotic populations (Crow, 1988). Secondly, it is well recognised that gender may affect the expression of the disorder (Castle & Murray, 1991). Thirdly, related individuals with schizophrenia are more likely to be of the same sex (Crow *et al*, 1991). In order to account for the involvement of sex chromosomes but the lack of obvious sex-linked inheritance, Crow *et al* (1989) suggested that the gene for schizophrenia is located in the pseudoautosomal region of the sex chromosomes. This is a segment of sequence homology between the X and Y chromosomes in which meiotic cross-over (recombination) can occur. Depending on its exact location, a gene situated within this region could be inherited either in an autosomal or in a sex-linked manner (hence 'pseudoautosomal'). Tentative evidence of linkage between markers in this region and schizophrenia has been documented (Collinge *et al*, 1991; d'Amanto *et al*, 1992), but other studies report no linkage (Asherson *et al*, 1992).

Genetic association studies

Association studies, which use genetic marker information at a population level as opposed to a family level, are a useful adjunct to linkage studies (see Emery, 1986). The objective of an association study is to detect any difference in the frequency distribution of marker alleles between samples of unrelated affected individuals and control samples (of unrelated, unaffected individuals). Allelic association is said to be present when a particular marker allele is found significantly more often in the affected individuals than in the controls. This might occur because the marker locus has a causative role in the disease or because the marker locus is so close to the disease locus that recombination between them at meiosis is extremely rare. However, spurious associations can also occur and most commonly reflect biased sampling and a failure to control for ethnic and socio-economic status between the affected and controls.

From a practical point of view, association studies are easier to conduct than linkage studies. They may also be more appropriate, as an initial strategy, for disorders which are caused by more than one disease gene. Thus, while linkage to a particular marker may be obscured by genetic heterogeneity (i.e. only a proportion of families are linked), genetic association between the disorder and marker polymorphism might still be apparent at a population level (Clerget-Darpoux, 1990). One disadvantage of these studies is that the association effects in the population rapidly diminish as the physical distance between a marker and disease locus enlarges (because recombination occurs). This means that association analyses should preferably be restricted to candidate loci.

Several early association studies of schizophrenia focused on HLA types as genetic markers. This was influenced both by the availability of these markers and by reports of a much lower than average risk of rheumatoid arthritis in patients with schizophrenia (Vinogradov *et al*, 1991). Findings have been conflicting but overall, there is some suggestion of an association between schizophrenia and the HLA A9 polymorphism (McGuffin & Sturt, 1986). This requires further clarification.

Neurochemistry

Dopamine

In its simplest form, the dopamine theory proposes that schizophrenia is the result of a hyperdopaminergic state. The theory's credibility rests on the following observations:

(i) The neuroleptic potency of drugs correlates strongly with their anti-psychotic effects. The anti-psychotic effect of drugs which have geometrical isomers (e.g. alpha and beta flupenthixol) is confined to the isomer with dopamine antagonist effects.

(ii) Drugs which cause dopamine release (e.g. amphetamines), dopamine agonists (e.g. bromocriptine) or dopamine precursors (e.g. L-dopa) have been observed to produce psychotic symptoms or worsen schizophrenic symptoms (see also page 1127).

These findings have led to a search to identify a specific abnormality of dopamine function in schizophrenia. Attempts to measure levels of dopamine and its metabolite, homovanillic acid (HVA) have until recently been confined to post-mortem tissues. However, the majority of subjects in such studies have been treated with neuroleptics when alive, an important confounding factor which may account for the inconsistent results. Although some studies reported raised concentrations of dopamine in the nucleus accumbens, caudate and amygdala and raised HVA in the caudate nucleus, nucleus accumbens and cortex (Davis *et al*, 1991), the significance of abnormal findings is unclear.

An indirect assessment of central dopamine turnover can be obtained by measurement of plasma HVA. However, HVA is also produced peripherally, which complicates the interpretation of results. Some studies of patients with schizophrenia have found a relationship between HVA levels and severity of psychosis (Davis *et al*, 1985), but other investigators have failed to replicate these findings. Pickar's group did not find a difference in HVA levels between schizophrenic and normal controls, but CSF HVA levels were negatively correlated with psychotic symptoms, whereas plasma HVA levels were positively correlated with psychotic symptoms (Pickar *et al*, 1990). These puzzling results have led investigators to consider dynamic tests, which assess changes in HVA levels following administration of neuroleptics, in the hope that these will be more sensitive to abnormalities in dopamine turnover. HVA levels rise dramatically after administration of neuroleptics, and after one week fall to below pretreatment levels. The fall in HVA levels has been shown to be associated with clinical response (Davidson *et al*, 1991).

Recent studies have confirmed the presence of at least six dopamine receptor subtypes. D_1 receptors, which are positively coupled to adenylyl cyclase, are found post-synaptically in the striatum. D_2 receptors are not coupled or are negatively coupled to adenylyl cyclase. Neuroleptic affinity to the D_2 receptor correlates most closely to their anti-psychotic potency. Several post-mortem studies have reported an increased density of D_1 and D_2 receptor sites in schizophrenic patients compared with normals. The problem of interpreting these studies is complicated by the selection of subjects; many of whom are elderly, have other illnesses and have received long-term anti-psychotic medication; and that the receptor measures are confined to the dopamine-rich basal ganglia, which are not sites of maximal interest in the aetiology of schizophrenia.

Some of the problems of post-mortem studies have been overcome by functional imaging of dopamine receptors using positron emission tomography (PET) and single photon emission tomography (SPET). PET scanning allows *in vivo* measurement of D_2 receptor affinity using specific ligands such as [11C] methylspiperone and [11C] raclopride. Although an initial study by Wong *et al* (1986) reported an increase in basal ganglia D_2 receptors in patients with schizophrenia compared with controls, larger meticulously designed studies by Farde and colleagues at the Karolinska Institute in Stockholm have failed to replicate this finding. They reported an asymmetry of binding, with higher D_2 receptor density in the left than right putamen, but not controls (Farde *et al*, 1987,1990).

The impressive results of clozapine in treatment resistant schizophrenia have led to interest in its *in vivo* activities. The results of PET and SPET studies show that affinity for the D_2 receptor does not account for the antipsychotic properties of the drug. The drug has a higher affinity for D_1 receptor, lower for D_2 receptors and higher D_1 affinity than conventional neuroleptics (Farde *et al*, 1989) and D_2 receptor blockade does not correlate with clinical response (Pilowsky *et al*, 1992).

These findings add to the evidence that blockade of D_2 alone does not account for the clinical efficacy of neuroleptic drugs. New discoveries about dopamine sub-receptors may be a promising avenue of investigation. It is now clear that there are at least five dopamine receptor subtypes. The D_3 and D_4 receptor subtypes are also known to have a high affinity for anti-psychotic drugs, and they are most densely distributed in the limbic forebrain areas, an area of theoretical interest in the aetiology of psychosis. The D_4 receptor is also of interest because of its high affinity for the atypical neuroleptic clozapine, and because there are different forms of the receptor in humans. This polymorphism raises the theoretical possibility that various forms of the receptor are functionally different and, in some cases, predispose to schizophrenia, or predict clinical response to different anti-psychotics (Shaikh *et al*, 1993). There is as yet no evidence to support this proposal. The simplest version of the dopamine theory is no longer tenable, but our increasing knowledge of the neurochemistry of dopamine has encouraged the formulation of more sophisticated hypotheses about the role of dopamine in schizophrenia which can be investigated using functional imaging and molecular genetics.

Noradrenaline

Noradrenaline neurones are widely distributed through the human brain. In the limbic system, noradrenergic neurones predominate over dopamine or serotonin. The importance of noradrenaline in schizophrenia is called into question by the observation that neuroleptic drugs have significant noradrenaline antagonist effects. The increased level of arousal in the acute psychotic phase can be related to noradrenergic activation of the reticular activating system, and the anti-adrenergic properties of neuroleptics may account for their tranquillising effects.

Post-mortem studies have reported increased noradrenaline levels in the brain stem and limbic forebrain areas of patients with schizophrenia (Hornykiewicz, 1982). Raised levels of the nor-adrenaline metabolite, 3-methoxy-4-hydroxyphenylglycol have also been reported in the CSF of patients with schizophrenia (Pickar *et al*,

1990). A serious limitation of a noradrenaline hypothesis is that the antipsychotic potency of the neuroleptics does not correlate well with their noradrenaline antagonist effects, and noradrenergic agonists (e.g. antidepressants) and antagonists (e.g. propranolol) do not have impressive effects on schizophrenic symptoms. Of course, the noradrenaline and dopamine systems are dynamically inter-related, and the abnormalities which have been detected in both these neurotransmitters may be expressions of the same underlying disturbance.

Serotonin

The serotonin (5-HT) hypothesis of schizophrenia has attracted renewed interest since the serotoninergic properties of the atypical neuroleptic clozapine were characterised. The 5-HT hypothesis is supported by the observation that 5-HT agonist drugs, such as LSD, may induce psychotic symptoms. However, the psychotropic effects of LSD, which mainly induces perceptual changes, bear little similarity to the positive symptoms of schizophrenia.

Post-mortem studies of 5-HT or its metabolite 5-hydroxyindolacetic acid (5-HIAA) have reported contradictory findings, which may be accounted for by the selection of patients, many of whom had extensive histories of medication or even psychosurgery (Bleich *et al*, 1988). The results of receptor binding assays using [3H]LSD or [3H]ketanserin have been equally inconsistent.

Probenecid-induced 5-HIAA accumulation in the CSF provides a crude measure of central 5-HT function. The association between decreased CSF 5-HIAA and suicidal behaviour which has been reported in depressed patients has also been reported in patients with schizophrenia (van Praag, 1986), but the majority of CSF studies have failed to demonstrate differences between patients with schizophrenia and normal controls.

Neuroendocrine challenge testing, such as the measurement of 5-HT-dependent prolactin release following administration of an agonist (e.g. fenfluramine), are one method of exploring central 5-HT function *in vivo*. Tests using this elegant technique are underway, but the small number of studies published so far (e.g. Iqbal *et al*, 1991) have been unhelpful as they are compromised by major methodological flaws, the most serious being the inclusion of medicated or recently-medicated patients.

Another relatively accessible model of central 5-HT function is the human platelet, which has a high-affinity active transport system for 5-HT. Studies of 5-HT uptake in schizophrenia have given inconsistent results. Platelet levels of 5-HT are increased in chronic schizophrenia, but the cause or significance of this finding is unknown (Bleich *et al*, 1988).

A number of small treatment studies with 5-HT precursors (e.g. tryptophan) and 5-HT depleting agonists (e.g. fenfluramine) have shown no consistent benefit. Drugs with $5\text{-}HT_2$ antagonist effects are currently the focus of much research interest. In a trial of chronic patients with schizophrenia, setoperone (a $5\text{-}HT_2$ and dopamine antagonist) appeared to be effective in reducing negative symptoms (Ceulemans *et al*, 1985). The $5\text{-}HT_2$ antagonist ritanserin has also been reported to have a specific effect on negative symptoms. These studies need to be replicated.

The investigation of 5-HT dysfunction in schizophrenia illustrates the challenge of neurochemical research in the disorder. The complex interaction between neurotransmitter systems means that observed disturbances may be epiphenomena of the disorder. The confounding effects of neuroleptic medications on neurotransmitter function causes major problems in the interpretation of abnormal results from clinical studies. The role of 5-HT dysfunction in schizophrenia remains unclear, but improving standards of research which make serious attempts to deal with confounding factors will help to clarify this issue.

Glutamate

The dopamine model of schizophrenia derives in part from observations on the psychotomimetic properties of amphetamine. Another drug which can induce psychotic symptoms is phencyclidine (PCP). This drug, initially used as an anaesthetic, was widely abused in the USA in the 1960s and '70s, hallucinations, delusions and agitation persisted in some users for weeks after ingestion (Rainey & Crowder, 1975). Psychotomimetic effects have also been noted in normal volunteers and schizophrenic subjects (Javitt & Zukin, 1991), which, unlike amphetamine-associated psychosis, include apathy, negativism, prominent disorganisation of thought and neuro-psychological deficits.

The PCP binding site is within the ion channel of a glutamate receptor subtype (the N-methyl-D-aspartate receptor complex: NMDA), leading to a disruption of glutamatergic neurotransmission. The limbic system contains the highest content of the glutamate in the mammalian brain. This excitatory neurotransmitter acts on several types of receptor, classified according to their sensitivity to exogenous ligands (e.g. NMDA, Kainate (KA) and quisqualate (QA)). Post-mortem studies in patients with schizophrenia and controls by Kerwin and colleagues have shown a possible reduction of KA and QA receptors in schizophrenia (Kerwin *et al,* 1988; 1990).

The therapeutic role of non-toxic agents which act on glutamate receptors has not yet been evaluated, but this is the direction which this research will now follow.

Neuropeptides

At least 70 endogenous neuropeptides have been identified in the mammalian brain, but although they are known to have important roles as neurotransmitters and neuromodulators, their role in the aetiology of schizophrenia is unknown. Bearing in mind the limitations of the technique, post-mortem studies have reported differences between patients with schizophrenia and controls in levels of cholecystokinin (CCK), Substance P, vasoactive-intestinal peptide, somatostatin, neurotensin, thyrotropin-releasing factor and endorphin levels (Nemeroff, 1991). Some of these findings have been supported by CSF studies. However treatment trials have failed to show any unequivocal benefits of drugs which alter neuropeptide function.

Neuropathology of schizophrenia

Neuropathology techniques can be used to measure neuronal number, volume and cytoarchitecture in more detail than is possible with MRI. There are, however, some difficulties with post-mortem studies. Post-mortem findings in the brain may be complicated by the cause of death, for example, cerebral anoxia due to myocardial infarction, coincident cerebral disease, or drugs such as cortico-steroids. Relating post-mortem changes to functional or clinical measures has to be performed retrospectively. Post-mortem brain shrinkage and swelling, fixation, processing and staining artifacts may further complicate findings.

Cerebral cortex and brain size

Cortical atrophy, particularly in cortical association areas was described in early non-quantitative studies (Southard, 1915). Some recent reports suggest reduced whole cortical volume and reduced neuronal density in frontal regions (Pakkenberg, 1987; Benes, 1991), however several other studies did not find such changes (Rosenthal & Bigelow, 1972; Heckers *et al,* 1991).

Recent quantitative studies have found that brains of patients with schizophrenia are lighter by 5–8% and shorter in antero-posterior length by 4% (Brown *et al,* 1986; Bruton *et al,* 1990). However one study found no difference in weight between brains of patients with schizophrenia and controls (Heckers *et al,* 1991).

Basal ganglia brain stem and thalamus

The dopaminergic hypothesis of schizophrenia has led researchers to look for structural abnormalities in brain regions rich in dopaminergic neurones, such as the basal ganglia. Some post-mortem studies provide evidence of altered structure of globus pallidus and striatum in catatonic schizophrenics. Volumes of these structures were decreased in patients with schizophrenia (Dom *et al*, 1981; Bogerts *et al*, 1990). However, the possible effect of medication on the size of basal ganglia structures has to be considered. The corpus striatum is enlarged in patients treated with neuroleptics for long periods (Heckers *et al*, 1991). These findings are confirmed by those using MRI (Jernigan *et al*, 1991). It is possible that blocked inhibitory dopaminergic input leads to striatal hyperactivity (Bogerts, 1993). Reduced substantia nigra volume due to smaller neurones has been reported (Bogerts *et al*, 1983).

In the noradrenergic system, Lohr & Jest (1988) found decreased neuropil in the locus ceruleus of schizophrenic brains, whereas numbers of cholinergic neurones in the pontine nuclei were increased (Karson *et al*, 1991).

Reduced neuronal number in the dorsomedial nucleus of the thalamus was described in one series of patients with schizophrenia but not in another (Treff & Hempel, 1958; Lesch & Bogerts, 1984). Some reduction in periventricular grey matter around the third ventricle has also been described (Lesch & Bogerts, 1984). This finding is consistent with those neuroimaging studies which report increased third ventricular size in schizophrenia. Clinical symptoms of patients with either thalamic lesions or enlargement of the third ventricle within the thalamus may resemble negative symptoms of schizophrenia (Lishman, 1987).

Temporo-limbic region

The majority of post-mortem studies have reported abnormalities of these regions in the brains of patients with schizophrenia. Indirect evidence of temporal lobe pathology came from the observation in brains of schizophrenics that the temporal horn of the left ventricle was enlarged. Such enlargement might be associated with tissue loss of surrounding medial temporal structures (Crow *et al*, 1989).

More direct evidence of temporo-limbic pathology in schizophrenia includes observations of: 1) reduced grey and white matter volume of hippocampus, amygdala and parahippocampal gyrus; 2) reduced neuronal number, size or abnormal arrangements in the hippocampus, parahippocampal gyrus and entorhinal cortex (Bogerts, 1993).

Despite the significant overlap between patients and controls in volume of limbic structures and cell numbers within them, and the subtle nature of changes observed, brain abnormalities in limbic regions probably contribute to the pathology of schizophrenia. The hippocampus and amygdala are key structures involved in sensory information processing and control of basic drives, both of which may be abnormal in schizophrenics. Schizophreniform reactions with delusions and auditory hallucinations may accompany diseases of the temporal lobe, for example, epileptic foci, tumours, and viral encephalitis. Links between temporo-limbic abnormalities of structure and function using neuroimaging techniques have already yielded useful data. Such data partly complement pathological changes observed in post-mortem brains. Most MRI studies show smaller left temporal lobes in patients with schizophrenia. Similarly, blood flow and metabolism in temporo-limbic regions in schizophrenics, determined by SPET and PET studies have pointed to increases (Liddle *et al*, 1992) and decreases (Cleghorn *et al*, 1992). Liddle's study purported to show that schizophrenia consisted of three distinct clinical syndromes: reality distortion; psychomotor poverty and disorganisation. The question remains whether such clinical syndromes are reflected in underlying brain pathology. Most neuro-pathological studies support a developmental aetiology of schizophrenia. Reactive gliosis of the brain begins after the second trimester of pregnancy, and absence of gliosis may indicate abnormal brain development. At least ten studies reviewed by Bogerts (1993) have found no evidence of gliosis in the medial temporal lobe, cingulate or thalamus despite cell loss, reduced volumes and disrupted cell orientation. Abnormally arranged neurones also probably indicate early disturbance of brain development. The finding of such abnormalities in hippocampi, frontal cortex and cingulate gyrus further supports a developmental aetiology.

Normal brain asymmetry consists of larger left planum temporale, longer left sylvian fissure and larger right frontal and temporal lobes. Brain asymmetry is thought to develop late in pregnancy. Therefore abnormally increased or decreased asymmetry in schizophrenia may indicate that something has interfered with normal brain growth. Abnormal brain asymmetry in schizophrenia is suggested by the findings of selective left temporal horn enlargement (Crow *et al*, 1989), predominantly left sided cytoarchitectural abnormalities (Jakob & Beckmann, 1986) and loss of sylvian fissure asymmetry (Falkai *et al*, 1992).

There is now much neuropathological evidence for structural brain abnormalities in patients with schizophrenia. However, interpretation of post-mortem findings is difficult. Without prospective follow-up data, not possible with post-mortem studies, it is difficult to know exactly how much of the changes observed might be due to degenerative processes. Useful information can however be obtained from the pattern of pathology and this tends to support problems of brain development in schizophrenia. Reduced brain weight, cortical loss and abnormalities in the basal ganglia and in the temporolimbic regions are paralleled by MRI *in vivo* findings. Combining information from neuropathology with that obtained from *in vivo* structural and functional imaging techniques may further our understanding of processes underlying the schizophrenic disease process.

Neuroimaging

An attempt to define the role of structural brain abnormalities in the aetiology of schizophrenia has been a subject of continuous research since Kraepelin's description of dementia praecox. Early research was confined to case reports of associations between gross neuro-pathological abnormalities and schizophrenia. Pneumoencephalography was the first technique to provide information on brain structure in living patients. These studies showed non-progressive ventricular enlargement in patients with schizophrenia (Huber, 1957, Huber *et al*, 1975). The development of non-invasive imaging techniques including computerised tomography (CT) and, more recently, magnetic resonance imaging (MRI) has led to a huge research effort to characterise the structural abnormalities present in the brains of patients with psychotic illnesses.

Several CT studies have reported increased ventricular volume or ventricle:brain ratio (VBR; which attempts to control for head size) in patients with schizophrenia compared with control subjects (e.g. Johnstone *et al*, 1976, Andreasen *et al*, 1982). Raised VBR has been associated with poor prognosis, including poor social adjustment and negative symptoms (van Os *et al*, 1995). It is unclear how specific these findings are to schizophrenia, but in one study which included a bipolar control group, the VBR of bipolar patients lay between that of patients with schizophrenia and controls (Harvey *et al*, 1990), and the study by van Os *et al* shows a weaker association between VBR and outcome.

Although the resolution of CT scans has improved since the application of the technology to schizophrenia research, the greater resolution and safety of MRI has meant that this technique is now the standard research tool in structural neuroimaging studies. For this reason, the remainder of this section will focus on the results of MRI studies in schizophrenia.

Principles of magnetic resonance imaging

Magnetic resonance imaging (MRI) is an *in vivo* technique for producing high resolution anatomical images. The MR signal results from the combined effect of resonating hydrogen protons in a magnetic field. This signal varies according to the relative contributions to it from different tissues, resulting in an anatomical image. Using computers it is now possible to outline cerebral anatomy and measure areas and volumes of the outlined structure. MRI does not expose patients to X-ray radiation, and as long as there are no contraindications, such as metallic foreign bodies, it is safer than CT.

MRI is the most sensitive technique for detecting small lesions such as small cerebral infarcts. It is possible to detect discrete lesions such as plaques in multiple sclerosis as well as diffuse changes such as leukoencephalopathy in AIDS. MRI may demonstrate cerebral atrophy before obvious cognitive decline in patients with dementing illnesses. Specific brain regions may also be more easily identified with MRI than CT.

MRI has been used in psychiatric research to expand on knowledge obtained from post-mortem and CT brain studies. The combination of structural MRI with other information including clinical, neuropsychological, neurophysiological and functional neuroimaging techniques provides a means of detecting important relationships between brain structure and function in psychiatry.

Ventricular size

It has been found consistently that patients with schizophrenia have enlarged ventricles compared with controls (Woodruff, 1994*a*). This confirms that abnormalities similar to those found in post-mortem brain studies occurred *in vivo*. The range of ventricular size is usually greater in schizophrenic than control groups (Johnstone *et al*, 1989; Andreasen *et al*, 1990). This observation may, in part, be due to the heterogeneity of patient groups selected for study. Fewer studies report 3rd and 4th ventricular enlargement in schizophrenia but those that do find such enlargement to be of a similar order to that of the lateral ventricles. For example, one study showed that lateral ventricular volume was 62% greater, and 3rd ventricular volume 73% larger in patients with schizophrenia, compared with normal controls (Kelsoe *et al*, 1988). Lateral ventricular volume tends also to be greater on the left-hand side and in the temporo-frontal regions, although this is not always the case (Degreef *et al*, 1992). Generally, ventricular enlargement, in common with other brain regions, is more pronounced in male as opposed to female patients with schizophrenia and control groups.

A number of recent studies report correlations between lateral and 3rd ventricular volumes and a variety of both positive and negative symptoms, for example, hallucinations, bizarre behaviour, affective flattening, attention deficit and anhedonia (Andreasen *et al*, 1990; Young *et al*, 1991; Degreef *et al*, 1992). Increased ventricular size has been related to poor outcome (Johnstone *et al*, 1989). Correlations with other variables including age of onset of schizophrenia, duration and number of hospital admissions, cognitive impairment or previous neuroleptic treatment have been largely negative (Andreasen *et al*, 1990).

The ventricular region is surrounded by areas such as the amygdala, hippocampus and parahippocampal gyrus. These structures contain neuronal networks concerned with a number of cortical activities, including selection, association and integration of sensory information, memory and control of basic drives and emotions. The structural and functional relationship between enlarged ventricles and surrounding brain regions is currently an active area of research. Evidence so far suggests that such relationships are not direct or straightforward (Kelsoe *et al*, 1988).

That ventricular enlargement is often found in patients shortly after their first psychotic illness suggests that these brain abnormalities are longstanding. The lack of correlation between ventricular size and duration of illness further suggests non-progression of structural brain abnormalities once symptoms develop (Young *et al*, 1991). As foetal brain tissue expands, the proportion of ventricle to brain volume decreases. Therefore increased VBR in schizophrenia *may* represent incomplete brain maturation. An alternative explanation is that ventricular enlargement in schizophrenia is secondary to progressive atrophy of ventricles or surrounding regions. There is some evidence for progressive enlargement of ventricles in schizophrenia (DeLisi *et al*, 1994).

Whole brain

A number of MRI studies have demonstrated significant reduction of cerebral size in schizophrenia (Woodruff, 1994*a*). This reduction is not necessarily accompanied by equal alterations of other brain regions. For example, Barta *et al* (1990) found a 2% decrease in whole brain as opposed to that of 7–10% in temporal lobes. In this study, mid-brain and pontine areas were actually increased in patients with schizophrenia by 8% and 11% respectively. Reduced brain or cortical volume is sometimes accompanied by increased cerebrospinal fluid in patients with schizophrenia (Harvey *et al*, 1993).

Frontal lobe

The frontal lobe has been the focus of much interest in schizophrenia. Patients with frontal lobe damage, in common with patients with schizophrenia with negative symptoms, may exhibit deficits of attention, abstract thinking, judgement, motivation, affect and emotion, impulse control, as well as decreased spontaneous speech, verbal fluency and voluntary motor behaviour. Furthermore, patients with schizophrenia may show impaired performance on neuropsychological tasks that require adequate frontal lobe function (Goldberg *et al*, 1990). Evidence from functional neuroimaging work suggests that there is frontal lobe underactivity during activation tasks in schizophrenia (Weinberger *et al*, 1992). The question is whether frontal lobe underactivity is reflected in abnormalities of underlying brain structure as has been shown in some preliminary studies (Woodruff *et al*, 1994*b*).

A few studies have demonstrated a statistically significant reduction of frontal lobe size in schizophrenia (Breier *et al,* 1992). However some individual patients with schizophrenia show markedly reduced frontal lobe size. The question is whether those individuals with reduced frontal lobes are those who also suffer from the deficits observed in frontal lobe function. Evidence is emerging that this may be the case. For instance, studies looking at neuropsychological measures of frontal lobe activity have found relationships between deficits and frontal lobe size (Seidman *et al,* 1994). Frontal lobe deficits may also arise from abnormalities in brain regions closely connected to the frontal lobe. For example, underactivity of dorsolateral prefrontal cortex in schizophrenia during tasks requiring working memory was related to hippocampal volume (Weinberger *et al,* 1992). There is a suggestion therefore that neural networks connecting these and other brain regions may be functionally defective in schizophrenia.

Temporal lobes, hippocampus and amygdala

The temporal lobes are of theoretical and practical importance in our understanding of schizophrenia. Within the dominant temporal lobe lie many of the auditory and language functions that may underlie abnormalities of thought, speech and auditory perception in schizophrenia. Post-mortem studies have found increased infero-temporal horn ventricular volume within the temporal lobes of patients with schizophrenia (Brown *et al,* 1986).

Out of 13 recent MRI studies that have compared temporal lobe volume between patients with schizophrenia and controls, 12 find less volume on the left (statistically significant in seven studies) and nine on the right (statistically significant in three studies). Three studies measured grey and white matter separately, all found grey matter reduction in patients with schizophrenia, one found white matter reduction bilaterally, one white matter reduction on the left and increased on the right (Woodruff, 1994*a*).

It has been argued that lateralisation of pathology to the left is central to the condition (Crow, 1990). It has also been argued that this observation supports disruption of developmental processes early in the developing brain. As the left temporal lobe normally develops later than the right, it might be more susceptible to early injury during foetal brain development.

Correlations between temporal lobe volume and that of neighbouring regions including the ventricles have been inconsistent (Suddath *et al,* 1990). It is therefore difficult at present to be certain about the exact nature of the processes that lead to these abnormalities.

Temporal lobe abnormalities in schizophrenia tend to be more pronounced in males (Bogerts *et al,* 1990*a*). There may also be a genetic association between temporal lobe abnormalities and schizophrenia. For instance, patients with familial schizophrenia also have smaller temporal lobes (Dauphinais *et al*, 1990).

Abnormal temporal lobe morphology is often seen at the time of first onset of psychosis and tends not to be related to exposure to neuroleptic medication and duration of illness (DeLisi *et al*, 1992).

Temporal lobe abnormalities may predispose patients with schizophrenia to develop certain symptoms. Barta *et al* (1990) demonstrated associations between reduction of left superior temporal gyrus volume and auditory hallucinations. Shenton *et al* (1992) found that degree of thought disorder was related to reduction in volume of the left posterior superior temporal gyrus.

Basal ganglia

MRI studies of the basal ganglia in schizophrenia have led to inconsistent findings. Enlargement of the caudate demonstrated by DeLisi *et al* (1992) and Breier *et al* (1992) were not confirmed in other studies (Kelsoe *et al*, 1988; Young *et al*, 1991). Enlargement of the lenticular nucleus and putamen has also been described (Jernigan *et al*, 1991). Explanations for these varied findings have to include the long-term effects of anti-dopaminergic medication.

The corpus callosum

The corpus callosum consists of myelinated axons that connect one hemisphere to the other. Since the 'split brain' experiments of Sperry the importance of the corpus callosum in providing the major means of inter-hemispheric transfer of conscious and unconscious information has become apparent. Theorists have long been attracted to the idea that in schizophrenia, one hemisphere might become 'disconnected' from the other. Evidence supporting such an idea comes from observations that patients with schizophrenia perform poorly on neuropsychological tests reliant on intact inter-hemispheric communication (David, 1987; Coger & Serafetinides, 1990).

Evidence of structural abnormalities of the corpus callosum in schizophrenia came from post-mortem and structural neuroimaging studies. Bigelow *et al* (1983) found enlargement of the corpus callosum in brains of patients with schizophrenia. Using CT and MRI, an association between psychosis and dysgenesis of the corpus callosum, first noted by Lewis *et al* (1988) was confirmed by others (Swayze *et al*, 1990). A developmental anomaly related developmentally to the corpus callosum is cavum septum pellucidum. Associations between the presence of cavum septum pellucidum and schizophrenia have also been described (Lewis & Mezey, 1985). It has been inferred from these associations that neurodevelopmental damage to the corpus callosum may predispose to the later onset of psychosis (Lewis *et al,* 1988).

Early MRI studies using linear measures of width and length mostly found no significant differences between patients with schizophrenia and controls, although there was a suggestion that length was increased. As a result of these and similar post-mortem studies the importance of taking account of the influences of gender and handedness on corpus callosum morphology became apparent. Increased widths predominate in female patients with schizophrenia (Nasrallah *et al,* 1986; Raine *et al,* 1990) whereas reduced corpus callosum area is mainly confined to male schizophrenics (Woodruff *et al,* 1993). Witelson (1989) found larger corpus callosum areas in right-handed individuals on post-mortem examination. Nasrallah *et al* (1986) found MRI measurements of the corpus callosum area greater in right-handed, compared with left-handed, male patients with schizophrenia.

The shape of the corpus callosum is extremely variable. Therefore area measures of the corpus callosum are probably more reliable than linear ones (Woodruff *et al,* 1993). Eight of the 12 studies that have measured corpus callosum area show it to be smaller in patients with schizophrenia compared with controls (three statistically significant) (Woodruff, 1994), confirmed in a recent meta-analysis study (Woodruff *et al,* 1995*a*).

It may be that clinical syndromes encompassed within those diagnosed as schizophrenic have different corpus callosum morphology. For instance, Gunther *et al* (1991) found positive symptoms associated with larger, and negative symptoms with smaller, corpora callosa in patients with schizophrenia. Another study of patients with schizophrenia found that corpus callosum area was especially reduced in the part that transmits fibres between the two superior temporal gyri, reduction of which has been associated with auditory hallucinations in schizophrenia (Barta *et al,* 1990).

Overall, evidence favours reduced area of the corpus callosum in schizophrenia, predominantly in males. There is also evidence of corpus callosum dysfunction in schizophrenia and an association between developmental abnormalities of the corpus callosum and psychosis. Deficient function due to neuronal loss, demyelination or failed development might account for altered corpus callosum size in this condition.

Conclusions

Post-mortem and early CT scan studies demonstrated diminished cerebral size and enlargement of the lateral ventricles. More detailed regional patterns of abnormalities have emerged with the use of MRI.

Consistent patterns include: generalised reduction of cerebral cortex, focal diminution of temporal lobes and possibly hippocampi, particularly on the left, and a greater tendency for male than female patients with schizophrenia to exhibit alterations of brain morphology. Deficiencies of grey and white matter have been demonstrated within regions such as the temporal lobes. White matter abnormalities in the corpus callosum have also been found. Detailed examination of the brain has improved our understanding of factors that influence brain structure, such as age and sex.

With this understanding of brain structure in schizophrenia the next step is to link brain structure to functional deficits and symptoms. An important example of early attempts at this include that of reduced superior temporal gyrus size and auditory hallucinations in schizophrenia.

Recent developments in MRI technology have reduced the time required to produce a scan, and measure changes in tissue oxyhaemoglobin: deoxyhaemoglobin ratio. These advances have led to the development of functional MRI, which allows investigators to obtain non-invasive images of changes in regional cerebral blood flow. Functional MRI is a technique which can be readily applied to psychiatric and neuropsychological research (David, 1994), and we are already seeing the technique applied in the study of the biological correlates of psychopathological phenomena and neuropsychological dysfunction in schizophrenia (Woodruff *et al*, 1995*b*).

Neuropsychology

This discipline examines the interface between brain and psychological abnormalities. In schizophrenia, two general approaches have been adopted. The first, usually using batteries of standard tests, looks for cognitive impairments in patients with schizophrenia similar to those in patients with known organic brain lesions (see also page 293). The second attempts to define cognitive processes which underlie schizophrenic symptoms and to link these to brain functioning; that is, testing of specific neuropsychological paradigms.

Despite numerous studies of the first classical neuropsychological type there is little agreement as to their significance. In addition to the confounding influences of drug treatment, institutionalisation, and diagnostic heterogeneity, interpretation of results is troublesome because subjects with schizophrenia perform badly on most tests. Also there is no sufficiently elaborate theory of normal cognitive functioning to know what a particular test result implies about underlying cognitive mechanisms and their subserving brain systems. Goldstein (1986) concluded that no-one has been able to derive a characteristic pattern of performance specific to schizophrenia based on standard neuropsychological tests. Discriminating between cognitive performance of patients with schizophrenia and those with other severe 'functional' disorders has proved difficult.

The problem of defining an appropriate control group was tackled in an innovative study examining performance of MZ twins pairs discordant for schizophrenia on a test battery (Goldberg *et al*, 1993). The affected twin scored worse on nearly all tests, but most markedly on vigilance, memory and concept formation, suggesting fronto-temporal dysfunction. Detailed investigation of memory and learning showed that the affected MZ twin was impaired on 'declarative memory' – story recall, paired associate learning and visual recall of designs, but relatively intact on recognition memory and 'procedural memory' – skill-based learning of motor tasks. The unaffected twins showed mild 'episodic' memory disturbances – immediate and delayed recall of a story, delayed recall of designs – and possibly problem-solving compared to a small group of normal MZ twin controls. It was concluded that the major neuropsychological impairments seen in the affected MZ twin were a consequence of having schizophrenia and not genetically explicable. However, the subtle cognitive dysfunctions seen in the unaffected discordant twins compared with normal controls raises the possibility that these constitute genetic abnormalities predisposing to the disorder.

In the second type of neuropsychological approach are studies using frameworks directly derived from experimental psychology. Performance on tests of sustained attention such as the Continuous Performance Test, has been of special interest. Impaired performance on versions of this test demanding high processing capacity might indicate vulnerability to schizophrenia since it occurs in remitted as well as ill patients, and in children of schizophrenic parents, a group at increased risk of developing the disorder (Neuchterlein & Dawson, 1984*a*,*b*; Neuchterlein & Zaucha, 1990). Also studied have been neuropsychological functions involving cerebral laterality or inter-hemispheric transfer, but findings have been inconsistent. Work involving attention and information processing is allied to psychophysiological studies; there are possible analogues in measures of 'arousal' or 'activation', and those used in quantitative EEG research, such as the late evoked potential response, the P300 (Dawson, 1990). A reduced P300 in schizophrenia is a fairly consistent finding and may reflect a reduced processing capacity or an inability to appropriately allocate processing demands (Grillon *et al*, 1990). Overall, the findings from this group of studies thus far are suggestive only.

Broader cognitive theories of schizophrenia have recently emerged where cognitive processes, explored afresh, are purported to underlie the patient's abnormal experiences on the one hand, and to link with demonstrated abnormalities of brain function on the other. This approach is symptom-based rather than disorder-based. Some of the cognitive functions studied, for example 'intentional acts', have evolved specifically in relationship to schizophrenia instead of being derived from work on patients with organic brain disease.

Two models of this kind have received substantial attention. Hemsley (1992, 1994) developed a theory derived from information processing in which schizophrenia corresponds to a breakdown in the normal relationship between stored material and current sensory input. Normal perception and cognition is dependent on the interaction between current stimuli and stored regularities in previous input. The latter contribute to appropriate expectancies, response biases, memories and interpretations of what is currently happening. In schizophrenia, past information is stored but the rapid assessment of its significance in a current context may be impaired. For example, redundant information may not be treated as such, consequently heightening information processing demands abnormally. Some experimental studies support the model. For example, the phenomenon of 'latent inhibition' involves the reduction in attention to a stimulus which is repeatedly presented but not reinforced. The 'stored regularity' is that the stimulus has no consequence. In acute schizophrenia, latent inhibition seems to be reduced; thus by continuing to attend to the stimulus, patients may perform better than normals at tasks usually impaired as a consequence of the phenomenon. Other experimental phenomena such as 'Kamin's Blocking Effect' and 'Negative Priming' indicate a different pattern of performance in schizophrenia and are also dependent on the integration of previously presented material with current sensory input (Hemsley, 1994).

The proposed fundamental cognitive disturbance could be linked with schizophrenic symptoms such as delusions and hallucinations. The former may arise from the perception of abnormal relationships between events because of the intrusion of redundant material, or because perceptions dramatically violate expectations thus leading to the need for new explanations. Further the cognitive disturbances can be linked to neural systems involving the hippocampus and related brain structures. This system may be central in comparing actual and expected stimuli, an aspect of 'past regularities' in interaction with current stimuli (Gray, 1982; Gray *et al*, 1991). Hemsley also points out that amphetamines or hippocampal damage impair latent inhibition in animals.

The second model, not inconsistent with the first, is of schizophrenia as a 'disorder of self-awareness' (Frith & Done, 1988; Frith, 1992). Fundamental to the model is a cognitive psychology of 'willed intentions' – self-generated actions arising from an individual's goals and plans. These are distinguished from stimulus-driven responses to the environment. The negative symptoms of schizophrenia are seen as corresponding to a defect in the initiation of spontaneous action. Positive symptoms reflect a defect further along the sequence – in an internal monitoring system for actions or thoughts (or internalised actions). The internal monitor receives feed forward information about intentions and compares these with actions actually instigated. Normally, discrepancies signal the need for alterations of goals or plans.

One consequence of a breakdown in this monitor might be a subject experiencing himself carrying out acts without awareness of an intention to perform them. Their origin thus becomes puzzling; symptoms such as delusions of control and thought insertion could be understandable consequences. Auditory hallucinations might represent a more extreme case since the subject does not recognise the location of an internal act as internal at all. Frith presents some experimental evidence concerning the operation of the internal monitor and its impairment in schizophrenia. Further, the generation of negative and positive symptoms can be mapped onto reasonably well-characterised brain systems. The prefrontal cortex is essential in planning and goal directed behaviour. The failure to generate spontaneous action (negative symptoms) could represent a malfunction somewhere in the pathways connecting the prefrontal lobes and the striatum. Further evidence suggests that the internal monitoring centre is related to the hippocampal system; as in Hemsley's model above this acts as a comparator of current sensory information with an internally generated model of the world so that actualities can be set against expectancies (Gray, 1982).

Positive symptoms may thus represent disruption of inputs from the prefrontal cortex (associated with willed intentions) to the hippocampus, possibly in the parahippocampal gyrus or cingulate cortex. As seen earlier, there is good evidence of structural and functional abnormalities of both brain areas in schizophrenia. A later addition to Frith's model is abnormalities in the awareness of others – sufferers have problems making inferences about the knowledge and intentions of others. This failure in awareness of the mental states of others seems to parallel deficits in self-awareness and may lead to paranoid thinking.

Frith's model is consistent with three syndromes arising from a number of factor analyses of schizophrenic symptoms – psychomotor poverty, disorganisation and reality distortion – and patterns of blood flow involving prefrontal cortex and medial temporal lobe revealed by early PET studies (Liddle *et al*, 1992).

Developmental factors

Psychoanalytic theories

Schizophrenia is now rarely regarded by analysts as entirely psychogenic. The position of Rosenfeld (1965) is probably representative. Trauma in infancy, he states, plays an important part:

"but similar traumas and problems related to the parents of our patients are known to us from our experience with neurotic patients and are not typical for schizophrenia. The examinations of a large number of parents and families of patients with schizophrenia have shown that the parents of patients with schizophrenia have no character traits which can be regarded as specific. One has to assume that a certain predisposition to the psychosis exists from birth".

This constitutional vulnerability is cast in psychoanalytic terms – a rudimentary ego with a tendency to fragmentation and splitting. Rosenfeld also comments on the need to consider "not only the influence of the mother on the child, but the reaction of the mother to a particularly difficult schizoid infant". This may include a diminished tolerance towards the projections of the infant, with the mother feeling disturbed and persecuted and consequently withdrawing feelings from the child. Psychoanalytic methods may thus illuminate understanding of the content of a patient's illness, but not its form – why schizophrenia rather than depression?

Early development

Retrospective studies in which patients with schizophrenia have been compared with normal controls as children, have shown differences. Watt (1978) using school records found a pattern of greater irritability, disagreeableness and defiance of authority in boys, while girls were more likely than controls to be insecure, inhibited and shy. Abnormalities were more striking in the boys.

Two cohort studies of strong design have confirmed the presence of significant differences in early life between children destined to develop schizophrenia compared with those who do not. Done *et al* (1994) used the 1958 British perinatal mortality survey cohort comprising 98% of births in England, Scotland and Wales during a single week. They were able to trace all adults from this cohort who were treated in hospital between 1974 and 1986 for psychiatric reasons. Forty were diagnosed with schizophrenia, 35 with affective psychosis and 79 with a neurotic disorder. Social adjustment ratings, made when the children were aged 7 and 11 years, were compared across these groups and with random normal controls. By the age of 7 years those who later developed schizophrenia were rated by their teachers as showing more social maladjustment, especially the boys. Boys were more likely to be rated as 'over-reactive' – 'anxious for acceptance', hostile to others, and engaging in 'inconsequential behaviours' (e.g. poor concentration, carelessness, lolling about, mischievous). The 'preschizophrenic' boys showed a similar pattern at 11 years, but the girls at that age had become more 'underreactive' – withdrawn, unforthcoming and depressed. The pattern in both sexes was quite different from children who later developed affective disorders.

In the second study, Jones *et al* (1994) examined a cohort representing a random sample of all births in England, Scotland and Wales during one week in 1946 (Medical Research Council National Survey of Health and Development). Cases of schizophrenia between the ages of 16 and 43 were identified from a variety of sources. Childhood variables collected between the ages of 6 weeks and 16 years were examined and compared with non-schizophrenic cohort subjects. Again more abnormalities were found in the 'pre-schizophrenic' group. These included delayed motor milestones; speech problems; low educational test scores at 8, 11 and 15 years; solitary play at 4 and 6 years; less social confidence at 13 years, and greater social anxiety at 15 years. There was no evidence of increased antisocial or aggressive behaviour. When the child was 4 years old, mothers were also more likely to be rated by health visitors as having below-average mothering skills. Thus differences were noted across a range of developmental domains.

Both cohort studies thus found childhood differences between those later developing schizophrenia and controls, including those developing other psychiatric disorders. There is some discrepancy in the precise nature of the differences, possibly reflecting in part the different examinations made.

Another perspective on early development emerges from studies on 'high-risk' subjects, for example, those genetically related to patients with schizophrenia. By following up a cohort of offspring of schizophrenic parents, for example, with periodic re-testing it is hoped to identify predictors of later illness. Findings to date have been limited. Background factors including early life events and disturbed family relations have shown little evidence of specificity for schizophrenia when controls such as offspring of parents with other psychiatric disorders have been studied (Erlenmeyer-Kimling & Cornblatt, 1987). However, a range of bio-behavioural 'markers' or 'traits' have been posited. Most studied has been attentional dysfunction, especially complex versions of the Continuous Performance Test as mentioned earlier. Impaired performance is found in schizophrenia even during remission, is more common in unaffected relatives (including at-risk children) than in controls, is heritable, and is predictive of later behavioural disturbances, such as social isolation, thought to be related to schizophrenia (Cornblatt & Keilp, 1994). Also studied have been eye-tracking dysfunction (e.g. smooth pursuit eye-movements), electrodermal responsivity (including both hyper- and hypo-responsiveness), and event-related brain potentials. Each has shown promise, but to date there is insufficient evidence that they predict the emergence of schizophrenia. Sample sizes tend to be relatively small while the same domains of functioning have not been similarly examined across studies. Thus results have not been generally replicated and inconsistencies have been common (for a review of a wide range of putative predictors see a special issue of *Schizophrenia Bulletin*, 1994, 20 (1)).

Premorbid personality

Reviewing studies of premorbid personality in schizophrenia, Cutting (1985) concluded that about a quarter of patients had a 'schizoid' personality and a further one-sixth were abnormal in other respects. Foerster *et al* (1991) interviewed mothers of 73 consecutively admitted patients with DSM–III schizophrenia or affective psychosis. Men with schizophrenia showed much greater premorbid schizoid and schizotypal traits than schizophrenic women, or patients with an affective disorder. The same applied to reported adjustment at secondary school age. Late childhood impairments were more predictive of schizophrenia than early impairments, while the poorer the premorbid adjustment, the earlier the age at first admission to hospital. A further study showed that patients with schizophrenia underachieved occupationally compared with their fathers, as did patients with an affective psychosis. However, only in the former was underachievement already evident before the illness began. In both groups decline was noted after illness onset (Jones *et al*, 1993). This suggests that subtle cognitive or social difficulties antedate obvious symptoms of the illness by many years.

The studies reviewed above indicate that abnormalities occur in those destined to develop schizophrenia and that some are evident from early childhood. The data are consistent with a neurodevelopmental basis for the disorder. A number of interpretations are possible concerning what the premorbid abnormalities represent. They might express a vulnerability to schizophrenia, the disorder occurring in the face of later provoking events. Jones *et al* (1994) discuss how the disturbances they detected might initiate a self-perpetuating cascade of progressively more abnormal function, culminating in the emergence of psychosis. Late adolescent abnormalities such as schizotypal personality disorder might represent a subclinical form (or formes fruste) of the disorder, possibly a phenotypic variant of the same genetic makeup. Such unexpressed liability is supported by the finding of a similar number of offspring with schizophrenia from both affected and unaffected MZ twin pairs (Gottesman & Bertelsen, 1989). Alternatively, at later stages of development abnormalities might represent early signs of the illness itself.

Social factors

Life events

The role of life events in the causation of schizophrenia has proven difficult to elucidate. Cutting (1985) concluded that there was little evidence that catastrophic, single events could cause schizophrenia. However, much of the data derive from uncontrolled wartime observations, including the effects of incarceration in concentration camps. It was noted that admissions for psychosis in England during the blitz did not increase, while the rate of hospitalisation for psychosis in US military personnel remained relatively constant over 40 years, independent of war or peace.

Steinberg & Durrell (1968) studied the impact of a specific major life event – recruitment to the US army. The subjects were young men aged 20–24 years and included both volunteers and draftees. Records of hospital admissions with a diagnosis of schizophrenia were studied. There was a striking increase in admissions during the first year after recruitment, especially in the first few months, compared with the second year. This could not be explained by pre-existent symptoms or a choice to join the army due to psychiatric illness. There was evidence of more schizoid traits in those developing schizophrenia early. The authors concluded that the demands for adaptation were greatest in the early months after entry and that the most predisposed broke down first.

The most common approach to studying life events derives from a seminal study by Brown & Birley (1968) which examined the frequency of a range of life events prior to the onset or relapse of a schizophrenic illness. Forty-six per cent of patients had a significant independent (see below) life event in the three weeks prior to onset compared to 12% during other three-week periods in the study period. Fouteen per cent of a group of normal controls experienced life events in a three week period. There was no difference in the rate of events between first onset cases and relapsing patients. Relapse was associated with life events especially in patients compliant with neuroleptic medication; those discontinuing relapsed anyway.

Further studies in this vein have contended with a variety of thorny issues (Norman & Malla, 1993b; Bebbington *et al*, 1995). These include:

(i) Establishing a valid measure of life events. Each person's experience of events is unique; a similar occurrence may have quite different meanings to different people. However, a patient's personal view about the seriousness of a life event might be exaggerated by an attempt to explain why they became ill ('effort after meaning') or might be coloured by being ill. Which dimension of stress should be emphasised is another problem – for example, threat or the requirement for change.

Newer life event instruments such as the Life Events and Difficulties Schedule (LEDS; Brown & Harris, 1978) involve a semi-objective approach. Each event is assessed by a research panel for the degree of threat it entails for the individual, rated in the context of other information about the person's life history and current situation (Brown & Harris, 1978).

(ii) Problems with recall. Biases due to differential recall may be introduced when two groups, for example, patients versus normals are compared. There may be a 'recency effect' where 3 months before the control's interview is compared with 3 months before the onset of illness (which may have been some time ago) in the patients. Similarly, recall of events in a specified period before illness onset may be favoured when compared to similar length periods in the more distant past.

(iii) Independence between the life events and illness. Suffering from schizophrenia leads to new life events such as unemployment, failed relationships, loss of home, and so on. Results of the illness may thus be erroneously regarded as causes. Measures now evaluate the likelihood that the life event is independent of the illness by scrupulous attention to timing.

(iv) Interpretation of causality. In determining whether life events might 'cause' schizophrenia much depends on who is selected for comparison – e.g. do patients with schizophrenia have more life events before an episode than a normal community sample, patients with other psychiatric disorders, or schizophrenia patients who do not relapse. There are further complications. Compared to normals, schizophrenia patients could have more life events (because of premorbid difficulties in first onset cases, or residual difficulties in relapsing ones) or fewer (because of a tendency to withdraw socially, perhaps self-protectively). They may also be especially vulnerable to life events – thus life events may exert a significant causal effect in sufferers, yet be no more severe or frequent than in normals. Longitudinal studies in patients in which both life events and symptoms are assessed repeatedly, and preferably prospectively, address this question. This can be combined with a control group studied in the same way.

In reviewing the role of life events in schizophrenia, Norman & Malla (1993*a*) group a dozen or so studies to answer three questions:

(i) Do patients with schizophrenia have more severe life events before illness onset than those suffering from other psychiatric disorders?

(ii) Do they have more life events than normal controls?

(iii) Is there a relationship in patients suffering from schizophrenia between life event stressors and severity of symptoms?

The studies examined varied substantially in methods and populations. None of eight studies showed more life events for schizophrenia than other psychiatric disorders. Five of 14 studies reported more life events for schizophrenia than normal controls; none found the opposite. Most studies of the third type found a peaking of life events before illness onset or worsening of symptoms. The authors concluded:

> "In general, there is considerably more evidence for variation in stressors being associated with changes in the course of symptoms for patients with schizophrenia than for patients with schizophrenia having been exposed to more external life event stressors than the general population or patients suffering from other psychiatric disorders".

The findings were not influenced by variation across studies in time periods studied, patient selection, or diagnostic criteria. There were also no differences between first episode patients and relapsers.

A later study from the Camberwell Collaborative Study (Bebbington *et al*, 1993) compared patients with three types of disorder: schizophrenia, mania and depressive psychosis, with a datable episode in the previous year. They were compared with each other as well as a normal community group for six months before onset. There was a significant excess of events in the cases compared to controls in the three months before onset, and to a lesser degree between four and six months. The excess was apparent for both severe and mild events. The most marked pre-onset peak occurred for depressive psychosis, but the number of subjects was small. This study is consistent with the conclusions of Norman & Malla (1993*a*), but strengthens the idea that before illness onset, schizophrenia patients experience more life event stressors than normals.

The interval over which excess events occur is unclear; in some studies this has been 3–4 weeks before onset; in others it has been up to 6 months. Most studies have focused on major life events. It is possible, however, that an accumulation of apparently trivial difficulties or 'hassles' might also be capable of precipitating the disorder. Also unclear is the interaction between life events and neuroleptic medication, especially whether those off medication are more likely to relapse in the absence of a major life event (Bebbington *et al*, 1995). The role of life events in the remote past is much more difficult to study. The possible role of social adversity has been discussed in the section dealing with epidemiology.

Family factors

Interest in family aspects of schizophrenia burgeoned after the Second World War. Initially, the influence of psychoanalytical theory was strong, including the notion of the 'schizophrenogenic mother'. Work in the 1950s and '60s by researchers such as Lidz failed to identify a specific 'schizophrenogenic' pattern. The focus shifted to relationship difficulties between the parents, and the way in which the patient was ensnared by them. This could extend to the patient having a role in stabilising the parental relationship. Bowen described problems of individuation in the family, especially due to projective mechanisms, possibly transmitted across several generations.

Bateson and co-workers focused on family communication, both verbal and non-verbal, leading to the idea of the 'double-bind', considered by them as an important mechanism in the genesis of schizophrenia. The recipient of the bind picks up contradictory messages at verbal and non-verbal levels, but because of dependency on the sender, is not able to comment on this inconsistency nor quit the relationship. A response to this situation could be the development of a communication disorder characteristic of schizophrenia. This group was also prominent in developing the idea of family homeostasis, and the ways in which a family may under certain circumstances achieve stability at the expense of the health of its members.

The 1960s saw many observational studies of families with a schizophrenic member, but few consistent findings emerged. Features such as family efficiency, flexibility, conflict, dominance, coalitions, and distorted communications, including the 'double bind', were studied. Variations in the overall framework of the research, the kinds of observations made, the measures used, and the definitions employed has made interpretation of the results difficult (Doane, 1978; Jacob & Grounds, 1978). Hirsch & Leff (1975), reviewing the findings, concluded that parents of patients with schizophrenia tend to be more psychiatrically disturbed than parents of normal children; that there may be more marital disharmony than in the parents of other psychiatric patients; and that mothers of patients with schizophrenia may show more concern and protectiveness than mothers of normals. However, they noted that none of these conclusions were strong and that no study provided evidence that parental abnormalities exerted a specific effect during the patient's formative years. There was evidence that the 'preschizophrenic' child frequently manifested physical ill-health or mild disability in early life, so that parental abnormalities might have been a consequence of these. Peculiarities in both parent and child might also of course share a common genetic basis.

In the 1970s research began to focus on two areas which have become subjects of enduring interest: 'communication deviance' and, particularly, 'expressed emotion'.

Communication deviance (CD)

This concept, developed by Wynne & Singer (1963*a,b*), refers to a subject's fragmented and disorganised communications, including poor ability to maintain a focus. They hypothesised that such communication styles could result in disturbed information processing and thinking in vulnerable offspring. Measures of CD were developed on the basis of parents' interpretation of projective tests. The researchers found it possible to differentiate between offspring with and without schizophrenia solely on the basis of parental CD. An important replication of this work was attempted by Hirsch & Leff (1975). They compared CD in relatives of patients suffering from schizophrenia with relatives of neurotic controls. CD was increased in the former group, but was accounted for by their greater verbosity. Hirsch & Leff concluded that the relationship between CD and schizophrenia was not supported; but it remains possible that increased verbosity might result from communication difficulties. It is also possible that CD is a genetic trait manifesting in parents and offspring, irrespective of any transactional component, or that it is a consequence of living with a youngster with schizophrenia.

In a unique prospective study (UCLA high-risk study) family factors were examined before the onset of schizophrenia (Goldstein, 1985). Fifty teenagers seen at a psychological clinic more than 15 years previously were followed-up and diagnoses made. At their original presentation, assessments had been made of CD, affective style (AS; ratings from transcribed family discussions measuring criticism and intrusiveness), and expressed emotion (EE). By the time of follow-up a sufficient number had developed schizophrenia or a schizophrenia-related disorder to examine prediction by the three family measures. Despite small numbers, 'schizophrenia-spectrum' disorders were significantly associated with high CD, negative AS, and high EE. Strongest prediction was by CD in association with negative AS. A degree of specificity was suggested because these family qualities related more closely to schizophrenia than to other psychiatric disorders. The family measures were not accounted for by the level of the adolescent's disturbance. This singular study needs replication, but suggests that family stressors may trigger the onset of schizophrenia in a vulnerable youngster.

Expressed emotion (EE)

Prompted by a finding that patients with schizophrenia fared worse when discharged to the family home with parents or spouses than to siblings or lodgings (Brown *et al*, 1958), a series of studies investigating family emotional climate was initiated (Brown, *et al*, 1972). From these arose the influential concept of EE. Early work examined the role of both positive and negative features, but later research narrowed the concept to negative or intrusive attitudes expressed by relatives about the patient.

EE is now assessed on the basis of a semi-structured, standardised interview, the Camberwell Family Interview (CFI; Brown *et al*, 1972), carried out with a relative. Ratings are made from audiotapes and are based on both content and vocal tone. The key ratings are:

(i)   Critical comments (CC) – a frequency count of statements of resentment, disapproval, or dislike, together with comments showing critical tone irrespective of content.

(ii) Hostility – criticism for what the person is rather than for what he does, or excessive generalised criticism.

(iii) Emotional overinvolvement (EOI) – unusually marked concern about the patient, such as constant worry over minor matters, overprotective attitudes, or intrusive behaviour.

Warmth and positive comments are also rated. A designation of 'high' EE is based on a score above a designated threshold level for CC, hostility, or EOI. For excellent reviews of EE and its implications see Kavanagh (1992), Lefley (1992) and Kuipers (1994).

Around 30 studies of EE, involving over 1500 patients, have focused on prediction of relapse. Bebbington & Kuipers (1994) carried out an aggregate analysis using data from 25 studies. With a high EE relative the relapse rate, usually assessed 9 months later, was 50%; for low EE it was 21%. EE was equally predictive for patients of both sexes. While frequent contact with a high EE relative increased the risk of relapse, low EE homes appeared protective. Medication independently reduced relapse in both high and low EE settings. The predictive validity of EE seems to be independent of patient symptom severity and history of illness, although a minority of studies have found that EE is higher when patients' symptoms are worse and their behaviour more disturbed (MacMillan *et al*, 1986).

EE is often seen as activating relapse through psychophysiological mechanisms. Centrally originating 'autonomic hyperarousal', measured for example by electrodermal activity, has been hypothesised to lead to schizophrenic symptoms in someone with a specific vulnerability, perhaps related to an impairment in the capacity for information processing (see above). This suggestion has led to studies examining the effects of parental EE on the patient's psychophysiology. There is a fairly consistent finding that under certain conditions patients respond to the presence of a high EE relative with higher levels of electrodermal activity than a low EE relative. However, a correlation between changes in electrodermal activity and EE over time has not been clearly shown (Tarrier & Turpin, 1992).

Most studies have assessed EE at the time of the patient's admission to hospital and then examined its ability to predict relapse over the next year or so. Assessing EE at admission introduces a possible 'reactive' contribution relating to relatives facing a crisis and the effectiveness with which they handle it, in addition to any ongoing aspect of the relationship it may reflect. In a study in which EE was assessed in stable schizophrenia out-patients over 5 years, the level of EE was stable in 63% of families (25% high; 38% low), but fluctuated between high and low in the remainder (McCreadie *et al*, 1993). Thus EE, though often steady, is not necessarily a 'static' attribute of a relative or a family and may vary with circumstances and treatment interventions.

Reductionist models where high EE causes relapse in a vulnerable patient, or alternatively, where EE is seen as an epiphenomenon of the behavioural disturbance of schizophrenia, are unlikely to prove satisfactory. Reciprocal interactions between patient and relatives make the processes more complex. It has been claimed, for example, that problem behaviours may lead to unsuccessful attempts at coping by relatives which may lead to the expression of high EE, which in turn may exacerbate the problem behaviours and symptoms. Smith *et al* (1993) found that high EE relatives experience more distress and burden, and perceive themselves as coping with life less well than low EE relatives. However, approximately one quarter of the low EE relatives reported high stress, burden, or impaired coping. A developmental, interactional view of EE is begining to emerge.

EE is able to predict relapse across cultures, including British, American (including both Anglo-American and Americans of Mexican descent), Spanish, Italian, Czechoslovakian, Japanese and Indian. Expressions of criticism and emotional overinvolvement are highly culturally determined (Jenkins & Karno, 1992), but apparently they can be reliably rated. A strength of the measure is its rating against standards appropriate to a specific culture. Levels of criticism and overinvolvement, and their relative contributions to high EE vary across cultures, yet within different ranges they have predictive validity. It has been suggested that cross-cultural differences in family structure and emotional atmosphere indexed by EE might contribute to the variability in outcomes for schizophrenia across the world.

EE and family interactions

EE is a remarkably simple, yet valid measure of the family emotional environment. Its relationship to what actually happens in the family is described by Kuipers (1994) as analogous to blood pressure as a measure of the state of the vascular system. Both say little about the underlying processes but they have important predictive value. How EE relates to family interaction is only begining to be explored. The evidence indicates that high EE is associated with a number of negative patterns. High EE relatives are probably less informed about schizophrenia, and are more likely to attribute difficult behaviour to personal characteristics of the patient rather than the illness, or to believe more control could be exercised (Brewin *et al*, 1991). High EE relatives are more likely to be unpredictable in their responses to the patient, while low EE relatives are often described as calm, empathic, and respectful of the patient's, often eccentric, needs.

High EE parents appear to be critical in direct interaction with their ill offspring and negative patterns of interaction have been identified. A study using a concurrent measure of affective style (AS) in which transcripts of direct interactions are rated for critical or intrusive statements, has shown that high EE critical parents are more likely to show the former, while high EOI is associated with the latter (Miklowitz *et al*, 1984). The patient's contribution to the interaction has also been examined. Hahlweg *et al* (1989) examined verbal and non-verbal sequences between a parent and patient. When discussing emotion-laden family problems, high EE critical parents exhibited more criticism, negative affect, and negative solution proposals. Low EE parents showed more positive and supportive statements. Patients with critical relatives displayed more negative non-verbal affect, more disagreement, and made more self-justifying statements. Sequential analyses showed sustained negative reciprocal patterns in critical families.

The EE concept has not proved popular with families, nor with relatives' organisations, being sometimes perceived as yet another means of blaming relatives for the patient's illness. A focus on the protective aspects of low EE has been urged by some as a counterbalance to the more common emphasis on determining what is detrimental about high EE (Lefley, 1992).

Conclusions

No necessary or sufficient cause of schizophrenia has so far been identified. However, there has been progress in implicating a variety of aetiological factors. Substantial evidence supports an important role for genetic influences. Technological advances in brain imaging reinforce the belief that schizophrenia, at least in a proportion of cases, is associated with structural brain abnormalities and represents a neurodevelopmental disorder. The impact of these processes may be already evident in early life; many people destined to develop schizophrenia in early adulthood show impaired psychological and social functioning in childhood. How these influences contribute to the pathogenesis of the disorder remains largely unknown, but new neuropsychological paradigms promise to elucidate links between symptoms, cognitive functions and brain systems. In addition to biological processes, social influences have also been shown to be significant, at least in triggering relapse, but possibly also in precipitating an initial episode of psychosis. These include adverse life events and exposure to specific social or family environments.

A widely accepted framework for integrating the factors so far identified has been termed the 'vulnerability-stress' model (Zubin, 1988). Vulnerability in an individual is considered to issue from genetic and early life influences (e.g. perinatal). These predispose to the disorder but its expression also requires environmental stress factors (e.g. adverse life events). The greater the degree of vulnerability, the less severe the stressors required to cause the disorder, and vice-versa. The search for vulnerability markers such as attentional dysfunctions has been discussed. In addition to vulnerability and stressors, some also postulate moderating or protective factors. These might include specific psychological characteristics and a stabilising social environment, but so far they remain largely undefined. Following the onset of the illness, a separate set of factors might enter the arena, serving to limit the episode or to promote chronicity. Expressed emotion may be one of these.

This paradigm is well illustrated in a Finnish adoption study, still in progress (Tienari, 1991). Adoptees with biological mothers with schizophrenia were compared with adoptees born of normal mothers. All were adopted by non-relative families, the majority before the age of two years. The adoptees in both groups, most now older than 20, received a detailed psychiatric assessment. In addition, the adoptive families were rated for disturbance on a number of dimensions of family functioning. Results to date show that offspring from mothers with schizophrenia are significantly more likely to show severe disturbance (psychosis or borderline psychosis) than offspring from the control mothers. When disorders in the offspring were related to levels of family disturbance, it was found that disturbance in the offspring increased with increasing family disturbance in both groups. However, the differences between the offspring of mothers with schizophrenia and the offspring of controls only became clear when the adoptive family showed significant disturbance; 46% of the adoptees of mothers with schizophrenia compared with 24% of the control adoptees showed a disorder when the family was rated as disturbed, but only 5% versus 3% when the family was rated as well-functioning. Thus a poorly functioning family enhances the expression of the genetic vulnerability while a healthy family may protect against such a development. A potential problem with this conclusion concerns the possible effect on family functioning of the disturbed youngster, but as this study also has a prospective component, this issue should be resolvable in the future.

Still bedevilling aetiological research in schizophrenia is the problem of heterogeneity. Although there is now impressive international agreement on operational definitions, it remains highly likely that more than one disorder is being studied. Related issues are the boundaries of the 'schizophrenic spectrum' concept, and the degree of specificity to schizophrenia of many of the abnormalities detected. Despite numerous false directions in the past, the last decade has witnessed renewed optimism that consistent advances are being, and will continue to be made.

Acknowledgements

We would like to thank Drs Cathy Walsh, David Castle, Ian Everall and Michael Isaacs for their helpful advice in preparing this chapter.

References

Andreasen, N. C., Endicott, J., Spitzer, R. L., *et al* (1977) The family history method using diagnostic criteria. *Archives of General Psychiatry*, **34**, 1229–1235.

——, Smith, M. R., Jacoby, C. G., *et al* (1982) Ventricular enlargement in schizophrenia, definition and prevalence. *American Journal of Psychiatry*, **139**, 292–296.

——, Erhardt, J. C., Swayze, V. W., *et al* (1990) Magnetic resonance imaging of the brain in schizophrenia, the pathophysiologic significance of structural abnormalities. *Archives of General Psychiatry*, **47**, 35–44.

Astrup, C. & Odegaard, O. (1961) Internal migration and mental illness in Norway. *Psychiatry Quarterly*, **34**, 116–130.

Barr, C. E., Mednick, S. S. A. & Munk-Jorgensen, P. (1990) Exposure to influenza epidemics during gestation and adult schizophrenia. *Archives of General Psychiatry*, **47**, 869–874.

Barta, P. E., Pearlson, G. D., Powers, R. E., *et al* (1990) Auditory hallucinations and smaller superior temporal gyral volume in schizophrenia. *American Journal of Psychiatry*, **147**, 1457–1462.

Bassett, A. S., Jones, B. D., McGillivray, B. C., *et al* (1988) Partial trisomy chromosome 5 cosegregating with schizophrenia. *Lancet*, *i*, 799–801.

Bebbington, P. E., Wilkins, S., Jones, P., *et al* (1993) Life events and psychosis. Initial results from the Camberwell Collaborative Psychosis Study. *British Journal of Psychiatry*, **162**, 72–79.

—— & Kuipers, L. (1994) The predictive utility of expressed emotion in schizophrenia, an aggregate analysis. *Psychological Medicine*, **24**, 707–718.

——, Bowen, J., Hirsch, S. R., *et al* (1995) Schizophrenia and psychosocial stresses. In *Schizophrenia* (eds S. R. Hirsch & D. Weinberg), pp. 585–602. Oxford: Blackwell.

Benes, F. M., McSparren, J., Bird, E. D., *et al* (1991) Deficits in small interneurons in prefrontal and cingulate cortices of schizophrenic and schizoaffective patients. *Archives of General Psychiatry*, **48**, 996–1001.

Bigelow, L. B., Nasrallah, H. A. & Rauscher, F. P. (1983) Corpus callosum thickness in chronic schizophrenia. *British Journal of Psychiatry*, **142**, 282–287.

Bleich, A., Brown, S. L., Kahn, R., *et al* (1988) The role of serotonin in schizophrenia. *Schizophrenia Bulletin*, **14**, 297–315.

Boddington, J. D. (1992) A comparison of diagnosis and treatment in black and white acute psychiatric patients, with particular reference to major psychotic illness. *Schizophrenia Research*, **6**, 102–103.

Bogerts B. (1993) Recent advances in the neuropathology of schizophrenia. *Schizophrenia Bulletin*, **19**, 431–445.

——, Hantsch, H. & Herzer, M. (1983) A morphometric study of the dopamine-containing cell groups in the mesencephalon of normals, Parkinson patients, and schizophrenics. *Biological Psychiatry*, **18**, 951–971.

——, Ashtari, M., Degreef, G., *et al* (1990*a*) Reduced temporal limbic structure volumes on magnetic resonance images in first episode schizophrenia. *Psychiatry Research, Neuroimaging*, **35**, 1–13.

——, Falkai, P., Haupts, M., *et al* (1990*b*) Post-mortem volume measurements of limbic system and basal ganglia structures in chronic schizophrenics. *Schizophrenia Research*, **3**, 295–301.

Bohman, M. & Sigvardsson, S. (1980) A prospective longitudinal study of children registered for adoption. A 15 year follow-up. *Acta Psychiatrica Scandinavica*, **61**, 339–353.

Bowler, A. E. & Torrey, E. F. (1990) Influenza and schizophrenia. *Archives of General Psychiatry*, **47**, 877.

Bradbury, T. N. & Miller, G. A. (1985) Season of birth in schizophrenia, A review of evidence, methodology, and aetiology. *Psychology Bulletin*. **98**, 569–594.

Breier, A., Buchanan, R. W., Elkashef, A., *et al* (1992) A magnetic resonance imaging study of limbic, prefrontal cortex, and caudate structures. *Archives of General Psychiatry*, **49**, 921–925.

Brewin, C. R., MacCarthy, B., Duda, K., *et al* (1991) Attribution and expressed emotion in the relatives of patients with schizophrenia. *Journal of Abnormal Psychology*, **100**, 546–554.

Brown, G. W., Carstairs, G. M. & Topping, G. C. (1958) The post hospital adjustment of chronic mental patients. *Lancet*, **2**, 685–689.

—— & Birley, J. L. T. (1968) Crises and life changes and the onset of schizophrenia. *Journal of Health and Social Behaviour*, **9**, 203–214.

——, —— & Wing, J. K. (1972) The influence of family life on the course of schizophrenic disorders, a replication. *British Journal of Psychiatry*, **121**, 241–258.

—— & Harris, T. (1978) *The Social Origins of Depression. A Study of Psychiatric Disorder in Women*. London: Tavistock.

Brown, R., Colter, N., Corsellis, J. A. N., *et al* (1986) Post-mortem evidence of structural brain changes in schizophrenia, Differences in brain weight, temporal horn area, and parahippocampal gyrus compared with affective disorder. *Archives of General Psychiatry*, **43**, 36–42.

Bruton, C. J., Crow, T. J., Frith, C. D., *et al* (1990) Schizophrenia and the brain, A prospective clinico-neuropathological study. *Psychological Medicine*, **20**, 285–304.

Castle, D. J. & Murray, R. M. (1991) The neurodevelopmental basis of sex differences in schizophrenia. *Psychological Medicine*, **21**, 565–575.

——, Wessely, S., Der G., *et al* (1991) The incidence of operationally defined schizophrenia in Camberwell 1965–1984. *British Journal of Psychiatry*, **159**, 790–794.

——, Scott, K., Wessely, S., *et al* (1993) Does social deprivation in utero or in early life predispose to schizophrenia? *Social Psychiatry and Psychiatric Epidemiology*, **28**, 1–4.

Ceulemans, D. S. L., Gelders, Y., Hoppenbrouwers, M. L., *et al* (1985) Effect of serotonin antagonism in schizophrenia, a pilot study with setoperone. *Psychopharmacology*, **85**, 3299–3232.

Cleghorn, J. M., Franco, S., Szechtman, B., *et al* (1992) Toward a brain map of auditory hallucinations. *American Journal of Psychiatry*, **149**, 1062–1069.

Clerget-Darpoux, F. (1990) *Genetic Approaches in the Prevention of Mental Disorders*. Berlin: Springer-Verlag.

Coger, R. W. & Serafetinides, E. A. (1990) Schizophrenia, corpus callosum, and inter-hemispheric communication: a review. *Psychiatry Research*, **34**, 163–184.

Collinge, J. S., DeLisi, L. E., Boccio, A., *et al* (1991) Evidence for a pseudoautosomal locus for schizophrenia using the method of affected sibling pairs. *British Journal of Psychiatry*, **158**, 624–629.

Cooper, J. E. Kendell, R. E., Gurland, B. J., *et al* (1972) *Psychiatric Diagnosis in New York and London*. Maudsley Monograph No. 20. London: Oxford University Press.

Cornblatt, B. A. & Keilp, J. G. (1994) Impaired attention, genetics, and the pathophysiology of schizophrenia. *Schizophrenia Bulletin*, **20**, 31–46.

Crow, T. J. (1983) Is schizophrenia an infectious disease? *Lancet*, **1**, 173–175.

—— (1988) Sex chromosomes and psychosis: the case for a pseudoautosomal locus. *British Journal of Psychiatry*, **149**, 419–429.

—— (1990) Temporal lobe asymmetries as the key to the etiology of schizophrenia. *Schizophrenia Bulletin*, **16**, 434–443.

——, DeLisi, L. E. & Johnstone, E. C. (1989) Concordance by sex in sibling pairs with schizophrenia is paternally inherited: evidence for a pseudoautosomal locus. *British Journal of Psychiatry*, **155**, 89–97.

——, Done, D. J. & Johnstone, E. (1991) Schizophrenia and influenza. *Lancet*, **338**, 116–117.

Cutting, J. (1985) *The Psychology of Schizophrenia*. Edinburgh: Churchill Livingstone.

d'Amanto, T., Campion, D., Gorwood, M., *et al* (1992) Evidence for a pseudoautosomal locus for schizophrenia II. *British Journal of Psychiatry*, **161**, 59–62.

Dauphinais, D., DeLisi, L. E., Crow, T. J., *et al* (1990) Reduction in temporal lobe size in siblings with schizophrenia: a magnetic resonance imaging study. *Psychiatry Research*, **35**, 137–147.

David, A. S. (1987) Tachistoscopic tests of colour naming and matching in schizophrenia: evidence for posterior callosal dysfunction? *Psychological Medicine*, **17**, 621–630.

—— (1994) Functional magnetic resonance imaging. *British Journal of Psychiatry* **164**, 2–7.

Davidson, M., Kahn, R. S., Knott, P., *et al* (1991) Effects of neuroleptic treatment on symptoms of schizophrenia and plasma homovanillic acid concentrations. *Archives of General Psychiatry*, **48**, 910–913.

Davis, K. L., Davidson, M., Mohs, R. C., *et al* (1985) Plasma homovanillic acid concentrations and the severity of schizophrenia. *Science*, **227**, 1601–1602.

——, Kahn, R. S., Ko, G., *et al* (1991) Dopamine in schizophrenia: A review and reconceptualization. *American Journal of Psychiatry*, **148**, 1474–1486.

Dawson, M. E. (1990) Psychophysiology at the interface of clinical science, cognitive science and neuroscience. *Psychophysiology*, **27**, 243–255.

de Alarcon, J., Seagroatt, V. & Goldacre, M. (1990) Trends in schizophrenia. *Lancet*, **335**, 852–853.

Degreef, G., Ashtari, M., Bogerts, B., *et al* (1992) Volumes of ventricular system subdivisions measured from magnetic resonance images in first-episode schizophrenic patients. *Archives of General Psychiatry*, **49**, 531–537.

DeLisi, L. E., Stritzke, P., Riordan, H., *et al* (1992) The timing of brain morphological changes in schizophrenia and their relationship to clinical outcome. *Biological Psychiatry*, **31**, 241–254.

——, Grimson, R., Kushner, M., *et al* (1994) Is there progressive brain change following a first hospitalization for schizophrenia? A 4 year follow-up. *Schizophrenia Research*, **11**, 135–136.

Der, G., Gupta, S. & Murray, R. M. (1990) Is schizophrenia disappearing? *Lancet*, **335**, 513–516.

Doane, J. A. (1978) Family interaction and communication deviance in disturbed and normal families: A review of research. *Family Process*, **17**, 357–376.

Dom, R., de Saedeler, J., Bogerts, B., *et al* (1981) Quantitative cytometric analysis of basal ganglia in catatonic schizophrenics. In *Biological Psychiatry* (eds C. Perris, G. Struwe & B. Jansson), pp. 723–726. Amsterdam: Elsevier.

Done, D. J., Crow, T. J., Johnstone, E. C., *et al* (1994) Childhood antecedents of schizophrenia and affective illness: Social adjustment at ages 7 and 11. *British Medical Journal*, **309**, 699–703.

Eagles, J. M., Hunter, D. & McCance, C. (1988) Decline in the diagnosis of schizophrenia among first contacts with psychiatric services in North-East Scotland, 1969–1989. *British Journal of Psychiatry*, **152**, 793–798.

Eaton, W. W. (1985) Epidemiology of schizophrenia. *Epidemiologic Reviews*, **7**, 105–126.

—— (1991) Update on the epidemiology of schizophrenia. *Epidemiological Review*, **13**, 320–328.

Elston, R. C. & Campbell, M. A. (1970) Schizophrenia: evidence for a major gene hypothesis. *Behavioural Genetics*, **1**, 3–10.

Emery, A. E. (1986) *Methodology in Medical Genetics: An Introduction to Statistical Methods* (2nd edn). Edinburgh: Churchill Livingstone.

Erlenmeyer-Kimling, L. & Cornblatt, B. (1987) High-risk research in schizophrenia: a summary of what has been learned. *Journal of Psychiatric Research*, **21**, 401–411.

Falconer, D. S. (1965) The inheritance of liability to certain diseases, estimated from the incidence among relatives. *Annuls of Human Genetics*, **29**, 51–76.

Falkai, P., Bogerts, B., Greve, B., *et al* (1992) Loss of Sylvian fissure asymmetry in schizophrenia: A quantitative post-mortem study. *Schizophrenia Research*, **7**, 23–32.

Faraone, S. V. & Tsuang, M. T. (1985) Quantitative models of genetic transmission of schizophrenia. *Psychological Bulletin*, **98**, 41–46.

Farde, L., Wiesel, F. A., Hall, H., *et al* (1987) No D2 receptor increase in PET study of schizophrenia. *Archives of General Psychiatry*, **44**, 671–672.

——, ——, Nordstrom, A. L., *et al* (1989) D1 and D2 dopamine receptors occupancy during treatment with conventional and atypical neuroleptics. *Psychopharmacology*, **99**, S28–S31.

—, —, Stone-Elander, S., *et al* (1990) D2 receptors in neuroleptic-naive schizophrenic patients: a positron emission study with [11C] Raclopride.*Archives of General Psychiatry*, **47**, 213–219.

Faris, R. E. L. & Dunham, H. W. (1939) *Mental Disorders in Urban Areas*. Chicago: Chicago University Press.

Foerster, A., Lewis, S., Owen, M., *et al* (1991) Premorbid adjustment and personality in psychosis: Effects of sex and diagnosis. *British Journal of Psychiatry*, **158**, 171–176.

Frith, C. D. (1992) *The Cognitive Neuropsychology of Schizophrenia*. Hove,: Laurence Erlbaum.

Frith, C. D. & Done, D. J. (1988) Towards a neuropsychology of schizophrenia. *British Journal of Psychiatry*, **153**, 437–443.

Giggs, J. A. & Cooper, J. E. (1987) Ecological structure and the distribution of schizophrenia and affective psychosis in Nottingham. *British Journal of Psychiatry*, **151**, 627–633.

Gill, M., McGuffin, P., Parfitt, E., *et al* (1993) A linkage study of schizophrenia with DNA markers from the long arm of chromosome 11. *Psychological Medicine*, **23**, 27–44.

Goldberg, E. M. & Morrison, S. L. (1963) Schizophrenia and social class. *British Journal of Psychiatry*, **109**, 785–802.

Goldberg, T. E., Raglan, J. D., Torrey, E. F., *et al* (1990) Neuropsychological assessment of monozygotic twins discordant for schizophrenia. *Archives of General Psychiatry*, **47**, 1066–1072.

—, Torrey, E. F., Gold, J. M., *et al* (1993) Learning and memory in mono-zygotic twin pairs discordant for schizophrenia. *Psychological Medicine*, **23**, 71–85.

Goldstein, G. (1986) The neuropsychology of schizophrenia. In *Neuropsychological Assessment of Neuropsychiatric Disorders* (eds I. Grant & K. M. Adams), pp. 147–171. New York: Oxford University Press.

Goldstein, M. J. (1985). Family factors that antedate the onset of schizophrenia and related disorders: the results of a fifteen year prospective longitudinal study. *Acta Psychiatrica Scandinavica*, **71** (suppl. 319), 7–18.

Gottesman, I. I. & Shields, J. (1967) A polygenic theory of schizophrenia.*Proceedings of the National Academy of Science*, **58**, 199–205.

— & — (1982) *Schizophrenia: The Epigenetic Puzzle*. New York: Cambridge University Press.

— & Bertelsen, A. (1989) Confirming unexpressed genotypes for schizophrenia. Risks in the offspring of Fischer's Danish identical and fraternal discordant twins. *Archives of General Psychiatry*, **46**, 862–872.

Grandy, D. K., Litt, M., Allen, L., *et al* (1989) The human dopamine receptor gene is located on chromosome 11 at q22–q23 and identifies a Taq1 RFLP.*American Journal of Human Genetics*, **45**, 778–785.

Gray, J. A. (1982) *The Neuropsychology of Anxiety: an Enquiry into the Function of the Septo-Hippocampal System*. Oxford: Oxford University Press.

—, Feldon, J., Rawlins, J. P. N., *et al* (1991) The neuropsychology of schizophrenia. *Behavioural Brain Science*, **14**, 1–20.

Grillon, C., Courchesne, E., Ameli, R., *et al* (1990) Increased distractibility in schizophrenic patients: electrophysiologic and behavioural evidence.*Archives of General Psychiatry*, **47**, 171–179.

Gunther, W., Petsch, R., Steinberg, R., *et al* (1991) Brain dysfunction during motor activation and corpus callosum alterations in schizophrenia measured by cerebral blood flow and magnetic resonance imaging. *Biological Psychiatry*, **29**, 535–553.

Hahlweg, K., Goldstein, M. J., Neuchterlein K. H., *et al* (1989) Expressed emotion and patient–relative interaction in families of recent onset schizophrenics. *Journal of Consulting & Clinical Psychology*, **57**, 11–18.

Hare, E. H. (1956) Mental illness and social conditions in Bristol. *Journal of Mental Science*, **102**, 349–357.

Harrison, G. (1991) Searching for the causes of schizophrenia, The role of migrant studies. *Schizophrenia Bulletin*, **16**, 663–671.

——, Owens, D., Holton, A., *et al* (1988) A prospective study of severe mental disorder in Afro-Caribbean patients. *Psychological Medicine*, **18**, 643–657.

Harvey, I., Williams, M., Toone, B. K., *et al* (1990) The ventricular-brain ration (VBR) in functional psychoses: the relationship of lateral ventricular and total intracranial area. *Psychological Medicine*, **20**, 55–62.

——, Ron, M. A., DuBoulay, G., *et al* (1993) Reduction of cortical volume in schizophrenia on magnetic resonance imaging. *Psychological Medicine*, **23**, 591–604.

Heckers, S., Heinsen, H., Heinsen, Y. C., *et al* (1991) Cortex, white matter and basal ganglia in schizophrenia: A volumetric post-mortem study. *Biological Psychiatry*, **29**, 556–566.

Hemsley, D. R. (1992) Cognitive abnormalities and schizophrenic symptoms. *Psychological Medicine*, **22**, 839–842.

—— (1994) Cognitive disturbances as the link between schizophrenic symptoms and their biological bases. *Neurology, Psychiatry and Brain Research*, **2**, 163–170.

Heston, L. L. (1966) Psychiatric disorder in foster home-reared children of schizophrenic mothers. *British Journal of Psychiatry*, **112**, 819–825.

Hindley, J. (1983) *DNA Sequencing: Laboratory Techniques in Biochemistry and Molecular Genetics.* Amsterdam: Elsevier Science Publishers.

Hirsch, S. R. & Leff, J. P. (1975) *Abnormalities in the Parents of Schizophrenics.* Oxford: Oxford University Press.

Holland, A. & Gosden, C. (1990) A balanced chromosomal translocation partially co-segregating with psychotic illness in a family. *Psychiatric Research*, **32**, 1–8.

Hollingshead, A. B. & Redlich, F. C. (1954) Schizophrenia and social structure. *American Journal of Psychiatry*, **110**, 695–701.

Hornykiewicz, O. (1982) Brain catecholamine in schizophrenia – a good case for noradrenaline. *Nature*, **299**, 484–486.

Huber, G. (1957) *Pneumoencephalograpische and psychopathologische Bilder bei endogen Psychosen.* Berlin: Springer-Verlag.

——, Gross, G. & Schutter, R. (1975) A long-term follow-up study of schizophrenia: psychiatric course of illness and prognosis. *Acta Psychiatrica Scandinavica*, **52**, 49–57.

Ineichen, B., Harrison, G. & Morgan, H. G. (1984) Psychiatric hospital admissions in Bristol: I. Geographical and ethnic factors. *British Journal of Psychiatry*, **145**, 600–604.

Iqbal, N., Asnis, G. M., Wetzler, S., *et al* (1991) The MCPP challenge test in schizophrenia: hormonal and behavioural responses. *Biological Psychiatry*, **30**, 770–778.

Jacob, T. & Grounds, L. (1978) Confusions and conclusions: A response to Doane. *Family Process*, **17**, 377–387.

Jakob, J. & Beckman, H. (1986) Prenatal developmental disturbances in the limbic allocortex in schizophrenics. *Journal of Neural Transmission*, **65**, 303–326.

Javitt, D. C. & Zukin, S. R. (1991) Recent advances in the phencyclidine model of schizophrenia. *American Journal of Psychiatry*, **148**, 1301–1308.

Jenkins, J. H. & Karno, M. (1992) The meaning of Expressed Emotion: theoretical issues raised by cross cultural research. *American Journal of Psychiatry*, **149**, 9–21.

Jernigan, T. L., Zisook, S., Heaton, R. K., *et al* (1991) Magnetic resonance imaging abnormalities in lenticular nuclei and cerebral cortex in schizophrenia. *Archives of General Psychiatry*, **48**, 881–890.

Johnstone, E. C., Crow, T. J., Frith, C. D., *et al* (1976) Cerebral ventricular size and cognitive impairment in chronic schizophrenia. *Lancet*, *ii*, 924–926.

——, Owens, D. G. C., Crow, T. J., *et al* (1989) Temporal lobe structure as determined by nuclear magnetic resonance in schizophrenia and bipolar affective disorder. *Journal of Neurosurgery and Psychiatry*, **52**, 736–741.

Jones, P. B. & Murray, R. M. (1991) The genetics of schizophrenia is the genetics of neurodevelopment. *British Journal of Psychiatry*, **158**, 615–623.

——, Bebbington, P., Foerster, A., *et al* (1993) Premorbid underachievement in schizophrenia: Results from the Camberwell Collaborative Psychosis Study. *British Journal of Psychiatry*, **162**, 65–71.

——, Rodgers, B., Murray, R., *et al* (1994) Child developmental risk factors for adult schizophrenia in the British 1946 birth cohort. *Lancet*, **344**, 1398–1402.

Karson, C. N., Garcia-Rill, E., Biedermann, J. A. *et al* (1991) The brain stem reticular formation in schizophrenia. *Psychiatry Research*, **40**, 31–48.

Kavanagh, D. J. (1992) Recent developments in expressed emotion and schizophrenia. *British Journal of Psychiatry*, **160**, 601–620.

Keith, S. J., Regier, D. A. & Rae, D. S. (1991) Schizophrenic disorders. In *Psychiatric Disorders in America* (eds L. N. Robins & D. A. Regier). New York: Free Press.

Kelsoe, J. R., Cadet, J. L., Pickar, D., *et al* (1988) Quantitative neuroanatomy in schizophrenia. *Archives of General Psychiatry*, **45**, 533–541.

Kendell, R. E. & Kemp, I. W. (1989) Maternal influenza in the aetiology of schizophrenia. *Archives of General Psychiatry*, **46**, 878–882.

Kendler, K. S. (1988) The genetics of schizophrenia: an overview. In *Handbook of Schizophrenia*, (vol 3) (eds M. T. Tsuang & J. C. Simpson), pp. 437–462. Amsterdam: Elsevier.

Kennedy, J. L., Giuffra, L. A., Moises, H. W., *et al* (1988) Evidence against linkage of schizophrenia to markers on chromosome 5 in a northern Swedish pedigree. *Nature*, **336**, 167–169.

Kerwin, R., Patel, S., Meldrum, B., *et al* (1988) Asymmetrical loss of a glutamate receptor subtype in left hippocampus in post-mortem schizophrenic brain. *Lancet*, *i*, 583–584.

——, —— & —— (1990) Quantitative auto-radiographic analysis of glutamate binding sites in the hippocampal formation in normal and schizophrenic brain post-mortem. *Neuroscience*, **39**, 25–32.

Kety, S., Rosenthal, D., Wender, P. H., *et al* (1968) The types and prevalence of mental illness in the biological and adoptive families of adopted schizophrenics. *Journal of Psychiatric Research*, **6**, 345–362.

Kety, S. S., Rosenthal, D., Wender, P. H. *et al* (1975) In *Genetic Research in Psychiatry* (eds R. Fieve, D. Rosenthal & H. Brill). Baltimore: Johns Hopkins Press.

Kohn, M. L. (1975) Social class and schizophrenia: A critical review and reformulation. In *Annual Review of the Schizophrenic Syndrome* (ed R. Cancro). New York: Brunner/Mazel.

Kringlen, E. (1967) *Heredity and Environment in the Functional Psychoses*. Oslo: Universitetsforlaget.

Kuipers, L. (1994) The measurement of expressed emotion: its influence on research and clinical practice. *International Reviews of Psychiatry*, **6**, 187–199.

Lander, E. S. (1988) Splitting schizophrenia. *Nature*, **336**, 105–106.

Lane, E. A. & Albee, G. W. (1966) Comparative birth weights of schizophrenics and their siblings. *Journal of Psychology*, **64**, 227–231.

Lefley, H. P. (1992) Expressed emotion: Conceptual, clinical, and social policy issues. *Hospital and Community Psychiatry* **43**, 591–598.

Lesch, A. & Bogerts, B. (1984) The dicencephalon in schizophrenia: Evidence for reduced thickness of the periventricular grey matter. *European Archives of Psychiatric Neurological Sciences*, **234**, 212–219.

Lewine, R. J. (1988) Gender and schizophrenia. In *Handbook of Schizophrenia* (vol. 3) (ed. H. A. Nasrallah). Amsterdam: Elsevier.

Lewis, G., David, A., Andreasson, S., *et al* (1992) Schizophrenia and city life. *Lancet*, **34**, 137–140.

Lewis, S. W. & Mezey, G. C. (1985) Clinical correlates of septum pellucidum cavities: an unusual association with psychosis. *Psychological Medicine*, **15**, 43–54.

—— & Murray, R. M. (1987) Obstetric complications, neurodevelopmental deviance, and risk of schizophrenia. *Journal of Psychiatric Research*, **4**, 413–421.

——, Reveley, M. A., David, A. S., *et al* (1988) Agenesis of the corpus callosum and schizophrenia: a case report. *Psychological Medicine*, **18**, 341–347.

Liddle, P. F., Friston, K. J., Frith, C. D., *et al* (1992) Patterns of cerebral blood flow in schizophrenia. *British Journal of Psychiatry*, **160**, 179–186.

Lishman, W. A. (1987) Cerebral tumours. In *Organic Psychiatry, the Psychological Consequences of Cerebral Disorder*, p.198. Oxford: Blackwell.

Littlewood, R. & Lipsedge, M. (1981) Acute psychotic reactions in Caribbean born patients. *Psychological Medicine*, **11**, 303–318.

Lohr, J. B. & Jeste, D. V. (1988) Locus ceruleus morphometry in aging and schizophrenia. *Acta Psychiatrica Scandinavica*, **77**, 689–697.

MacGillivray, I., Campbell, D. M. & Thompson, D. (1988) *Twinning and Twins*. Chichester: Wiley.

Machon, R. A., Mednick, S. F. & Schulsinger, F. (1983) The interaction of seasonality, place of birth, genetic risk and subsequent schizophrenia in a high-risk sample. *British Journal of Psychiatry*, **143**, 383–388.

MacMillan, J. F., Gold, A., Crow, T. J., *et al* (1986) Expressed emotion and relapse. *British Journal of Psychiatry*, **148**, 133–143.

Malzberg, B. & Lee, E. S. (1956) *Migration and Mental Disease: A Study of First Admissions to Hospitals for Mental Disease in New York 1939–1941*. New York: Social Science Research Council.

Mankoo, B., Sherrington, R., Brynjolfsson, J., *et al* (1991) New microsatellite polymorphisms provide a highly polymorphic map of chromosome 5 bands q11. 2–q13. 3 for linkage analysis of Icelandic and English families affected by schizophrenia. *Abstract in Psychiatric Genetics*, **2**, 17.

Matthysse, S. W. & Kidd, K. K. (1976) Estimating the genetic contribution to schizophrenia. *American Journal of Psychiatry*, **133**, 185–191.

McCreadie, R. G., Robertson, L. J., Hall, D. J., *et al* (1993) The Nithsdale Schizophrenia Surveys. XI. Relatives' expressed emotion. Stability over five years and its relation to relapse. *British Journal of Psychiatry*, **162**, 393–397.

McGue, M., Gottesman, I. I. & Rao, D. C. (1985) Resolving genetic models for the transmission of schizophrenia. *Genetic Epidemiology*, **2**, 99–110.

—— & Gottesman, I. I. (1990) *Genetic Approaches in the Prevention of Mental Disorders*. Berlin: Springer-Verlag.

McGuffin, P. & Sturt, E. (1986) Genetic markers in schizophrenia. *Human Heredity*, **36**, 65–88.

——, Farmer, A. & Gottesman, I. I. (1987) Is there really a split in schizophrenia? *British Journal of Psychiatry*, **150**, 581–592.

——, Sargeant, M., Hett, G., *et al* (1990) Exclusion of a schizophrenia susceptibility gene from the chromosome 5q11–13 region: new data and a reanalysis of previous reports. *American Journal of Human Genetics*, **47**, 524–535.

Mednick, S. A., Machon, R. A., Huttenen, M. O., *et al* (1998) Adult schizophrenia following prenatal exposure to an influenza epidemic. *Archives of General Psychiatry*, **45**, 189–192.

——, ——, ——, *et al* (1990) Influenza and schizophrenia. *Archives of General Psychiatry*, **47**, 875–877.

Miklowitz, D. J., Goldstein, M. J., Falloon, I. R. H., *et al* (1984) Interactional correlates of expressed emotion in the families of schizophrenics. *British Journal of Psychiatry*, **144**, 482–487.

Moises, H. W., Gelernter, J., Giuffra, L., *et al* (1991) No linkage between D2 dopamine receptor gene region and schizophrenia. *Archives of General Psychiatry*, **48**, 643–647.

Murray, R. M., O'Callaghan, E., Castle, D. J., *et al* (1992) A neurodevelopmental approach to the classification of schizophrenia. *Schizophrenia Bulletin*, **18**, 319–332.

Nasrallah, H. A., Andreasen, N. C., Coffman, J. A., *et al* (1986) A controlled mangetic resonance imaging study of corpus callosum thickness in schizophrenia. *Biological Psychiatry*, **21**, 274–282.

Nemeroff, C. B. (1991) Neuropeptides and schizophrenia. In *Advances in Neuropsychiatry and Psychopharmacology* (eds C. A. Tamminga & S. C. Schulz). New York: Raven Press.

Neuchterlein, K. H. & Dawson, M. E. (1984*a*) Information processing and attentional functioning in the developmental course of schizophrenic disorders. *Schizophrenia Bulletin*, **10**, 160–203.

—— & —— (1984*b*) A heuristic vulnerability/stress model of schizophrenic episodes. *Schizophrenia Bulletin*, **10**, 300–312.

—— & Zaucha, K. M. (1990) Similarities between information processing abnormalities of acutely symptomatic schizophrenic patients and high-risk children. In *Schizophrenia: Concepts, Vulnerability and Intervention* (eds E. Straube & K. Halweg). Berlin: Springer-Verlag.

Norman, R. M. G. & Malla, A. K. (1993*a*) Stressful life events and schizophrenia. I: A review of the research. *British Journal of Psychiatry*, **162**, 161–165.

—— & —— (1993*b*) Stressful life events and schizophrenia. II: Conceptual and methodological issues. *British Journal of Psychiatry*, **162**, 166–174.

O'Callaghan, E., Gibson, T., Colohan, H., *et al* (1991*a*) Season of birth effect in schizophrenia. *British Journal of Psychiatry*, **158**, 764–769.

——, Sham, P., Takei, N., *et al* (1991*b*) Schizophrenia after prenatal exposure to 1957 A2 influenza epidemic. *Lancet*, **337**, 1248–1250.

O'Rourke, D. H., Gottesman, I. I., Suarez, B. K., *et al* (1982) Refutation of the general single-locus model for the aetiology of schizophrenia. *American Journal of Human Genetics*, **34**, 325–333.

Odegaard, O. (1932) Emigration and insanity. *Acta Psychiatrica Scandinavica*, suppl. 4.

Ott, J. (1985) *Analysis of Human Genetic Linkage*. Baltimore: Johns Hopkins University Press.

Owen, M. & McGuffin, P. (1991) DNA and classical genetic markers in schizophrenia. *European Archives of Psychiatry and Clinical Neuroscience*, **240**, 197–203.

——, Lewis, S. W. & Murray, R. M. (1988) Obstetric complications and cerebral abnormalities in schizophrenia. *Psychological Medicine*, **18**, 331–340.

Pakkenberg, B. (1987) Post-mortem study of chronic schizophrenic brains. *British Journal of Psychiatry*, **151**, 744–752.

Pickar, D., Breier, A., Hsiao, J. K., *et al* (1990) Cerebrospinal fluid and plasma monoamine metabolites and their relation to psychosis. *Archives of General Psychiatry*, **47**, 641–648.

Pilowsky, L. S., Costa, D. C., Ell, P. J., *et al* (1992) Clozapine, single photon emission tomography, and the D2 dopamine receptor blockade hypothesis of schizophrenia. *Lancet*, **340**, 199–202.

Puck, T. T. & Kao, F. T. (1982) Somatic cell genetics and its applications to medicine. *Annual Review of Genetics*, **16**, 225–272.

Pulver, A. E., Liang, K. Y., Brown, C. H., *et al* (1991) Risk factors in schizophrenia. *British Journal of Psychiatry*, **160**, 65–70.

Raine, A., Harrison, G. N., Reynolds, G. P., *et al* (1990) Structural and functional characteristics of the corpus callosum in schizophrenics, psychiatric controls, and normal controls. *Archives of General Psychiatry*, **47**, 1060–1063.

Rainey, J. M. & Crowder, M. K. (1975) Prolonged psychosis attributed to phencyclidine: report of three cases. *American Journal of Psychiatry*, **132**, 1076–1078.

Redlich, F. C, Hollingshead, A. B., Roberts, B. H., *et al* (1953) Social structure and psychiatric disorders. *American Journal of Psychiatry*, **109**, 729–734.

Reich, T., Cloninger, C. R. & Guze, S. B. (1975) The multifactorial model of disease transmission. *British Journal of Psychiatry*, **127**, 1–10.

Rosenfeld, H. (1965) *Psychotic States: A Psychoanalytical Approach*. London: Karnac.

Rosenthal, D., Wender, P. H., Kety, S. S., *et al* (1971) The adopted-away offspring of schizophrenics. *American Journal of Psychiatry*, **128**, 307–311.

—— & Bigelow, L. B. (1972) Quantitative brain measurements in chronic schizophrenia. *British Journal of Psychiatry*, **121**, 259–264.

Rutter, M., Bolton, P., Harrington, R., *et al* (1990) Genetic factors in child psychiatric disorders: I. A review of research strategies. *Journal of Child Psychology and Psychiatry*, **31**, 3–38.

Sartorius, N., Jablensky, A., Korten, A., *et al* (1986) Early manifestations and first-contact incidence of schizophrenia in different cultures. *Psychological Medicine*, **16**, 909–928.

Scarr, S. & Carter-Saltzman, L. (1979) Twin method: Defense of a critical assumption. *Behavioural Genetics*, **9**, 527–542.

Seidman, L. J., Yurgelun-Todd, D., Kremen, W. S., et al (1994) Relationship of prefrontal and temporal lobe MRI measures to neuropsychological performance in chronic schizophrenia. *Biological Psychiatry*, **35**, 235–236.

Shaikh, S., Collier, D., Kerwin, R. W., *et al* (1993) Dopamine D4 receptor subtypes and response to clozapine. *Lancet*, **341**, 116.

Sham, P., O'Callaghan, E., Takei, N., *et al* (1992) Schizophrenia following prenatal exposure to influenza epidemics between 1939 and 1960. *British Journal of Psychiatry*, **160**, 461–466.

Shenton, M. E., Kikinis, R., Jolesz, F. A., *et al* (1992) Left-lateralized temporal lobe abnormalities in schizophrenia and their relationship to thought disorder. A computerized, quantitative MRI study. *New England Journal of Medicine*, **327**, 604–612.

Sherrington, R., Brynjolffson, J., Petursson, H., *et al* (1988) Localisation of a susceptibility locus for schizophrenia on chromosome 5. *Nature*, **336**, 164–167.

Silverton, L. & Mednick, S. (1984) Class drift and schizophrenia. *Acta Psychiatrica Scandinavica*, **70**, 304–309.

Smith, M., Wasmuth, J., McPherson, J. D., *et al* (1989) Cosegregation of an 11q22–9p22 translocation with affective disorder: proximity of the dopamine D2 receptor gene relative to the translocation breakpoint. *American Journal of Human Genetics*, **45** (suppl.), A220.

Smith, C. (1974) Concordance in twins: methods and interpretation. *American Journal of Human Genetics*, **26**, 456–466.

Smith, J., Birchwood, M., Cochrane, R., *et al* (1993) The needs of high and low expressed emotion families: a normative approach. *Social Psychiatry and Psychiatric Epidemiology*, **28**, 11–16.

Southard, E. E. (1915) On the topographic distribution of cortex lesions and anomalies in dementia praecox with some account of their functional significance. *American Journal of Insanity*, **71**, 603–671.

St Clair, D., Blackwood, D., Muir, W., *et al* (1989) No linkage of chromosome 5q11–q13 markers to schizophrenia in Scottish families. *Nature*, **339**, 305–309.

——, ——, ——, *et al* (1990) Association within a family of a balanced autosomal translocation with major mental illness. *Lancet*, **336**, 164–167.

Steinberg, H. R. & Durrell, J. (1968) A stressful social situation as a precipitant of schizophrenic symptoms: an epidemiological study. *British Journal of Psychiatry*, **114**, 1097–1105.

Strang, J. & Gurling, H. (1989) Computerized tomography and neuropsychological assessment in long-term high-dose heroin addicts. *British Journal of Addiction*, **84**, 1011–1019.

Suddath, R. L., Christison, G. W., Torrey, E. F., *et al* (1990) Anatomical abnormalities in the brains of monozygotic twins discordant for schizophrenia. *New England Journal of Medicine*, **322**, 789–794.

Swayze, W., Andreasen, N. C., Erhardt, J. C., *et al* (1990) Development abnormalities of the corpus callosum in schizophrenia: an MRI study. *Archives of Neurology*, **47**, 805–808.

Takei, N., O'Callaghan, E., Sham, P., *et al* (1992) Winter birth excess in schizophrenia: its relationship to place of birth. *Schizophrenia Research*, **6**, 102.

Tarrier, N. & Turpin, G. (1992) Psychosocial factors, arousal, and schizophrenic relapse. The psychophysiological data. *British Journal of Psychiatry*, **161**, 3–11.

Tienari, P. (1991). Interaction between genetic vulnerability and family environment: The Finnish adoptive study of schizophrenia. *Acta Psychiatrica Scandinavica*, **84**, 460–465.

—— (1992) Implications of adoption studies on schizophrenia. *British Journal of Psychiatry*, **161** (Suppl. 18), 52–58.

——, Lahti, I., Sorri, A., *et al* (1987) The Finnish adoptive family study of schizophrenia. *Journal of Psychiatric Research*, **21**, 437–484.

Treff, W. M. & Hempel, K. J. (1958) Die Zelidichte bei Schizophrenen und klinisch Gesunden. *Journal fur Hirnforschung*, **4**, 314–369.

Tsuang, M. T. & Farrone, S. V. (1990) *The Genetics of Mood Disorders*. Baltimore: The Johns Hopkins University Press.

Turner, R. J. & Wagenfeld, M. O. (1967) Occupational mobility and schizophrenia: An assessment of the social causation and social selection hypothesis. *American Sociology Review*, **32**, 104–113.

van Os, J., Fahy, T. A., Jones, P., *et al* (1995) Increased intracerebral cerebrospinal fluid spaces predict unemployment and negative symptoms in psychotic illness. A prospective study. *British Journal of Psychiatry*, **166**, 750–758.

van Praag, H. M. (1986) Biological suicide research: outcome and limitations. *Biological Psychiatry*, **21**, 1305–1323.

Vinogradov, S., Gottesman, I. I., Moises, H., *et al* (1991) Negative association between schizophrenia and rheumatoid arthritis. *Schizophrenia Bulletin*, **17**, 669–678.

Watt, N. F. (1978) Patterns of childhood social development in adult schizophrenics. *Archives of General Psychiatry*, **35**, 160–165.

Weinberger, D. R., Berman, K. F., Suddath, R., *et al* (1992) Evidence of dysfunction of a pre-frontal-limbic network in schizophrenia: A magnetic resonance imaging and regional cerebral blood flow study of discordant monozygotic twins. *American Journal of Psychiatry*, **149**, 880–897.

Wender, P. H., Rosenthal, D. & Kety, K. (1968) A psychiatric assessment of the adoptive parents of schizophrenics. In *The Transmission of Schizophrenia*. (eds D. Rosenthal & S. Kety). Oxford: Pergamon Press.

——, ——, ——, *et al* (1974) Cross fostering: a research strategy for clarifying the role of genetic and experimental factors in the aetiology of schizophrenia. *Archives of General Psychiatry*, **30**, 121–128.

Wessely, S., Castle, D., Der G., *et al* (1991) Schizophrenia and Afro-Caribbeans: A case-control study. *British Journal of Psychiatry*, **159**, 795–801.

Wetherall, D. (1992) *The New Genetics and Clinical Practice* (3rd edn). Oxford: Oxford University Press.

Witelson, S. F. (1989) Hand and sex differences in the isthmus and genu of the human corpus callosum. *Brain*, **112**, 799–833.

Woerner, M. G., Pollack, M. & Klein D. F. (1971) Birth weight and length in schizophrenics personality disorders and their siblings. *Brittish Journal of Psychiatry*, **118**, 461–464.

Wong, D. F., Wagner, H. N., Tune, L. E., *et al* (1986) Positron emission tomography reveals elevated D2 dopamine receptors in drug-naive schizophrenics. *Science*, **234**, 1558–1563.

Woodruff, P. W. R. (1994) Structural magnetic resonance imaging in psychiatry – the functional psychoses. In *Cambridge Medical Reviews: Neurobiology and Psychiatry 3* (eds R. Kerwin, D. Dawbarn, J. McCulloch, *et al*). Cambridge University Press.

——, Pearlson, G. D., Geer, M. J., *et al* (1993) A computerized magnetic resonance imaging study of corpus callosum morphology in schizophrenia. *Psychological Medicine*, **23**, 45–56.

——, Howard, R., Rushe, T., *et al* (1994) Frontal lobe volume and cognitive estimation in schizophrenia. *Schizophrenia Research*, **11**, 133–134.

——, McMannus, I. C. & David, I. S. (1995*a*) A meta-analysis of corpus callosum size i schizophrenia. *Journal of Neurology, Neurosurgery and Psychiatry*, **58**, 457–461.

——, Branmmer, M., Mellers, J., *et al* (1995*b*) Auditory hallucinations and peception of external speech. *Lancet*, **346**, 1035.

Wynne, L. & Singer, M. (1963*a*) Thought disorder and family relations of schizophrenics. I. Research strategy. *Archives of General Psychiatry*, **9**, 191–198.

—— & —— (1963*b*) Thought disorder and family relations of schizophrenics. II. A classification of forms of thinking. *Archives of General Psychiatry*, **9**, 199–206.

Young, A. H., Blackwood, D. H. R., Roxborough, H., *et al* (1991) A magnetic resonance imaging study of schizophrenia: brain structure and clinical symptoms. *British Journal of Psychiatry*, **158**, 158–164.

Youseff, H. A., Kinsella, A. & Waddington, J. L. (1991) Evidence for geographical variations in the prevalence of schizophrenia in rural Ireland. *Archives of General Psychiatry*, **48**, 254–258.

Zubin, J. (1988) Chronicity versus vulnerability. In *Handbook of Schizophrenia: Nosology, Epidemiology and Genetics* (vol 3) (eds M. T. Tsuang & J. C. Simpson), pp. 463–480. Elsevier: Amsterdam.

9 The drug treatment of schizophrenia

David Cunningham Owens

Terminology • Antipsychotic drugs • Clinical management • The acute phase • The post-acute phase • The maintenance phase • Dose equivalence • Pregnancy and lactation • Treatment resistance • Interactions • Other drug treatments of schizophrenia • The treatment of post-psychotic depression • Adverse effects of antipsychotic drugs • Non-neurological adverse effects • Neurological adverse effects

---

"Dr Tyerman had tried shaving the head, blisters to the nape or vertex, occasional local depletion, once arteriotomy, calomel followed by purgatives, hot and cold shower baths during severe paroxyms, tonics ..." *Commissioners in Lunacy Annual Report, 1847 (Quoted A.T. Scull 'Museums of Madness')*

It is sobering in psychiatry to realise how little some things have changed. Substitute for each of the above (mercifully redundant) procedures, the name of an antipsychotic drug, and Dr Tyerman's efforts acquire an alarming air of modernity!

The introduction of antipsychotics into clinical psychiatric practice was what textbooks often refer to as 'serendipity'. Phenothiazine is an analogue of the aniline dye methylene blue and was in fact first synthesised over a century ago. It was used for a time as an antiseptic and an antihelminthic in veterinary practice but it was the discovery of antihistamine activity in 1937 that provided the impetus for development of this class of drugs at the Rhone-Poulenc Laboratories in Paris. Promethazine was the major product of this programme and because of its strong sedative properties it was tried in schizophrenics but was found to be no more effective than barbiturates. It did however potentiate barbiturates and caught the attention of a surgeon, Henri Laborit, who was investigating operative premedications. His so-called 'lytic (i.e. sympatho-/parasympatholytic) cocktail', of which promethazine became a part in 1949, was designed to reduce post-operative shock by reducing anxiety, decreasing the amount of general anaesthetic required, and speeding post-operative recovery.

In 1950 a chemist at Rhone-Poulenc, Paul Charpentier, synthesised a new phenothiazine derivative, chlorophenothiazine. This was less antihistaminic than promethazine, yet produced a greater reduction in autonomic activity. This in itself made it an excellent 'lytic' agent from a surgical point of view. However, Laborit further noted that it prompted a curious calm, unemotional indifference to the environment. This crucial observation led him to suggest that this new drug – renamed chlorpromazine – might be of interest to psychiatrists. Laborit's suggestion was not met with unbridled enthusiasm by the psychiatric community, but colleagues at the Val-de-Grace military hospital did try it. Their experience with a 24-year-old manic man was presented to the Societe Medico-Psychologique in February 1952 and published in the Society's Annals the following month. Jean Delay and Pierre Deniker of the L'Hopital St. Anne, also in Paris, reported their results at the prestigious Centennial of the Societe in May of 1952 and as a result priority is usually, somewhat incorrectly, attributed to them. But the modern era of psychopharmacology actually began on 28 December 1951, when J. Sigwald started chlorpromazine alone in a 57-year-old psychotic lady, "Madame Gob".

The introduction of chlorpromazine into psychiatry was therefore not really serendipity. It was certainly empirical but was based on the careful observations of a skilled clinician. The problem for psychiatrists is coming to terms with the fact that one of the major advances in our speciality rests on the keen observations of a surgeon!

Terminology

Many names have been given to the family of drugs used in the treatment of schizophrenia and other psychotic conditions. The antiquated term 'psycholeptics' is redundant and 'ataraxics' is, perhaps unfortunately, seen as old-fashioned. 'Antischizophrenics' is inaccurate as it is clear the beneficial effects of these preparations are non-specific and not confined solely to that form of psychosis we call schizophrenia. The term 'major tranquillisers' is still to be found, but is inappropriate. It implies an action that is merely secondary to sedation, which is not the case, and by analogy with 'minor tranquillisers' confuses the public with all the ills that these preparations have fallen victim to.

The most widely used term is 'neuroleptics', coined by Delay in 1955. It literally means 'seizing or acting on the nervous system' and has been strongly advocated as the appropriate term in view of the diversity of CNS actions it implies. When this class of drugs was named it was widely believed that their beneficial effects on psychotic symptomatology were necessarily linked to the production of extrapyramidal signs, a view that fell into disrepute by the 1960s. In addition, not all the standard screening properties of classical 'neuroleptic' action, e.g. the production of catalepsy in laboratory animals, are possessed by all the compounds which are clinically effective against psychosis. And of course, any number of drugs, from antidepressants to analgesics, have any number of CNS actions yet are classified on the basis of their major clinical function. Increasingly, the simple descriptive term 'antipsychotics' seems most appropriate and this term will be used in this chapter.

Antipsychotic drugs

Classification and structures

The major classifications of the antipsychotic drugs and the preparations currently available in the United Kingdom are shown in Table 9.1.

Phenothiazines

A large number of phenothiazines have been synthesised although only a few have become available clinically. Chlorpromazine, because of its long use, is regarded by many as the reference antipsychotic drug, although pharmacologically speaking it is a 'dirty' drug and, particularly in the United States, more pharmacologically 'pure' preparations (e.g. haloperidol) have been advocated as the standard against which new treatments should be tested.

All phenothiazines share the same tricyclic structure from which they gain their name – two benzene rings (PHENO-) linked by a central ring containing a sulphur (THIO-) and a nitrogen (-AZO-) atom (Appendix 1, page 450). Compounds differ in the substitutions at positions 2 (the R1 position) and 10 (the R2 position). Substitution at the R1 position is necessary to enhance antipsychotic activity. For example promazine, which has weak antipsychotic activity, and chlorpromazine differ only in the latter's R1 halogen substitution; and the potent trifluoperazine differs from the clinically weak prochlorperazine only in its R1 trifluoromethyl (-CF$_3$) substitution.

Phenothiazines are however classified on the basis of the chemical nature of the R2 substituted side chains. The major groups are *aliphatic*, *piperidine* and *piperazine*.

Aliphatic compounds tend to be sedative and of relatively low potency. Piperidine compounds are roughly equipotent with their aliphatic counterparts but are more sedative. Piperazine compounds are of high potency, with relatively little autonomic activity but enhanced potential for producing extrapyramidal effects.

Thioxanthenes

These were developed in Denmark in the late 1950s and are structurally closely related to the phenothiazines (Appendix 1, page 451). They differ in that the nitrogen of the phenothiazine central ring (Position 10) is substituted by a double bond. As a result these compounds exhibit

Table 9.1 Antipsychotic drugs available in the UK (1995)

Phenothiazine	Aliphatic	Chlorpromazine	Largactil
		Promazine	Sparine
		Methotrimeprazine	Nozinan
	Piperidine	Thioridazine	Melleril
		Pericyazine	Neulactil
		Pipothiazine	Piportil*
	Piperazine	Trifluoperazine	Stelazine
		Perphenazine	Fentazine
		Fluphenazine	Modecate*
			Moditen
Butyrophenone		Haloperidol	Serenace
			Fortunan
			Dozic
			Haldol*
		Droperidol	Droleptan
		Trifluperidol	Triperidol
	Diphenylbutyl-piperidine	Pimozide	Orap
		Fluspirilene	Redeptin(*)
Thioxanthene		Flupenthixol	Depixol*
			Fluanxol
		Zuclopenthixol	Clopixol*
			Clopixol
			Acuphase (*)
Atypical	Substituted Benzamide	Sulpiride	Dolmatil
			Sulpitil
		Remoxipride	Roxiam ++
	Dibenzoxazepine	Loxapine	Loxapac
	Dibenzodiazepine	Clozapine	Clozaril ++
	Indolylazine	Oxypertine	Integrin
	Benzisoxazole	Risperidone	Risperdal

*Denotes long acting depot preparation, (*) See text, ++ Restricted use only.
The Phenothiazine Prochlorperazine ('Stemetil') and the Butyrophenome
Benperidol ('Anquil') are not conventionally used for antipsychotic purposes.

stereoisomerism – that is, the side chains attach in two 'mirror image' forms. This has a bearing on their clinical pharmacology. Although several thioxanthenes are commercially available in other countries, only flupenthixol, the thioxanthene analogue of fluphenazine, and clopenthixol, the analogue of perphenazine, are available in the UK.

Butyrophenones (and diphenylbutylpiperidines)

Butyrophenones were developed in Belgium around the same time as the thioxanthenes, and emerged from a programme exploring the analgesic properties of pethidine analogues. They are chemically quite unrelated to the phenothiazines (Appendix 1). They are of high potency and because of their relatively selective receptor actions, produce few of the general side-effects associated with phenothiazines. However they have a marked propensity to produce extrapyramidal side-effects (EPS) which may relate to their limited anticholinergic activity. The most potent butyrophenone, spiroperidol (or spiperone) is not used clinically but has widespread research application, particularly in receptor binding studies. The diphenylbutylpiperidines are basically butyrophenones with a modification in the side chain. This results in compounds with some of the longest biological half-lives found with antipsychotics.

Atypical antipsychotics

A chemically disparate group of compounds has been developed over the last 20 years or so which, although possessing antipsychotic properties, do not behave like the 'classical' antipsychotics on a range of laboratory tests by which these drugs have traditionally been defined. These are usually referred to collectively as 'atypical' antipsychotics, the most prominent of which are the substituted benzamides and clozapine although the recently licensed risperidone could also be considered under this heading.

Of the benzamides, only sulpiride and remoxipride are currently available in the UK but a range of these compounds has been synthesised, e.g. amisulpiride, sultopride, tiapride. These drugs are substituted amides of benzoic acid (Appendix 1) and were developed from the antiarrhythmic compound procainamide, via metoclopramide. Substituted benzamides have a strikingly different pharmacokinetic profile from 'classical' anti-psychotics, characterised by a low volume of distribution and relatively short half-life. Pharmacologically they are more selective in their receptor actions and have been reported as possessing a lesser potential for producing extrapyramidal side-effects. Clozapine is a dibenzazepine derivative (Appendix 1). In other words, it is chemically similar to imipramine and was in fact developed as a result of German clinicians' desire for new (tricyclic) antidepressants. The central ring is 7 membered rather than 6, and the side chain piperazine in type. Clozapine was found to have little antidepressant activity but was an effective antipsychotic. Unfortunately its development was dramatically curtailed in 1974 following reports from Scandinavia of eight deaths as a result of agranulocytosis. However, interest was once again stimulated by the results of a large multicentre study from the US demonstrating its efficacy in treatment-resistant schizophrenia (Kane *et al*, 1988). Clozapine is a novel compound with a unique pharmacological profile. It is strongly anticholinergic which may account for the apparent absence of major EPS with its use.

Risperidone, a benzisoxazole compound, is the first drug to emerge from a deliberate reversal of the strategy of producing new antipsychotics that are highly selective D_2 antagonists (e.g. such as the benzamides). It is a potent $5HT_2$ antagonist with lesser (x25) D_2 blocking ability. It also interacts with histamine H_1 and a_1 and a_2 adrenoreceptors. Initial evidence suggests that although not devoid of EPS, its potential for such is less than standard drugs (Owens, 1994).

Metabolism and pharmacokinetics

The study of antipsychotic pharmacokinetics has proved extremely difficult for several reasons. Firstly, wide inter-individual variations in blood levels (20-fold or more) have been found between subjects on similar regimes especially after oral administration (Alfredsson *et al*, 1984). Variations are less marked after intramuscular than after oral administration, which suggests that they reflect differences in the extent of pre-systemic metabolism. Secondly, specific genetic factors may also be important. About 10% of Caucasians exhibit a genetic polymorphism in the oxidation of debrisoquine and sparteine. These 'slow metabolisers' are deficient in the cytochrome isoenzyme P450 dbl on which some tricyclics and antipsychotics such as thioridazine and perphenazine depend for their elimination (see also page 176). This deficiency may lead to an accumulation of the parent drug and/or metabolites (Brosen & Gram, 1989) and may be a factor in varying tolerability as well as in variability of plasma levels. Thirdly, because of their lipophilicity and consequent wide distribution, antipsychotics are for the most part only present in very low – often nanomolar – concentrations in plasma, and detection has pushed present technology to the limits.

The main methods of measurement are gas-liquid chromatography (GLC) which is both sensitive and specific but is expensive; high performance liquid chromatography (HPLC) which enables metabolites to be studied but is less sensitive; radioimmunoassay (RIA) which is better for small volume samples, but lacks specificity; radioreceptor assay (RRA) which measures total dopamine blocking activity, but lacks both sensitivity and specificity.

A fourth reason for poor understanding of body handling is simply its sheer complexity. For example, textbooks often quote the half-life of chlorpromazine as 6–8 hours, which would result in virtually complete clearance within 48 hours. Yet it is known that evidence of ingestion can be detected up to two years after discontinuing phenothiazines (Forrest *et al*, 1964). The 6–8 hour figure appears to represent a distributional half-life – that is the fall from peak to trough resulting from tissue uptake during active ingestion. As most of this tissue localisation is reversible, cessation of treatment leads to slow leakage back into plasma. The terminal phase half-life of chlorpromazine, reflecting whole body decline, is around 60 days – which is compatible with detection of drug-related material for up to two years (Curry, 1986).

Oral administration

Most orally administered antipsychotics share common pharmacokinetic properties, the major exception being the substituted benzamides, which will be considered separately.

Classical antipsychotics are all well absorbed, although details of patterns and rates of absorption are unknown. All, especially phenothiazines, undergo extensive first-pass metabolism – that is metabolism in gut wall, lumen, and liver prior to an orally administered preparation reaching the systemic circulation. As a result, classical antipsychotics have low systemic availability, ranging from around 30% for chlorpromazine to 60% for haloperidol (Forsman & Ohman, 1976; Dahl & Strandjord, 1977). Furthermore, systemic clearance is high because of a high hepatic extraction ratio. Despite this, elimination half-lives are in the intermediate range, around 20 hours or more, largely because, as a result of their lipophilicity, they have a high apparent volume of distribution. Peak levels are attained 2–4 hours after oral administration although wide discrepancies have been reported for haloperidol (0.5–6 hours) (Jorgensen, 1986).

Typical, non-benzamide drugs are all over 90% protein bound, some more than 98%. Binding is reversible and dynamic, the major protein being albumen, although alpha-1-glycoprotein is also involved. This is important in two ways. Firstly, only the free fraction is available for receptor activity, and secondly, states associated with alterations in plasma protein levels (for example intercurrent illness, old age) will influence the proportion of unbound drug. These compounds readily cross the blood–brain barrier, presumably because of their lipophilicity although other physico-chemical properties may also operate. CSF concentrations have not been extensively studied but appear to show less inter-individual variation than those in plasma. Levels do, however, vary widely among preparations and formulations, ranging from 3–4% of plasma levels for chlorpromazine and haloperidol administered orally (Jorgensen, 1986), to around 50% for fluphenazine decanoate (Wiles & Gelder, 1980).

Metabolism is, in general, extensive with little or no parent drug excreted unchanged. Theoretically 168 metabolites have been postulated for chlorpromazine, although thankfully only a fraction have been identified. Haloperidol by contrast produces few metabolites. For phenothiazines and thioxanthenes, the major metabolic steps involve ring sulphoxidation and N-dealkylation in the side-chain. Some metabolites are conjugated, mainly with glucuronic acid, while others remain unconjugated.

Butyrophenones undergo primarily oxidative N-dealkylation which cleaves the molecule into two moieties. Aliphatic and aromatic alcohols are also formed.

The contribution that active metabolites make to the therapeutic effect and therapeutic blood levels is largely unknown. Some compounds have not yet been shown to produce any metabolites with intrinsic antipsychotic activity (e.g. flupenthixol, pimozide) but some commonly used drugs do produce metabolites with considerable *in vitro* binding activity and proven clinical efficacy. Examples include chlorpromazine sulphoxide, 7-hydroxychlorpromazine, and thioridazine-2-sulphoxide and 2-sulphone. A further complication is that plasma concentrations of metabolites may bear little relation to concentrations in brain. For example, both the side chain metabolites of thioridazine have more potent D_2 receptor affinities *in vitro* than the parent and the sulphoxide has in addition been reported as present in higher plasma concentrations. But as far as total drug components in the brain are concerned, the parent overwhelmingly predominates. Lipid solubility tends to decrease further down the metabolic pathway, which may help explain relatively poor brain penetrance of metabolites and perhaps a lesser therapeutic role than plasma levels might suggest. However, against this is the fact that metabolites tend to be less protein bound than parent compounds.

Benzamides differ in their pharmacokinetics from the classical antipsychotics. Of the two preparations currently available in the UK, sulpiride is marketed as a 1:1 mix of (+) and (-) sulpiride with the bulk of the antipsychotic efficacy attributable to the (-) enantiomer, while remoxipride is marketed as pure (-) enantiomer.

Bioavailability of sulpiride is low, with a calculated figure of 27%. Substantial amounts are recoverable from faeces and the drug appears to be subject to little first pass effect. Hence low availability appears to result from poor absorption. Remoxipride, by contrast seems to be rapidly and almost completely absorbed but likewise undergoes little first pass metabolism, so bioavailability is high at around 90% (Von Bahr *et al*, 1990). Both compounds are substantially less protein bound than classical drugs, with the free-fraction for remoxipride about 20%, and sulpiride as high as 60%. Peak plasma concentrations are reached after 2–6 hours, with remoxipride at the lower end. Half-life values for sulpiride are widely discrepant (Jorgensen, 1986), with an average of 8 hours suggested, while for remoxipride they are in the range 4–7 hours. Benzamides are subject to a number of metabolic steps, but despite this they are to a large extent excreted unchanged in urine. No antipsychotic action has been attributed to any of the metabolites.

The bioavailability of clozapine is on average 50–60%, although with some wide variations reported. It is subject to extensive first pass metabolism, with formation of N-desmethyl and N-oxide metabolites of low pharmacological activity. The percentage protein binding of clozapine is unclear, although apparent volume of distribution is lower than most other antipsychotics which suggests less tissue uptake. Peak levels are attained after an average of two hours and the nominal elimination half-life is about 12 hours. Steady state should be reached after about one week on stable twice-daily regimes.

Risperidone is well absorbed with plasma levels peaking at two hours. Its bioavailability is about 66%, indicating some first pass effects. Approximately 88% of the parent drug is protein bound. Risperidone's metabolism is of interest. It readily undergoes hydroxylation to 9-hydroxyrisperidone which has antipsychotic activity. Since metabolism is cytochrome P450 dbl dependent the proportion of parent to metabolite varies substantially depending on the patient's phenotype. However, the overall 'antipsychotic fraction' – the combination of both parent and metabolite – remains the same in 'fast' as in 'slow' metabolisers.

Depot administration

Depot antipsychotics are manufactured by esterification of their hydroxyl group to a long chain fatty acid, the resulting esters being dissolved in vegetable oil. The characteristics of the oil are important since one of the main factors contributing to the sustained release property is the oil/water partition co-efficient. Most manufacturers use sesame oil, although flupenthixol decanoate and zuclopenthixol decanoate are dissolved in a proprietary low viscosity trigylceride called Viscoleo, which appears to be degraded more rapidly than sesame oil. This may be a factor in why fluphenazine is generally detectable for a longer period after last injection than flupenthixol. There is evidence from animal studies that chronic intramuscular injection of these oils may lead to lymphatic absorption with the possible risk of pulmonary oil microembolisms, although it seems unlikely that this represents a clinically significant problem.

Once injected, esters slowly diffuse from the oil to be rapidly hydrolysed by plasma esterases, thus releasing the active drug. The rate limiting step in release is therefore diffusion of the esterified compound from the oil vehicle. The nature of the fatty acid used to some extent determines the rate of release. For example, zuclopenthixol esterified with acetic acid (Clopixol Acuphase) gives plasma concentration curves closer to those obtained following intramuscular injection of aqueous solutions than those following injection of the same drug esterified with decanoic acid (Clopixol). Although escape of esters from the oil vehicle is usually described as occurring by diffusion, the process is probably more complex involving dispersal of the oil and perhaps even its partial metabolism.

The slow release of active drug with long-acting depots profoundly affects their pharmacokinetics which are rate-limited not by the rate of metabolism, as with oral preparations, but by the rate of absorption (i.e. release) (Jann *et al*, 1985). In other words, the absorption rate constant

Table 9.2 Some characteristics of depot antipsychotics

Preparation	Time to peak plasma level	'Disappearance' half-life (approx.)
Fluphenazine decanoate	2–18 hours	7–10 days
Pipothiazine palmitate	?	7–12 days
Flupenthixol decanoate	4–10 days	*
Clopenthixol decanoate	4–7 days	20 days
Haloperidol decanoate	1–3 days	20 days

* Widely divergent figures reported in different subjects minimum 5 days, maximum 112 days (average 49.6 days)

is less than the elimination rate constant, and a so-called 'flip-flop' pharmacokinetic model pertains. Consequently curves of decline in plasma levels are difficult to interpret as they reflect not simply metabolism but also continuing absorption.

There are two main kinetic consequences of depot presentation of antipsychotics. The first is that by being given intramuscularly they avoid first pass effects and this may lead to lower concentrations of circulating metabolites than when oral drugs are used. Secondly, they require longer to reach steady state after starting treatment and then to disappear from plasma after the cessation of treatment. These differences have obvious and important clinical implications.

The first long-acting antipsychotic was produced by esterification of the side chain of fluphenazine hydrochloride with heptanoic acid to produce fluphenazine enanthate ('Moditen'). Although still available this is now little used, having been largely supplanted by fluphenazine decanoate (Modecate). The decanoate is unique among depots in producing a sharp, transient post-injection peak in blood levels maximal from 2 to 24 hours, after which the levels return to about one-third peak levels, with a subsequent slow decline (Jann *et al*, 1985). The reasons for this phenomenon are unclear. One possible cause may be the unique property of fluphenazine to bind to muscle at the injection site, rendering it particularly susceptible to initial hydrolysis by plasma esterases. Other depots show a slower rise to peak levels followed by a gradual decline (Jann *et al*, 1985). Some characteristics are shown in Table 9.2.

Most depots require approximately three months to attain steady state after commencing treatment, although with fluphenazine decanoate this may occur somewhat earlier (about 4–6 weeks). Zuclopenthixol acetate has, as noted, pharmacokinetic properties more akin to those of an injected aqueous solution, with peak levels obtained in about 24 hours and plasma concentrations one-third peak at approximately 72 hours.

Fluspirilene is not a depot as the term has been used, but a diphenylbutylpiperidine with a long half-life (three weeks) characteristic of this group. It is insoluble in water, but is administered as a particle suspension which forms, in effect, a 'reservoir' at the injection site, from which active drug is released. Peak levels are reached after 4–8 hours, reflecting the aqueous formulation.

Blood levels

The potential value of identifying therapeutic blood levels includes monitoring compliance, avoidance of toxicity, evaluating non-response, titration of a therapeutic range and investigation of medico-legal issues involving antipsychotics. The fabled 'therapeutic window' remains a Holy Grail whose whereabouts is a mystery even for the most intensively studied drugs, chlorpromazine and haloperidol. The most optimistic appraisals indicate that correlations between outcome and plasma levels account for only about 10–25% of the variance in response, even when metabolites are considered (Lader, 1979; Midha *et al*, 1987). This work to date has produced nothing that is of value in routine clinical practice. The management of schizophrenia is about achieving a clinical balance between improvement and tolerability by empirical methods, in which 'therapeutic' drug monitoring as yet plays no part.

Pharmacological actions

Antipsychotics are a diverse group of compounds which interact with a wide range of peripheral and central transmitter systems. Peripheral actions are relevant only with regard to side-effects, although a number of adverse effects generally attributed to peripheral blockade (e.g. hypotension) may also have important central components. The major clinical issue relates to the use of low potency phenothiazines, especially chlorpromazine, which have marked anti-adrenergic actions and can result in disturbance of vasomotor tone and consequent hypotension. Because of this, such drugs must never be given intravenously and care should be exercised with their use in drug-naive patients, the physically debilitated and the elderly.

It is, however, the central pharmacology of these drugs which is of far greater importance. As would be expected of such a diverse group of compounds, the pattern of central receptor blockade associated with individual preparations varies widely, and although some drugs are 'relatively' selective in their actions, it is important to bear in mind that none have pure receptor actions (Fig. 9.1).

Despite this pharmacological diversity, antipsychotics share in common one crucial function – the ability to block central dopaminergic neurotransmission. Evidence from two sources indicates the importance of this in their therapeutic actions. In the laboratory, the affinity of antipsychotics for dopamine receptors correlates closely with their ability to block a range of dopamine-related behaviours, such as amphetamine-induced stereotypy in rodents, and more importantly, their affinity for tritiated neuroleptic binding sites correlates closely with their clinical potency. Clinically, the crucial role of dopamine blockade has been shown in a study of the isomers of flupenthixol. The cis (or Z) isomer of this compound has approximately 1000 times greater dopamine blocking ability than the trans (or E) isomer. In a double-blind, placebo controlled study comparing the effectiveness of the two isomers in acute schizophrenics, Johnstone *et al* (1978) showed that antipsychotic benefits were restricted to the cis isomer, the trans being clinically no more effective than placebo.

Thus the evidence is strong that the therapeutic benefits of antipsychotics are mediated by central dopaminergic blockade. The site of this action is not clear but it is likely to lie within the mesolimbic

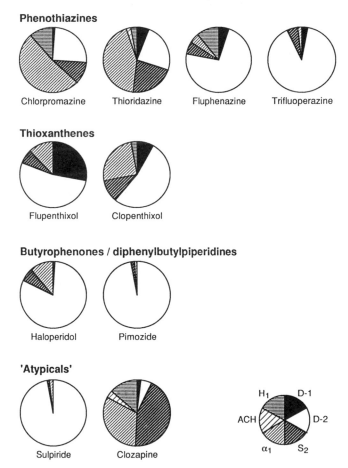

Fig. 9.1 Receptor binding profiles of some commonly used antipsychotic drugs (data from Hyttel *et al*, 1985)

dopamine system (Crow *et al*, 1977). Such simple statements, however, undoubtedly mask a complex reality. Two main types of dopamine receptor have been firmly established for a number of years – the D_1 receptor associated with stimulation of adenylate cyclase, and the D_2 receptor, either inactive or inhibitory on this enzyme. Antipsychotic efficacy has so far been related mainly to D_2 receptor blockade, leaving the D_1 as an entity of uncertain function although there is evidence to suggest that D_1 and D_2 may not operate in isolation but in some linked or cooperative fashion (Carlsson, 1988; Waddington, 1988). However, molecular biological techniques have recently identified several subtypes, or isomorphs, of the dopamine receptor and it is now more correct to consider the original classification as representing 'families' of receptors – those which are D_1-like (i.e. D_1 and D_5) and those which are D_2-like (i.e. D_2 long and short varieties, D_3 and D_4). The importance of this may be in the variable affinities that different antipsychotic drugs appear to have for different receptor subtypes. D_2 dopamine receptors do also exist presynaptically (so-called autoreceptors) and these may also be relevant to antipsychotic actions in some as yet unknown way.

Dopamine systems do not of course act in isolation and while dopamine blockade may be an important, and possibly essential, component of antipsychotic action, it is likely that this is only the necessary 'first step'. Dopamine blockade, as inferred from a rise in serum prolactin, can be shown to occur within 24–72 hours of classical antipsychotic administration with a plateau in prolactin levels evident in 4–7 days (Meltzer & Fang, 1976), yet clinically, resolution of psychotic symptomatology does not usually begin until the second or third week or even longer (Davis & Garver, 1978). Some of this delay may be attributable to the interposing adverse effects of coincidentally administered anticholinergics but it seems likely that dopamine receptor blockade is a necessary prerequisite of other, longer-term changes elsewhere.

Other changes implicated relate to actions on serotonergic (especially $5\text{-}HT_2$), alpha-1-noradrenergic and possibly glutaminergic systems.

Efficacy

Three questions must be posed when considering the efficacy of antipsychotic drugs in the management of schizophrenia: their role in the management of the acute phase, the management of the negative features, and maintaining well-being.

Antipsychotic drug efficacy in acute schizophrenia

There is now abundant evidence that antipsychotic drugs are beneficial in the management of acute schizophrenic episodes – that is, that they are effective treatments for the florid, productive or 'positive' mental state features and the behavioural disturbances which characterise these states. This is not merely an action secondary to sedation as it is not shared by other classes of drugs having sedative properties (e.g. barbiturates or benzodiazepines).

The best and most quoted study of this question is the multicentre trial conducted by the National Institute of Mental Health Collaborative Study Group, published in 1964. This large double-blind placebo controlled trial looked at the efficacy of three different phenothiazines, chlorpromazine, thioridazine and fluphenazine, over a 6 week treatment interval. In summary, its findings were:

(1) Antipsychotics produced a significantly greater improvement in acute schizophrenic symptoms over the trial period than placebo.

(2) Response was variable – overall significant improvement in group mean scores concealed the fact that while 75% were 'much' or 'very much' improved, 20% improved only minimally, and 5% not at all. However no patient on active medication worsened.

(3) Although the trial drugs differed in potency and ability to produce side-effects they did not differ in efficacy.

(4) Some patients on placebo improved – 23% were noted as showing moderate or marked improvement.

Points 1 and 2 are relevant to all antipsychotics currently available in the UK as is, with one important qualification, point 3. (See section on 'Treatment resistance' for further discussion of clozapine.)

It has also been shown that these drugs are superior to psychodynamic interventions. In an elegant study in California in the mid-60s, Philip May compared five different treatment approaches in first episode patients. The treatments consisted of antipsychotics alone; individual psychotherapy alone; antipsychotics plus individual psychotherapy; ECT; or 'milieu' (i.e. ward environment).

Compared with those receiving psychotherapy alone or 'milieu' treatment, antipsychotics and ECT speeded up the rate of discharge, decreased the duration of hospitalisation and decreased the need for additional treatments, for example other sedatives (May, 1968).

Thus there is clear evidence for the efficacy of antipsychotics in the great majority of patients suffering from acute episodes of schizophrenia, whether they are first episodes or exacerbations of established illness. It must be remembered, however, that these effects are non-specific, similar beneficial actions being evident on productive psychotic symptomatology from whatever cause.

Antipsychotic drug efficacy in 'negative' states

Negative features are considered in detail in chapter 7. Most of the arguments surrounding the efficacy of antipsychotics in their treatment relate to Crow's hypothesis that schizophrenia could be considered as comprising two syndromes (Crow, 1980). The Type I Syndrome, characterised by 'positive' symptomatology, was hypothesised as having a pathophysiology based on underlying disturbance of dopaminergic function, while the Type II Syndrome, characterised by 'negative' symptomatology, was proposed as emanating from structural brain change. This hypothesis has proved highly influential, not least because of its inference that Type II ('negative') features are unlikely to respond or will only respond poorly to antipsychotic medication.

A number of reports have disputed this inference – often robustly – and claimed that 'negative' symptomatology does indeed respond favourably to antipsychotics (Goldberg, 1985; Meltzer *et al*, 1986; Breier *et al*, 1987). The problem, however, arises from the way one conceptualises 'negative' symptomatology. This fundamental question is fraught with methodological difficulties (Sommers, 1985) which in practice hinge on whether measures of negative symptoms are measuring only negative features and not other associated features. The so-called 'secondary negative states' (Carpenter *et al*, 1985) associated with intrusive or overwhelming productive features, the psychomotor retardation of depression and other dysphoric states, the bradykinesia of Parkinsonism and the effects of social dislocation, can all cloud the differential and thereby the evaluation of the efficacy of antipsychotics on the authentic (or primary) negative syndrome.

As a theoretical construct Crow's hypothesis still stands. The evidence to date does not support the view that antipsychotics in general exert any fundamental benefit on genuine 'negative' schizophrenic features. Likewise suggestions of particular benefits from specific classes of drugs, such as diphenylbutylpiperidines and substituted benzamides, have not weathered the rigours of the controlled clinical trial. Whether the newer compounds offer better prospects remains to be clarified. In view of their somewhat more favourable side-effect profile however, benefits reported for risperidone and in particular for clozapine may spring more from the absence of a counter-therapeutic action than from the presence of a therapeutic one.

Antipsychotic drug efficacy in long-term maintenance

There is also sound evidence that antipsychotics prevent the recrudescence of florid, productive schizophrenic symptoms following recovery from an acute episode of illness (for review, see Kane & Lieberman, 1987). The term 'prophylaxis' is often applied in this context and is clinically useful, but it must be appreciated that schizophrenia is for most sufferers a chronic disorder. While long-term medication may prevent symptomatic exacerbations it does not provide prophylaxis in the sense of preventing relapse in a disorder that has been previously cured. Furthermore, it is

Table 9.3 Representative relapse rates in drug and placebo treated schizophrenics

Maintenance interval	Drugs	Placebo
1 year [1]	30%	65%
2 years [2]	53%	75%
>3 years [3]	65%	87%

1. Davis (1975).
2. Average Hogarty *et al* (1976) and Crow *et al* (1986).
3. Estimate Hogarty & Ulrich (1977).

important to be aware that studies of long-term maintenance have not in general been extended beyond two years, and in most studies the follow-up intervals have been much less.

Davis (1975) suggested that in the studies he reviewed the percentage relapse in drug-treated groups (about 30%) was less than half that in groups maintained on placebo (about 65%). Baldessarini (1985) reviewed 28 studies, most with a 3–6 month follow-up and found a highly significant drug/placebo difference in favour of antipsychotics. There is some consensus that after stabilisation ('remission') about 5–10% of placebo treated patients will relapse each month, at least for the first 12 months (Davis, 1975; Baldessarini, 1985) with a modal point at between 3–5 months (Hirsch, 1986). It is clear that drugs diminish this figure substantially, by a factor of around two or three (Baldessarini, 1985). Figures up to 2 years are still scant but indicate firstly, a continuing benefit from medication but secondly, a steady relapse rate in actively treated samples (Table 9.3).

Beyond 2 years, the question of efficacy is more speculative, with conclusions based largely on statistical projections. These are nonetheless of interest. Their prediction that about 13% of patients remain well over many years without medication is very similar to the figures for permanent 'relief' reported long before the introduction of physical forms of treatment. The fact that the rate of exacerbations with long-term treatment corresponds to the 12 month placebo rate suggests that for most patients antipsychotics may only be delaying for a few years, not actually preventing, acute flare-ups. The most sobering implication is that long-term control may only be achieved in about 20% of cases.

First schizophrenic episodes – early versus delayed treatment?

Schizophrenia is not a diagnosis that clinicians impart lightly and when confronted with a first episode of illness, especially if of mild or atypical presentation, many will feel it legitimate to 'wait and see' rather than begin treatment immediately. There are few facts available to help decide on the better course of action, but two observations are worth bearing in mind.

Analysis of follow-up data from May's study, mentioned above, showed that those who had received physical treatment initially – and hence earlier – spent strikingly less time in hospital subsequently (May *et al*, 1976) and after 2 years those who had been treated with drugs during their first illness were spending twice as much time in remunerative employment as those who received only psychotherapeutic approaches initially (May *et al*, 1981). The ECT-treated patients did not fare so well in this regard as the drug-treated ones. The implication is that regardless of treatment strategies subsequently, early antipsychotic treatment may lead to a more favourable long-term outcome.

A similar point emerged from a study of long-term maintenance following first episodes conducted at Northwick Park Hospital. The only factor predictive of relapse was time from onset of illness to point of treatment. Those ill for longer than one year prior to admission were significantly more likely to relapse than those ill for less than one year (Crow *et al*, 1986). This could be interpreted simply as those with relatively bad prognosis illnesses taking longer to get to medical attention, but it does again raise the possibility that early intervention has long-term benefits. Indeed in a recent review, Wyatt concluded that data so far indicated that "early intervention with neuroleptics in firstbreak schizophrenia patients increased the likelihood of an improved long-term course" (Wyatt, 1991).

The second point to bear in mind however is a possible caveat. This relates to how one defines a favourable outcome. The Northwick Park Study referred to above found that of those who had obtained a definite academic, occupational or professional achievement in the follow-up period, significantly more were in the placebo than in the active treatment group (Johnstone *et al*, 1990). The numbers were small but this does raise the point that improved outcome in terms of stable employment, as May's study indicated, is not the same as academic or professional advancement, especially in a young population in whom a degree of such advancement could reasonably be anticipated.

Clinical management

In the drug treatment of schizophrenia it is useful to consider three phases; the acute phase, the post-acute phase, and the maintenance phase. These phases are not discrete, nor do they have predictable components or durations, but they can provide a general structure to management. Their delineation should be based on judgements regarding the activeness of the illness, as gauged for example by the degree to which psychotic symptomatology dominates the picture; whether or not insight is developing; preoccupation with past psychotic experiences; the affective state; the patient's behavioural status and possibly dangerousness; psychological functioning; and the patient's own, as well as the nursing and medical, assessment of progress and well-being.

Admission versus non-admission

There is no concensus on the merits and demerits of admission for patients suffering acute schizophrenic episodes. Certainly it is unnecessary to admit all acutely psychotic patients. Long-standing patients, especially if well known to the service, who suffer a relapse or others, whose relapses are detected early, can often be managed quite adequately as out-patients. The same is true for those with slowly evolving, relatively late onset paranoid illnesses dominated by delusions of reference/misinterpretation/ persecution. On the other hand there are certain situations where admission is strongly advisable or mandatory (Box 9.1). Admission is generally advisable for the first episode, due to several reasons.

Adequate observation and assessment

Diagnosis is only one part of assessment, and diagnostic work should not cease when a particular psychopathology is revealed during the initial contact, even if this is sufficient for a reasonable working hypothesis. Schizophrenia is invariably a rich symptomatic tapestry whose threads can rarely be unravelled at a single glance. A sound knowledge of the extent of the initial mental state disorder is also essential for evaluating

---

Box 9.1 Schizophrenia – situations where admission is indicated

Dangerousness
Marked affective change - suspiciousness, anger, hostility
Imperative hallucinations to harm self or others
Severe depression / hopelessness
Specific suicidal ideation
Gross behavioural disturbance / disorganisation
Inability to comprehend recommendations
Likelihood of non-compliance
Inadequate social support
Vagrancy / severe personal neglect
Secondary medical issues
  - intercurrent physical illness
  - alcohol/drug abuse

---

the course of the illness, its response to treatment and the significance of apparent set-backs which may occur later.

Establishing a relationship

Junior doctors on rotational training schemes tend to forget that young consultants and young schizophrenics grow old together. Establishing a sound and trusting relationship will stand you in good stead long-term and can usually best be fostered with the patient 'on the premises', and with a high medical profile.

Stabilisation of medication

The idea of medication often goes against the grain for patients and considerable tact and perseverance may be required to get them to accept the need for it and to persist with it in the longer term. Adverse effects ranging from the disagreeable to the terrifying can rapidly sabotage your efforts. Side-effects are particularly likely to damage rapport when they are not readily acknowledged and promptly dealt with. Medication on which the patient is stabilised initially is likely to be the drug of first choice for that particular patient during any subsquent episodes, so it is crucial to establish maximum tolerance limits early on.

Unpredictability

Acute psychotic shifts can produce symptomatology which has a changing impact on the patient. Uncertainties can rapidly crystallise to certainties and friends transform to foes. It is often not possible to predict such developments, nor, more importantly, to exclude them with confidence.

Asylum

Patients and their families are often at their wits end by the time (first) illnesses reach specialist attention. Admission, by offering stability and calm in a supportive, but emotionally neutral environment, can provide a necessary breathing space for all concerned.

The concept of illness

Schizophrenia is an illness – and a major one at that. Hospital, in our society, is where people go when they have major health problems, and that includes psychiatric health problems. The offer of admission demonstrates from the start that the doctor perceives the condition as a medical disorder.

The acute phase

Preliminaries

There is no 'first-line' drug in the treatment of schizophrenia but several general points are worth considering.

The issue of compliance recurs throughout the treatment of schizophrenia. The reasons for non-compliance are many including denial of illness, outright antipathy to medical intervention, and simple oversight – but top of the list is inability or unwillingness to persist with, or in some cases even start medication, because of side-effects. In one survey of mainly experienced patients, 35% of those who refused medication cited side-effects as their reason, while doctors, on the other hand, thought side-effects were an issue in only 7% of refusers (Hoge *et al*, 1990) – a striking indication of the different perceptions of medication between those who have to take it, and those who need only talk about it!

Compliance is usually perceived as a patient problem, but in fact the physician can exert considerable influence on most of the major variables that contribute to it. Reluctance to accept medication should be readily acknowledged and reasons for recommending it explained: regimes should be kept as simple as possible; and the issue of side-effects must be confronted. When acutely unwell, patients are unlikely to be able to assimilate much detailed explanation and in anxious, somatically preoccupied subjects, a well-intentioned explanation may become the basis for spurious and confusing somatic overlay. So explanations should be kept simple. However, patients often have remarkable resilience to adverse drug effects provided they have confidence in the doctor and in his/her willingness to discuss drug recommendations and side-effects at any time.

If a patient has had previous episodes of illness it is always worthwhile enquiring about their past experience of medication. Many patients with long-standing illnesses are skilled psychopharmacologists! Drugs that have helped in the past should be the first choice for acute relapses. By the same token it is prudent to avoid medication that has not been well tolerated previously or in which the patient has no confidence.

In your own practice, it is advisable to acquire 'in depth' experience with a few preparations encompassing the range of classes and to acquire confidence in the use of these, particularly in the recognition of side-effect profiles, rather than trying one drug in one patient, one in another and so on. It is also helpful to familiarise nursing colleagues, and others who work in the team, of your particular preferences and of the underlying rationale.

Debate continues as to whether low potency sedative drugs are superior in excited or agitated patients and high potency ones preferentially beneficial in those exhibiting withdrawal or retardation. The research evidence to date does not support such a clear distinction, with numerous studies indicating equal efficacy for high or low potency preparations in both types of patient (Kane, 1987).

This undoubtedly valid conclusion from the literature must nonetheless be viewed critically for routine implementation. Schizophrenic patients participating in clinical trials are probably a rather atypical breed. They are likely to be more biddable and compliant than the average and more accepting of medical intervention, and they certainly receive more intensive and structured patterns of care. So extrapolating findings from such subjects to the generality of patients must be tempered with pragmatism. In the face of gross behavioural disturbance, to soldier on with just non-sedative, high potency drugs for the two to three weeks it will take for antipsychotic efficacy to filter through, would seem to require nerves of steel or a mode of practice punctuated by long absences from the ward!

Treatment: aims and methods

The acute phase of illness is characterised by change. Florid psychotic symptoms have either emerged for the first time or re-emerged after a period in abeyance, alongside which are variable degrees of non-specific symptomatology and behavioural disorganisation. The aims of treatment in this phase are fourfold, as follows.

The management of non-specific symptomatology

Alleviation of symptoms such as anxiety, restlessness and especially insomnia is a priority, which often follow from the pursuit of other aims. Their persistence may cause the patient to reconsider their decision to accept medical recommendations and may become a source of escalating conflict on the ward. Their prompt alleviation on the other hand can be held up as signs of progress. Benzodiazepines can be used, but since the basic problem shares common cause with the psychosis, sedative antipsychotics are more logical, although the two may be usefully combined.

The establishment of adequate, tolerable regimes

In the management of the acute phase, 'tolerable regimes' are not the same as regimes free from side-effects. They are quite simply regimes the patient is prepared to tolerate. Side-effects are common – perhaps even inevitable – in treatment of the acute symptoms especially in first episode, drug naive patients, or those where rapid containment of excitement or violence is a priority, but listening to patients' complaints and, most importantly, reassuring them may go a long way in helping the patient to cooperate with the medical recommendations. Prompt intervention is always required for acute dystonias, symptomatic postural hypotension and signs of allergy.

If compliance appears to be in jeopardy, or the patient's goodwill to the treatment programme is diminishing, side-effects should be managed specifically, e.g. with anticholinergics (see below) or non-specifically with dose reduction and/or transfer to a preparation of a different class.

The establishment of stable control of psychotic symptomatology

This is the major aim of acute phase treatment. The management approach adopted initially is best determined more by the presence or absence of behavioural disturbance, than by the mental state itself.

Patients with behavioural disturbance.   This includes those whose mental state disorder is characterised by severe anxiety, perplexity or bewilderment, suspiciousness, lability and other symptoms that result in behaviour which is restless and agitated, excitable, hostile and combative, withdrawn or generally disorganised and volatile.

In these cases a low potency drug is preferred: in practice chlorpromazine (CPZ) is usually the first choice. In first episodes, initial doses in the range 300–600 mg per day are most often sufficient. There is little point in starting with less than 300 mg daily and most drug-naive patients can tolerate this. Even if the patient is initially sedated this will rapidly habituate. Slightly lower introductory doses (~150 mg per day) may be indicated for the elderly and the physically debilitated. Those experiencing exacerbations of established illness and who have a past treatment history, especially if they have been receiving maintenance medication, will generally tolerate higher doses than the drug-naive, but even for these cases 600 mg daily is usually adequate, although guidance should be sought from the patient's past experience.

The last dose should be given before retiring and it is often helpful to give a larger amount then, to help insomnia and obviate excessive day time sedation. It is important to appreciate that the pharmacokinetics of most antipsychotics are such that equal efficacy probably accrues from single (nocte) dosing as from divided dose regimes. However, as low potency drugs are selected in order to capitalise on their sedative side-effects, divided dosage during the daytime is more logical, at least initially.

As well as regular medication, an 'as required', or prn, dose can be prescribed (e.g. CPZ 100 mg) to be administered at the nurses' discretion. This will help the staff to contain distress or disturbance as it occurs and measuring the amount used will be helpful in determining the size of subsequent increments. However clear written guidance *must* be given on the administration of prn medication. The maximum number of doses in 24 hours must be specified (three should be sufficient) and a single mode of administration for each single dose stated. Doses should not be written up as a range, e.g. 50–150 mg chlorpromazine, to be given oral/ i.m. This is sloppy and only leads to confusion. If a range of options in both dosage and mode of administration is deemed appropriate each should be written up separately.

The essential element in the early management of patients with behavioural disturbance is daily review. There is no point in starting an introductory regime in someone swinging from the curtain rails and retiring for a week to await some response. If the initial regime produces little or no effect within 24–48 hours, the dose should be increased, a process that should continue until some impact is evident. Increments should take into account nursing reports as well as the amount of prn required since last assessment, and should continue until excited, aggressive or otherwise disturbed behaviour begins to resolve, anxiety eases and a sleep pattern, assessed from sleep charts, of at least 6 hours at night with no more than 1–2 hours in the day, is established. A plateau can thereafter be maintained with doses held steady. Even at this stage increments should not be withheld – and doses most definitely *not* reduced – on the basis of an apparent early resolution of psychotic features. At this stage any such improvement is likely to be a non-specific response.

The range of dosage at which a stable plateau will be achieved varies enormously and it is pointless to provide guidelines which would be meaningless. These must be derived empirically in each individual patient. Maximum doses of chlorpromazine are often regarded as open-ended, which from the safety point of view may have a certain validity. From the therapeutic point of view however, if little response is evident after 3–4 weeks with doses in the 1000–1200 mg per day range, substantial benefits with further increments are unlikely to accrue, and in these instances it is better to change preparation or add a second drug of a different class, for example a butyrophenone. Polypharmacy is rightly criticised when, without justification, it becomes the norm but in selected cases where, after an adequate trial of a single drug, disturbing symptomatology remains stubbornly entrenched, addition of a second drug of a different class is legitimate. However, the rule is always to aim for single drug treatment when possible.

Once the non-specific features are contained as indicated above, the dose plateau should be held for 2–3 weeks while awaiting genuine movement in the psychotic symptomatology. If after this time acute features remain stubbornly florid or active, further increases should be made, but more slowly than before (e.g. once or twice weekly) as worsening side-effects may jeopardise compliance. It may be possible at this stage to reduce the frequency of drug administration from q.d.s. to b.d. or even once daily.

Although there is little reference to it in the literature, for patients who are on low potency drugs, the period of specific symptom resolution is often heralded by complaints of increasing sedation and sleep, both nocturnal and daytime, among those who were previously composed but alert. This may serve as a useful clue to specific antipsychotic actions beginning but requires careful handling. Reductions at this stage to accommodate side-effects should always be very cautious as the risk of florid exacerbation is substantial.

Patients without behavioural disturbance.   Some patients, especially those whose illnesses have evolved relatively slowly, will show little in the way of objective distress or disturbance and non-specific symptomatology. For them, the goal of treatment is control of their psychotic symptomatology, and the sedative side-effects of low potency drugs may be a disadvantage. High potency preparations should be the first option. For those without previous antipsychotic drug exposure low doses should be used initially, e.g. trifluoperazine 10mg or pimozide 4mg nocte. For those with a previous history, past drug experience should serve as a guide.

Increments should rarely be more frequent than twice weekly and likewise should be cautious, e.g. no more than 50%. The reason for restraint is simply that most patients will not require high dose regimes. As has been explained, antipsychotic benefits usually take time (around 2–3 weeks) to emerge. The limiting factor in the use of high potency drugs is EPS. Emergence of these is commonly delayed after starting, and tends to lag behind dose increments. Pushing to large doses too quickly may impair compliance by promoting side-effects in advance of therapeutic benefits.

It should rarely be necessary to go beyond 20–40 mg trifluoperazine per day (with pimozide the CSM has made specific recommendations, see below) and higher doses should be avoided. It is the author's impression that unnecessarily high doses of antipsychotics continue to be used. It is mandatory to treat schizophrenia adequately but studies indicate that for the average patient, doses in the range of 400–600 mg chlorpromazine or its equivalent are usually sufficient (Kane, 1987), even though the therapeutic effect may not appear for some time.

Prevention or containment of psychiatric emergencies

It is axiomatic that psychiatric emergencies should if possible be prevented. Unrestrained psychotic violence is an awesome sight and although not as common as the lay public believes, it should be viewed as a potential development in all acutely disturbed psychotic patients. Some incidents are of course unavoidable, but one of the more important responsibilities of the psychiatrist is the prompt identification and management of such situations.

Trust your instincts. If you detect brooding resentment, increasing tension, suspicious hostility, respond to your 'gut reaction'.

Know when to back off. If intervention by others, including doctors, is making the patient increasingly restless and agitated, withdraw.

Know when to intervene and be prepared to act quickly and decisively. Increasing unprovoked restlessness, unamenability, verbal hostility, etc. should not be ignored.

Pay heed to the mental state content. Diagnostically form is of greater weight, but in anticipating probable violence look to the content.

Provide liberal reassurance. If disturbance is based on fear or suspicion do not treat this with contempt by ignoring it. Statements that the patient is safe, that you are there to help them, and so forth may sound platitudinous, but may be just what the patient longs to hear.

Define the limits. All social behaviour has boundaries and that includes the behaviour of schizophrenics. By being unduly tolerant the physician may fail other patients and unwittingly foster resentments that may later explode into conflict.

There is no standard regime for dealing with potential or actual emergencies, but several strategies are outlined below.

Low potency antipsychotics – oral or i.m.

In practice this means chlorpromazine given as syrup or suspension or by i.m. injection. This remains a popular approach in the UK because of its justifiable reputation for safety. Nonetheless, it is often forgotten that chlorpromazine must be treated with respect, especially in the drug-naive. It must *never* be given i.v. and even i.m. should be used sparingly, at least initially. Occasionally inexperienced doctors still authorise the use of 200 mg of chlorpromazine i.m. In someone never before exposed, this is potentially a lethal dose.

Plan 1

Rx   Chlorpromazine. 100mg oral or i.m. stat. (75–50mgm in the elderly, frail or debilitated)

Monitor sedation. If heavily sedated, order close nursing observation

Monitor BP. If heavily sedated, every half hour till peak blood levels at 3–4 hours post administration. Note: If BP cannot be taken because of continuing disturbance, this suggests it does not need to be taken because significant hypotension is unlikely.

If further sedation is required but supine BP fails strikingly (systolic <100 mm Hg) switch to an alternative, e.g. haloperidol. If falls are slight (<20 mm Hg systolic) the above can be repeated after 2–4 hours.

In drug-naive patients, repeats are seldom necessary for the simple reason that chlorpromazine in these patients is usually highly sedative.

However sedative effects rapidly undergo tolerance and so they cannot be relied on, particularly in previously treated patients.

High potency antipsychotics - Oral/i.m./i.v.

Haloperidol has achieved its status as the world-wide 'market leader' antipsychotic largely because of its parenteral use in US emergency rooms. Because of their weak anti-adrenergic actions, and hence minimal hypotensive effects, butyrophenones are particularly suited to intravenous administration. They appear safe in high dosage and repeated administration is possible at relatively short intervals. Droperidol (up to 20mg oral, 15mg i.v. and 10mg. i.m.), which is more sedative and shorter acting than haloperidol, is also useful.

> *Plan 2*
> Rx Haloperidol 10–20 mg stat i.m. or i.v.
> Check sedation level
> Check BP at one hour
> Can be repeated as required
> Be alert to the possibility of acute extrapyramidal symptoms

Other approaches

Diazepam. Psychiatrists' therapeutic decisions tend to be diagnosis-bound and as benzodiazepines are not antipsychotics, these drugs are seldom used in the management of psychotic emergencies. This is a great pity, because diazepam on its own, or as an adjunct to any of the above strategies, is rapid-acting, effective and safe, and while perhaps not quite repeatable 'ad infinitum', can usually be given sufficiently frequently to control most emergency situations.

> *Plan 3*
> Rx Diazepam 10–20 mg i.v., repeatable
> Diazemuls

Clopixol Acuphase. Zuclopenthixol esterified with acetic acid and dissolved in Viscoleo has a rapid onset producing detectable sedation in 15–90 minutes. Peak levels are attained in 24–36 hours and it is supposedly effective up to 72 hours. Claims that it produces an antipsychotic effect over its three day period of action must be interpreted with caution, and the precise role of this drug in psychiatric emergencies has yet to be evaluated.

Emergency situations arising from acute schizophrenic disturbance test every professional's nerve and skill. This is no time for the doctor to be busily doing something else or to be anywhere but on the ward. The management of such situations should not be delegated solely to nursing staff. Some emergencies can be defused by reason and negotiation but even these situations are best finalised with an adequate dose of (liquid) medication.

While psychiatric emergencies may inevitably require to be managed with often high doses of medication, it must be remembered that the sedated state is a potentially risky one, and psychiatrists would do well to treat its induction and supervision with care.

Rapid neuroleptisation

'Crash tranquillisation', subsequently referred to as 'rapid neuroleptization' became popular in the US in the 1970s. Implementation of this was confused but essentially involved frequent dosing (up to hourly) and/or high daily intake within the first few days of hospitalisation. Spectacular daily doses were sometimes reported (for example 3.6 g chlorpromazine, 160 mg haloperidol orally). Enthusiasm for such heroic efforts was backed by uncontrolled observations but subsequent controlled studies failed to demonstrate any benefits for rapid, high dose regimes (Neborsky *et al*, 1981). This will come as no surprise to those familiar with the delay in onset of antipsychotic efficacy. Side-effects on the other hand were predictably "virtually inevitable" (Neborsky *et al*, 1981). 'Rapid neuroleptisation' as routine practice is yet another psychiatric oddity that should be consigned to the dustbin of history.

The post-acute phase

There are no absolute rules as to how long it takes to achieve the three primary aims of acute treatment, but signs of stabilisation should be evident in the majority of patients by about 4–6 weeks. The aims of the post-acute phase are consolidation; rationalisation of treatment; establishment of adequate but non-intrusive regimes; consideration of long-term management issues; and starting active rehabilitation (as described in chapter 10).

Consolidation

A common error is for doctors to give in to pressure from patients for dose reduction at the first tentative signs of improvement. The priority once acute symptomatology stabilises is consolidation. Improvements achieved in the hospital ward must be shown to generalise to the outside world, for example by increasingly long and successful periods of leave. Furthermore all schizophrenic symptomatology does not resolve comprehensively, all at the same time. Improvements continue to develop progressively over weeks or even months during the post-discharge period and these should be closely monitored.

Rationalisation of treatment

Having consolidated the position for 3–4 weeks the drug regime should be rationalised to something the patient has a chance of complying with on discharge. The aims are two-fold:

(1) to switch as far as possible to a single preparation, particularly when more than one has been used for acute management. If both a low and a high potency drug have been prescribed concurrently, the high potency drug is preferred in the longer term.

(2) to reduce the frequency of administration to a minimum, and if possible to achieve a single daily dose, preferably at night. The expectation that discharged patients will be able to cope with several different drugs administered at different times is fanciful nonsense.

Establishment of adequate, non-intrusive regimes

In this context 'adequate' means doses sufficient to maintain progress, while 'non-intrusive' refers to achieving this with minimal or no side-effects. These goals can usually be attained together with a degree of rationalisation, although reductions in the post-acute phase should rarely be substantial. Most patients will be content with 25–30% overall reductions which for them will reflect progress and should free the majority from the most obtrusive side-effects. Even among those initially disturbed patients who required heavy doses, substantial reductions at this stage are seldom necessary or advisable.

Perhaps of more importance than the absolute reduction, is the rate at which it is done. Because of the pharmacokinetics of antipsychotics, exacerbations in mental state disturbances may not reflect the most recent dose reductions but those effected some time before. Likewise benefits in side-effect profiles will take some time (perhaps a week or two) to filter through. Hence reductions ideally should only be recommended weekly or fortnightly.

Antipsychotic side-effects are in general dose-dependent but a threshold effect seems to operate in the patients' subjective experience of the resolution of certain side-effects. Progressive, constant reductions may produce little improvement until a certain strategic point when awareness of side-effects such as sedation, slowness or Parkinsonian stiffness seems to suddenly diminish disproportionately.

In gauging how far to proceed with dose reduction at this stage, the benchmark is not primarily the re-emergence of specific psychotic features, but rather the recurrence of non-specific symptomatology (e.g. anxiety, agitation, irritability, insomnia or any change in sleep pattern) which may be a much more sensitive index of incipient exacerbation. If such features re-emerge, medication should be increased to the previous level and held for a month or two before a subsequent, more restrained attempt is undertaken.

The recurrent theme in successful management at this stage is *caution*. Relapse at this point is deeply demoralising and is to be avoided at all costs. Furthermore, there is an impression that florid symptomatology recurring in the post-acute period is more intractable to treatment than the original acute episode, with higher doses for longer periods being needed to re-establish stability.

Consideration of long-term management issues

The post-acute phase is also the time to discuss issues of long-term treatment with the patient. Around this time, many patients will request discontinuation of their medication and considerable time and expertise may be needed to persuade them to continue – which they certainly should, as the high early relapse rates noted above, emphasise.

Medication should be maintained for at least 6 and preferably 12 months before the question of discontinuation is discussed in detail. This will allow patients to regain confidence and independence and settle as far as possible into previous routines with the minimum risk of relapse. During this period the 'bonus' of further reductions, every one or two months, will help gain acceptance. Thereafter, slightly different principles should inform advice to first episode patients compared to those who have had previous episodes.

First episode patients

For most patients, a drug-free trial following resolution of a first schizophrenic episode is a legitimate, planned option. Around 25% of patients will do badly from the start, when the question of stopping medication does not arise. Around 25% will not relapse at all or will at least achieve a substantial period, perhaps years, of well-being before they do so. This leaves the majority (50%) with a relapsing and remitting course, with exacerbations most likely in the first 12 months (see above). It is clear that even the most optimistic odds are strongly against remaining well off drugs. The patient should nonetheless be given the opportunity of deciding – but on the basis of fact, not hope.

Although the option of discontinuing can be discussed with most first episode patients, a small minority should always be advised, unequivocally, to maintain on long-term medication. These are patients who against expectations have made a good recovery from severe protracted illnesses; those who behaved dangerously towards others and whose illnesses had major forensic implications; and those who committed serious self-harm.

Patients with previous episodes

These patients usually require long-term maintenance. It is not necessary (or perhaps possible) to define 'long-term' at this stage, though for most this is likely to mean life-long. There is no evidence to suggest that one mode of administration of maintenance antipsychotics is better than the others, and many patients prefer continuing with oral preparations. However, in acknowledgement of the very real problems of compliance in this situation, the author always raises the option of depot injections and commends them.

There is a rare exception to the rule of recommending maintenance after second and subsequent episodes. If the patient has made a good symptomatic recovery, with a reasonable period of a year or two between episodes during which time they appear to have functioned competently, and if they are also relatively insightful in terms of accepting they have an illness, an alternative recommendation might be intermittent treatment by targeting of early symptoms. Schizophrenic episodes tend to run true to form so the evolution of symptoms tends to be characteristic with each episode. If the patients (or their relatives) can be made sensitive to their own pattern and can be relied upon to present at the first signs of prodromal features re-emerging, prompt treatment with oral medication can be successful in aborting full-blown exacerbations.

Follow-up

The question of medical follow-up is controversial and only a personal view can be offered. There are several reasons to support this being by the psychiatrist.

If *you* make a recommendation for indefinite potent psychotropic medication, *you* should be prepared to provide monitoring.

If the patient requires specialist services, these can be accessed directly at any time without involving third parties.

A relationship established with the patient when well will provide an invaluable basis for trust in relapse.

Awareness of the patient's functioning at its best provides essential information in assessing the significance of recurrent psychopathology.

Patients like it! In a survey of out-patients at Northwick Park Hospital, London almost 60% preferred solely specialist follow-up, while 20% preferred that this was from their GP. Less than 10% wished for follow-up by CPN alone.

The cessation of medication, whether by mutual agreement or against medical advice must not be taken as an opportunity for discharge but rather as a cue for increased vigilance. The next 12–18 months will usually prove crucial and this is just the time when you should offer maximum support. Long-term follow-up is particularly important for patients discontinuing depots. Because of their pharmacokinetics, relapse following cessation of depot treatment is likely to be considerably delayed compared to patients stopping orals.

The maintenance phase

The aims here are to maintain maximal well-being and psychosocial functioning for as long as possible on as low a dose of medication as possible; to monitor long-term medication; and to complete active rehabilitation and re-integration (described in chapter 10).

Maintenance of well-being

The aims of maintenance may be obvious to the doctor but are not necessarily so to the patient. It is worth explaining that the purpose is to keep them well but not to make well patients 'super-well'.

Doctors often fail to distinguish between post-acute and maintenance treatment. This is a mistake. The philosophies that lie behind the management of these two phases are very different. In post-acute management the point is to try and hold the patient on as much medication as practicable; during maintenance, the goal is to achieve as low a dose as possible. Failure to make this distinction is an important reason why so many patients are maintained on unnecessarily high doses of antipsychotics, with all the later risks of neurological sequelae, quite apart from the on-going torpor. In most cases radical reductions should eventually be possible during the course of maintenance but these must be effected gradually. If such reductions are not undertaken the psychiatrist will never gain any impression of minimum dose requirements.

Although oral medication is the more appropriate mode of antipsychotic administration in the management of acute illnesses, depot preparations are the ideal for maintenance mainly because of the compliance issue. However the change-over should be gradual. As was pointed out earlier, depots do not reach steady state for some three months (perhaps a little earlier with fluphenazine decanoate), and so orals should not be stopped immediately after the first injection. It is advisable to attempt no more than a 50% reduction in oral dosage during the first three months of depot treatment, with discontinuation over the subsequent 3–6 months. The watchword again is *caution*.

Several studies have looked at the efficacy of 'standard' versus 'low' dose depot maintenance (for review see Kane, 1987). While exacerbations seem clearly more common with low doses, there appear to be advantages with this approach in terms of a decrease in side-effects and improvement in some measures of well-being (cf. earlier – efficacy). Hence the patient may have to be given a choice – but this should include the option of gradual attainment of low maintenance dosage which may accommodate both the concerns about exacerbation as well as those surrounding level of functioning.

Effective drug intake with depot formulations can be altered in two ways – either by changing the milligram dose or by varying the inter-injection interval. When it comes to reductions, patients will usually prefer the latter for obvious reasons, but in practice it is better to alternate between the two, as thus far the phamacokinetic data provide no guidelines as to which is clearly more appropriate. The aim is for the lowest dose and longest interval compatible with well-being.

Yet again, non-specific symptomatology (i.e. anxiety, agitation, impaired concentration, impaired quality and/or quantity of sleep) is the most sensitive indicator of the adequacy of your management. Should such features re-emerge at any point you must consider (1) immediate containment and (2) the long-term implications.

For immediate containment re-introduction or increase of persisting oral medication is the best recommendation. While a booster depot can also be used, the advantages of depots also hold the seeds of their disadvantages in this situation – the protracted period for change to become effective. Orals should be held for at least 6–8 weeks after stability is re-established before attempts at gradual reduction are made once again. Such insignificant exacerbations must not be ignored by doctor or patient. There is good evidence that they can be relatively simply contained and full-blown relapse aborted (Marder *et al*, 1987).

The long-term implication of a relapse following on from dosage reduction may be that previous levels of maintenance have been barely adequate and although it may be possible to postulate that exceptional life circumstances might have been the trigger, it is prudent to recommend an increase in depot to the previous level associated with well-being.

Monitoring long-term medication

Antipsychotics are powerful, centrally acting drugs, exposure to which can be associated with major neurological adverse effects. Long-term administration requires long-term monitoring. There is evidence that psychiatrists involved in routine clinical work overlook a considerable amount of drug-related neurological abnormality (Weiden *et al*, 1987). This is regrettable. Psychiatrists must be skilled in comprehensive patient assessment – and that includes neurological assessment. Evaluation of neurological status in 'at risk' psychiatric patients is a quality of care issue, that must be addressed by routine examination at least annually and preferably every six months.

Dose equivalence

Although many impressive and authoritative-looking tables have been published listing relative antipsychotic potencies (Davis, 1976*a*; Wyatt, 1976) it is important to appreciate that these are only approximations. Equivalence values are not established on the basis of some objective scientific test, but rather from information from clinical studies which incorporated flexible dosing schedules. There is particular lack of agreement on dose equivalence for the more potent compounds. In practice when making conversions much greater reliance should be placed on dosage ranges than on absolute values (Table 9.4).

Conversions from orals to depots are even more problematic. In practice, oral dose equivalence tables usually need to be used first to convert a particular oral treatment to the equivalent of the oral form of the drug proposed to be given as a depot, after which an oral–depot conversion can be applied. This probably compounds the inaccuracies! Schultz *et al* (1989) have looked at the question of oral–depot conversions in the light of pharmacokinetic considerations and have demonstrated quite marked discrepancies between guidelines that adopt this approach and those supplied by manufacturers which are largely clinically based (Table 9.5).

Equivalence and conversion tables are only of value if they are viewed as providing a rough guide to the sort of levels to aim at for continued well-being and relative lack of side-effects.

Pregnancy and lactation

The data sheet recommendations for the use of antipsychotics in pregnancy are cautious – as well they might be. In clinical practice however, the absolute imperative is to try and maintain optimum psychiatric well-being throughout pregnancy and into the puerperium. There is no evidence that any of the 'classical' antipsychotics are teratogenic in humans even when given through the first trimester,

Table 9.4 Some antipsychotic dose equivalences (mg)

Drug	Average	Range
Chlorpromazine	100	
Promazine	200	100–250
Thioridazine	100	50–120
Pericyazine	18	10–20
Fluphenazine	2	1–5
Perphenazine	10	6.5–20
Trifluoperazine	5	3.5–7
Flupenthixol	1.5	1.25–2.5
Haloperidol	2	1.5–5
Pimozide	1.5	1.25–2
Sulpiride	200	200–350

After Rey *et al* (1989) and Foster (1989).

Table 9.5 Guidelines for conversion from oral to depot anti-psychotic formulations

	Manufacturers' guidelines		Guidelines calculated from pharmacokinetic considerations	
	Oral dose	Depot dose	Oral dose	Depot dose
Haldol	x 20	= 4 weeks	x 23	= 4 weeks
Modecate	x 2.5	= 3 weeks	x 6	= 3 weeks
Depixol[1]	x 10–20	= 2–4 weeks	x 5	= 2 weeks
Clopixol	x 4	= 2 weeks	x 4.9	= 2 weeks
Piportil			x 17	= 4 weeks

1. E:Z isomers ratio in oral formulation accounted for.
After Schultz *et al* (1989).

although there is evidence of teratogenicity in animal studies. There is likewise no evidence implicating 'atypical' or newer antipsychotic compounds in foetal maldevelopment, but because of their relatively limited use, they are best avoided in favour of more established preparations.

The data sheet advice for use of depots is variable, though for some, for example flupenthixol, it is proscriptive. The author has continued the use of flupenthixol during pregnancy but it is best to tail off depot preparations during the last trimester and substitute a standard oral drug in equivalent dosage. This is because a depot can contribute to protracted labour and a 'flat' baby with low Apgar score. Hence the aim should be a brief drug-free interval around delivery, and this is only attainable with orals.

The last depot should be given at about the 28th week. A high potency oral preparation should be introduced around the time when the next depot would have been due and increased to roughly dose equivalence. Thereafter, for these patients, and those maintained throughout on orals, medication should be held until the two weeks before expected delivery at which point discontinuation should be started, with the aim of having the patient drug-free for 48–72 hours prior to the onset of labour.

The issue of breast feeding is complex, and whenever possible should be discussed early in pregnancy and not for the first time in the postnatal ward. The puerperium is an unpredictable period with a high risk of florid relapse which you will wish to avoid by rapidly reinstating medication once again. Antipsychotics are excreted in breast milk, and although present in much lower concentrations than in plasma, acute dystonias and tremors have been reported in neonates in this situation. These reactions can readily be confused with fits which will cause great distress all round. In addition, antipsychotics may make the infant slow to suckle. Thus, while doctors need to acknowledge patients' deep-seated wishes to breastfeed, a general recommendation to avoid this while receiving antipsychotic treatment is prudent.

If depots are restarted postnatally, 6–12 weeks (depending on preparation) will be required to achieve steady state, so orals should be restarted at the same time. Outside bodies, such as the social services, as well as the patient and her family will be concerned to ensure mental state stability, so it is doubly important that any intervention at this time is both swift and effective, and that subsequent follow-up is comprehensive.

Treatment resistance

Antipsychotic drugs will produce therapeutic benefits in the majority of schizophrenic patients, as the NIMH Collaborative Study, mentioned earlier, demonstrated. Despite their proven efficacy, however, around 30% of patients respond poorly (Davis, 1976b) and about 6–8% can be classified as total non-responders (Tuma & May, 1979). The management of this group remains a challenge, and with the exception of clozapine, there is insufficient information to permit the formulation of clear alternative strategies.

Assuming the diagnosis is sound, the first step should be a total review of medication. Some patients may have been left on conventional doses that are inadequate and if this is the case it is worth pushing to high doses (>1 g chlorpromazine or its equivalence), and holding for 4 weeks. However, the opposite is more often the case – namely that patients have had medication progressively increased and have failed to respond to regimes that have become too high and complex almost by default, a situation to be avoided in view of recent concern about the possible risks of high dose regimes (Thompson, 1994). In this situation it may be worth radically *reducing* medication and in particular considering the patient's total anticholinergic load. Patients on high doses of certain (especially low potency) antipsychotics, combined with an anticholinergic, which juniors may prescribe in unnecessarily high dosage, and perhaps even a tricyclic antidepressant, will be receiving a hefty anticholinergic intake. Rarely this may produce toxicity whose specific features are often missed because they are buried in the more general mental state and behavioural disturbance. Of greater potential significance however is, firstly, the bowel stasis that may result from this, which may unpredictably alter absorption of parent drug and/or metabolites formed in the bowel, and secondly, the fact that anticholinergics have been shown to interfere with antipsychotic drug efficacy, their introduction being associated with a demonstrable exacerbation in 'positive' symptomatology (Johnstone *et al*, 1983). The mechanism for this is unclear but it does not appear to result from toxicity or a straightforward pharmacokinetic interaction. Thus the total anticholinergic intake should be reduced.

Although there is no evidence that most antipsychotics differ overall in efficacy (but see below), they have widely differing receptor binding profiles, even those of similar chemical classes (Fig. 9.1). It is therefore well worth trying different preparations from different classes if the first choice in adequate dose for a sufficient time has not worked. A maximum of two alternative drugs in full dosage for at least 4 weeks should be tried.

A further strategy is to introduce a depot. Because of their pharmacokinetics, depots are not in general a suitable presentation of antipsychotic medication for treating acute schizophrenic symptomatology unless everyone involved is possessed of exceptional patience. Initial benefits are probably non-specific, but in a few treatment-resistant cases depots can be effective although improvement may take some weeks to develop. Whether this is the result of a definite advantage from parenteral administration or whether the improvement might have occurred with greater persistence with orals is uncertain.

The one alternative strategy in treatment-resistant schizophrenia that does appear to have scientific validity is clozapine. In an elegant mutlicentre study, Kane *et al* (1988) recruited schizophrenic patients who had failed to respond to at least three different antipsychotics in adequate dose, and entered them in a 6 week, single-blind treatment period with haloperidol. Those patients who remained unimproved then entered a 6 week double-blind phase ($n = 268$) when they received either clozapine up to 900 mg per day or chlorpromazine up to 1800 mg per day. Of the clozapine treated group, 30% were classed as responders, compared to only 4% in the chlorpromazine group. Subsequent evidence has suggested that the response rate with clozapine may rise to 50–60% if treatment is extended to 6 months or more. Thus clozapine may be the first antipsychotic with enhanced therapeutic efficacy compared to other drugs, although to what extent patients who fail to respond to standard treatments have 'more severe' or simply 'different' illnesses remains unclear. Clozapine is not a miracle drug but in severely ill patients who fail to respond to conventional approaches it should be tried. It is of course a potentially dangerous – indeed lethal – drug for some (Baldessarini & Frankenburg, 1991). In the UK, it is only licensed for use in treatment-resistant schizophrenia or where sensitivity to the extrapyramidal side-effects of other drugs precludes optimal dosing. Patients must be registered with the Clozaril Patient Monitoring Service for regular haematological evaluation before it can be prescribed.

Interactions

Antipsychotics interact with a wide variety of other drugs but these seldom cause management problems (Table 9.6). Because patients have to be maintained on an antipsychotic for many years, a variety of incidental

Table 9.6 Antipsychotic interactions

Class	Drug	Effect of antipsychotic interaction
Psychotropics	Alcohol Sedative/hypnotics Narcotics	Potentiation of CNS depressant effects
	Tricyclics	Increased tricyclic levels
	MAOIs	Potentiation of hypotension
	Lithium	Neurotoxicity reported with haloperidol. Caution with combination. Esp. keep to low doses haloperidol and avoid Li toxicity
Anticonvulsants	Phenytoin	Variable, usually decreased phenytoin levels from hepatic enzyme induction
	Carbamazepine	Decreased antipsychotic levels
Dopamine	L-Dopa Bromocriptine	Receptor antagonism
Cardiovascular agents	Antihypertensives	Potentiation from α-adrenergic blockade Phenothiazines: antagonise guanethidine decreased propranolol levels (hepatic enzyme competition)
	Digoxin	Increases bioavailability from reduced GI motility
	Quinidine	Delayed intraventricular conduction leads to cardiac arrhythmias
Anticoagulants		Potentiation from hepatic enzyme competition
Contraceptives		Enhanced hyperprolactinaemia with oestrogen containing preparations
Corticosteroids		Increased bioavailability from reduced GI motility
Sympathomimetics		Inhibition of α-adrenergically mediated pressor effects

Note: Chlorpromazine may interfere with certain laboratory measures
Overestimate: Cholesterol; CSF protein; Urinary ketones; Urinary steroids
Underestimate: Haptoglobin

illnesses may occur and so it is important to be aware of the more important drug interactions.

Other drug treatments of schizophrenia

Propranolol

Following initial favourable reports in the early 1970s (Yorkston *et al*, 1974) propranolol was much discussed as either an adjunctive treatment in chronic patients with on-going productive symptomatology or as the sole treatment of acute episodes of illness. Formal trial results have however been contradictory, but in general unfavourable (Hirsch, 1986; Manchanda & Hirsch, 1986). Overall, any benefits that accrue from adding propranolol to standard antipsychotics in chronic patients are marginal. They certainly do not justify the high-dose regimes reported, which are potentially hazardous.

Lithium

In the first report of the efficacy of lithium salts in mania, John Cade also noted "no fundamental improvement" in six patients with 'dementia praecox'. Cade did note, however, that three of these patients who were "usually restless, noisy and shouting nonsensical abuse" did seem to become "quiet and amenable" (Cade, 1949). Over the years a body of support built up for lithium having antipsychotic as well as normothymic properties (Delva & Letemendia, 1982).

Johnstone *et al* (1988) studied 120 patients who rated positively on any of the psychotic items of the Present State Examination but were not otherwise formally diagnosed. Patients were randomly assigned on the basis of the presence or absence of mood change to an antipsychotic (pimozide), lithium, both, or neither and followed for four weeks. While the beneficial effects of the antipsychotic were evident across retrospectively applied diagnostic categories, those associated with lithium were entirely attributable to its effects on mood, indicating that its usefulness in schizophrenia has probably been overstated.

Carbamazepine

The tricyclic anticonvulsant carbamazepine has been reported as useful in certain patients (Christison *et al*, 1991) but so far there is insufficient information to know whether it has a definite role, although there is a suggestion that it may be helpful in aggressive or violent subjects. Some studies suggest improvement is more likely in the presence of an abnormal

EEG, but in others even those with normal EEGs have responded (Hakola & Lautumaa, 1982).

The treatment of post-psychotic depression

The majority of schizophrenic patients are likely to experience depressive features at some point. The evidence now strongly supports the view that this is directly related to the illness rather than 'pharmacogenic', i.e. antipsychotic related. Of particular importance is depression occuring in the post-acute or maintenance period, so-called 'post-psychotic' or 'post-schizophrenic' (ICD–10) depression. This affects about 25% of patients (Siris, 1991) and may be the major reason for readmission to hospital (Falloon *et al*, 1978).

Despite its prevalence and importance, post-psychotic depression has been poorly researched, especially in terms of its response to conventional treatment. The evidence has not been encouraging overall suggesting a poor response to standard antidepressants. These rather pessimistic conclusions undoubtedly reflect the quality of the earlier studies rather than the quality of the treatment! Recent work, using operationally defined criteria for depression has clearly demonstrated the benefits of tricyclic antidepressants (imipramine) not only in the treatment of depression in the post-psychotic period but also in long-term prophylaxis (Siris *et al*, 1994). Hence a depressive syndrome occurring in this situation is as much an indication for vigorous (tricyclic) antidepressant therapy as such a syndrome in any other context. The value of newer classes of antidepressants must await clarification.

There is a suggestion that tricyclics may exacerbate the productive features of schizophrenia, especially during active phases of illness. In the more symptomatologically stable, post-acute and maintenance phases however, this does not appear to present a practical problem (Siris *et al*, 1994).

Depression is of course, no more a homogenous entity among schizophrenic patients that it is in non-psychotic groups and in some cases approaches other than simply drug therapy may be indicated. This may be particularly the case when demoralisation and hopelessness ensue from an appreciation of the nature of the illness and its consequences.

Adverse effects of antipsychotic drugs

Antipsychotics are remarkably safe. Mortality in overdose, if ingested alone, is low. They are, however, powerful drugs which affect many different organ and neurotransmitter systems. Side-effects therefore are common. Adverse effects can be classified as non-neurological and neurological.

Non-neurological adverse effects

Pharmacological

General

Most antipsychotics can produce dry mouth, blurred vision, constipation and urinary problems. These are usually viewed as anticholinergic effects but probably also reflect anti-adrenergic actions as well. Hence they can be found with preparations which apparently have little intrinsic anticholinergic activity. Likewise sexual difficulties, such as anorgasmia in females, and especially erectile impotence and ejaculatory dysfunction in males, probably reflect a complex interaction of central and peripheral mechanisms. Disturbances of sexual function are more common than is realised, although are reversible and probably dose-related. Priapism has been reported infrequently. Table 9.7 summarises the non-neurological adverse effects.

Cardiovascular system

Antipsychotics increase basal heart rate, although this is usually clinically insignificant. They can, however, cause significant hypotension both supine and postural. This is particularly the case with low potency phenothiazines which possess significant anti-adrenergic activity. It tends to habituate with continued exposure.

ECG changes include increase in the QT interval, depression of the ST segment, T-wave flattening and possibly the emergence of U-waves. The prevalence of such changes appears greater with low potency preparations. Thus approximately 50% of patients on chlorpromazine or thioridazine will show some of these changes, a figure which rises to 70% with high dosage thioridazine (up to 900 mg/day) (Lipscomb, 1980). The comparable figure for trifluoperazine is about 16%. These changes appear largely benign, although lengthening QT interval, indicative of delayed ventricular repolarisation, may be associated with the development of arrhythmias particularly in those with pre-existing cardiac disease, especially conduction disorders. Ventricular arrhythmias are however rarely a problem in practice. They appear to be dose-related, and are most frequently associated with thioridazine. They have nonetheless been implicated in the sudden death syndrome (see below). Since thioridazine in particular is often used preferentially in the elderly, routine pre-treatment and treatment ECG monitoring is prudent in this group if practicable, especially when higher doses are contemplated.

The question of sudden death occurring in patients on antipsychotics remains controversial and has received prominence following a circular from the Committee on Safety of Medicines in1990 concerning 13 cases who were taking pimozide. Such reports usually involve younger,

Table 9.7 Summary of non-neurological adverse reactions to antipsychotics

Adverse reaction		Frequency	Comment
General	Sedation	++	Esp. with low potency drugs
	'Torpor' (Ataraxy)	+++	
	Dry mouth	+	
	Blurred vision	+	Conventionally viewed as peripheral
	Constipation	+	anticholinergic effects. Some probably
	Urinary difficulties	+	include adrenergic actions
	Impaired sexual function	+	
	Weight gain	+++	May have endocrine component
Cardio-vascular	Incr. heart rate	+++	Not clinically significant
	Hypotension	++	Can be fatal – caution with early exposure to low potency drugs
	ECG changes	++	Quinidine-like effect: rarely causes ventricular tachyarrhythmias particularly with thioridazine
Endocrine	Hyperpro-lactinaemia	+++	Universal effect (except clozapine)
	– Galactorrhoea	Rare	
	– Amenorrhoea	+	
	Gynaecomastia	Rare	Rarely clinically significant
	Hyper/hypogly-caemia	Rare	
	Inappropriate ADH	Rare	
Hepatic function	Impaired liver	++	Transient changes common. Jaundice esp. with chlorpromazine
Dermato-logical	Skin rashes	++	
	– Erythematous	++	Especially with chlorpromazine
	– Urticarial	Rare	
	– Contact	Rare	
	Photosensitivity	++	Can result in serious burning. Temp. less important than brightness
	Pigmentation	?Rare	Infrequently reported nowadays
Haemato-logical	Neutropenia	Rare	But note – with clozapine: reversible
	Agranulocytosis	Rare	neutropenia (~ 2%) Can progress to agranulocytosis if drug maintained
	Thrombocytopenia	V. rare	
	Haemolytic anaemia	V. rare	
Ophth-almic	Lenticular deposits	Rare	Reversible with early detection
	Pigmentary retin-opathy		High dose, long-term thioridazine only

apparently fit patients treated with relatively high antipsychotic doses for severe or protracted illnesses. It is impossible to determine what part autonomic (vagal) over-activity or other sequelae of profound mental state disturbance may play in this, and how much can legitimately be attributed to a drug effect (Simpson *et al*, 1987). There is some evidence however that phenothiazines, and in particular thioridazine may be disproportionately associated with this phenomenon (Mehtonen *et al*, 1991), although this observation must await clarification. There is at this stage no evidence that pimozide is uniquely hazardous in this regard, but the CSM guidelines recommend:

pretreatment ECG
initial maximum dose of 4 mg per day ('acute situations' 10 mg)
increments of no more than 4 mg weekly
maximum dose of 20 mg/day
routine ECG monitoring above 16 mg daily.

Sudden death in antipsychotic-treated patients is exceedingly rare but because it represents the ultimate tragedy, all doctors must be aware of the phenomenon, although the precise role of the drugs in such cases remains uncertain.

Endocrine changes

With the exception of clozapine, all antipsychotic drugs produce sharp rises in serum prolactin from blockade of tuberoinfundibular hypothalamic dopamine (D_2) receptors. The raised prolactin is usually not associated with any clinical changes but may cause galactorrhoea (in either gender). It may also contribute to amenorrhoea, although the causes of this in psychoses are undoubtedly multiple. Gynaecomastia, which can rarely develop following long-term exposure, appears to relate more to androgen/oestrogen ratios rather than hyperprolactinaemia *per se*. Breast enlargement combined with amenorrhoea may lead to the erroneous belief that the patient is pregnant. A theoretical concern has been that antipsychotics, by their ability to increase serum prolactin, may predispose to the development of hormone-dependent breast cancer, although so far no such link has been established.

Phenothiazines can unpredictably interfere with glucose metabolism, especially high dose chlorpromazine, which may inhibit insulin secretion, although only rarely does this contribute to instability of diabetic control. Suppression of corticotrophin, growth hormone, thyroid stimulating hormone, follicle stimulating hormone and luteinising hormone have been observed, but the clinical significance, if any, of these effects is unclear. Inappropriate ADH secretion can occur, and this may be one factor in the oedema sometimes encountered.

Patients on antipsychotics frequently complain of weight gain, which can be dramatic. The mechanisms are unclear and probably multiple, such as endocrine changes including fluid retention, interference with hypothalamic 5-HT systems regulating appetite, diminished 'output' from inactivity, carbohydrate craving, etc. Weight gain, or even fear of weight gain, is a major cause of non-compliance, especially in women, and must be taken seriously not only for its cosmetic, but also for the more important medical risks.

Allergic/toxic effects

Liver

Minor, usually transient elevations in hepatic enzymes, especially early in exposure to antipsychotics, are not uncommon and usually do not warrant any action. Marked elevations and clinical jaundice can probably occur with all antipsychotics but remain largely a problem with phenothiazines, particularly chlorpromazine. The prevalence of chlorpromazine-induced jaundice is around 1–2% (Regal *et al*, 1987), which represents a decline since the drug was first introduced, the reasons for which are unclear.

It is conventionally taught that this is a hypersensitivity type problem, because most cases are not dose-related. However, the data actually suggest an admixture of allergic and toxic aetiologies. Thus, the onset may be instant or delayed for over one year; a hypersensitivity syndrome (e.g. fever, chills, malaise, myalgia, arthralgia, etc.) may or may not occur, and biopsy, which characteristically shows cholestatic damage, may also reveal scattered hepatic necrosis. Furthermore, it is clear that some patients (perhaps up to 40%) will not develop jaundice on subsequent exposure (Regal *et al*, 1987).

Phenothiazine-induced jaundice is usually benign. Although symptoms may sometimes subside with continued therapy, the offending medication should be withdrawn after which liver function usually returns to normal in 2–8 weeks. A small number of patients have gone on to develop a syndrome resembling primary biliary cirrhosis, although the prognosis for the drug-induced condition is better than for the idiopathic disorder. Cross-sensitivity among phenothiazines is rare, and a straight dose equivalent switch to another antipsychotic is usually without incident.

Dermatological

Skin rashes are rare with non-phenothiazines, but occur in 5–10% of those on chlorpromazine. These are fairly typical of any drug-related allergic reaction, developing suddenly within two weeks of first exposure and characterised by a widespread, hot, itching erythematous eruption. Rarely urticarial rashes and contact dermatitis can occur. Skin rashes seldom inhibit management and require only a change of antipsychotic and possibly symptomatic treatment with antihistamines or topical lotions.

Photosensitivity is another problem associated mainly with chlorpromazine. Dermatologists believe it to be relatively uncommon (about 3%), but this may be an underestimate especially if mild reactions presenting solely as prickly, itching discomfort in exposed areas are included. It is caused by a combination of phototoxicity (or chemical injury) and photoallergy, due to light (not heat) in the UVA band of the spectrum. Patients on chlorpromazine should be advised to avoid bright – although not necessarily hot – direct sunshine. Topical barrier creams are helpful.

Long-term exposure to chlorpromazine may also promote development of a blue-grey or brown pigmentation especially on exposed areas. Women are supposedly more frequently affected. The cause is unknown although it may be associated with generalised pigmentary deposition, including in the internal organs.

Haematological

Antipsychotics can interfere with marrow production and agranulocytosis and thrombocytopaenic purpura have been described, although they seem to be very rare with classical antipsychotics. Most are probably allergic, but some reported cases were seen to have been dose-dependent, and may have been toxic. Haemolytic anaemia has also been infrequently recorded.

The impact of early fatalities from agranulocytosis on the development of clozapine has already been mentioned. Clozapine appears to cause a neutropenia in about 2–3% of cases. On average, onset is after 8 weeks of treatment but the range is wide – from a few days to 6 months. This appears to be reversible with early detection and immediate discontinuation. Clozapine is only suitable for patients who can cope with the rigorous haematological monitoring procedures (weekly blood tests for the first 18 weeks, samples every fortnight thereafter).

In November 1993, eight cases of aplastic anaemia, two of which were fatal, were reported in association with remoxipride use and this drug is currently only available for use in the UK on a 'named patient' basis, with a requirement for routine haematology monitoring (FBCs weekly for 6 months, monthly thereafter). Remoxipride cannot therefore be considered a 'first line' drug at present, though its position may change as more information becomes available.

Eyes

Impairment of accommodation is common, and although inconvenient it is only likely to pose a problem in patients with undiagnosed closed-angle glaucoma. In diagnosed patients, low potency drugs with marked anticholinergic effects should be avoided. Two other ophthalmic problems are of potentially greater significance. Long-term use of phenothiazines can be associated with the development of lenticular and corneal deposits. They probably relate to dose, or perhaps more accurately, total drug intake and may be associated with generalised pigmentary deposition. While these may progress to impair vision they are largely benign and certainly, if detected early, appear reversible.

Of more sinister import is pigmentary retinopathy which can seriously impair vision. This disorder appears to be particularly associated with patients treated for long periods with high dose (> 1 g) thioridazine. For this reason thioridazine in doses of greater than 600 mg per day should not be used for other than short-term (i.e. up to 4 weeks) treatment.

Neurological adverse effects

These are the most frequent and important side-effects associated with antipsychotic use, and will be considered in two groups, general and extrapyramidal.

General neurological effects

Sedation and drowsiness and the peculiar emotional detachment of torpor (or 'ataraxy') have already been alluded to. There has been much debate about the relationship between antipsychotic administration and the development of depression. Early opinion, still held by some (Galdi, 1983) was that these drugs, especially in depot form, could promote depression. However, depression can be an integral part of schizophrenic symptomatology, affecting 50–60% of patients at admission (Knights *et al*, 1979; Moller & Von Zerssen, 1982) and 25–30% at some point in the post-psychotic period, when it can be sufficiently pronounced to fulfil operational criteria for major depression (Siris *et al*, 1981). The evidence to date is that antipsychotics do not cause depressed mood *per se* (Knights & Hirsch, 1981; Moller & Von Zerssen, 1982). They may of course produce subjective slowing, lack of interest and initiative and inefficiency of thinking which has been rather confusingly referred to as 'akinetic depression' (Van Putten & May, 1978), but this relates to their extrapyramidal actions (i.e. Parkinsonism) rather than to primary effects on mood.

Antipsychotics alter the EEG. The general effect is slowing with decreased alpha and increased theta and delta activity. Fast beta activity may be evident, but with chronic therapy synchronisation occurs along with increasing slow wave activity, amplitude and superimposition of spikes and sharp waves. Paroxysmal discharge patterns similar to those found in seizure disorders may emerge – hence the importance of knowing the patient's drug history when interpreting the EEG. At a clinical level they can lower the seizure threshold and may promote fits. The risk may be increased among those with a history of epilepsy, or previous drug-induced fits, head trauma and other brain pathology but can occur without any prior predisposition. The evidence suggests the risk is greatest with chlorpromazine, intermediate with trifluoperazine and lowest with thioridazine, pimozide, haloperidol and fluphenazine (Cold *et al*, 1990). High doses, rapid increments, sudden dose changes and polypharmacy should be avoided where fits may be suspected or become evident. The frequency is no more than 1% of cases (Cold *et al*, 1990) and seizures do not represent an absolute contraindication to continued antipsychotic treatment. Should they emerge, they can be treated conventionally with anticonvulsants and if appropriate, gradual change to a preparation with lower potential. Epileptiform EEG abnormalities appear to be more common with clozapine, which has a reported fit frequency of 4%, a phenomenon that appears to be dose dependent (Baldessarini & Frankenburg, 1991).

Temperature control: hypothermia

Antipsychotics can interfere with temperature control. Phenothiazines, especially chlorpromazine, can promote hypothermia by a combination of hypothalamic and peripheral vasomotor actions. A particularly dangerous scenario is the chronic schizophrenic who goes on an alcoholic 'bender' and spends the night outside, comatose. The combination of drug-related hypothermia and heat loss from alcohol-induced vasodilation can readily prove fatal.

Neuroleptic malignant syndrome (NMS)

Much greater attention has been devoted to the opposite problem in recent years – namely the so-called neuroleptic malignant syndrome. This term has been applied to the sudden development of fever (sometimes qualifying as hyperpyrexia), rigidity, confusion and autonomic instability, usually within a few weeks of starting antipsychotics. Serum creatinine phosphokinase (CK) is often dramatically raised. Most reports have concerned young men, and permanent neurological damage or a fatal outcome has frequently ensued, though the reported mortality appears to have declined (Shaler *et al*, 1989).

Regretfully, the author is not in a position to impart his experience of this problem to the reader, for after 20 years of practice, specialising in schizophrenia, he has never seen a case. It will come as no surprise therefore, to be told that he finds the reported prevalance of up to 2.4% (Addonizio *et al*, 1986) highly perplexing and in need of explanation. Psychotic illness associated with hyperpyrexia, neurological signs including catalepsy and rigidity, autonomic dysfunction such as tachycardia, diaphoresis and labile BP, and a rapidly fatal outcome has been described for over a century under a variety of names (Mann *et al*, 1986). These include Bell's mania, mortal catatonia, acute delirious mania, delirium acutum, delire aigu and Scheid's cyantoic syndrome. It is perhaps now usually remembered as Stauder's lethal catatonia described in 1934. So the first point is that this syndrome clearly existed long before the introduction of antipsychotic medication.

Diagnostic techniques were, of course, less refined then and it is likely that many of these cases had some undetected intercurrent physical illness. The second point is, how little things have changed! In a review of the modern literature on 'neuroleptic malignant syndrome', Levinson & Simpson (1986) concluded that physical conditions such as pneumonia and dehydration could have accounted for the clinical presentation in 65% of cases, and other extenuating factors could be implicated in a further 23%.

It must be concluded that neuroleptic malignant syndrome is extremely rare when all other potential causes of a similar presentation are excluded – and diagnosis must be by exclusion. Proposed diagnostic criteria (Keck *et al*, 1989) are very wide and could easily be fulfilled by patients with, for example, inadequately treated Parkinsonism.

Patients on antipsychotics who do develop fever must be thoroughly investigated along conventional lines for foci of infection – CXR, WBC, MSU etc. If extrapyramidal signs also become evident for the first time or dramatically worsen it is prudent to reduce or stop antipsychotics temporarily. Anticholinergics should not be withheld in the presence of a hypokinetic-rigid syndrome, but should be used thoughtfully as in excess they may contribute (indeed have contributed) to pyrexia by impairment of sweating, and to increasing confusion. All other non-essential medication, especially that with significant anticholinergic activity such as tricyclics, should also be stopped. Benzodiazepines can be used as required to control disturbed behaviour. It is also essential to detect and correct dehydration, by i.v. infusion if necessary. It is for situations such as this that psychiatrists are firstly physicians and these skills must be exercised rigorously.

In cases where signs persist or progress, dopamine agonists such as bromocriptine have been advocated (Levinson & Simpson, 1986) as there is evidence that stimulation of hypothalamic dopamine receptors in rats can result in a lowering of core temperature, though any benefits from this approach may arise as much from effects on muscle rigidity as on central thermoregulation. Dantrolene, a potent peripheral muscle relaxant, has been advocated empirically on the basis of its use in treating malignant hyperthermia, a rare condition which can follow general anaesthesia in predisposed individuals. Both this and bromocriptine are heroic strategies of unproven efficacy.

Once the condition has settled, antipsychotics can be reintroduced cautiously. In particular, the rate of increase should be tempered. Fever has been reported as recurring in this situation without demonstrable cause, in which case it may still be possible to treat with a drug of a different class.

Extrapyramidal side-effects (EPS)

These are the most important side-effects associated with antipsychotic drug use, and should be regularly sought and never ignored.

Descriptively EPS embrace two broad syndromes, the hyperkinetic and the bradykinetic, which may co-exist. Conventionally EPS are classified on the basis of the relationship of their onset to the duration of drug exposure. Three main types are described: acute (onset within hours or days); intermediate (onset within days or weeks, sometimes months); and late (onset sometimes within months, usually after years).

Acute extrapyramidal effects

The acute extrapyramidal effects of antipsychotic use are hyperkinetic movement disorders of sudden onset – that is, they are acute dyskinesias. Most commonly, although not invariably, they are clinically dystonias. All dystonias share two characteristics – they are involuntary movements which have a twisting or rotational quality and which are sustained for a variable period at the point of maximal contraction (Owens, 1990). The result is postural distortion. With acute dystonias the sustained component is prominent and prolonged so these are examples of myostatic dystonias (as opposed to the kinetic types where constant movement predominates).

Clinical features.   The range of dystonic presentations is infinite and all lists, including Table 9.8, should be viewed as outlines only.

Like all dystonias acute drug-related disorder tends to be more generalised and severe in children and adolescents (Ayd, 1961; Marsden *et al*, 1975). Although any involuntary muscles can be affected, in adults, neck muscles are most frequently involved (30%) followed by tongue/ jaw (15–17%), while extraocular involvement is relatively uncommon (approximately 6%) (Swett, 1975). When unassociated with other neuro-psychiatric disturbance, deviation of the eyes on its own is insufficient disorder to be characterised as an oculogyric 'crisis', and the simple descriptive term 'oculogyric spasm' is more appropriate (Owens, 1990).

Mild or early disorder may only present as subjective stiffness and loss of function or aching discomfort without objective signs. These features should not be ignored as full-blown dystonia can rapidly ensue. It is also important to bear in mind that in addition to the physical component acute dystonias have a clear affective component. Even when objective signs are few, this can result in distress which appears out of all proportion. The often bizarre presentation of acute dystonias and this affective component may explain why even nowadays, these disorders are still mistakenly diagnosed as 'hysterical'.

With the possible exception of anxiety, no specific precipitating factors have been identified. The majority of examples (90%) occur within the first 4–5 days of exposure or dose increment (Ayd, 1961). Reports have, however, suggested both an earlier and a delayed onset following depot administration compared with orals. These findings are not necessarily contradictory. The onset of most dystonias within 12 hours of depot administration was reported from the US at a time when the only depots available there were of fluphenazine. As has already been mentioned, fluphenazine decanoate produces a unique, rapid, post-injection peak which could explain an earlier onset of acute dystonias with this formulation. The pharmacokinetics of other depots however, may indicate the later onset reported elsewhere.

Table 9.8 Clinical features of acute dystonias

Presentation	Affect
Neck	Retrocollis Torticollis Laterocollis Anterocollis
Tongue	Rotation Protrusion Retraction
Jaw	Forced opening Lateral deviation Trismus
Extraocular	Upward (± lateral) deviation
Trunk	Scoliosis Opisthotonos
Limbs	Full range of dystonic postures – Hyperpronation of arms – Wrist flexion – Metacarpal-phalangeal flexion/ extension – Extension of lower limbs – Adductor spasm – Plantarflexion-inversion – Dorsiflexion-eversion

Untreated, the natural course of acute dystonias is either persistence over hours or even days, or alternatively, a waxing and waning with periods of intense symptoms interspersed with relative relief. Again this must not be taken as evidence of psychogenic causation.

Prevalence.   The widely quoted figure of 2.3% (Ayd, 1961) is certainly an underestimate because of the way in which it was calculated (Owens, 1990). A more realistic figure of 25–36% has been reported from both recent retrospective and prospective studies (Addonizio & Alexopoulos, 1988; Singh *et al*, 1990; Chakos *et al*, 1992).

An inverse relationship with age exists, with acute dystonias uncommon in the elderly (< 2% for those over 60 years of age). However, the generally held view that young men are at greater risk seems more likely to have reflected heavier treatment regimes in this group than in their female counterparts, as evidence from prospective studies has not supported male gender *per se* as being a predisposing factor (Singh *et al*, 1990).

Pathophysiology.   The pathophysiology of acute dystonias is not understood but part of the problem may involve overactivity of striatal dopamine systems at both pre- and post-synaptic sites. The disorder most frequently occurs early in exposure at a time that is particularly dynamic for dopaminergic systems adapting to blockade. This is when the early adaptive response, increased dopamine turnover, is fading though still present but the long-term response, post-synaptic receptor supersensitivity, is also emerging (Marsden & Jenner, 1980; Marsden *et al*, 1986).

Treatment.   Many different treatments have been reported as effective in acute dystonias (e.g. barbiturates, benzodiazepines, antihistamines) but they have been supplanted by the anticholinergics. In the presence of established disorder, slow i.v. administration of procyclidine 10 mg stat. is safe and effective within minutes.

After a first dystonic episode antipsychotics should be held unchanged or even reduced for a few days before attempting further increments. If symptoms or signs recur, routine oral anticholinergics can be started for 1–2 weeks while antipsychotic dose increases, but should be discontinued thereafter. Sometimes after depot injections patients complain of feeling uncomfortable for a few days. This can often be helped by a small dose of anticholinergic (e.g. procyclidine 5 mg daily or b.d.) for 3–7 days post-injection, but this practice should be limited to cases where clear benefit is demonstrated and no alternative, such as change of dose, injection interval, or depot, has worked.

Intermediate extrapyramidal effects

Parkinsonism.   Parkinsonism associated with antipsychotic drugs is sometimes referred to as 'pseudoparkinsonism' to distinguish it from the idiopathic disorder. Although there are often striking differences in clinical presentation, the core features of bradykinesia, rigidity and tremor can be found in both the idiopathic and drug-induced Parkinsonian states.

Bradykinesia (also known as hypokinesia/akinesia) refers to loss of voluntary motor activity. This shows itself as a decrease in associated or background movement, slowing of voluntary movements, and interruption to the normal flow of movement. This is the commonest manifestation of Parkinsonism in patients treated with anti-dopaminergic medication.

Rigidity refers to an increase in resting muscle tone evident on passive movement. Both so-called 'cog-wheel' and 'lead-pipe' types are equally important in drug-related cases. Cogwheeling is a jerky pattern of resistance that is intermittently broken and re-established throughout the range of passive movements. This pattern probably results from the combination of rigidity with tremor. Lead pipe is rigidity uniformly sustained throughout the range of passive movements. Rigidity is usually mild in drug-related disorders and may require reinforcement to elicit it.

Tremor is the regular involuntary movement of a body part about a joint. Tremors can be classified on the basis of their frequency and amplitude, or simply in terms of the situations in which they occur. In Parkinsonism two main types may develop – the classical resting tremor, of low frequency and high amplitude (~6 Hz), and a postural or action tremor of high frequency and low amplitude (~15–20 Hz) usually best seen in the hands with arms outstretched. In drug-related Parkinsonism, action tremor is a common and early sign, while the resting tremor characteristic of idiopathic disease is a relatively less frequent and later development.

In addition, disturbances of postural reflexes develop, along with gait and autonomic abnormalities.

Clinical features. It is often forgotten in the face of striking objective abnormality that Parkinsonism presents major subjective problems for the sufferer. Especially in mild or early cases these symptoms can be difficult to distinguish from features associated with mental state – e.g. weakness, listlessness, stiffness, aching discomfort especially on rising in the morning – but such vague subjective symptoms should be sought.

With more established disorder, the features of Parkinsonism can seriously impinge on the patient's everyday life. Progressive loss of dexterity can lead to major problems with everyday domestic and occupational tasks. Neurologists evaluate subjective disability by rating the so-called Activities of Daily Living, and while most patients with drug-related disorder will not (or should not) progress to serious impairment in these areas, a thorough assessment should always include enquiry into the subjective impact of symptomatology.

The objective signs of Parkinsonism are multiple (Table 9.9) and patients present diverse clinical pictures. Loss of arm swing is, in the author's experience, one of the earliest and most sensitive indicators of antipsychotic exposure and should always be sought. Contrariwise, marked postural or gait abnormalities are uncommon and if they develop, dosage schedules should be seriously reconsidered.

Onset is usually gradual over anything from days to months although speed of evolution probably depends on a combination of patient factors such as age and individual susceptibility, and physician factors e.g. type of drug, dosage, rate of increments. Most cases (90%) are evident in the first 10 weeks (Ayd, 1961). The condition may have a fluctuating course, and in some patients, once established, can to some extent remit spontaneously after some months on stable regimes. As with idiopathic disease, a 2:1 female excess has been found. This may reflect a genuine gender difference or incidental factors such as age or the different prescribing practices reported between the sexes (Laska *et al*, 1973).

Table 9.9 Clinical features of Parkinsonism

Feature	Comment
Posture: Flexion	In drug related disorder slight hyper-extension of spine more common
Hypomimia	'Masked' expression / loss of facial contours
Sialorrhoea	May be failure to swallow rather than excessive production – drooling
Seborrhoea	
Loss of background body movement	Decreased gesture and interactive postural movements
Loss of pendular arm swing	Early, sensitive sign
Tremor: resting : action/postural	~ 6 Hz relatively uncommon, late sign ~15–20 Hz common, early sign
Rigidity	Rarely marked
Loss of dexterity	May impair independent living/self-care. Caution with driving/operating machinery
Micrographia	Reduction in vertical and horizontal size
Impairment of speech	Loss of pitch and power – soft monotonous speech – inarticulate
Impaired initiation of voluntary activity	
Instability	
Disturbance of gait	Reduced length and height of step – shuffling/festination

It is accepted wisdom that drug-related Parkinsonism invariably resolves once the offending medication has been withdrawn. This has never been conclusively demonstrated, and there are undoubtedly some patients whose symptoms persist indefinitely. In such cases drugs may have released a latent tendency to idiopathic disorder.

Prevalence. A consensus on prevalence is hard to establish. The reasons for this include the variable effects in different populations of differing drug potencies, dose schedules, durations of treatment and age. The most important determinants of prevalence are simply how closely you look and what you call abnormal – in other words, the comprehensiveness and sensitivity of the assessment.

The literature suggests a prevalence of 15–20% (Ayd, 1961; Kennedy *et al*, 1971). This is probably reasonable for patients showing sufficient abnormality to qualify for a clinical Parkinson's syndrome. However, if prevalence is based on the presence of isolated features, insufficient in type or degree to qualify as a full syndrome, the figure is undoubtedly higher. It could be argued that virtually all adequately treated patients followed closely enough will show some Parkinsonian features at some time.

Pathophysiology. The pathophysiology of Parkinsonism is the easiest of the drug-related extrapyramidal abnormalities to conceptualise. By analogy with Parkinson's disease it is seen as resulting from blockade of nigro-striatal dopaminergic pathways. However, it is likely that individual susceptibility – i.e. the patient's individual dopaminergic 'endowment' – is important in the expression of the disorder.

Treatment. The treatment of drug-related Parkinsonism is not as easy as is often thought. The commonest strategy, of adding anticholinergics, is largely empirical, and while these drugs may help the subjective 'stiffness' and the unpleasant awareness of slowed, ponderous movement, overall their effects can be disappointing. In particular, objective signs often persist.

Anticholinergics are overprescribed. There is no justification for the widespread practice of automatically prescribing anticholinergics when starting antipsychotics. They should only be added if Parkinsonian features become significant, as assessed by (1) the nature and severity of individual signs; (2) the multiplicity of signs, and (3) the subjective complaint of distress and/or incapacity.

In view of its established, as opposed to its empirical efficacy, procyclidine is probably the drug of choice, in an oral dosage of 5 mg t.i.d. Dosages should be kept conservative. Little further improvement is likely with doses above 20 mg per day that was not evident with lower doses.

After one month the t.i.d. regime can be reduced to b.d. and response assessed. Overall, anticholinergics should be held for 3–4 months, after which a definite attempt at discontinuation should be made, as there is evidence that in the majority of cases Parkinsonian features will not recur (Orlov *et al*, 1971). If resurgence of features necessitates maintenance beyond three months, further attempts to discontinue should still be made at three-monthly intervals.

If response to anticholinergics proves less than satisfactory, then one should consider reduction of antipsychotic dose – mental state permitting – and/or transfer to a drug of a different class, though this should in fact always be considered as an alternative to simply adding an anticholinergic.

Akathisia.   Akathisia literally means 'an inability to sit still'. The term 'tasikinesia' has been applied to 'an inability to stand still' but this is probably not a separate entity. Akathisia was described from the beginning of the century as a paradoxical restlessness that could afflict patients with Parkinson's disease. As traditionally understood, it is not a movement disorder. There is nothing abnormal about the patients' movements which are a voluntary and coordinated, if purposeless (i.e. non-goal directed), response to the intensely unpleasant affect that is the cornerstone of the disorder. Having said that the movement is voluntary, it is the 'voluntary' activity of someone with a pistol at their head! This forced or 'driven' quality is characteristic.

Clinical features. The cardinal features are an intense, unpleasant inner restlessness, and a need to move in an attempt – usually vain – to relieve the subjective distress. The common presentations are shown in Table 9.10.

As with drug-related Parkinsonism, 80–90% of cases are evident in the first 6–10 weeks of treatment and females are reported as being affected twice as frequently as males, though as with Parkinsonism, this may not reflect a genuine gender difference.

Akathisia is an extremely distressing condition for patients and a major source of their non-compliance with medication. It has also been associated with violent behaviour and suicide. Thus it must always be sought and taken seriously.

The major diagnostic dilemma with akathisia is, of course, its close phenomenological similarity to psychomotor agitation. The trap is that the treatment of the two disorders is diametrically opposite. Akathisia worsens with increased antipsychotic medication whereas agitation may improve, hence dosage reduction may be one way of clarifying the diagnosis. A further distinction is that with akathisia, some patients may be able to localise the source of their restlessness to the lower part of the body and in particular to their legs.

Prevalence. The prevalence of akathisia has usually been found to be between 21% (Ayd, 1961) and 32% (Kennedy *et al*, 1971), and is likely to be dependent on the same variables (e.g. drug potency, dose and rate of increment) noted as being relevant to Parkinsonism.

Pathophysiology. The frequent co-existence of Parkinsonism and akathisia and their strikingly similar epidemiologies suggest both a common mechanism and a paradox. The common mechanism is likely to be blockade of dopaminergic neurotransmission, but the paradox is how such dominating restlessness can occur at the same time as a condition whose cardinal feature is motor poverty. One obvious explanation is a different site for the two pathophysiologies. In line with this, akathisia has been proposed as resulting from blockade of mesocortical dopamine neurones (Marsden *et al*, 1986). This system has been implicated on the inhibitory side of the motor equation and hence blockade could be associated with both 'release' of non-goal directed behaviours and, conceivably, a distressingly subjective awareness. However, this hypothesis remains speculative.

Treatment. Treatment of akathisia is unsatisfactory. Reducing dosage may be the most useful first option, and because high potency preparations are more likely to be causal (Munetz & Cornes, 1983) switching to a low potency preparation is a good second choice, but this may not always be possible. Most clinicians seem to opt for specific additional medication, in particular anticholinergics. Even though these are often prescribed there is little evidence for their efficacy. Benzodiazepines may modify akathisia non-specifically, due to their anxiolytic activity, or more specifically by facilitating GABA-ergic transmission, which is inhibitory on dopaminergic systems. Recently, β-blockers have been reported to be effective in patients with akathisia (Adler *et al*, 1986), and where additional medication is deemed necessary, propranolol 20–60 mg/day should now be the first option.

Late extrapyramidal effects

Tardive dyskinesia. This problem was probably first identified in 1959 by Sigwald and colleagues but was more clearly defined by Uhrbrand &

Table 9.10 Clinical features of akathisia

Feature	Comment
Anxious, tense expression	
Restlessness on sitting	Hands fidgety
	'Sitting up' repeatedly
	Side to side movement
	Rocking – backwards/forwards
	Swinging legs
	Crossing/uncrossing legs
Inability to sit	Standing (e.g. in mid-sentence)
Inability to stand still	Shifting weight from foot to foot
	Pacing (with 'driven' quality)

Faurbye in Denmark in 1960. They described a syndrome consisting of mainly, but not exclusively, orofacial involuntary movements in 33 diagnostically heterogeneous long stay patients, who had all been treated with a range of physical treatments including prolonged exposure to antipsychotic medication, which the authors considered the likely causative factor (Uhrbrand & Faurbye, 1960). Because this syndrome appeared to come on later in the course of antipsychotic exposure than the other known extrapyramidal syndromes, it was subsequently designated tardive dyskinesia (Faurbye *et al*, 1964) – 'dyskinesia' being simply the generic neurological term for 'any abnormal movement'.

At first the descriptive term 'orofacial dyskinesia' and the aetiological one 'tardive dyskinesia' were used interchangeably (Crane & Naranjo, 1971) but it soon became clear that orofacial movements could be found in patients never exposed to antipsychotic medication. Also comprehensive studies using detailed recording instruments have shown no body part to be immune, so movements anywhere, not just in the face, must be included. Any type of involuntary movement – chorea, dystonia, tics, myoclonus, etc. – can, with one exception, comprise the syndrome. The exception is tremor which is specifically excluded (Marsden *et al*, 1975). The time criterion, however, remains arbitrary. Originally, an exposure period of 2 years was proposed, though it is now clear that abnormal movements, especially chronic dystonia, may occasionally appear after only a few weeks or months of treatment. In general therefore 'tardive' is perhaps best reserved for movements emerging after on average one year.

The term tardive dyskinesia can only be used to infer a role for (antidopaminergic) medication in producing the movement disorder – which at this stage, effectively means treatment with antipsychotics, non-antipsychotic phenothiazines and the benzamide, metoclopramide. To talk of 'spontaneous tardive dyskinesia' is clearly to betray an ignorance of the concept which the present reader has mercifully been spared!

Clinical features. Textbooks often present the features of tardive dyskinesia as a regular progression, but it is unlikely things are quite so neat. Certainly, vermicular or worm-like movements of the tongue without its displacement are usually accepted as the earliest orofacial sign and appear to be the premonitory features of lingual choreoathetosis, but tongue movements may sometimes be mild in the presence of striking disorder elsewhere.

The oral/perioral musculature is the most commonly affected, often as a group, and the term bucco-linguo-masticatory (BLM) triad is often applied to this 'en masse' involvement. These movements are descriptively referred to as 'choreoathetoid' in type but it should be noted that in their characteristics they are usually complex, repetitive and coordinated – quite the opposite of the rudimentary, non-repetitive and uncoordinated

Table 9.11 Clinical features of tardive dyskinesia

Presentation	Effect
Tongue	No displacement 　'Vermicular' movements 　Twisting: horizontal/longitudinal axis Displacement 　Sweeping buccal surface: 'bon bon' sign 　Irregular jerky protrusion: 'Fly catcher' sign 　'Tromboning' on voluntary protrusion
Lips	Puckering Pouting Puffing Smacking Lateral retraction: 'bridling'
Jaw	Mouth opening Clenching ('Trismus') Grinding ('Bruxism') Forward/lateral protrusion
Facial expression	Tics Grimacing Blepharoclonus Blepharospasm Irregular eyebrow elevation Frowning
Neck	Torti-/Retro-/Latero-/Antero-Collis 　(Kinetic (spasmodic) or static)
Trunk	Unilateral dystonia: 'Pisa syndrome' Hyperextension of spine (bilateral dystonia) Axial hyperkinesis: 'copulatory' movements
Upper limbs	Shoulder tics Hyperpronation Choreoathetoid finger/wrist movements
Lower limbs	'Restless' legs Squirming: 'outsplaying' of toes Ankle rotation Eversion/inversion Stamping
Oropharynx	Dysphagia
Diaphragm/ Intercostals	Irregular respiration/grunting

characteristics conventionally attributed to chorea. Interestingly the movements of the BLM triad simulate normal eating-related behaviours which suggests that the entire cerebral engram modulating such actions has been released from inhibitory control.

The list of features in Table 9.11 is only a guide. Many patients will illustrate examples of bizarre movements that defy rational classification.

One descriptive subtype of tardive dyskinesia, tardive dystonia, is uncommon but deserves special attention. It has a generally younger age of onset than classical tardive dyskinesia, produces much greater functional disability and subjective distress, and may have somewhat different treatment characteristics (Owens, 1990). Although the literature suggests that only about 2% of tardive syndromes are dystonic in type, this may be an underestimate.

In common with many extrapyramidal syndromes, the movements of tardive dyskinesia are intimately related to the mental state and this should always be taken into account when performing assessments. Thus they are more pronounced, or indeed may only emerge, when the patient is alert or excited (i.e. 'aroused'), ease during periods of composure, and disappear during sedation or sleep. They can be suppressed for variable periods by voluntary effort and may disappear during intense concentration. Voluntary activity in another body part may exacerbate them (i.e. activation), but if writing is selected as the way of demonstrating this, it is important to be aware that the concentration required by some patients to write even simple things may produce an unpredictable response, in some cases worsening the movements but in others diminishing them.

Factors suggested in retrospective studies as predisposing to tardive dyskinesia are shown in Table 9.12. None of the drug-related variables has been conclusively implicated, although this may partly reflect the problems of quantifying such data accurately. Episodic 'on-off' exposure, with 'offs' longer than 1–3 months, does have a theoretical basis in the electrophysiological principle of 'kindling' (Jeste *et al*, 1979) and if confirmed prospectively would have major clinical implications. Increasing age is the single non-drug variable clearly established, though evidence that a prior history of EPS and the recently reported association with diabetes mellitus (Ganzini *et al*, 1991) look convincing. The much quoted female excess (1.6:1) may reflect interposing influences as much as a gender predisposition. Reports of associations with an affective diagnosis (American Psychiatric Association, 1984) seem less robust than a decade ago and require confirmation, as do those linking tardive dyskinesia to 'negative' schizophrenia (Owens & Johnstone, 1980; Waddington & Youssef, 1986; Johnstone *et al*, 1989). This is nonetheless of interest in relation to the observation that such movements may be found in schizophrenics never exposed to antipsychotics (Owens *et al*, 1982). It may be that for some patients, antipsychotics are promoting a tendency to movement disorder inherent in their psychiatric disorder.

Recent prospective work has found a relationship between the development of tardive dyskinesia and antipsychotic dose (Morgenstern & Glazer, 1993), and although this requires replication it would be prudent to take it as a cautionary signal for routine practice.

Tardive movements may be exacerbated temporarily, for a month or so, following antipsychotic reduction or discontinuation ('release' or 'withdrawal' phenomenon) and can be suppressed, at least for a time, by dose increment. Hence the need for stable regimes when performing repeated assessments. Reversibility is age-related and is more likely following discontinuation in those under 40 years of age (Seeman, 1981). Nevertheless it would seem sensible to view irreversibility as a potential outcome in all patients.

The long-term course of tardive dyskinesia has been difficult to establish but initial pessimism suggesting inexorable progression has not been borne out. Some cases appear to resolve, but the majority reach a plateau after which their signs seem to remain relatively stable, at least for a few years.

Prevalence. Pooled data suggests a prevalence for involuntary movements of around 20% overall, about 5–7% of which is attributable to spontaneous abnormality, leaving approximately 13–15% related to drugs (Jeste & Wyatt, 1981; Kane & Smith, 1982). More recent studies which have applied standardised, comprehensive recording techniques, and so probably pick up milder cases, have found prevalences in the 30–40% range.

Pathophysiology. Carlsson (1970) proposed that blockade of post-synaptic dopamine receptors resulted in the development of super-sensitivity of these sites, in a similar manner to denervation supersensitivity which is known to occur in the peripheral and autonomic nervous systems. An increase in striatal receptor numbers following chronic antipsychotic administration was subsequently demonstrated.

Table 9.12 Proposed predisposing factors for tardive dyskinesia (retrospective data)

Drug-related factors	Non-drug variables
Type of drug (potency)	Age
Maximum daily exposure	Gender
Duration of exposure	Organicity
Cumulative exposure	Past physical treatment
Polypharmacy	Leucotomy
Antipsychotic – free intervals	Insulin coma
Previous extrapyramidal side-effects	ECT
Anticholinergics	Age at onset of psychosis
	Mental state disorder
	Diabetes mellitus

Table 9.13 Treatment of tardive dyskinesia – double-blind studies

Treatment (pharmacological type)	Percent improved
Dopaminergic inhibitors	67.3
Cholinergic inhibitors	0
Dopaminergic potentiators	10.3
Cholinergic potentiators	32.1
GABA-ergic potentiators	54.8

Jeste & Wyatt (1979)

In line with this, the conventional theory of the pathophysiology of tardive dyskinesia invokes striatal post-synaptic dopamine receptor supersensitivity. In simplified terms, normal motor function is seen as a balance between cholinergic and dopaminergic actions in the striatum. Reduction on the dopaminergic side results in cholinergic predominance and this causes motor poverty as in Parkinsonism. Anticholinergics act to restore the balance, albeit at a reduced absolute level. Supersensitivity is seen as tipping the balance towards the dopaminergic side, resulting in hyperkinesis. Hence tardive dyskinesia is viewed by this model as the pathophysiological 'opposite' of Parkinsonism.

It is important to bear in mind that the dopamine supersensitivity hypothesis of tardive dyskinesia is only a theory which explains some, but not all, the clinical facts.

Treatment. No additional type of drug has been conclusively shown as successful in the treatment of tardive dyskinesia. In a detailed review of double-blind trials of tardive dyskinesia treatment, Jeste & Wyatt (1979) (Table 9.13) found that the most successful drugs in producing improvement were those which supposedly caused the condition in the first place!

The suppression phenomenon noted above could account for this finding, but antipsychotic dose increment cannot be recommended as a routine management strategy. This carries the theoretical risk of a breakthrough of the symptoms, possibly with increased severity, at a later date. This method should only be used in exceptional (e.g. life-threatening) circumstances, such as the presence of severe dysphagia with the risk of inhalation, progressive cachexia, and a raised CK and myoglobinuria as signs of muscle breakdown.

The management of tardive dyskinesia (Box 9.2) should always begin with a thorough review of the necessity for continuance of antipsychotic agents. Indications for their use should be strictly delineated. Dose schedules must be constantly justified with the aim of reduction to the minimum compatible with therapeutic efficacy. Patients on depots should, whenever possible, be switched to orals as the 'fine tuning' of dose reduction is far easier. Empirically the author's first choice is pimozide. It is possible, however, that a less pure D_2 blocker may be better because of evidence that D_1 antagonism may be antidyskinetic (Waddington, 1988), although this has not as yet been established clinically. With classical (i.e. choreiform/choreoathetoid) dyskinesia, the anticholinergic load should be reduced as far as possible, but where the clinical picture is of a relatively pure dystonia, it may be worth trying a slow, progressive increase in anticholinergics (e.g. benzhexol up to 20 mg/day or more) as there is now evidence that this may help chronic idiopathic dystonias (Burke *et al*, 1986). However, a careful watch should be kept for the emergence of choreiform movements. Presynaptic depleting agents, such as tetrabenazine can help idiopathic dystonia but in psychiatric patients they may cause depression and sometimes an unacceptable degree of bradykinesia. Even so they may permit a reduction in antipsychotic dosage.

Diazepam is also worth considering in all types of dyskinesia as its anxiolytic properties should help to reduce the severity of disorder by calming mental state while its GABA-facilitatory action may promote more specific antidyskinetic effects. Valproate, with similar GABA-ergic effects, may be a reasonable alternative.

Noradrenergic antagonists have been reported as beneficial in some patients (Jeste *et al*, 1988) although these drugs – such as clonidine (0.15–0.45 mg/day) and propranolol in high dose (up to 800 mg/day) – need more careful handling.

In line with a general interest in the pathogenic effects of free radicals, alpha-tocopherol or vitamin E, a free radical scavenger, has been reported as effective in the treatment of tardive dykinesia (Lohr *et al*, 1987; Adler *et al*, 1993). Although a clear role for this requires elucidation, it is a relatively safe treatment that may be worth considering.

Clozapine is certainly well worth trying when other measures have not helped (Lieberman *et al*, 1991), even if its function is only to hold mental state stable for long enough to permit some degree of resolution of the movement disorder.

Tardive akathisia. Akathisia as defined previously has both a subjective and an objective component. Recently it has been suggested that after long-term treatment patients can lose the distressing subjective restlessness (the affective component) while retaining the objective manifestations of purposeless, non-goal directed behaviours. This has been termed tardive akathisia (Simpson, 1977; Munetz & Cornes, 1983). Such a concept represents a substantial shift from the original notion of akathisia and places considerable burdens of choice on examiners to distinguish restlessness of this type from apparent restlessness resulting from dyskinesias such as chorea and dystonia, and from manneristic or catatonic behaviours.

Box 9.2 Outline for management of tardive dyskinesias

'Classical' tardive dyskinesia
  Justify antipsychotic use
  If on depots, switch to orals (dose equivalence)
  Aim for gradual but maximal reduction
  Reduce anticholinergic load
  Consider diazepam (GABA facilitatory & anxiolytic actions)
  or valproate
  Consider Vitamin E
  Consider noradrenergic antagonist (e.g. clonidine)
  Consider clozapine

Pure tardive dystonia
  Justify antipsychotic use
  If on depots, switch to orals (dose equivalence)
  Aim for gradual but maximal reduction
  Try gradual, progressive increase in anticholinergics to
  tolerance
  Consider presynaptic depleting agent, e.g. tetrabenazine
  Consider diazepam
  Consider clozapine

Extrapyramidal side-effects represent the major problem with the use of antipsychotic drugs. Their appearance may limit optimal therapeutic dosing and present a major barrier to compliance. Furthermore, it must be pointed out that the medico-legal position, especially with regard to tardive syndromes, has not, as yet, been clarified. In the US, when medical culpability has been established, it has been largely on the basis of a perceived ignorance or indifference by practitioners to the problem. Psychiatrists in the UK would do well to learn this lesson and become educated in recognition and diligent in assessment.

Conclusions

It sometimes seems that health care professionals view schizophrenia as a rather unchallenging condition. Nothing could be further from the truth. Because of its complexities, schizophrenia takes time, and because of the long-term nature of its disabilities, it demands commitment. That much of this time and commitment should be medical seems axiomatic. Medical input is complementary, not alternative, to that provided by other disciplines. Maximising this potential means that doctors require a sound understanding of the therapeutic tools at their disposal, and so management of schizophrenia also needs homework.

Patients with schizophrenia are not always easy to deal with but given time, commitment and homework, the condition can be commended as a fulfilling and fascinating field of medical practice.

References

Addonizio, G., Susman, V. L. & Roth, S. D. (1986) Symptoms of neuroleptic malignant syndrome in 82 consecutive in-patients. *American Journal of Psychiatry*, **143**, 1587–1590.

—— & Alexopoulos, G. S. (1988) Drug-induced dystonia in young and elderly patients. *American Journal of Psychiatry*, **145**, 869–871.

Adler, L. A., Angrist, B., Peselow, E., *et al* (1986) A controlled study of propranolol in the treatment of neuroleptic-induced akathisia. *British Journal of Psychiatry*, **149**, 42–45.

——, Peselow, E., Rotrosen, J., *et al* (1993) Vitamin E treatment of tardive dyskinesia. *American Journal of Psychiatry*, **164**, 448–458.

Alfredsson, G., Bjerkenstedt, L., Edman, G., *et al* (1984) Relationship between drug concentrations in serum and CSF clinical effects and monoaminergic variables in schizoprehnic patients treated with sulpiride or chlorpromazine. *Acta Psychiatrica Scandinavica*, **69** (Suppl. 311), 49–74.

American Psychiatric Association (1984) *Tardive Dyskinesia and Affective Disorders* (eds G. Gardos & D. E. Casey). Washington, DC: American Psychiatric Press.

Ayd, F. J. (1961) A survey of drug-induced extrapyramidal reactions. *Journal of the American Medical Association*, **175**, 1054–1060.

Baldessarini, R. (1985) *Chemotherapy in Psychiatry: Principles and Practice*. Cambridge, Mass.: Harvard University Press

—— & Frankenburg, F. R. (1991) Clozapine. A novel antipsychotic agent. *New England Journal of Medicine*, **324**, 746–754.

Breier, A. B., Wolkowitz, O. M., Doran, A. R., *et al* (1987) Neuroleptic responsivity of negative and positive symptoms in schizophrenia. *American Journal of Psychiatry*, **144**, 1549–1555.

Brosen, K. & Gram, L. F. (1989) Pharmacokinetic and clinical significance of genetic variability in psychotropic drug metabolism. In *Clinical Pharmacology in Psychiatry* (Psychopharmacology Series 7) (eds S. G. Dahl & L. F. Gram), pp. 192–200. Berlin: Springer Verlag.

Burke, R. E., Fahn, S. & Marsden, C. D. (1986) Torsion dystonia: a double-blind, prospective trial of high-dosage trihexyphenidyl. *Neurology*, **36**, 160–164.

Cade, J. F. J. (1949) Lithium salts in the treatment of psychotic excitement. *Medical Journal of Australia*, **36**, 349–352.

Carlsson, A. (1970) Biochemical implications of dopa-induced actions on the central nervous system with particular reference to abnormal movements. In *L-dopa and Parkinsonism* (eds A. Barbeau & F. H. McDowell). Philadelphia: Davis.

—— (1988) The current status of the dopamine hypothesis of schizophrenia. *Neuropsychopharmacology*, **1**, 179–186.

Carpenter, W. T., Heinrichs, D. W. & Alphs, L. D. (1985) Treatment of negative symptoms. *Schizophrenia Bulletin*, **11**, 440–452.

Chakos, M. H., Mayerhoff, D. I., Loebel, A. D., *et al* (1992). Incidence and correlates of acute extrapyramidal symptoms in first episode of schizophrenia. *Psychopharmacology Bulletin*, **28**, 81–86.

Christison, G. W., Kirch, D. G. & Wyatt, R. J. (1991) When symptoms persist: choosing among alternative somatic treatments for schizophrenia. *Schizophrenia Bulletin*, **17**, 217–245.

Cold, J. A., Wells, B. G. & Froemming, J. H. (1990) Seizure activity associated with antipsychotic therapy. *DICP Annals of Pharmacotherapy*, **24**, 601–606.

Crane, G. E. & Naranjo, E. R. (1971) Motor disorders induced by neuroleptics: A proposed new classification. *Archives of General Psychiatry*, **24**, 179–184.

Crow, T. J. (1980) Molecular pathology of schizophrenia: More than one disease process? *British Medical Journal*, **280**, 66–68.

——, Deakin, J. F. W. & Longden, A. (1977) The nucleus accumbens – possible site of antipsychotic action of neuroleptic drugs. *Psychological Medicine*, **7**, 213–221.

——, McMillan, J. F., Johnson, A. L., *et al* (1986) The Northwick Park study of first episodes of schizophrenia. II. A randomised controlled trial of prophylactic neuroleptic treatment. *British Journal of Psychiatry*, **148**, 120–127.

Curry, S. H. (1986) Applied clinical pharmacology of schizophrenia. In *The Psychopharmacology and Treatment of Schizophrenia* (eds P. B. Bradley & S. R. Hirsch), pp. 103–131. Oxford: Oxford University Press.

Dahl, S. G. & Strandjord, R. E. (1977) Pharmacokinetics of chlorpromazine after single and chronic dosage. *Clinical Pharmacology and Therapeutics*, **21**, 437–448.

Davis, J. M. (1975) Overview: maintenance therapy in psychiatry. I. Schizophrenia. *American Journal of Psychiatry*, **132**, 1237–1245.

—— (1976*a*) Comparative doses and costs of antipsychotic medication. *Archives of General Psychiatry*, **33**, 858–861.

—— (1976*b*) Recent developments in the drug treatment of schizophrenia. *American Journal of Psychiatry*, **133**, 208–214.

—— & Garver, D. L. (1978) Neuroleptics: clinical use in psychiatry. In *Handbook of Psychopharmacology* (eds L. Iverson, S. Iverson & S. Snyder), pp. 129–164. New York: Plenum Press.

Delva, N. J. & Letemendia, F. J. J. (1982) Lithium treatment in schizophrenia and schizo-affecive disorders. *British Journal of Psychiatry*, **141**, 387–400.

Falloon, I., Watt, D. C. & Shepherd, M. (1978) A comparative controlled trial of pimozide and fluphenazine deconoate in the continuation therapy of schizophrenia. *Psychological Medicine*, **8**, 59–70.

Faurbye, A., Rasch, P. J., Petersen, P. B., *et al* (1964) Neurological symptoms in pharmacotherapy of psychoses. *Acta Psychiatrica Scandinavica*, **40**, 10–27.

Forrest, I. S., Green, D. E. & Udale, B. P. (1964) In vivo metabolism of chlorpromazine. *Proceedings of the Western Pharmacology Society*, **7**, 35–38.

Forsman, A. & Ohman, R. (1976) Pharmacokinetic studies on haloperidol in man. *Current Therapeutic Research*, **20**, 319–336.

Foster, P. (1989) Neuroleptic equivalence. *Pharmaceutical Journal*, **243**, 431–432.

Galdi, J. (1983) The causality of depression in schizophrenia. *British Journal of Psychiatry*, **142**, 621–625.

Ganzini, L., Heintz, R. T., Hoffman, W. F., *et al* (1991) The prevalence of tardive dyskinesia on neuroleptic-treated diabetics. *Archives of General Psychiatry*, **48**, 259–263.

Goldberg, S. C. (1985) Negative and deficit symptoms in schizophrenia do respond to neuroleptics. *Schizophrenia Bulletin*, **11**, 453–456.

Hakola, H. P. A. & Lautumaa, V. A. (1982) Carbamazepine in treatment of violent schizophrenics. *Lancet*, i, 1358.

Hirsch, S. R. (1986) Clinical treatment of schizophrenia. In *The Psychopharmacology and Treatment of Schizophrenia* (eds P. B. Bradley & S. R. Hirsch), pp. 286–339. Oxford: Oxford University Press.

Hogarty, G. E., Goldberg, S., Schooler, N., *et al* (1974) Drugs and sociotherapy in the aftercare of schizophrenic patients. II. 2-year relapse rates. *Archives of General Psychiatry*, **31**, 603–608.

—— & Ulrich, R. F. (1977) Temporal effects of drug and placebo in delaying relapse in schizophrenic out-patients. *Archives of General Psychiatry*, **34**, 297–301.

Hoge, S. K., Appelbaum, P. S., Lawlor, T., *et al* (1990) A prospective, multicentre study of patients' refusal of antipsychotic medication. *Archives of General Psychiatry*, **47**, 949–956.

Hyttel, J., Larsen, J-J., Christensen, A. V., *et al* (1985) Receptor-binding profiles of neuroleptics. In *Dyskinesia – Research and Treatment* (Psychopharmacology Suppl. 2) (eds D. E. Casey, T. N. Chase, A. V. Christensen, *et al*), pp. 9–18. New York: Springer-Verlag.

Jann, M. W., Ereshefsky, L. & Saklad, S. R. (1985) Clinical pharmacokinetics of the depot antipsychotics. *Clinical Pharmacokinetics*, **10**, 315–333.

Jeste, D. V. & Wyatt, R. J. (1979) In search of treatment for tardive dyskinesia – a review of the literature. *Schizophrenia Bulletin*, **5**, 251–293.

—— & Wyatt, R. J. (1981) Changing epidemiology of tardive dyskinesia: an overview. *American Journal of Psychiatry*, **138**, 297–309.

Jeste, D. V., Lohr, J. B., Clark, K., *et al* (1988). Pharmacological treatments of tardive dyskinesia in the 1980s. *Journal of Clinical Psychopharmacology*, **8**, 38s–48s.

——, Potkin, S. G. , Sinha, S., *et al* (1979) Tardive dyskinesia: reversible and persistent. *Archives of General Psychiatry*, **36**, 585–590.

Johnstone, E. C., Crow, T. J., Frith, C. D.,*et al* (1978) Mechanism of the antipsychotic effect in the treatment of acute schizophrenia. *Lancet*, i, 848–851.

——,——, Ferrier, I. N., *et al* (1983) Adverse effects of anticholinergic medication on positive schizophrenic symptoms. *Psychological Medicine*, **13**, 513–527.

——, ——, Frith, C. D., *et al* (1988) The Northwick Park "Functional" psychosis study: diagnosis and treatment response. *Lancet*, **2**, 119–125.

——, Owens, D. G. C., Bydder, G. M., *et al* (1989) The spectrum of structural brain changes in schizophrenia: Age of onset as a predictor of cognitive and clinical impairments and their cerebral correlates. *Psychological Medicine*, **19**, 91–103.

——, Macmillan, J. F., Frith, C. D.,*et al* (1990) Further investigation of the predictors of outcome following first schizophrenic episodes. *British Journal of Psychiatry*, **157**, 182–189.

Jorgensen, A. (1986) Metabolism and pharmacokinetics of antipsychotic drugs. In *Progress in Drug Metabolism, Vol. 9.* (eds J. W. Bridges & L. F. Chasseaud), pp. 111–174. New York: Taylor and Francis.

Kane, J. M. (1987) Treatment of schizophrenia. *Schizophrenia Bulletin*, **13**, 133–156.

—— & Smith, J. M. (1982) Tardive dyskinesia: Prevalence and risk factors 1959–1979. *Archives of General Psychiatry*, **39**, 473–481.

—— & Lieberman, J. A. (1987) Maintenance pharmacotherapy in schizophrenia. In *Psychopharmacology. The Third Generation of Progress* (ed. H. Y. Meltzer), pp. 1103–1109. New York: Raven Press.

——, Honigfeld, G., Singer, J., *et al* (1988) Clozapine for the treatment-resistant schizophrenic: A double-blind comparison with chlorpromazine. *Archives of General Psychiatry*, **45**, 789–796.

Keck, P. E., Pope, H. G., Cohen, B. M., *et al* (1989) Risk factors for neuroleptic malignant syndrome. A case-control study. *Archives of General Psychiatry*, **46**, 914–918.

Kennedy, P. F., Hershon, H. I. & McGuire, R. J. (1971) Extrapyramidal disorders after prolonged phenothiazine therapy. *British Journal of Psychiatry*. **118**, 509–518.

Knights, A., Okasha, M. S., Salih, M., *et al* (1979) Depressive and extrapyramidal symptoms and clinical effects. A trial of fluphenazine versus flupenthixol in maintenance of schizophrenic out-patients. *British Journal of Psychiatry*, **135**, 515–523.

—— & Hirsch, S. R. (1981) 'Revealed' depression and drug treatment for schizophrenia. *Archives of General Psychiatry*, **38**, 806–811.

Lader, M. (1979) Monitoring plasma concentrations of neuroleptics. *Pharmacopsychology*, **9**, 170–177.

Laska, E., Verga, E., Wanderling, J., *et al* (1973) Patterns of psychotropic drug use for schizophrenia. *Diseases of the Nervous System*, **34**, 294–305.

Levinson, D. F. & Simpson, G. M. (1986) Neuroleptic-induced extrapyramidal symptoms with fever. *Archives of General Psychiatry*, **43**, 839–848.

Lieberman, J. A., Saltz, B. L., Johns, C. A., *et al* (1991) The effects of clozapine on tardive dyskinesia. *British Journal of Psychiatry*, **158**, 503–510.

Lipscomb, P. A. (1980) Cardiovascular side-effects of phenothiazines and tricyclic antidepressants: a review with precautionary measures. *Postgraduate Medicine*, **67**, 189–196.

Lohr, J. B., Cadet, J. L., Lohr, M. A., *et al* (1987) Alpha-tocopherol in tardive dyskinesia. *Lancet*, 1, 913–914.

Manchanda, R. & Hirsch, S. R. (1986) Does propranolol have an antipsychotic effect? A placebo-controlled study in acute schizophrenia.*British Journal of Psychiatry*, **148**, 701–717.

Mann, S. C., Caroff, S. N., Bleier, H. R., *et al* (1986) Lethal catatonia. *American Journal of Psychiatry*, **143**, 1374–1381.

Marder, S. R., Van Putten, T., Mintz, J., *et al* (1987) Low – and conventional – dose maintenance therapy with fluphenazine decanoate. *Archives of General Psychiatry*, **44**, 518–521

Marsden, C. D., Tarsy, D. & Baldessarini, R. J. (1975) Spontaneous and drug-induced movement disorders in psychotic patients. In *Psychiatric Aspects of Neurological Disease* (eds D. F. Benson & D. Blumer), pp. 219–266. New York: Grune and Stratton.

—— & Jenner, P. (1980) The pathophysiology of extrapyramidal side-effects of neuroleptic drugs. *Psychological Medicine*, **10**, 55–72.

——, Mindham, R. H. S. & Mackay, A. V. P. (1986) Extrapyramidal movement disorders produced by antipsychotic drugs. In *The Psychopharmacology and*

Treatment of Schizophrenia (eds P. B. Bradley & S. R. Hirsch), pp. 340–402. Oxford: Oxford University Press.

May, P. R. A. (1968) *Treatment of Schizophrenia: A Comparative Study of Five Treatment Methods*. New York: Science House.

—, Tuma, A. H., Yale, C., *et al* (1976) Schizophrenia: A follow-up study of results of treatment. II. Hospital stay over 2 to 5 years. *Archives of General Psychiatry*, **33**, 481–486.

—. — & Dixon, W. J. (1981) Schizophrenia: a follow-up study of results of five forms of treatment. *Archives of General Psychiatry*, **38**, 776–784.

Mehtonen, O-P., Aranko, K., Malkonen, L., *et al* (1991) A survey of sudden death associated with the use of antipsychotic or antidepressant drugs: 49 cases in Finland. *Acta Psychiatrica Scandinavica*, **84**, 58–64.

Meltzer, H. Y. & Fang, V. S. (1976) The effect of neuroleptics on serum prolactin in schizophrenic patients. *Archives of General Psychiatry*, **33**, 279–286.

—, Sommers, A. A. & Luchins, D. J. (1986) The effect of neuroleptics and other psychotropic drugs on negative symptoms in schizophrenia. *Journal of Clinical Psychopharmacology*, **6**, 329–338.

Midha, K. K., Hawes, E. M., Hubbard, J. W., *et al* (1987) The search for correlations between neuroleptic plasma levels and clinical outcome: a critical review. In *Psychopharmacology: The Third Generation of Progress* (ed. H. Y. Meltzer), pp. 1341–1351. New York: Raven Press.

Moller, H-J. & Von Zerssen, D. (1982) Depressive states occurring during the neuroleptic treatment of schizophrenia. *Schizophrenia Bulletin*, **8**, 109–117.

Morgenstern, H. & Glazer, G. W. M. (1993) Identifying risk factors for tardive dyskinesia among long-term outpatients maintained with neuroleptic medications. *Archives of General Psychiatry*, **50**, 723–733.

Munetz, M. R. & Cornes, C. L. (1983) Distinguishing akathisia and tardive dyskinesia: A review of the literature. *Journal of Clinical Psychopharmacology*, **3**, 343–350.

National Institute of Mental Health Psychopharmacology Service Center Collaborative Study Group (1964) Phenothiazine treatment in acute schizophrenia. *Archives of General Psychiatry*, **10**, 246–261.

Neborsky, R., Janowsky, D., Munson, E., *et al* (1981) Rapid treatment of acute psychotic symptoms with high- and low-dose haloperidol. *Archives of General Psychiatry*, **38**, 195–199.

Orlov, P., Kasporian, G., Dimascio, A., *et al* (1971) Withdrawal of antiparkinson drugs. *Archives of General Psychiatry*, **25**, 410–412.

Owens, D. G. C. (1990) Dystonia – a potential psychiatric pitfall. *British Journal of Psychiatry*, **156**, 620–634.

— (1994) Extrapyramidal side-effects and tolerability of risperidone: a review. *Journal of Clinical Psychiatry*, **55** (Suppl. 5), 29–35.

— & Johnstone, E. C. (1980) The disabilities of chronic schizophrenia: their nature and the factors contributing to their development. *British Journal of Psychiatry*, **136**, 384–395.

—, — & Frith, C. D. (1982) Spontaneous involuntary disorders of movement: their prevalence, severity and distribution in chronic schizophrenics with and without treatment with neuroleptics. *Archives of General Psychiatry*, **39**, 452–461.

Regal, R. E., Billi, J. E. & Glazer, H. M. (1987) Phenothiazine-induced cholestatic jaundice. *Clinical Pharmacy*, **6**, 787–794.

Rey, M-J., Schultz, P., Costa, C., *et al* (1989) Guidelines for the dosage of neuroleptics. I: Chlorpromazine equivalents of orally administered neuroleptics. *International Clinical Psychopharmacology*, **4**, 95–104.

Schultz, P., Rey, M-J., Dick, P., *et al* (1989) Guidelines for the dosage of neuroleptics. II: Changing from daily oral to long-acting injectable neuroleptics. *International Clinical Psychopharmacology*, **4**, 105–114.

Scull, A. T. (1982) *Museums of Madness*. Harmondsworth: Penguin.

Seeman, M. (1981) Tardive dyskinesia: two-year recovery. *Comprehensive Psychiatry*, **22**, 189–192.

Shaler, A., Hermesh, H. & Munitz, H. (1989) Mortality from neuroleptic malignant syndrome. *Journal of Clinical Psychiatry*, **50**, 18–25.

Simpson, G. M. (1977) Neurotoxicity of major tranquillisers. In *Neurotoxicology* (eds L. Roizen, H. Shiraki & N. Grceic). New York: Raven Press.

Simpson, G. M., Jefferson, J., Davis, J., *et al* (1987) *Report of the Apa Task Force on Sudden Death*. Washington, DC: American Psychiatric Association.

Singh, H., Levinson, D. F., Simpson, G. M., *et al* (1990) Acute dystonia during fixed-dose neuroleptic treatment. *Journal of Clinical Psychopharmacology*, **10**, 389–396.

Siris, S. G. (1991) Diagnosis of secondary depression in schizophrenia: implications for DSM–IV. *Schizophrenia Bulletin*, **17**, 75–98.

——, Harmon, G. K. & Endicott, J. (1981) Postpsychotic depressive symptoms in hospitalised schizophrenic patients. *Archives of General Psychiatry*, **38**, 1122–1123.

——, Bermanzohn, P. C., Mason, S. E., *et al* (1994) Maintenance imipramine therapy for secondary depression in schizophrenia: A controlled trial. *Archives of General Psychiatry*, **51**, 109–115.

Sommers, A. A. (1985) "Negative symptoms": conceptual and methodological problems. *Schizophrenia Bulletin*, **11**, 364–379.

Swett, C. (1975) Drug-induced dystonia. *American Journal of Psychiatry*, **132**, 532–534.

Thompson, C. (1994) The use of high dose antipsychotic medication. *British Journal of Psychiatry*, **164**, 448–458.

Tuma, A. H. & May, P. R. A. (1979) And if that doesn't work, what next? A study of treatment failures in schizophrenia. *Journal of Nervous and Mental Disease*, **167**, 566–571.

Uhrbrand, L. & Faurbye, A. (1960) Reversible and irreversible dyskinesia after treatment with perphenazine, chlorpromazine, reserpine and ECT. *Psychopharmacologia*, **1**, 408–418.

Van Putten, T. & May P. R. A. (1978) 'Akinetic depression' in schizophrenia. *Archives of General Psychiatry*, **35**, 1101–1107.

Von Bahr, C., Movin, G., Yisak, W-A., *et al* (1990) Clinical pharmacokinetics of remoxipride. *Acta Psychiatrica Scandinavica*, **82** (suppl. 358), 41–44.

Waddington, J. L. (1988) Therapeutic potential of selective D-I dopamine receptor agonists and antagonists in psychiatry and neurology. *General Pharmacology*, **19**, 55–60.

—— & Youssef, H. A. (1986) Late onset involuntary movements in chronic schizophrenia: Relationship of 'tardive' dyskinesia to intellectual impairment and negative symptoms. *British Journal of Psychiatry*, **149**, 616–620.

Weiden, P. J., Mann, J. J., Haas, G., *et al* (1987) Clinical non-recognition of neuroleptic-induced movement disorders: a cautionary study. *American Journal of Psychiatry*, **144**, 1148–1153.

Wiles, D. H. & Gelder, M. G. (1980) Plasma fluphenazine levels by radioimmuno-assay in schizophrenic patients treated with depot injections of fluphenazine decanoate. In *Advances in Biochemical Psychopharmacology*. Vol. 24 (ed. F. Cattabeni), pp. 599–602. New York: Raven Press.

Wyatt, R. J. (1976) Biochemistry and schizophrenia (Part IV). The neuroleptics – their mechanism of action: a review of the biochemical literature. *Psychopharmacology Bulletin*, **12**, 5–50.

—— (1991) Neuroleptics and the natural course of schizophrenia. *Schizophrenia Bulletin*, **17**, 325–351.

Yorkston, N., Zakin, S. A., Malifk, M. K. U., *et al* (1974) Propranolol in the control of schizophrenic symptoms. *British Medical Journal*, **4**, 633–635.

Appendix. Classes and chemical structures of antipsychotic drugs currently available in the UK (1994)

1. The basic Phenothiazine structure and class members

Compound	R_1 substitution	R_2 substitution
Aliphatic		
Promazine	H	$-CH_2-CH_2-CH_2-N\begin{smallmatrix}CH_3\\CH_3\end{smallmatrix}$
Chlorpromazine	Cl	$-CH_2-CH_2-CH_2-N\begin{smallmatrix}CH_3\\CH_3\end{smallmatrix}$
Methotrimeprazine (Levomepromazine)	$-OCH_3$	$-CH_2-CH-CH_2-N\begin{smallmatrix}CH_3\\CH_3\end{smallmatrix}$ CH_3
Piperidine		
Thioridazine	$S-CH_3$	$-CH_2-CH_2-\bigcirc_{N-CH_3}$
Pericyazine	CN	$-CH_2-CH_2-CH_2-N\bigcirc-OH$
Pipothiazine	$SO_2N\begin{smallmatrix}CH_3\\CH_3\end{smallmatrix}$	$-CH_2-CH_2-CH_2-N\bigcirc-CH_2-CH_2-OH^*$
Piperazine		
Trifluoperazine	CF_3	$-CH_2-CH_2-CH_2-N\bigcirc N-CH_3$
Perphenazine	Cl	$-CH_2-CH_2-CH_2-N\bigcirc N-CH_2-CH_2-OH$
Fluphenazine	CF_3	$-CH_2-CH_2-CH_2-N\bigcirc N-CH_2-CH_2-OH^*$

*Esterification site in depot formulations

2. The basic Thioxanthene structure and class members

Compound	R₁ substitution	R₂ substitution
Clopenthixol	Cl	$-CH-CH_2-CH_2-N\underset{}{\bigcirc}N-CH_2-CH_2-OH^*$
Flupenthixol	CF₃	$-CH-CH_2-CH_2-N\underset{}{\bigcirc}N-CH_2-CH_2-OH^*$

*Esterification site in depot formulations

3. The basic Butyrophenone structure and class members

Compound	R
Haloperidol	
Droperidol	
Trifluperidol	

*Esterification site in depot formulations

4. The basic Diphenylbutylpiperidine structure and class members

Compound	R
Pimozide	
Fluspiriline	

5. Atypical antipsychotics
a. Substituted Benzamides

Sulpiride

Remoxipride

b. Other 'atypical' compounds

Loxapine

Clozapine

Oxypertine

10 The psychological and social management of schizophrenia

Frank Holloway

A brief history of care • Understanding disability in schizophrenia •
Meeting need in schizophrenia • Managing acute episodes •
Psychological treatment approaches • Family management •
Organisation and delivery of services • The psychiatrist's role

---

Until the introduction of antipsychotic medication in the 1950s the management of schizophrenia depended on social measures and ineffective physical treatments. Antipsychotics, although they are effective against positive symptoms in the acute situation, have little impact on negative symptoms and the social consequences of serious mental illness. Psychosocial approaches to treatment are particularly important in the long-term management of psychoses and serve to complement medication in the prevention of relapse (Birchwood & Shepherd, 1992). This chapter focuses on psychosocial approaches to individual patients and should be read in conjunction with chapter 27 which deals with the organisation of psychiatric services.

A brief history of care

The current network of psychiatric services in Britain and the United States of America, until recently based on the large mental hospitals, originated as a humane response to the needs of 'pauper lunatics'. Before the 19th century people with severe mental illnesses were cared for by their families or survived by begging. The behaviourally disturbed were kept in workhouses, bridewells and gaols that catered for all varieties of the indigent. People with means who became 'mad' were looked after at home or in private establishments, which were generally run by a 'mad-doctor' (a term used to describe those members of the medical profession who claimed some expertise in the treatment of the mentally ill). A handful of institutions specifically provided care for the insane poor, notably the Bethlem Royal Hospital in London (Allderidge, 1990). Concern over conditions in private establishments led to the passing of the Madhouses Act 1774, which allowed for the inspection of asylums. This was strengthened by a Madhouses Acts of 1828 which set up the Metropolitan Commissioners in Lunacy with a brief to visit madhouses four times a year and the power to release any patient wrongly confined.

At the end of the 18th century and during the early 19th century a number of asylums functioned as therapeutic institutions. 'Moral treatment' in small, humanely run asylums resulted in impressive discharge and cure rates (Bockhoven, 1954). "Humanity, reason and kindness animated [the] philosophy" of moral treatment (Porter, 1987), which in practice meant asylums with high staff–patient ratios where the inmates were encouraged to return to normal social function. The role of the superintendent of the asylum was crucial in setting the values and practices of the institution, and successful asylums owed much to the work of a handful of outstanding individuals.

The Lunatics Act 1845 set up a central Lunacy Commission with jurisdiction across the country and mandated the building of lunatic asylums in each county. However, from the middle of the century onwards the increasingly extensive network of local asylums, each containing an ever-expanding population, entered its 'long sleep'. During the subsequent era of custodial care, cost containment became a major priority, as the asylums became repositories for the insane poor (Scull, 1979). Some interest in the care of patients released into the community remained and the Mental Aftercare Association was founded in 1879 to provide homes for discharged patients. The focus of mental health legislation in the late 19th century was to place tight legal restrictions on admission to the asylum, with relatively little concern once the inmate was incarcerated.

The expansion of institutional care for the mentally ill, a world-wide phenomenon, was first halted in Britain and the USA in the mid 1950s. The reasons for the decline in hospital beds are complex and ill-understood. Major factors were a shift in professional attitudes back towards the active social treatment of mental illness and increasing public acceptance of the mentally ill. Attitudes towards care for the mentally ill were already changing during the 1920s. The Mental Treatment Act 1930 had made voluntary admission to hospital possible and encouraged the development of out-patient and aftercare services. Many traditional mental hospitals were transformed during the decade after 1945 as the concept of the 'therapeutic community', developed by military psychiatrists during World War II, and the 'Open door' movement, influenced psychiatric practice. In the pre-war mental hospital all the doors were locked and there was litle interchange between the hospital and the community. Within the more advanced hospitals active schemes were introduced for the rehabilitation of long-stay patients, while from the 1940s onwards an increasing proportion of patients treated were managed by relatively brief and often repeated in-patient stays on acute wards, with out-patient follow-up available after discharge.

The introduction of effective antipsychotic drugs and the rise of the District General Hospital psychiatric unit reinforced a medical model of psychiatric treatment within local services. This was based on optimistic assumptions about the possibility of a cure for major mental illnesses.

The Mental Health Act 1959 gave sanction to the medical approach to mental illness by taking hospital admission out of the legal arena. Informal admission became the norm while compulsory detention in hospital was permitted on the recommendation of registered medical practitioners.

During the 1950s and 1960s the potentially damaging effect of institutions on their inmates was increasingly recognised (Goffman, 1961; Wing & Brown, 1970). Crude extrapolation of the decline in bed numbers led to the prediction that large mental hospitals would quite rapidly close. The White Paper, *Better Services for the Mentally Ill* (Department of Health and Social Security, 1975), identified the components of a comprehensive psychiatric service to be organised around the local general hospital psychiatric unit. Subsequently the major thrust of professional practice and Government policy has been to provide care for the mentally ill (and indeed other groups, including the elderly, people with a physical disability and people with a mental handicap) in non-institutional settings.

In the USA Community Mental Health Centres (CMHCs) were developed as a comprehensive alternative to the state mental hospital system, with disappointing results, as they concentrated on the out-patient care of patients with minor psychiatric morbidity and ill-directed attempts at the primary prevention of mental illnesses. The phenomenon of 'upmarketing', whereby services drift away from the more difficult and demanding groups towards provision for the 'worried well', seems to dog community mental health services. Rapid contraction of the state hospitals resulted in a large number of patients being 'transinstitutionalised' into profit-making 'board and care homes' and nursing homes of dubious quality, and in some large cities a crisis of homeless mentally ill people on the streets.

In Britain a series of scandals in mental illness and mental handicap hospitals further undermined confidence in institutional provision at a time when the thinking of the 'antipsychiatrists' such as Laing (1960) and Szasz (1961) was fashionable. The Mental Health Act 1983 was introduced after a debate focused on concern for the protection of the rights of the decreasing minority of patients detained in hospital against their will. It marked a return to legalistic constraint of psychiatric practice and the revival of a Mental Health Act Commission charged with the oversight of the welfare of detained patients (Jones, 1991). The user movement and the concept of patient advocacy, which originated in the USA, began to have an impact on services during the 1980s.

The need to contain health and social care spending in the face of apparently infinite demand has led to a search for more effective and cheaper alternatives to hospital care for the mentally ill. The steady decline in hospital beds that began in 1954 was not, however, matched by developments in community services. Critics of community care blamed these policies for a visible problem of homeless mentally ill people living rough in major cities, an unacceptably heavy burden on families and other informal carers, poor quality of life for discharged patients and the inappropriate diversion of the mentally ill into the criminal justice system. These complaints represent an oversimplification of complex issues. However, follow-up of psychotic patients discharged from inner city psychiatric services showed that while continuing contact with psychiatrists or general practitioners (GPs) was the norm, patients received very little help with the more practical aspects of daily life (Melzer *et al*, 1991). The quality of community services seemed to have changed little since the early 1960's (Brown *et al*, 1966). Community care services have been hopelessly fragmented among a host of agencies and individuals without any clearcut responsibility for policy-making or individual care.

The first large mental hospitals actually closed in the 1980s. This process is set to gather momentum in the next decade. Initial evidence suggests that the majority of long-stay patients can successfully be resettled in community-based residential units.

Contemporary policy on care for the mentally ill in Britain was spelt out in the 1989 White Paper *Caring for People* (Secretary of State, 1989). This stressed the importance of enabling people to live within the community. Responsibility for the organisation and delivery of community care was placed on Social Services Departments, although health authorities retain a residual duty to provide the 'health' component of care. 'Care management' and the 'Care Programme Approach' were introduced in an attempt to overcome the fragmentation of community services. These changes together with the more recent NHS reforms are described in chapter 27.

Understanding disability in schizophrenia

The basic impairments of schizophrenia are manifested clinically as positive and negative symptoms and by a range of abnormalities in psychological functioning, such as poor attention and concentration and failure to recognise and act on social or affective cues (see Chapter 7). Typical disabilities that are encountered include poor interpersonal skills, difficulty coping with finances and inability to carry out domestic chores. Chronic mental illness often results in social handicaps, for example poverty, unemployment and homelessness. These handicaps may be compounded by poor premorbid social adjustment and adverse personal reactions to the illness by the sufferer. Adverse reactions to the illness, sometimes called 'secondary handicaps', include depression, despair and loss of motivation for self-help. They may be exacerbated by despair among professional and lay carers.

Psychiatrists tend to focus on the current mental state to the exclusion of social functioning. By definition the treatments available for the underlying impairments of chronic mental illness are unsatisfactory. Management strategies must therefore directly address issues of disability and social handicap.

Box 10.1 Impairment, disability and handicap

Impairment is defined as any loss or abnormality of psychological, physiological or anatomical structure or function
Disability is a restriction in functioning or lack of ability to
perform normal activities
Handicap is a disadvantage for a given individual (resulting
from impairment or disability) that limits or prevents the
fulfilment of a role that is normal for that individual

Psychiatric rehabilitation involves encouraging an optimal level of social
adaptation both by therapeutic interventions aimed at maximising the
patient's social functioning and by providing appropriately supportive
environments (Shepherd, 1991).

A pychosocial model of schizophrenia

The psychosocial approach to schizophrenia is based on the assumption
that the onset, course and outcome of major mental disorders are the
result of an interaction between biological, environmental and behavioural
factors. The 'vulnerability–interactionist' model of schizophrenia
(Birchwood *et al*, 1988) hypothesises an intrinsic vulnerability to the
development of schizophrenic symptoms. Acute episodes can be
precipitated by psychosocial stress. A psychotic relapse will have a range
of adverse social and psychological effects on the sufferer, the family and
other carers. These adverse effects will in turn make relapse more likely
by increasing the stresses experienced by the patient. The model predicts
that improving the coping ability and competence of the sufferer, the
family and other carers will reduce the capacity of stressors to precipitate
a relapse and will also result in a decrease in stressors. Interventions aimed
at minimising the adverse consequences of the illness by environmental
manipulation (for example, by providing supportive housing, day activities
and ready access to welfare benefits) should also reduce stressors. With
optimal care the likelihood of relapse should decrease, and what might
be a vicious cycle could be broken.

One factor that must be added to the 'vulnerability–interactionist' model
is the apparent balance between positive and negative psychotic
symptoms. Negative symptoms (notably social withdrawal and under-
activity) may be a protective mechanism against the emergence of positive
psychotic symptoms. Overenthusiastic attempts at rehabilitation may result
in an exacerbation of positive symptoms while understimulation
powerfully promotes the development of negative symptoms. This difficult
balance is one of the major dilemmas of psychiatric rehabilitation practice.

This model does not deny the biological basis of schizophrenia, and it can comfortably accommodate medical approaches to treatment. However, the 'vulnerability–interactionist' model offers hope for sufferers, family members and staff that help is possible when medication is incompletely effective.

Meeting need in schizophrenia

British Government policy for community care places assessment of need as a "cornerstone of high quality care" (Secretary of State, 1989). Diagnosis is not in itself a useful predictor of need. There is no generally accepted view of the needs of people with a severe mental illness, and numerous competing models of need have been developed. These include the often quoted hierarchy of needs described by Maslow (1954), which extends from basic physiological needs through needs for safety, love and self-esteem to 'self-actualisation' needs; the strictly clinical view of the MRC Needs for Care Schedule (Brewin *et al*, 1987), where need is defined as a problem requiring specific psychiatric treatment or care; the normalisation/social role valorisation perspective (Wolfensberger, 1983), which identifies the central goal of services as "the creation, support and defense of valued social roles"; a psychodynamic approach (Harris & Bergman, 1987) that stresses intrapsychic needs; and concentration on needs identified by the patient and their strengths.

Lehman *et al* (1982) described eight 'quality of life' domains: living situation, finances, personal safety, family relationships, general social relationships, work, leisure activities, and health. These domains are relevant both to the general population and the chronically mentally ill.

Box 10.2 What mental health services should be providing

Identification of people in need
Optimal control of psychiatric symptoms and prevention of relapse (using pharmacological, social and psychological treatments)
General health care
Promotion of independent living skills
Support and education of carers
Intervention in crises
Welfare rights advice
Appropriately supportive accommodation (including hospitals)
Opportunities for work and other structured day activities
Opportunities for leisure activities
Development of supportive social networks
Case management

Most people with a chronic mental illness are unemployed and dependent on welfare benefits. Impoverishment may be extreme: patients may leave hospital after decades with no personal possessions at all. Homelessness or grossly unsatisfactory housing conditions are common, particularly in inner city psychiatric services. Patients may have realistic fears for their personal safety and the security of their property. Chronic mental illness often results in alienation from family and progressive shrinkage of social networks: loneliness, isolation and sexual frustration may result.

Stein & Test (1980) identified a set of requirements that would enable patients disabled by a functional psychosis to remain out of hospital in the face of their disability. These were material resources (food, shelter, clothing); general and psychiatric medical care; coping skills to meet the demands of community living; motivation to persevere in the face of life difficulties; freedom from pathologically dependent relationships, for example with parents; and an assertive support system that would follow the patient when they ceased contact and act rapidly and effectively in time of crisis.

Box 10.2 sets out some of the priorities for psychiatric services. The problems of the mentally ill are so complex that cooperation between agencies and professionals is essential. The importance of motivating the patient is crucial. Patients and carers should feel respected by staff. Continuity of care, with a clearly identified point of contact in an emergency, is crucial. Disorganised and severely socially disabled patients may require structure and prompting if they are not to "rot with their rights on". A small minority of patients will be a danger to themselves or others, or present behaviours that are grossly socially unacceptable, and consequently require care within a hospital environment, either in the acute situation or (rarely) in the long term.

Managing acute episodes

Presentation to services

The events surounding the first contact with services, the diagnosis of schizophrenia and the initiation of treatment will have a profound effect on the relationship between the patient and carers and the services for years to come. Despite its importance the process of engagement with treatment is poorly understood. The GP is the major provider of psychiatric care in Britain, and usually the point of first contact with services (see chapter 28). However, in the inner city patients often receive treatment after dramatic presentations to emergency departments, the courts and the police. Some patients, particularly those with paranoid states who function well socially, never become engaged with services. Treatment may be postponed until the death or incapacity of a carer.

Obtaining treatment is often a painful process for the patient and their carers. Front line services, in particular the GP and the Social Services department (which has a statutory duty to undertake mental health assessments) frequently prove unhelpful. A message that "nothing can be done" may be given by primary care workers and first contact with the psychiatrist is often delayed until crisis point is reached. Prolonged delay in receiving help reflects the inaccessibility of many psychiatric services. This can be improved by closer liaison between psychiatry and primary medical care, social services and other community agencies. Delay in presentation will also be contributed to by the patient's lack of insight, negative family attitudes (which may have denial as their basis) towards the stigma of a mental illness explanation for their relative's problems, poor premorbid social adjustment and an insidious onset. Difficulty in accessing services in time of crisis is a major source of frustration for carers, who often do not know who to turn to even when the patient has had a long psychiatric career. Lack of resources, notably in-patient beds and highly supportive alternatives to in-patient care, add to the delay in providing help as may legal constraints on compulsory admission.

It is important that at the initial presentation a thorough assessment is made of the psychiatric and social history, current social situation, the presenting phenomenology and premorbid level of functioning. These data may be vital later when as the patient's psychiatric career develops the history becomes a catalogue of contacts with services and the phenomenology is obscured by repetition to a host of doctors. During the initial assessment both patients and carers will value information on what is happening and the management plans. Opinion differs about imparting the diagnosis to the relatives and patient: it is becoming increasingly common practice to reveal the diagnosis of schizophrenia early on. There are a number of difficulties with this practice, notably the potential for misdiagnosis in the acute situation and the lack of specificity attached to the diagnosis in terms of symptoms and prognosis. The author's practice is to be clear about the morbid nature of the phenomena the patient experiences and the rationale for the treatment being offered. Direct discussion about the diagnosis and its meaning are more appropriate once the course of the disorder has become apparent or in answer to direct questions.

Information for distressed relatives and patients whose information processing capacities are impaired must be presented simply and repeatedly. Handouts explaining the rationale for and side-effects of medication may be particularly helpful. Staff should take into account the illness beliefs held by the patient and family and enter into a dialogue rather than adopt a didactic stance. The aim should be that from the outset there is an atmosphere of cooperation between the patient, carers and the services. This can be very difficult to achieve in practice.

Indications for hospital admission

Conventional wisdom suggests that all newly-presenting schizophrenics should be assessed in hospital (see also page 398). Even in the current era of community care and severe bed shortages most patients with schizophrenia are admitted to hospital at some stage, although there is some research evidence demonstrating the efficacy of day care, home treatment and respite care (Hoult, 1986). It is important to recognise that the hospital/community dichotomy is unhelpful. The in-patient unit remains a key component of the comprehensive mental health service, not a last resort when all else has failed.

Admission generally occurs as a result of a breakdown in social supports following a deterioration in mental state. This may in turn be due to a failure of compliance with medication. There are a number of positive indications for admission beyond compulsory treatment (which can only occur in Britain in hospital). These include the management of dangerous behaviour, suicidal behaviour and complicating physical illness; the assessment and reassessment of diagnosis, level of functioning and social circumstances; refinements of drug management; and the implementation of treatment programmes that are impossible outside hospital (Stein & Test, 1980). Often admission occurs when the burden of caring becomes too great for families and community support systems, although non-hospital respite care provision may well be a feasible (less stigmatising and cheaper) alternative in these circumstances. If the patient is well known to the service the referring doctor and the ward team should identify clear reasons for hospital admission.

In-patient care

The development of a therapeutic milieu within the in-patient unit owes much to the application of therapeutic community principles to general psychiatry. The aim is to provide a "stable and coherent social organisation which facilitates the development and application of an individual comprehensive treatment plan", sets limits on disturbed behaviour and fosters the development of psychosocial skills (Leeman, 1986). In classic 'Milieu therapy', the unit is sustained by a variety of meetings: a daily ward report; a community meeting involving all staff and patients; a series of patient discussion and activity groups; ward rounds and discharge planning conferences; regular staff meetings and educational meetings. The unit will be aiming to offer containment, structure and support for patients while attempting to involve them in their care.

Wing & Brown (1970) described an ideal therapeutic environment for patients with chronic schizophrenia as one where, as far as possible, patients do things for themselves. They also emphasised the importance of high staff morale and positive staff attitudes towards patients.

The author's experience suggests that psychiatric in-patient units for both acute and long-stay patients should provide a supportive and low-key environment. A cohesive staff team should be working consistently to a care plan that is negotiated with the patient and focuses on real-life difficulties. Increasingly nursing teams are organised so that a primary nurse takes overall responsibility for the care planning of an individual patient, in collaboration with nursing colleagues and the multi-disciplinary team.

Acutely psychotic patients should be neither over- or understimulated. Intrusive psychotherapeutic groups and individual psychotherapy are contraindicated. However, there should be clear expectations of patients to maintain a degree of social competence, and the care plan should consider their social functioning. The ward should be equipped to allow patients to look after themselves as much as is feasible, with ready access to a kitchen and washing machine. The ward routine should provide structure without the imposition of institutional practices. Occupational therapy (OT), both on the ward and in the OT department, can offer a graded range of structured activities as well as the opportunity to assess social and interpersonal functioning.

Little is known about in-patient admission from the patient's perspective. Relationships with hospital staff and other patients are subjectively important in the process of recovery (Lieberman & Strauss, 1986).

The management of disturbed behaviour

Violence, and the threat of violence, is ever-present in many in-patient units. Recently particular concern has been expressed over sexual harassment of women on mixed-sex wards. Violent incidents are related both to patient characteristics and environmental factors. One study found that perpetrators of violence in a psychiatric hospital were younger, more commonly male, suffering from schizophrenia, and had more frequently previously exhibited verbally aggressive and threatening behaviour and damaged property than a control group of non-violent patients (Noble & Roger, 1989). Violent acts are generally preceded by behavioural changes, and assaults tend to be repetitive. The best predictor of future violence is past violence, although psychiatrists are poor predictors of dangerousness. While nursing staff are the commonest reported victims of violence, incidents involving patient victims are much less likely to be recognised and reported.

Among patients with schizophrenia, violence will be more likely if there is evidence of an antisocial premorbid personality and coexisting drug abuse. Violent behaviour may be psychotically motivated (for example, attacking the perceived source of auditory hallucinations and passivity experiences) or reflect disinhibition, when interpersonal difficulties flare up into physical attacks. The seriousness of the index incident, lack of provocation, lack of remorse, evidence of premeditation, poor response to medication and a negative attitude to treatment are all indicators of possible future dangerousness.

Behavioural disturbance is related to environmental factors. Violence is more common in inner city psychiatric units, presumably mirroring the pattern in the local community. Disturbed behaviour in these units, which now generally admit only severely ill psychotic patients, tends to occur when the unit is under particular strain. In one study the frequency of violent episodes increased during periods when a higher proportion of agency (locum) nursing staff were employed on the wards (James *et al*, 1990). Disturbance can be minimised if there is a well-trained staff group who work as a cohesive team that adopts a consistent approach to patients and sets clear limits on behaviour (James *et al*, 1990). There is some evidence that bored patients are more likely to be verbally and physically aggressive and provocative to others. Aggression can also be a means of gaining attention when staff otherwise interact little with their patients. Occasionally patients will display dramatic or aggressive behaviour in order to deliberately obtain attention at a time when staff are dealing with some other crises on the ward. Expectations of violence may become a self-fulfilling prophesy. Particular concern has been expressed over the stereotyping of patients from ethnic minorities as violence-prone. Occasionally staff members may provoke violence by their attitudes towards a patient.

On a practical level it is important for in-patient units to have clear policies governing the prevention and management of violence. Further details of these are given in Kidd & Stark (1995). Staff working in out-patient settings and the community must also be aware of the risks of violence, particularly when the patient is unknown to services or has a past history of dangerous behaviour.

If an incident occurs help will be vital. An emergency team, led by the nurse in charge of the ward, may be summoned if the incident is serious. Physical restraint, which will require adequate numbers of trained staff working to the unit policy, may be necessary. If the patient has a weapon staff should retreat and call the police. Emergency sedation may be required (see page 405). Some units have a seclusion room, in which patients may be isolated from the rest of the ward, without risk of harm to themselves or others. Seclusion is "the supervised confinement of a patient alone in a room which may be locked..." (*Code of Practice, Mental Health Act 1983*; Department of Health & Welsh Office, 1993). There is a lack of research evidence on the use of seclusion, which must follow locally agreed policies, should be strictly time-limited and must be reviewed regularly by nursing and medical staff particularly if patients have been heavily medicated, as deaths have occurred in these circumstances. An outline seclusion procedure is contained in the Code of Practice.

Clinical experience suggests that seclusion may bring disturbed behaviour rapidly under control, although its long-term effects on the ward environment and the attitudes of patients towards their treatment may be less desirable. It is important to distinguish seclusion, which by definition is an unplanned response to an emergency, from time-out, which is a psychological technique for managing disruptive behaviour (Hogg & Hall, 1992). In essence time-out is the brief (15 minutes at most) exclusion of the patient from positive reinforcement following inappropriate behaviour, generally by moving the patient to a quiet room. Time-out is one of a range of behavioural techniques being deployed to manage "challenging behaviour". Success demands persistence since programmes that involve withdrawing reinforcements for problematical behaviours will often result in an initial increase in the frequency, severity and duration of target behaviours (Hogg & Hall, 1992).

Following a serious incident the staff team should get together for a debriefing session to facilitate the ventilation of feelings, have a critical review of the way that policies were implemented and consider a revision of the patient's care plan. Cognitive–behavioural assessment of the antecedents and consequences of problematic behaviours may be valuable, medication may have to be reviewed and on occasion the involvement of the police or the forensic psychiatric services is necessary. The needs of the victim of an assault should be considered, and appropriate counselling offered.

Discharge planning

"Planning for discharge is probably the most important process in the in-patient hospitalisation of persons suffering from chronic illness. It involves planning the management of the patient's illness over a lifetime..." (Talbott & Glick, 1986).

In Britain health authorities have to develop a 'Care Programme Approach', with the aim of ensuring all vulnerable patients leaving hospital receive multidisciplinary assessment and are allocated a key worker responsible for coordinating follow-up.

Discharge planning should begin soon after admission. Plans should address the needs already described in this chapter, focusing particularly on practical issues such as income maintenance, appropriate accommodation and arrangements to continue physical and psychological treatments. Long-term planning and continued involvement by the treatment team is equally important for patients whose acute episodes are managed in the community (Stein & Test, 1980).

Psychological treatment approaches

Psychotherapy

For several decades the major form of specific psychological treatment for schizophrenia was psychodynamic psychotherapy. The research literature offers no good evidence that insight or growth oriented approaches to treatment are of any value, either as an alternative or in addition to psychotropic medication (Mueser & Berenbaum, 1990). Over-enthusiastic attempts at insight-oriented psychotherapy may be positively harmful, but psychodynamic concepts can be useful in helping patients cope with the human issues raised by having a chronic disability, and dealing with the normal psychological problems common to all. In particular, patients (and family members) with a severe schizophrenic illness continually experience loss. Depression in schizophrenia is common and suicide an ever-present risk.

Supportive psychotherapy has a significant role in the management of schizophrenia, provided that it focuses on resolving the patient's personal and environmental problems and addresses needs for rehabilitation. The positive effects of such 'sociotherapy' on social functioning may not begin to appear until the second year after an acute episode (Hogarty *et al*, 1974). Professional help that encourages a feeling of self-worth and mastery, instils hope and recruits the patient as an active collaborator in treatment and rehabilitation may contribute significantly to long-term improvement in schizophrenia (Davidson & Strauss, 1992).

Both direct care staff and managers need to understand the psychodynamic implications of working with patients who are 'difficult to treat', often perceived as unrewarding and distressing to be with, can react with hostility towards well-intentioned carers and can induce powerful negative feelings in carers. Conflict in the relationship between care staff and patients is common and particularly destructive in residential settings: adequate staff supervision and support is needed if unacceptable practices are to be avoided.

Behaviour therapy

Early alternative psychological approaches involved the use of operant conditioning techniques to decrease psychotic behaviours and encourage socially acceptable behaviour. In the 'token economy' a ward environment was designed within which reinforcers (plastic tokens which could be exchanged for privileges) were systematically applied to modify patients' behaviour. The balance of research evidence suggests that token economies are effective in the short term, but that gains may generalise poorly to other settings. It is likely that the efficacy of the token economy unit was largely due to the social reinforcement provided by interaction with staff, although there is some evidence that more tangible reinforcers are initially required by very severely disabled patients (Hogg & Hall, 1992).

The token economy has not become part of mainstream psychiatric services. However, behavioural principles have become influential in the design of treatment programmes for patients with long-term impairments and 'challenging behaviour'. Skills training approaches use modelling, rehearsal, practice and feedback to facilitate the acquisition of daily living and interpersonal skills. When the primary problem is motivational rather than a skills deficit, analysis of the antecedents and consequences of behaviour will be required but motivational defects respond poorly to treatment. Reinforcement techniques are also relevant to the management of challenging behaviours, with selective reinforcement of positive behaviours used to balance non-reinforcement of problematic behaviours.

Assessment

Adequate assessment of the nature of problem behaviour or experiences, their antecedents and consequences forms the basis of successful psychological intervention. Interviews with patients and their carers seek to elicit details of the problem(s), its history and previous attempts at a solution and current coping resources (Hogg & Hall, 1992). This information should be complemented by details of personal strengths and social circumstances. Often it is useful to develop an individualised recording chart or checklist, to be filled in by the patient or care staff. Behavioural treatments can be monitored by repeated assessments using individualised scales that allow the rating of problem areas, for example, fear of certain situations or preoccupation with delusions.

Standardised rating scales can also be helpful. The REHAB Scale (Baker & Hall, 1983), which measures deviant behaviour (verbal and physical aggression and other socially unacceptable behaviour) and general behaviour (social functioning), provides a rapid assessment of long-term psychiatric patients. It is a broad-brush measure of disability and is useful for identifying problem areas that should be focused on in treatment and for monitoring progress. Cognitive assessment may be relevant in care planning, particularly when there is a suspicion that the patient is dementing or has focal neurological problems. Many standardised instruments are available for the assessment of symptoms, behaviour, social functioning and burden on relatives.

Treatment strategies for delusions and hallucinations

The clinical management of a psychotic patient is demanding. Traditional psychiatric practice concentrates on eliciting the form of symptoms rather than paying attention to their content. However, patients are concerned about their beliefs and what the voices are actually saying. Clinicians should be respectful and interested in these preoccupations and express sympathy about their impact, but rarely if ever collude with delusional beliefs: agreeing to disagree about the reality of abnormal experiences and beliefs is generally the best strategy. Medication may be presented as a treatment that helps patients cope with the distress that they are experiencing, or to 'help keep the voices at bay'.

Although medication is the mainstay of treatment for positive psychotic symptoms, it is ineffective in a significant minority of patients, is often refused, and frequently causes severe and occasionally unacceptable side-effects. Positive psychotic symptoms are exacerbated by stress and, at a general level, social interventions aimed at reducing stress (including hospital admission) will be appropriate. In addition a variety of promising specific psychological treatment strategies are being developed for the management of delusions and hallucinations (Box 10.3). These psychological treatments will for the forseeable future only be offered as an adjunct to medication and general social measures, or be tried when medication has failed.

Most patients spontaneously adopt coping strategies to control or master their symptoms or minimise the distress they cause. Distraction (watching TV, listening to music), relaxation or withdrawal (e.g. trying to go to sleep), talking to oneself, arguing directly with the voices, appealing to God and taking medication are all commonly reported coping strategies. Cognitive–behavioural treatments have been developed that identify and build on the patient's coping stategies (Tarrier, 1992).

Psychological theories of hallucinations suggest that modification of the auditory input could decrease the severity of the hallucinations. Subvocal counting, ear plugs or a portable cassette player may have some effect in intractable cases (Nelson *et al*, 1991). The personal cassette player is already a popular coping mechanism.

An emerging treatment for delusions is belief modification (Chadwick & Lowe, 1991). Patients are encouraged to view their beliefs as a reaction to and a way of making sense of specific experiences. During therapy a delusional belief is examined and the patient asked to consider arguments in support of the belief and those against it. Challenging a delusion must be done extremely carefully since direct confrontation of abnormal beliefs may actually result in an increase in the strength of the belief. Some delusions serve an important psychological function, and will be particularly resistant to change (for example delusions of pregnancy that are encountered among long-stay patients who have lost the opportunity

---

Box 10.3 Psychological approaches to the treatment of delusions and hallucinations

Enhance natural coping strategies
Belief modification
Stimulus control
Exposure
Thought stopping
Problem-solving
Modification of auditory input

Box 10.4 Elements of problem-solving (After Falloon, 1984)

Identification of the patient's problems
Identification of the patient's assets and supports
Agreeing target problems
Generating potential solutions to the problems
Evaluation of alternative solutions
Selecting the best solution
Planning implementation
Reviewing progress – modifying tasks and goals accordingly

---

of child-rearing). There is little value in attempting to alter beliefs that are neither distressing to the patient nor interfering with functioning.

Other cognitive–behavioural approaches to delusions and hallucinations have been tried. When patients can identify factors that bring on symptoms, stimulus control techniques may be adopted, for example in the use of relaxation exercises in patients whose hallucinations are worsened by anxiety. Exposure therapy may be useful if social situations are being avoided as a result of persecutory delusions. Thought stopping has been tried with persecutory delusions and thought insertion.

Problem-solving (Box 10.4) is an important general approach to helping people manage personal issues (Hawton & Kirk, 1989). Training in problem-solving skills is a potentially powerful method of improving the level of coping of patients and their families.

Functional and social skills training

Patients with chronic schizophrenia often lack interpersonal skills and the skills of daily living. Skills training seeks to reverse these deficits by the systematic application of "basic principles of human learning" (Liberman, 1988). Social skills training is usually offered in a group setting (Box 10.5). Core skills are identified (for example, starting a conversation, responding to a complaint or asking for help) and broken down into specific behavioural components. A task that is relevant for the patient may then be chosen and rehearsed, with feedback about performance from the therapist. Videotape can also be used for feedback. Homework exercises are provided to encourage *in vivo* rehearsal.

Instrumental skills, such as shopping, budgeting and grooming, can quite readily be taught either by nursing staff or occupational therapists. These skills tend not to be lost when patients are in contact with services that continue to make functional demands, in contrast with institutional provision that only demands subservience to a routine. Interpersonal skills, even if successfully acquired within a treatment setting, often do not generalise into behavioural change in the outside world. The 'generalisation problem' lends support to treatments that involve working with patients in their environment of need (Stein & Test, 1980). Supportive social environments that provide opportunities for normal social functioning may be more valuable than specific treatment sessions. Very satisfactory results can be obtained by offering chronically disabled patients the opportunity to care for themselves, join in cooking sessions and utilise community resources. Skilled therapists naturally utilise behavioural techniques of modelling, rehearsal, practice, feedback and social reinforcement.

Negative symptoms and 'challenging behaviour'

The classic three hospitals study demonstrated the importance of the social environment on the development and maintenance of negative symptoms, and that enrichment of the social environment, with increased levels of meaningful activity, could result in their improvement (Wing & Brown, 1970). The ideal therapeutic environment will offer consistency of staffing and a friendly low-key atmosphere. There should be positive expectations for appropriate behaviour and patients should have individual programmes that provide structure to their day. This structure must be balanced with opportunities for leisure, recreation and a degree of social withdrawal when pressures become excessive.

The token economy, social skills training, life skills training, cognitive–behavioural therapy and problem-solving have all been applied to negative symptoms. Negative symptoms are characterised by a lack of motivation on the patient's part, and treatment often requires the introduction of reinforcement for desired behaviours (Hogg & Hall, 1992). If a patient is severely impaired it may be extraordinarily difficult to identify reinforcers, and the patient may have to be introduced to new experiences that can later be used as sources of reinforcement. Initially tangible reinforcers

---

Box 10.5 Basic techniques of skills training (After Liberman, 1988)

Clear definition of the problems
Identification of assets
Establishment of a therapeutic alliance
Goal setting
Behavioural rehearsal
Positive reinforcement
Shaping
Prompting
Modelling
Homework and *in vivo* practice

may be required (e.g. a cigarette, a cup of tea), although social reinforcement (conversation about a favourite football team, praise) is ultimately likely to be more effective.

A small minority of patients present so-called "challenging behaviour". This may include aggression (to people, property or self), antisocial behaviour (shouting, swearing, stealing, vomiting, smearing of faeces), sexually inappropriate behaviour and bizarre behaviour (stereotypies, odd speech appearance and gait, polydypsia) (Hogg & Hall, 1992). Effective management demands an adequately staffed and appropriately designed care setting within which stressors are kept to a minimum. Challenging behaviour often quite understandably provokes a punitive response. Techniques for reducing unwanted behaviour include both altering the contingencies of behaviour (for example, time-out) and differential reinforcement of incompatible types of behaviour.

Promoting collaboration with medical treatment

Psychotic relapse following non-compliance with antipsychotic medication is a frequent clinical problem. Patients are often reluctant to engage in other forms of treatment, and may aspire to independent living when this is beyond their coping capacities. A key clinical skill is to establish a positive working relationship with the patient and their carers. Barriers to treatment adherence include the side-effects of medication and complex treatment regimes; ignorance about the illness and the role of medication among patients and carers; a poor relationship between the patient and clinicians; and aspects of the service system, such as prolonged waits in the clinic, difficulties with clerical staff and poor service coordination (Corrigan *et al*, 1990).

These problems are surmountable if addressed systematically. The decision not to accept treatment represents the individual's analysis of risk and benefit, and may be understandable in the light of unacceptable side-effects. Clinicians must be aware of and attempt to minimise side-effects. Akathisia is particularly distressing and often poorly recognised. In the longer term weight gain and interference with sexual functioning frequently concern patients. Depot antipsychotic medication may increase compliance, although some patients are well managed on low doses of high potency oral antipsychotics. Education for patients and carers about schizophrenia is important, although simply providing the standard psychiatric explanations of schizophrenia will be ineffective. Education should take account of the patient's health beliefs. The importance of a positive relationship between the psychiatrist and the patient and carers cannot be overemphasised. Regular out-patient visits may be crucial to maintain continuing community tenure, and attention should be paid to making the clinic visit as positive an experience as possible. (The author's depot clinic serves tea to attenders, who are encouraged to chat to one another as they wait and can also get a free lunch in the adjacent day hospital.)

There has been recent interest in involving the patient and carers in the management of medication, monitoring the mental state and identifying prodromal symptoms prior to a psychotic relapse (Birchwood *et al*, 1992). The clinical reality is that lack of insight into the illness is a major problem. One useful exercise is to enquire about the most recent hospital admission and the patient's experiences and behaviour at the time. Persistence and inventiveness may result in even the most difficult patient becoming engaged with treatment. Over a period of time, often several years, even patients severely lacking in insight gradually make the link between their cessation of medication and their repeated readmissions to hospital and so eventually modify their behaviour and take medication.

Family management

The impact of schizophrenia on the family

The majority of people with schizophrenia begin their psychiatric career within a family. As the disorder progresses there may be a gradual stripping away of family supports. The difficulties experienced by carers and patients during the early stages of the illness have aready been discussed. Families learning to accept the reality of long-term disturbance may pass through recognisable stages. Denial, guilt and blaming are commonly encountered early reactions, to be followed by feelings of loss, sorrow and regret. Eventually some form of chronic adjustment may be reached.

The burden that community care places on families has long been recognised. It is useful to distinguish between objective and subjective aspects of burden. Objective burdens consist of the effects that the patient and the illness have on family life, the impact on family finances and employment opportunities, the effects of social stigma and social isolation on carers, the behavioural disturbance presented by the patient and the problems of dealing with a fragmented, ill-coordinated service system. Subjective burden represents the distress experienced by the family and its impact on the physical and psychological health of family members.

Relatives are often dissatisfied with the help that they get. The importance of information has already been emphasised. The family often feel excluded from decision-making about treatment and future management. Advice on how to deal with difficult behaviour is rarely given. Families may feel that they have become an inexpensive alternative to adequate community services. Lack of resources such as day care, residential provision and transport can be a justified source of complaint. Poor continuity of care may result in inadequate support at a time of crisis. However, experimental studies have found that good quality community services that offer assertive outreach and continuity of care can decrease family burden and increase satisfaction with care when compared with more traditional hospital-based services (Hoult, 1986).

Family management of schizophrenia

The effect of the family environment on the course of schizophrenia has been reviewed in chapter 7. The initial observation that patients living with families rated as high expressed emotion (EE) were much more likely to relapse than those rated as low EE (Vaughan & Leff, 1976) led to a series of intervention studies. To date these have shown that attempts to alter the family atmosphere and/or reduce the amount of face-to-face contact between the relative and high EE families can succeed in reducing the frequency of relapse roughly to the levels of patients in low EE households. Pooling of data from intervention studies show a two year relapse rate following therapy of 30% compared with 70% for high EE controls (Kavanagh, 1992).

A number of common themes emerge from the intervention literature. Carrying out these interventions is a skill that has to be acquired by supervised clinical practice. A positive attitude towards families and acknowledgement of their difficulties is vital. Education about schizophrenia, although ineffective on its own in altering EE, is a useful basis for the initiation of family treatment. It involves providing information about the diagnosis, symptoms and causes of schizophrenia and the available treatments. Sessions should also allow relatives to raise their own questions. The focus of active treatment should be on the family's current problems, helping relatives and patients adopt more successful coping strategies. The components of the family problem-solving approach are described in detail by Falloon *et al* (1984). A relatives' group, facilitated by a professional, can reduce the stigma, isolation and loneliness experienced by carers and in addition lead to change in coping patterns and reduction in EE. Engagement with treatment may be a particular problem with the group approach, and "assertive outreach" may have to be extended to carers. Relapse rates can also be decreased by individual sessions with patients aimed at improving their skills in reducing family conflict (Hogarty *et al*, 1986). This approach also emphasises the process of individuation, with patients and relatives being encouraged to enhance their level of contact outside the family.

The EE literature has focused largely on patients presenting with acute symptoms. Successful adaptation to long-term disability is a matter of balance. High expectations from family members may be associated with good social functioning, but resignation and acceptance of disability will reduce the level of stress experienced by relatives and patients. Clinicians should be aware of the strengths of each family's style of adaptation to the illness, and help should aim to build on curent coping styles. Explicit or implicit criticism should be avoided.

The psychiatrist should be prepared to devote a considerable amount of time, often spread over several years, to family members, particularly the parents. This should be done regardless of EE status because those families with low EE scores may be just as distressed as those with high EE scores albeit with a lesser tendency to show their unhappiness. Often parents will accompany the patient on their regular visits to the clinic and on these occasions the psychiatrist should offer the parents a brief but separate interview – not only to asssess the patient's progress but also to offer support and sometimes advice as the parents are usually the principal carers.

Family management should not be restricted solely to high EE families. All carers experience difficulties that deserve help from services. Putting the results of recent research in family management into practice represents a major challenge for services, requiring a major investment in training.

Organisation and delivery of services

Components of care

The development of effective psychiatric services (Thornicroft & Bebbington, 1989; Bennett & Freeman, 1991; Pilling, 1991) requires leadership and clarity of vision and, above all else, cooperation between the providers of health and social care. Service planning should bring together community care agencies, involving front-line workers as well as the purchasers of care. Rational planning requires information systems that identify people who have had contact with the services and are in continuing need. Planning also requires knowledge about what monies are being spent on whom and to what benefit. Resource constraints, which will over the next decade get worse, make it imperative that finances are targeted to those most in need.

Optimal symptom control should be provided by the full range of psychological, pharmacological and social treatments described in this book. People with chronic mental illnesses have a high prevalence of general medical problems (and a significantly raised mortality rate). This chapter has discussed methods of improving and maintaining interpersonal and functional skills and has emphasised the importance of education and support for carers. Relatives in particular demand rapid and effective intervention in crises.

The majority of patients with a chronic disability depend on welfare benefits. Problems with benefit are a frequent cause of distress. Caring professionals may have to become involved in advocacy on behalf of their clients. Contemporary mental health services are also encouraging the development of client advocacy projects, with a stress on an independent 'user' voice in service planning and provision.

The key service components of accommodation, day care and case management are discussed below. The quality of services will depend on the staff and their training, supervision and support. Training for community care is particularly poorly developed, and should be focused on ensuring that staff have the knowledge and skills to carry out their job. Working with people with severe mental illnesses is personally demanding and staff burnout is a frequent problem. Burnout is characterised by apathy towards work, resentment of service users, absenteeism and high staff turnover. It is less likely to occur when staff are clear about their roles, participate actively in the developing of policies and procedures of their workplace, take part in care planning, have access to training, and feel that senior management take their share of the direct care and represent the interests of the setting in the wider service system.

Accommodation

Most patients either live independently or with families. A minority, because of the disabilities associated with their illness, require temporary or permanent supportive accommodation. Accommodation for the mentally ill is provided by health authorities, the local authority social services and housing departments, housing associations, and private and voluntary sector providers of residential and nursing home care. As the numbers of hospital beds decrease there is an increasing emphasis on use of the non-statutory sector and care for people in their own homes.

Residential services should be based on a number of principles. The degree of support should match the level of disability. Services should as far as possible be non-stigmatising, offer a homely environment and promote choice and independence for residents. Institutional practices, such as block treatment, lack of personal possessions for residents and social distance between care staff and residents should be avoided. There should be flexibility to cope with changing needs, either by altering the level of support or by offering a more appropriate alternative. One constant dilemma in residential care is balancing the rights of the individual and the promotion of independence against the need to provide a safe and structured environment for people with very severe disabilities. Another common difficulty is the unrealistic aspirations of patients who may be unwilling to recognise that they cannot cope independently.

In the past many patients left the large British psychiatric hospitals for a room in a boarding house in a seaside resort. More recently surveys have demonstrated considerable unmet housing need among patients discharged from acute psychiatric wards (Melzer *et al*, 1991). Many patients now leave inner city hospitals for temporary bed-and-breakfast accommodation, and a few soon end up sleeping on the streets. There is a considerable lack of accommodation that provides any form of support, and the shortage of highly supported provision is acute.

The traditional forms of residential care available were the group home (a minimally staffed shared house); the more highly staffed hostel, which could either offer 'rehabilitation' with an expectation that the resident would move on into less supported accommodation or provide a permanent home; and for the most disabled a long-stay hospital bed. There is now considerable need for more independent accommodation that nevertheless can provide supervision and support. One way of providing this is the 'core and cluster' model within which a central highly staffed unit (possibly offering day care) supports residents who live in a cluster of surrounding independent properties. An alternative is the extension of the sheltered housing model into the mental illness sector. Some residents require only occasional visits from a housing worker or social work aide to ensure that minimum standards are being met and the rent is paid. In adult fostering and boarding out schemes landladies offer patients considerable practical assistance with daily living and monitor their mental state within their own home.

Recent experience with hospital closure programmes indicates that even highly disabled long-stay patients can live successfully in ordinary housing with the support of non-professional care staff. Services espousing the ordinary housing model tend to adhere to the principles of normalisation, which, with its emphasis on the significance of stigma as a cause of social disability, can prove at odds with the realities of caring for people with severe psychiatric disabilities. Such projects require backup from a multidisciplinary psychiatric team that acts in a consultative capacity. Chronically disabled patients may also be discharged into elderly persons residential care homes and nursing homes, often far from their local area. Although the physical environment of such homes is often excellent, levels of activity among residents are often very low. For patients discharged into the private sector close follow-up is essential.

The most thoroughly evaluated form of residential provision is the hospital hostel, a specialised residence for 'new long-stay' patients (Garety & Morris, 1984). Hospital hostels can offer individually planned (often behaviourally oriented) interventions in an intensively staffed setting that is also a homely environment. Improved functioning and quality of life has been demonstrated for patients who would otherwise have been resident on hospital wards or inappropriately placed in acute units; despite the high staffing levels hospital hostels can be cost-effective compared to these unsatisfactory alternatives.

There are some patients who cannot be managed even within this highly supported environment. This small residual group of patients who exhibit challenging behaviour went almost unnoticed in the large mental hospitals and no generally agreed service model has emerged in the era of deinstitutionalisation. One suggestion has been the 'Haven' concept (Wing & Furlong, 1986), which seeks to recapture the positive aspects of the asylum without recourse to institutional care practices.

Day care

Day care forms a vital component of any good quality community-oriented psychiatric service. Controlled trials have shown that the day hospital can be an effective alternative to in-patient admission, even for patients with acute psychoses (Creed *et al*, 1990). Day care can provide support, supervision and monitoring for patients just discharged after a period in hospital, and therefore help decrease the length of in-patient stays. Brief intensive treatment can be provided within a day setting for patients whose needs cannot be met by out-patient or domiciliary services. Finally, and importantly, day treatment centres can act as a source of long-term structure and support for patients with chronic disabilities. In terms of preventing readmission of patients with schizophrenia, a controlled trial found that day centres with low readmission rates were characterised by a low-key atmosphere, slower patient flows and an emphasis on recreation and occupation rather than therapy (Linn *et al*, 1979).

British Government policy stipulates two types of day unit: the day hospital, which should provide a short-term treatment-oriented service within a medical setting, and the day centre, which should provide longer-term supportive and social care. Unfortunately this neat distinction between the 'health' and 'social' components of day care cannot readily be identified in practice. Many day hospitals, particularly those located in inner city catchment areas or associated with a large psychiatric hospital, serve a mainly long-term clientele. From the users' perspective, long-term day care plays a psychological role akin to the 'latent' functions of work. Users stress the importance of having somewhere to go, the support of staff and fellow attenders and the availability of activities in favour of any therapeutic function.

Patients often find evenings and weekends particularly difficult, and some services are now available out of working hours. Voluntary organisations can be particularly successful at providing informal 'drop-ins' which can complement the more formal statutory day care. Access to leisure activities is a major problem for some patients who may be restricted by lack of money, social anxiety, impaired social skills and lack of motivation. One important aspect of day care is that it provides users with a ready-made social network. It is important that this artificial social network encourages appropriately socially skilled behaviour. Ideally services should be encouraging patients to maintain or develop social networks that have nothing to do with the mental health system. Professional support systems should also be making use of generic resources. Adult Education courses and local leisure centres are particularly valuable forms of generic provision.

The influential 'Fountain House' model of psychosocial rehabilitation, which originated in New York in the 1950s, emphasises the significance of productive activity and the opportunity for gainful employment. Until recently interest in sheltered work was waning. It is now generally recognised that work is in itself potentially highly therapeutic, as well as bringing financial benefits and access to wider social networks. A range of provision is required. This will include work assessment and training, careers counselling, sheltered work, sheltered placements in ordinary firms and access to open employment (Harding *et al*, 1987).

The ideal day care service involves a network of facilities within a locality that cooperate to provide an accessible community support service. The service should ensure that patients' needs are regularly and systematically reviewed and that there is some form of central coordination.

Case management

Community care results in a fragmentation of mental health services, and the need for some form of coordinating mechanism is now recognised. Case management systems are intended to provide this coordination and offer vulnerable patients long-term flexible support (Holloway *et al*, 1991). The core case management activities are: (1) the assessment of need; (2) the development of a comprehensive service plan; (3) the arrangement of service delivery; and (4) the monitoring and assessment of what is provided. In principle, case management places an emphasis on tailoring services to patient need, rather than fitting patients into existing facilities. Some case management systems devolve budgetary responsibility to individual case managers, who then purchase services from local care providers. British Government policy is for a system of care management, within which care managers working to a cash-limited budget allocate and supervise the social care that clients are to receive.

Case management has evolved during the 1980s to become a major element of the mental health care system in the USA. Two contrasting models may be distinguished. Paraprofessional case managers may act as service brokers, responsible for, but not necessarily providing, the assessment and implementation of a package of care. Alternatively, in clinical case management a skilled psychiatric professional is directly concerned with all aspects of the patient's physical and social environment. The clinical case manager not only arranges access to appropriate services but also works directly with the patient offering a range of interventions. These include supportive psychotherapy, training in community living skills, family and patient psychoeducation and support during crises (Kanter, 1989). Ideally, clinical case managers should be anticipating impending crises and taking appropriate action: success in dealing effectively with relapses and other difficulties can give both patient and carers a sense of confidence and control over events (Harris & Bergman, 1987). Clinical case management is very similar to the traditional case-work approach in social work.

Case management systems must be targeted towards a clearly defined client group whose needs are adequately understood by the participants in the services. The service goals and operational policies must be clear and the case management service should work smoothly as a component of the overall local health and welfare system. Effective case management requires multidisciplinary and multi-agency working. The needs of the mentally ill are so complex and demanding that long-term continuity of care can only realistically be provided by a team. The existence of a team protects staff from the burden of sole responsibility, allows coordination of care from a group of relevant professionals, can improve workload management and may facilitate the establishment of common priorities. Where severely disabled patients are being targeted, staff–patient ratios may have to be very high (in the region of one staff member to 10 patients).

An extension of the case management concept is the multidisciplinary continuous treatment team, which strives to fulfil the core case management functions within a defined catchment area. The team aims to coordinate the other components of the long-term care system. The role of the primary health care team, the community psychiatric nurse and the generic social worker in this supportive network has not been fully defined. The GP is an undervalued resource in community care. Case management and the continuing care team are not a substitute for the range of services that the mentally ill require, and the cost-effectiveness of this approach is yet to be proven.

The psychiatrist's role

Given the complexity of the problems that patients with schizophrenia experience, the psychiatrist will only be fully effective as a member of a multidisciplinary treatment team and as part of a more extended network of supporting services. The development and maintenance of a functioning multidisciplinary team requires skill and persistence. The psychiatrist should not automatically assume a leadership role within every team, but will always look to ensure the smooth running, expertise and morale of the team.

The psychological and social management of schizophrenia places considerable demands on the psychiatrist, who will have a key role in the design and delivery of the patient's treatment and care. An understanding of the principles of psychological and physical treatments must be matched with empathy for the predicament of the patient and their carers. In the hard-pressed out-patient clinic it will be important to recall the key service elements identified in Box 10.2. The psychiatrist may not be able personally to ensure that the patient is receiving all available welfare benefits or that opportunities for social interaction are available to the patient but should be going through a mental checklist of critical patient care issues during the consultation. When deficiencies are identified appropriate help should be organised.

The clinician should actively be seeking to instil hope for the future, encouraging the patient and family to build on their existing strengths, devising interventions aimed at controlling symptoms and maximising social functioning and ensuring that patients are provided with appropriately structured and supported environments. Above all, the consultant psychiatrist should be providing a long-term perspective on the disorder and engaging both the patient and family in a therapeutic alliance with the services.

References

Allderidge, P. (1990) Hospitals, madhouses and asylums: cycles in the care of the insane. In *Lectures on the History of Psychiatry. The Squibb Series* (eds R. M. Murray & T. H. Turner), pp. 28–46. London: Gaskell.

Baker, R. & Hall, J. N. (1983) *REHAB: The Rehabilitation Evaluation*. Aberdeen: Vine.

Bennett, D. H. & Freeman, H. L. (eds) (1991) *Community Psychiatry. The Principles*. Edinburgh: Churchill Livingstone.

Birchwood, M., Hallett, S. & Preston, M. (1988) *Schizophrenia. An Integrated Approach to Research and Treatment*. London: Longman.

——, Macmillan, F. & Smith, J. (1992) Early intervention. In *Innovations in the Psychological Management of Schizophrenia* (eds M. Birchwood & N. Tarrier), pp. 115–146. Chichester: Wiley.

Bockhoven, J. S. (1954) Moral treatment in American psychiatry. *Journal of Nervous and Mental Diseases*, **124**, 167–194.

Brewin, C. R., Wing, J. K., Mangen, S. P., *et al* (1987) Principles and practice of measuring needs in the long-term mentally ill: the MRC needs for care assessment. *Psychological Medicine*, **17**, 955–971.

Brown, G. W., Bone, M., Dalison, B., *et al* (1966) *Schizophrenia and Social Care*. London: Oxford University Press.

Chadwick, P. & Lowe, F. (1991) The measurement and modification of delusional beliefs. *Journal of Consulting and Clinical Psychology*, **58**, 225–232.

Corrigan, P. W., Liberman, R. P. & Engel, J. D. (1990) From noncompliance to collaboration in the treatment of schizophrenia. *Hospital and Community Psychiatry*, **41**, 1203–1211.

Creed, F., Black, D., Anthony, P., *et al* (1990) Randomised controlled trial of day patient versus inpatient psychiatric treatment. *British Medical Journal*, **300**, 1033–1037.

Davidson, L. & Strauss, J. S. (1992) Sense of self in recovery from severe mental illness. *British Journal of Medical Psychology*, **65**, 131–145.

Department of Health & Social Security (1975) *Better Services for the Mentally Ill*. Cmnd 6233. London: HMSO.

Department of Health & Welsh Office (1993) *Code of Practice. Mental Health Act 1983*. London: HMSO.

Falloon, I. R. H., Boyd, J. L. & McGill, C. W. (1984) *Family Care of Schizophrenia*. New York: Guilford Press.

Garety, P. & Morris, I. (1984) A new unit for long-stay patients: organisation, attitude and quality of care. *Psychological Medicine*, **14**, 183–192.

Goffman, E. (1961) *Asylums: Essays on the Social Conditions of Mental Patients and Other Inmates*. New York: Doubleday.

Harris, M. & Bergman, H. C. (1987) Case management with the chronically mentally ill: a clinical perspective. *American Journal of Orthopsychiatry*, **57**, 296–302.

Hawton, K. & Kirk, J. (1989) Problem-solving. In *Cognitive Behaviour Therapy for Psychiatric Problems* (eds K Hawton, P. M. Salkovskis, J. Kirk *et al*). Oxford: Oxford University Press.

Harding, C. M., Strauss, J. S., Hafez, H. *et al* (1987) Work and mental illness. I. Toward an integration of the rehabilitation process. *Journal of Nervous and Mental Disease*, **175**, 317–325.

Hogarty, G. E., Goldberg, S. C., Schooler, N. R. and the Collaborative Study Group (1974) Drugs and sociotherapy in the aftercare of schizophrenic patients. III. Adjustment of non-relapsed patients. *Archives of General Psychiatry*, **31**, 609–618.

——, Anderson, C. M., Reiss, D. J., Kornblith, S. J., *et al* (1986) Family psycho-education, social skills training and maintenance chemotherapy in the aftercare treatment of schizophrenia. I. One year effects of a controlled study on relapse and expressed emotion. *Archives of General Psychiatry*, **43**, 633–642.

Hogg, L. & Hall, J. (1992) Management of long-term impairments and challenging behaviour. In *Innovations in the Psychological Management of Schizophrenia* (eds M Birchwood & N Tarrier), pp. 171–204. Chichester: Wiley.

Holloway, F., McLean, E. & Robertson, J. A. (1991) Case management. *British Journal of Psychiatry*, **159**, 142–148.

Hoult, J. (1986) Community care of the acutely mentally ill. *British Journal of Psychiatry*, **149**, 137–144.

James, D. V., Finberg, N. A., Shah, A. K., *et al* (1990) An increase in violence on an acute psychiatric ward. A study of associated factors. *British Journal of Psychiatry*, **156**, 846–852.

Jones, K. (1991) Law and Mental health: Sticks and Carrots? In *150 Years of British Psychiatry. 1841–1991* (eds G. E. Berrios & H. Freeman), pp. 89–102. London: Gaskell.

Kanter, J. (1989) Case management: Definition, principles and components. *Hospital and Community Psychiatry*, **40**, 361–368.

Kavanagh, D. J. (1992) Recent developments in expressed emotion and schizophrenia. *British Journal of Psychiatry*, **160**, 601–620.

Kidd, B. & Stark, C. (1995) *Management of Violence and Aggression in Health Care*. London: Gaskell.

Laing, R. D. (1960) *The Divided Self*. London: Tavistock.

Leeman, C. P. (1986) The therapeutic milieu. In *Inpatient Psychiatry. Diagnosis and Treatment* (ed. L. I. Sederer), pp. 222–233. Baltimore: Williams and Wilkins.

Lehman, A. F., Reed, S. K. & Possidente, S. M. (1982) Priorities for long-term care: comments from board-and-care residents. *Psychiatric Quarterly*, **54**, 181–189.

Liberman, P. (ed) (1988) *Psychiatric Rehabilitation of Chronic Mental Patients*. Washington: American Psychiatric Association Press.

Lieberman, P. B. & Strauss, J. S. (1986) Brief hospitalization: what are its effects? *American Journal of Psychiatry*, **143**, 1557–1562.

482 *Holloway*

Linn, M. W., Caffey, E. M., Klett, J., *et al* (1979) Day treatment and psychotropic drugs in the aftercare of schizophrenic patients. *Archives of General Psychiatry*, **36**, 1055–1066.

Maslow, A. (1954) *Motivation and Personality*. New York: Harper and Row.

Melzer, D., Hale, A. S., Malik, S. J., *et al* (1991) Community care for patients with schizophrenia one year after hospital discharge. *British Medical Journal*, **303**, 1023–1026.

Mueser, K. T. & Berenbaum, H. (1990) Psychodynamic treatment of schizophrenia: is there a future? *Psychological Medicine*, **20**, 253–262.

Nelson, H. E., Thrasher, S. & Barnes, T. R. E. (1991) Practical ways of alleviating auditory hallucinations. *British Medical Journal*, **302**, 327–328.

Noble, P. & Roger, S. (1989) Violence by psychiatric in-patients. *British Journal of Psychiatry*, **155**, 384–390.

Pilling, S. (1991) *Rehabilitation and Community Care*. London: Routledge.

Porter, R. (1987) *Mind-Forg'd Manacles*. London: Athlone Press.

Scull, A. T. (1979) *Museums of Madness*. Harmondsworth: Penguin.

Secretary of State for Health and Social Security (1989) *Caring for People. Community Care for the Next Decade and Beyond*. London: HMSO.

Shepherd, G. (1991) Psychiatric rehabilitation for the 1990s. In *Theory and Practice of Psychiatric Rehabilitation* (eds F. N. Watts & D. H. Bennett), pp. xiii–xviii. Chichester: Wiley.

Stein, L. I. & Test, M. A. (1980) Alternative to mental hospital treatment. *Archives of General Psychiatry*, **37**, 392–397.

Szasz, T. S. (1961) *The Myth of Mental Illness: Foundations of Theory of Personal Conduct*. New York: Deel.

Talbott, J. A. & Glick, I. D. (1986) The inpatient care of the chronically mentally ill. *Schizophrenia Bulletin*, **12**, 129–140.

Tarrier, N. (1992) Management and modification of residual positive psychotic symptoms. In *Innovations in the Psychological Management of Schizophrenia* (eds M. Birchwood & N. Tarrier), pp. 147–170. Chichester: Wiley.

Thornicroft, G. & Bebbington, P. (1989) Deinstitutionalisation – from hospital closure to service development. *British Journal of Psychiatry*, **155**, 739–753.

Vaughan, C. E. & Leff, J. P. (1976) The influence of family and social factors on the course of psychiatric illness: a comparison of schizophrenic and depressed neurotic patients. *British Journal of Psychiatry*, **129**, 125–137.

Wing, J. K. & Brown, G. W. (1970) *Institutionalism and Schizophrenia*. London: Cambridge University Press.

—— & Furlong, R. (1986) A haven for the severely disabled within the context of a comprehensive psychiatric community service. *British Journal of Psychiatry*, **149**, 449–457.

Wolfensberger, W. (1983) Social role valorization: a proposed new term for the principle of normalization. *Mental Retardation*, **21**, 234–239.

11 Schizoaffective, paranoid and other psychoses

Clive Mellor

History of the atypical psychoses • *Schizoaffective disorder* • *Cycloid psychosis* • *Reactive (psychogenic) psychoses* • *Schizophreniform disorder* • *Paranoid (delusional) disorders*

This chapter describes a miscellaneous group of non-organic psychoses. The factor common to these conditions is that they do not seem to belong to the two major Kraepelinian groups of non-organic psychoses: the schizophrenias and the affective psychoses.

Kraepelin's division of the non-organic psychoses into these two groups attracted criticism from the beginning. One objection was that cases often occurred which were not typical of schizophrenia or affective psychosis. These cases of 'atypical' psychosis have produced some nosological confusion. Different names have been used for similar disorders and the same name may be used for dissimilar clinical conditions.

The 'atypical' psychoses fall, like the typical ones, into two groups. In the schizoaffective group there are symptoms of schizophrenia and affective psychosis during the same illness. The second group, the paranoid disorders, is characterised by delusions in the absence of other features of psychosis.

The 'atypical psychoses' are listed in Box 11.1, together with the authorities principally responsible for defining them. Where dissimilar conditions have the same name, they are listed separately.

History of the atypical psychoses

The student of psychiatry viewing Box 11.1 might sympathise with the psychiatrist Hoche. Eighty years ago, he compared his contemporaries' repeated attempts at classification to "a great number of diligent workmen, most energetically engaged in clarifying a turbid fluid by pouring it busily from one vessel into another" (Lewis, 1934). The history of the different approaches to the nosological problem of the atypical psychoses enables us to understand the contemporary efforts to find a solution.

Kraepelin

The atypical psychoses have a pre-Kraepelinian history which is of academic interest, but not relevant to current thinking. Their history originates from and reflects changing diagnostic fashions in the criteria for identifying

---

**Box 11.1 Non-organic psychoses not typical of
schizophrenia or of affective psychosis**

Schizoaffective group

Schizoaffective disorder	Kasanin.
Schizoaffective disorder	ICD–10.
Schizoaffective disorder	DSM–IV
Schizophreniform	Langfeldt
Schizophreniform	DSM–IV
Psychogenic psychoses	Faegerman
Brief psychotic disorder	DSM–IV
Cycloid psychoses	Kleist, Leonhard
Atypical psychoses	Mitsuda
Periodical psychoses	Hatotani
Bouffée délirante	Mangan
Acute polymorphic psychotic disorder	ICD–10
Non-systematic schizophrenias	Kleist, Leonhard

Paranoid (delusional) disorders

Paranoia	Kahlbaum, Kraepelin
Acute delusional psychotic disorder	ICD–10
Persistent delusional disorder	ICD–10
Delusional disorder	DSM–IV
erotomanic	
grandiose	
jealous	
persecutory	
somatic	
Induced delusional disorder (folie à deux)	

---

schizophrenia and the affective psychoses. Contemporary classification began with Kraepelin's division of the non-organic psychoses into dementia praecox (schizophrenia) and manic–depressive disorder (affective psychoses). By definition, the atypical psychoses lie outside the diagnostic boundaries he set. Kraepelin (1919), in discussing the differential diagnosis of dementia praecox from manic–depressive insanity, stressed the total clinical picture. The diagnosis cannot be based on a single symptom or rest solely on a cyclical course. Outcome is the diagnostic arbiter. Complete recovery with good insight after the acute phase of the illness is diagnostic of manic–depressive insanity. Patients with dementia praecox did not recover, and he estimated that only 13% were eventually able to lead an independent existence. Most of them also had residual symptoms and personality change.

Kraepelin believed that there were few cases that could not be diagnostically accommodated within these two psychoses. The paranoid psychoses have a different history which is discussed later.

Four post-Kraepelinian approaches to the atypical psychoses will be considered:

(1) The concepts of Jaspers and Schneider which reinforced the dichotomy.
(2) The description of schizoaffective disorder by Kasanin and the subsequent development of this concept in the USA.
(3) The German school which originated with Wernicke, and whose successors Kleist and Leonhard identified the cycloid psychoses and the non-systematic schizophrenias.
(4) The Scandinavian concept, initiated by Wimmer, of psychoses which were produced by psychic stresses and had a benign course.

Jaspers and Schneider

Jaspers' (1963) hierarchical classification of psychiatric disorders and Schneider's (1959) identification of first rank symptoms of schizophrenia reinforced the division of the non-organic psychoses into two groups. Jaspers' hierarchical classification was based on the premise that it was only necessary to diagnose one illness if all the patient's symptoms could be explained by that illness. Although some of the patient's symptoms could occur in other conditions, one does not make a second diagnosis unless the evidence is overwhelming. (This is a medical application of Occam's razor – preference should be given to the most economical explanation.) Jaspers based his hierarchy on the diagnostic specificity of symptoms typical for each group of psychiatric disorders. Symptoms typical of the neuroses, for example, can occur in affective psychoses, schizophrenia and organic mental disorders. However, symptoms typical of these other conditions are not found in the neuroses. Therefore, neuroses lie at the lowest level of the hierarchy. The organic mental disorders are at the highest level because their typical symptoms are not found in other psychiatric disorders. Therefore, when the specific symptoms of an organic mental disorder are present, this diagnosis takes precedence over all others. Only after an organic illness has been excluded do neuroses, affective psychoses and schizophrenia become diagnostic possibilities. Jaspers, like most of his contemporaries, gave schizophrenia precedence over the affective psychoses. Therefore, if typical schizophrenic symptoms are present, the diagnosis is schizophrenia in spite of the presence of affective symptoms. This diagnostic hierarchy appears in Table 11.1; diagnostic hierarchies are further discussed on page 1246.

Table 11.1 Diagnostic hierarchy based on the specificity of the typical symptoms of each diagnostic category

Diagnosis	Presence of typical symptoms			
	Organic	Schizophrenic	Affective	Neurotic
Organic disorders	yes	possible	possible	possible
Schizophrenia	no	yes	possible	possible
Affective psychoses	no	no	yes	possible
Neuroses	no	no	no	yes

Unlike Kraepelin, Schneider believed that the patient's current mental state, rather than the course of the disorder should take priority for diagnostic purposes. Possibly this was because Schneider used Jaspers' phenomenological method, which had refined the mental state examination. Schneider's (1959) promotion of first-rank symptoms of schizophrenia over the symptoms of manic–depressive disorder is an application of the Jasperian hierarchy. Schneider believed that it was usually possible to diagnose either schizophrenia or affective psychosis in patients with 'atypical psychoses'. However, when this was not possible, he termed such cases 'zwischen-fallen' (cases in-between). In spite of criticism, this hierarchical view has continued to influence European thinking on psychiatric nosology. However, Jaspers' hierarchy was changed in DSM–III (APA, 1980) by promoting affective disorders over schizophrenia.

Kasanin and subsequent developments in the USA

The revolution against the European hierarchical view of nosology came from the USA. Kasanin (1933) in *The Acute Schizoaffective Psychoses* described nine patients who had psychiatric disorders exhibiting a mixture of schizophrenic and affective symptoms. Although the patients were diagnosed as having dementia praecox, their outcome was better than expected. They were young, had good premorbid personalities, and had been severely stressed before becoming ill. Unfortunately, it is difficult to determine from Kasanin's descriptions exactly what mental symptoms were present.

Kasanin and his contemporaries viewed schizoaffective disorder as a variant of schizophrenia. DSM–I and DSM–II (APA, 1968) continued to define schizoaffective disorder as a subtype of schizophrenia in which elation or depression was prominent. The outcome in such cases was said to be the same as that for schizophrenia.

There was a marked shift in American thinking about schizoaffective disorder in the 1970s. This followed a series of investigations using follow-up and family studies which concluded that schizoaffective disorder should be included with the affective disorders (see review by

Clayton, 1982). The identification of depressive and manic subtypes of schizoaffective disorder emphasised this notion. At the same time, the concept of schizophrenia, which had been essentially Bleulerian, was narrowed and that of affective disorder widened. These changes were reflected in DSM–III, in which schizophrenia became an illness of at least six months duration. Psychoses which were neither organic nor affective became brief reactive psychoses if they lasted less than a month, and schizophreniform psychoses if they had a duration of up to six months. Previously, both would have been diagnosed as schizophrenia. Many of the typical symptoms of schizophrenia, such as Schneider's first-rank symptoms, were now considered to be consistent with a diagnosis of affective disorder, particularly mania.

Cerebral localisers: Meynert, Wernicke, Kleist and Leonhard

The great neuro-pathologist psychiatrists Meynert and Wernicke approached psychiatric disorders from the position that mental illnesses were brain diseases. Their models were the hereditary–degenerative conditions such as Freidreich's Ataxia. The more precisely they could define syndromes in psychiatry, they believed, the greater the possibility of identifying the brain system pathology which caused them. Kraepelin's simple dichotomy of the non-organic psychoses was incompatible with this approach. Kleist, Wernicke's pupil, studied the effects of World War I head-wounds and drew comparisons between symptoms of schizophrenia and those attributable to specific brain lesions. This led Kleist (1928) to an elaborate classification of the non-organic psychoses, further developed by Leonhard (1979). In his system, the psychoses are divided into four main groups: the phasic psychoses group containing manic–depressive psychosis, the systematic schizophrenias, the cycloid psychoses and the non-systematic schizophrenias.

Scandinavian concepts of schizophreniform and reactive psychoses

Scandinavian psychiatry has differed from conventional psychiatry in its acceptance of two diagnostic concepts – the reactive psychoses and the schizophreniform psychoses. This tradition started with Wimmer, Professor of Psychiatry in Copenhagen, whose work in 1916 was not published in any major language and remained largely unknown outside Scandinavia. He described a group of psychoses that he believed were reactions to an 'affective shock'. Subsequent developments of this concept are associated with Faegerman, Stromgren and Retterstol. Langfeldt (1982) used the term 'schizophreniform psychosis' in a series of monographs on the prognosis in schizophrenia.

Summary

The history of the atypical psychoses reflects a variety of nosological approaches. Schneider denied that the proportion of such cases was significant, Leonhard denied that schizophrenia and affective psychosis were diagnostic entities, the Scandinavians focused on the role of stress, and the Americans have subdivided the group largely on the basis of outcome. It is important to maintain this historical perspective, and not be swayed by changing diagnostic fashions.

Schizoaffective disorder

Definition

Opinions on the nature of schizoaffective disorder are contingent upon its definition, as well as the definitions of schizophrenia and affective disorder. However, as many as 23 different definitions of schizoaffective disorder have been identified. Brockington & Leff (1979) used eight of them to classify a group of psychotic patients. They found a low level of agreement (kappa = 0.19) for the diagnosis of schizoaffective disorder, indicating that the definitions did not yield a clinically homogeneous group. The definitions provided by ICD–10 (WHO, 1992) and DSM–IV (APA, 1994) are generally used, and are compared in Table 11.2. In research the definitions provided by the Research Diagnostic Criteria (Spitzer *et al*, 1978) are frequently used.

Epidemiology

The definitions of schizoaffective disorder have varied so much that data on the frequency of this disorder are of limited value. The best estimates point to an annual incidence of 2 per 100 000, similar to that of mania and a quarter that of schizophrenia (Brockington & Meltzer, 1983). The frequency of schizoaffective disorder in psychiatric admissions has been variously estimated to be in the range of 2–11% (Levinson & Levitt, 1987).

> *Case example*
> SB, a married 38-year-old woman was admitted to psychiatric care after taking a tricyclic antidepressant overdose. Two months before admission, she became depressed with diurnal variation of mood. She had loss of libido and appetite, with three kilograms weight loss. She had been in hospital three times during the previous two years, with a diagnosis of major depression, and had improved with antidepressants and neuroleptics. However, her husband stated that following the first episode, she had never fully regained the interests that she once enjoyed. Her symptoms of depression, including suicidal ideation were confirmed in hospital and antidepressants were restarted. Five days after admission, she became withdrawn and suspicious and repeatedly looked at herself in the mirror. On mental examination, she had first-rank symptoms of schizophrenia, 'made' bodily experiences and auditory hallucinations of voices 'discussing' and 'commenting'. The bodily

experiences consisted of strange, unpleasant pulling and prickling sensations in the area of the lower jaw, chest, and perineum. She believed that her face was changing into that of a dog, and her body into that of a man. She could see early signs of these changes in the mirror, but could not describe them. These experiences, she believed, were imposed from the outside by the devil and his helpers who were changing her into a dog-headed man. She failed to improve with tricyclic antidepressants, neuroleptics and lithium but recovered following treatment with ECT combined with a neuroleptic. Her husband confirmed that following discharge, she was "the best she had been for years".

This case illustrates some of the difficulties in making a diagnosis of schizoaffective disorder. The patient met the inclusion criteria for an ICD–10 diagnosis of a severe depressive episode and the DSM–IV criteria for major depression. She also had persistent psychotic symptoms typical of schizophrenia. The diagnosis rests upon the answer to the question: "Did the schizophrenic and depressive symptoms always occur together?" If they did, then the ICD–10 diagnosis is schizoaffective disorder and the DSM–IV diagnosis is major depression with mood-incongruent psychotic features. If she had experienced the schizophrenic symptoms for at least two weeks without depressive symptoms, then the DSM–IV diagnosis is schizoaffective disorder and the ICD–10 diagnosis is schizophrenia! In practice, this question was difficult to answer. The patient was depressed when she had schizophrenic symptoms, but this seemed appropriate in a woman who believed that the devil was changing her into a dog-headed man. The response to treatment was not diagnostically helpful.

Validation of the concept of schizoaffective disorder

Conceptual hypotheses

Various hypotheses have been put forward about the nature of schizoaffective disorder. These include:

(1) It is a diagnostic 'waste basket' for patients, with symptom clusters which defy conventional categorisation.

(2) Schizoaffective disorder is a subtype of schizophrenia.

(3) Schizoaffective disorder is a variant of manic–depressive disorder.

(4) Schizoaffective disorder is the third psychosis; a disease entity independent from schizophrenia and affective psychosis.

(5) There is only one psychosis, the 'unitary psychosis'. Schizophrenia and manic-depressive psychosis are constructs which lie at opposite ends of the psychosis continuum, with schizoaffective disorder occupying an intermediate position.

(6) Schizoaffective disorder is a combination of two inherited diseases, schizophrenia and manic-depressive psychosis.

Table 11.2   Diagnostic criteria for schizoaffective disorder:
DSM–IV and   ICD–10

	ICD–10	DSM–IV
Symptoms	Schizophrenic and affective simultaneously present, both prominent.	Major depressive, or manic concurrent with criteria A schizophrenic symptoms[1]. At least two weeks of delusions and hallucinations without prominent mood disorder.
Course	Recurrent manic – defect unusual depressive – defect sometimes	Not included in criteria, but in preamble – better than schizophrenia, worse than mood disorder. Tends to chronicity
Types	Manic[2], mixed[2], depressive[2] includes affective type of schizophreniform psychosis	Bipolar, depressive
Exclude	Patients with separate episodes of schizophrenia and affective disorder	Organic disorders, schizophrenia, psychotic mood disorders

1. See chapter 7 on schizophrenia.
2. At least one, preferably two, typical schizophrenic symptoms.

Methodology

The strategies for validating the concept of schizoaffective disorder have defined the condition according to one of the sets of clinical criteria. They have then related it to external criteria such as the course of the illness, response to specific treatments, family studies and biological investigations.

Outcome

Harrow & Grossman (1984) reviewed outcome studies in schizoaffective disorder. In earlier investigations, schizoaffective disorder appeared to be a variant of schizophrenia, but later studies suggested that schizoaffective disorder was a variant of affective disorder. They concluded that in good prospective studies, schizoaffective disorder occupied an intermediate position, between the poor outcome of schizophrenia and the better outcome of affective psychosis. More recently, Moller *et al* (1988) confirmed these findings. However, outcome appears to vary with the type of clinical course. Maj & Perris (1990) have replicated earlier studies in which schizoaffective disorder – bipolar type had a good outcome, while in the depressive type of schizoaffective disorder the outcome was relatively poor.

Family studies

The possibility that schizoaffective disorder results from the combined inheritance of both schizophrenia and affective psychosis is small. The likelihood of inheriting the genes for these two relatively uncommon conditions is about 1 in 10 000. Abrams (1984) reviewed early USA studies which had found no evidence that schizoaffective disorder 'bred true'. The proportion of schizoaffective first-degree relatives of schizoaffective probands was small. However, mentally ill first-degree relatives had greater than expected rates of both schizophrenia and affective disorder, with the latter the higher of the two. More recently, Maj *et al* (1991) in a blind, controlled study found that the risk in families for schizophrenia was the same irrespective of whether probands had schizoaffective disorder or schizophrenia. This finding was reproduced by Tsuang (1991) who found that the risk for affective disorder with a schizoaffective proband was intermediate between that for families with schizophrenic probands and affective disorder probands.

Biological investigations

A variety of biological measures have been studied in the hope that they would yield a specific test for schizophrenia or affective disorder. This goal has not so far been realised, although some tests with a modest degree of specificity have been found. These include hormonal, biochemical and neurophysiological investigations. Meltzer *et al* (1984) reviewed the findings from such tests in schizoaffective disorder. Similarities were found between schizoaffective disorder and affective disorder with regard to decreased platelet 5-hydroxytryptamine (5-HT) uptake, shortened REM latency and a blunted growth-hormone response to clonidine. However, schizoaffective patients were more like the schizophrenic group in that they had increased cerebrospinal fluid norepinephrine and increased platelet 5-HT. Results of the Dexamethasone Suppression Test (DST) have been reviewed by Krishnan *et al* (1990) and the overall finding was that the proportion of non-suppressing schizoaffectives was midway between that for affective disorder and schizophrenia. More recently, Wahby *et al* (1990, 1991) used two state-markers for depression, the DST and the suppression of prolactin by thyrotropin-releasing-hormone, and concluded that schizoaffective disorder was more like schizophrenia than affective disorder.

Specific treatment effects

The use of treatment response as an external validating criterion for a diagnosis requires that the treatment effect is specific. Unfortunately, psychiatric treatments lack such specificity. There is good evidence that the response to lithium prophylaxis in bipolar or manic schizoaffective (schizomanic) disorder is similar to that of bipolar disorder. On the other hand, schizodepressive patients do not do well with antidepressant therapy unless it is combined with a neuroleptic.

Conclusion

Attempts to validate schizoaffective disorder as a disease entity lead to the conclusion that it is a heterogeneous group of conditions. Schizoaffective manic disorder has a close relationship to manic–depressive or bipolar disorder, while schizoaffective depressive disorder seems closely related to schizophrenia. If patients with schizophrenia and bipolar disorder can be excluded from the schizoaffective group, the residue may be a homogeneous group with true schizoaffective disorder, or the 'third psychosis'. An empirical approach which involves the constant revision and testing of definitions needs to continue.

Diagnosis and differential diagnosis

The diagnosis of schizoaffective disorder is made after first excluding an organic mental disorder, schizophrenia and affective disorder. The presence of equally severe typical symptoms of both schizophrenia and of a manic, mixed, or depressive episode is then sufficient to make the ICD–10 diagnosis of schizoaffective disorder. The difficulties that attend the DSM–IV diagnosis have already been discussed. The management is determined by the subcategory of schizoaffective disorder and it should therefore be qualified as either manic, mixed, or depressive type.

Differential diagnosis

The disorders that have to be differentiated from schizoaffective disorder are: schizophrenia with depressed or elated mood, mania, psychotic depression, and organic mental disorders. An organic psychosyndrome, due to drugs or other physical causes, superimposed on a typical non-organic psychosis will produce an atypical clinical picture.

(1)   *Schizophrenia with depression.* This condition frequently occurs. It is diagnosed by giving weight to clinical features common in schizophrenia, but unusual in schizoaffective disorder. These are negative schizophrenic symptoms, lengthy episodes of illness with slow and incomplete recovery and extended periods of treatment with neuroleptics.

(2)   *Schizophrenia with elation.* Heightened mood states in schizophrenia differ from those in schizoaffective disorder. They are short-lived and usually accompanied by evidence of affective disorganisation such as incongruity of affect. Schizophrenic elation

usually evokes feelings of discomfort in the examiner rather than empathic good humour. Other evidence which helps to differentiate schizophrenia from schizoaffective disorder is given in the preceding paragraph.

(3) *Affective disorder with psychotic symptoms.* When delusions are mood-congruent the differentiation of this condition from schizoaffective disorder is not difficult. Delusions in depressed patients will have themes such as guilt, poverty, disease and nihilism. However, affective disorders with mood-incongruent psychotic symptoms have attracted the interest of American psychiatrists and been given official recognition in DSM–III. DSM–IV notes that these symptoms include "persecutory delusions (not directly related to depressive themes), thought insertion, thought broadcasting and delusions of control" which the text suggests are associated with a poorer prognosis. Kendler (1991) has provided an e x t e n s i v e review of this concept. Distinguishing between affective disorder with mood-incongruent psychotic symptoms and schizoaffective disorder is a problem which derives from the diagnostic criteria, ICD–10 or DSM–IV, and not from symptomatic differences. These have already been discussed in the case of SB described above.

(4) *Organic mental disorders.* These may resemble schizoaffective disorder but should present little diagnostic difficulty as specific organic symptoms will be evident. However, the misuse of stimulant drugs such as cocaine, amphetamines, and methylphenidate may produce paranoid symptoms and elation when the patient is 'high', and depression after drug withdrawal. The resemblance between these states and schizoaffective disorder is strengthened because there is no clouding of consciousness. Other drug intoxications which can produce schizoaffective-like mental states are phencyclidine, L-dopa and corticosteroids. Therefore, in cases of atypical psychosis, particularly those with an acute onset, drug intoxication should be suspected.

Treatment

The treatment of schizoaffective disorder depends on the subcategory, bipolar or depressive, to which the patient belongs. Lithium prophylaxis appears to be as effective for schizoaffective manic disorder as it is for mania. Evidence that lithium is of value in acute treatment is limited. Studies are few, and the number of subjects small. Probably the best course at present is to treat schizoaffective mania similarly to mania. Valproate and carbamazepine, as in mania, have been used as alternative or adjunctive treatments to lithium but their efficacy in schizoaffective disorder is not known.

Treatment of schizoaffective depressive disorder with lithium is no more effective than it is in schizophrenia. Tricyclic antidepressants and neuroleptics are each more effective than lithium, and have a greater efficacy when used in combination (Brockington *et al*, 1978). In one of the few double-blind studies, Mattes & Nayak (1984) found that fluphenazine was more effective than lithium in preventing a relapse, a finding confirmed by Maj (1988). Therefore, the long-term prophylactic treatment of these patients is the same as that for schizophrenia.

There is good evidence that schizoaffective disorder does well with ECT and that its efficacy in schizoaffective depressives is greater than tricyclic–neuroleptic combinations. Therefore, ECT should be considered if there has been no response to medication. The risk of suicide is as great as in the affective psychoses.

Cycloid psychosis

This group of psychoses, perhaps more than any other, may qualify as the 'third psychosis'. Perris (1988) made a case for the cycloid psychoses being nosologically distinct from schizophrenia and the affective disorders. His case rests on their having a distinctive symptomatology, a bipolar form, a recurrent course with complete remissions, and a strong familial tendency. Cycloid psychoses constitute about 10% of admissions for functional psychoses (Lindvall *et al*, 1990).

Leonhard (1979) described three types of cycloid psychosis. All have a bipolar form, and the name identifies the predominant symptom. Any symptom which occurs in an affective disorder or schizophrenia, may appear during the illness. Leonhard's types of cycloid psychosis are:

(1)   anxiety–happiness psychosis in which affective symptoms predominate
(2)   excited–inhibited confusion psychosis in which thought disorder is dominant
(3)   hyperkinetic–akinetic psychosis has motor disorder as the predominant feature.

It is often difficult to assign cases to these subcategories because the patient's symptomatology changes so quickly and frequently. Leonhard later came to acknowledge this difficulty.

Diagnosis

Diagnostic guidelines for the cycloid psychoses were published by Perris & Brockington (1981):

(1)   An acute psychotic condition, not related to the administration or misuse of any drug, or to brain injury, occurring for the first time in subjects aged 15–50 years.
(2)   The condition has a sudden onset with a rapid change from a state of health to a full–blown psychotic condition within a few hours, or at the most a few days.

(3)   At least four of the following must be present:
  (i)   confusion of some degree, mostly expressed as perplexity or puzzlement
  (ii)   mood-incongruent delusions of any kind, mostly with a persecutory content
  (iii)   hallucinatory experiences of any kind, often related to themes of death
  (iv)   an overwhelming, frightening experience of anxiety, not bound to particular situations or circumstances (pan-anxiety)
  (v)   deep feelings of happiness or ecstasy, most often with a religious colouring
  (vi)   motility disturbances of an akinetic or hyperkinetic type which are mostly expressional
  (vii)   a particular concern with death
  (viii) mood swings in the background, and not so pronounced as to justify a diagnosis of affective disorder.
(4)   There is no fixed combination of symptoms; on the contrary, the symptoms may change frequently during an episode and s h o w bipolar characteristics.

These criteria are similar to those used by ICD–10. There is, however, a difference in nomenclature and the term 'cycloid psychosis' is replaced by 'acute psychotic disorder with or without symptoms of schizophrenia'. When making the diagnosis of cycloid psychosis, the polymorphous nature of the symptoms is of greatest value. The symptoms can be any of those which occur in schizophrenia (including first-rank symptoms) and in manic–depressive disorder. These symptoms usually change rapidly and occur in unusual combinations. The clinical diagnosis requires repeated mental examinations in order to recognise the variability and inconstancy of the clinical picture.

> *Case example*
> EP is a 38-year-old housewife, whose first attack of mental illness at age 19, led to her compulsory admission to hospital with a diagnosis of schizophrenia. Afterwards she recovered fully, resumed work, married, and remained well for seven years. Then, over the next 12 years, she had seven distinct episodes of psychosis, variously diagnosed as manic–depressive illness, schizophrenia and schizoaffective disorder. Each episode was followed by a complete remission. She presented for admission five weeks after an uncomplicated hysterectomy with a five-day history of severe insomnia and anxiety. On admission, she had marked psychomotor retardation, but later that day her mutism changed to echolalia. At night, she frequently screamed 'They are going to kill me!' and appeared to be having auditory hallucinations. The following day she was active, restless, and walked in a bizarre way on the balls of her feet (manneristic catatonia). Her mood was

cheerful and she repeatedly sang a TV advertising jingle. This behaviour lasted about two hours, before anxiety dominated the clinical picture again. At various times over the next two weeks, she had intermittent auditory hallucinations; both complex, such as voices, and simple, such as bangs and whistles. She experienced first-rank symptoms: 'made thoughts', 'made bodily experiences', and 'audible thoughts', all of which occurred episodically. Anxiety remained the dominant symptom, but it fluctuated in severity, and was sometimes associated with perplexity and ideas of reference. She recovered completely after four weeks and has remained well for the past two years on prophylactic treatment with lithium and carbamazepine. She fulfilled the ICD–10 criteria for acute polymorphic psychotic disorder with symptoms of schizophrenia. Although motor symptoms were evident at the onset of this psychosis, affective symptoms predominated and a diagnosis of anxiety–happiness psychosis was made.

Management

In managing the acute phase of the illness, neuroleptics appear to be the drugs of choice. Perris (1988) advocates rapid introduction of neuroleptics, for example with haloperidol followed by the addition of lithium. If there is severe anxiety which does not respond to neuroleptics, clonazepam may be helpful. The cycloid psychoses resemble the puerperal psychoses in their symptomatology, and like them may show a dramatic improvement with ECT. Long-term prophylactic treatment with lithium or depot neuroleptics has been advocated. The use of valproate and carbamazepine for this purpose appears promising.

Conditions related to the cycloid psychoses

Non-systematic schizophrenia

Leonhard (1979) describes these conditions as the 'evil relatives' of the cycloid psychoses. The symptomatology also tends to be polymorphous in type, but not as variable in time. The onset is less abrupt, and the outcome worse. The chance of a complete remission is the same as in schizophrenia. There are three types of non-systematic schizophrenia, which correspond in their dominant symptomatology to the cycloid psychoses:

Affect-laden paraphrenia resembles the anxiety–elation psychosis. Fluctuations in mood between anxiety and ecstasy dominate the clinical picture in the early stages. Ideas of self-reference, illusions and hallucinations appear and are congruent with the affective abnormalities. However, congruency tends to disappear as the patient's condition deteriorates.

Cataphasia (schizophasia) like the confusional cycloid psychosis, has excited and inhibited forms of thought disorder, but of greater severity.

Periodic catatonia resembles the motility psychosis in having both hyperkinetic and akinetic forms of motor activity. Both forms can occur at the same time in conjunction with other catatonic symptoms such as parakinesis and manneristic behaviours.As the name suggests, this condition usually runs an intermittent course, but without complete remissions between episodes. R. Gjessing's use of thyroid extract as treatment in the 1930s followed extensive metabolic studies of catatonic patients, and provided a model for the future development of biological psychiatry. See Gjessing (1974) for a review.

Boufée délirante

The French psychiatrist Mangan first described these disorders as psychoses of acute onset, a fluctuating clinical picture, recurrent course, and a tendency to occur in successive generations of the same family. His concept was adopted by Wernicke and these disorders became the cycloid psychoses. Modern French psychiatry still recognises them, qualifying the diagnosis as 'genuine' if there is no psychological stressor, and 'reactive' if there is (Pull *et al*, 1985).

Mitsuda's atypical psychoses and Hatotani's periodical psychoses

The Japanese were influenced by German psychiatry and Wernicke's concepts are apparent in the work of Mitsuda and Hatotani. They have described conditions which closely resemble the cycloid psychoses. Mitsuda (1965) has published genetic evidence that these conditions 'breed true' and Hatotani has attempted to establish their nosological identity through biological studies.

Reactive (psychogenic) psychoses

The diagnosis of reactive or psychogenic psychosis is widely employed in Scandinavia. This condition accounts for 15–20% of all first-time admissions for psychotic illness in Denmark (Rettersol, 1978).

Reactive psychoses, also termed psychogenic psychoses by Faegerman (1963) are considered to be psychotic reactions to external stresses. Rettersol (1986), in a summary of Scandinavian opinion, stated that the psychic trauma must be of such significance that the psychosis would not have appeared in its absence. In addition, there must be a temporal connection between the trauma and the onset of the psychosis, and the content of the psychotic symptoms must reflect the traumatic experience. In most cases, after weeks or months, the patient regains a normal level of functioning.

Rettersol also pointed to the ways in which the Scandinavian concept of reactive psychosis differed from those chosen by ICD–9 (WHO, 1978) and

DSM–III. Both stipulated that the onset of the psychosis should follow closely after the stress. This view of reactive psychosis remains unchanged in ICD–10 (acute and transient psychotic disorder with associated acute stress) and DSM–IV (brief psychotic disorder). In the ICD–10, the diagnosis incorporates stress only if the psychosis follows within about two weeks of the stressful event. The Scandinavian position is that the time between these events is not critical.

ICD–10 states that the event or events "would be markedly stressful to almost anyone in the person's culture". DSM–IV describes one subtype of brief psychotic disorder 'with marked stressors', but also describes a group 'without marked stressors' and a third group with 'postpartum' onset. The Scandinavians also view 'stress' differently. They take into account the weight given to the stress by the patient's culture as well as its specific effect on the individual. Such a definition of stress is difficult to define operationally, but appears closer to thinking in clinical practice.

The duration of the reactive psychosis is not so critical from the Scandinavian viewpoint as it is in ICD–10 (2–3 months) and DSM–IV (4 weeks). However, for all three, there is agreement that the outcome is good.

The Scandinavians define three forms of reactive psychosis, which together with their relative frequencies are emotional reactions (65%), paranoid reactions (20%), and disorders of consciousness (15%).

Case example
CP, a single 18-year-old woman, had lived all her life in a small fishing community. She had seven older brothers, and was the only child left at home with middle-aged indulgent parents. She had left school at age 16, and never been able to find work. She moved to a city a thousand miles away with a new boyfriend, intent on finding employment. She found work on three occasions, but left because it was too stressful. Two months after leaving home, she was admitted to hospital with acute anxiety and confusion. She believed that she was pregnant and could feel an animal moving around inside her abdomen and she could hear its cries. Other auditory hallucinations included voices talking about her pregnancy. No physical cause, including drug abuse, was found. She was treated with neuroleptics, transferred to a hospital closer to her home where only mild anxiety was observed, and the neuroleptics were gradually withdrawn. She then became acutely disturbed, restless, and repeatedly absconded from hospital. Her delusions of pregnancy returned, she felt that people were trying to kill her, and that her thoughts were being interfered with. Following reintroduction of treatment her hallucinations slowly diminished as did her delusions of pregnancy. She remained anxious and convinced that people were trying to kill her. At her parents' insistence, she was discharged home. Following this, she rapidly improved, and one month later she was asymptomatic and

off all medication. Four months later, her family reported that she was "back to her normal self".

This patient's illness conforms to the Scandinavian concept of reactive psychosis of the paranoid type and to the ICD–10 concept of acute and transient psychotic disorder, but the temporal relationship between the stressor and the appearance of the psychotic symptom is too long to qualify the diagnosis as 'with associated acute stress'. This patient also illustrates the problem of defining stress. The move away from home would not be regarded as a major stressor in her community, but was uniquely stressful for her. The duration of the illness is too long for the DSM–IV category of brief psychotic disorder and a diagnosis of schizophreniform disorder would be made.

Treatment

Treatment of these conditions is symptomatic since they are, by definition, self-limiting. If psychotic symptoms predominate, short-term neuroleptic treatment is indicated. In milder cases, anxiolytics alone may suffice. The persistence of the condition, or the failure to make a complete recovery, indicates that the diagnosis of reactive psychosis is wrong.

Schizophreniform disorder

The term 'schizophreniform' was first used by Langfeldt in 1937 to identify those patients with schizophrenic symptoms who had a good prognosis. This position is clear from the comments he made on the use of the term in DSM–III (Langfeldt, 1982): "My proposal is that only psychotic cases characterized by quite typical symptoms associated with a poor prognosis should be diagnosed as typical schizophrenias. All other psychoses similar to schizophrenia should be diagnosed as schizophreniform psychoses."

All of the conditions discussed in this chapter would qualify as schizophreniform psychoses according to Langfeldt. In addition, he included organic psychosyndromes with clinical features of schizophrenia. The term 'schizophreniform', therefore, may be used according to Langfeldt as a general description or, as in DSM–IV to define a specific syndrome.

Bergem *et al* (1990) reclassified Langfeldt's schizophreniform patients using ICD–9 and DSM–III–R and raised doubts about the validity of his concept. They found that one third of the patients had schizophrenia and that most of the remainder had affective or adjustment disorders. Only 14% fulfilled the DSM–III–R criteria for schizophreniform disorder.

DSM–III took the term schizophreniform and used it to identify cases which were symptomatically typical of schizophrenia, but recovered. The

DSM–IV criteria are the same as for schizophrenia except that the total duration of the illness (prodrome, active phase, and recovery) should not last more than six months. DSM–IV also provides for the identification of prognostic features. For a good prognosis, the patient should have two of the following features:

(1)   psychotic symptoms appear within four weeks of the onset of the illness

(2)   confusion, disorientation and perplexity

(3)   good premorbid or social functioning

(4)   the absence of blunted or flat affect.

Beiser *et al* (1988) have claimed that it might be possible to differentiate schizophrenia from schizophreniform disorder before the six-month outcome is known. Patients with schizophreniform disorder have higher ratings on the DSM–III Axis 5 (their general level of functioning is better); are less ill than schizophrenic patients; do not have a flattened affect; and have a better rapport with the examiner. The confusion, disorientation, and perplexity which sometimes occur at the height of the schizophreniform illness may be associated with an acute onset. These particular symptoms may be caused by the patient's difficulty in living with a sudden psychotic experience.

Treatment

Schizophreniform disorder is treated in the same way as schizophrenia. Initially, large doses of neuroleptics may be required. If schizophreniform disorder is suspected, the medication should be gradually reduced. If the symptoms return, then the diagnosis should be revised to schizophrenia.

Paranoid (delusional) disorders

History

Psychiatrists have come to view the term paranoia and its adjective paranoid with suspicion, as these words have acquired a variety of meanings (Lewis, 1970). To the Greeks, who originated the word paranoia, it meant to be 'beside one's self'. They used it as a general term for insanity.

The modern use of 'paranoia' started with Kahlbaum. He applied it to a group of chronic conditions which had delusions as the major symptom. Kraepelin endorsed this definition and psychiatrists generally accepted it. Kahlbaum's concept of paranoia appeared virtually unchanged in ICD–9.

Unfortunately, paranoia and paranoid have been applied to other psychiatric conditions. 'Paranoid' was used to describe the type of schizophrenia in which delusions, of any kind, predominate. Later, in Anglo–American literature, paranoid became synonymous with delusions of persecution, as they are the commonest type of delusion in paranoid schizophrenia. The meaning of paranoid was further extended to include non-delusional ideas of persecution and self-reference. In this sense it describes personality traits and makes a nosological appearance as paranoid personality disorder. Finally, the lay public found it too useful a word to be left to the psychiatrists and 'paranoid' has entered everyday language.

This semantic confusion led the authors of DSM–III–R to replace both paranoia and paranoid disorder with the term 'delusional disorder', which remains in DSM–IV; this condition is defined as "the presence of a persistent, non-bizarre delusion that is not due to any other mental disorder, such as schizophrenia, schizophreniform disorder, or a mood disorder". ICD–10 has followed DSM–IV, and the paranoia of ICD–9 has become persistent delusional disorder. Although DSM–IV and ICD–10 give similar definitions, there are differences in emphasis. The ICD–10 states that it is a group of heterogeneous conditions with variable aetiology and stipulates that the delusion must be present for at least three months.

Kraepelin believed that a condition similar to paranoia with persistent hallucinations was a different disorder, which he named paraphrenia.

Epidemiology

The figures for the frequency of paranoid disorder are probably an underestimate, as it usually requires markedly abnormal behaviour to bring patients to psychiatric attention. The prevalence is thought to be about 0.03% and the life-time risk 0.05–0.1% for the general population. The onset is usually in the range of 40–55 years, but it can occur in adults of any age.

Theories of causation

There are two basic theories about the cause of delusional disorders. One postulates an abnormal personality development in which the development of the delusions is understandable and inevitable. The second attributes the delusion to a 'process', a pathophysiological change in the brain. This could be associated with a physical insult or schizophrenia. How the delusion is formed is not understandable although the content in terms of the patient's personality and life experience will be.

Kraepelin appears to have preferred the personality development theory, but it was Gaupp and Kretschmer who presented supporting evidence. A famous case cited as an example of psychologically understandable paranoia was that of the mass-murderer Wagner.

Case example
Gaupp (1974) described a sensitive, intelligent, self-critical man who, in his youth, was troubled by the moral and physical damage he

had sustained by masturbating. Later in life, while working as a schoolmaster in a small village, he committed bestiality. No one else knew, but he was convinced that the villagers were aware of his crime and mocked him for it. He then moved, but over the next seven years, plotted the destruction of these villagers. His papers revealed that he waited four more years before acting. He first killed his wife and children, then set fire to the village and shot the inhabitants as they fled, killing eight and seriously wounding 12 others.

Kretschmer's theory of the development of sensitive ideas of reference appeared as a monograph in 1927. Kretschmer (1974) described a particular type of personality, the sensitive, who was liable to develop delusions. Significant emotional complexes are consciously retained and worked over by such personalities, who are unable to discharge their feelings. Given a particular set of life experiences, and one key experience, such people develop delusions of self-reference particularly when mentally or physically exhausted.

Case example
JW was a 33-year-old man referred by a urologist, to whom he had repeatedly taken his complaint of a small penis. The patient believed that this was common knowledge and discussed by his neighbours. Changes of residence provided only temporary relief. The beliefs began at the age of 13, when he was taking a communal shower at school. Another lad had laughed at him because his genitalia were small and recruited other boys to join in the teasing. This distressed him greatly for a short period of time, and was largely forgotten. Following conscription into the army, he felt homesick and miserable, and recognised in the barracks the boy who had teased him at school. He was with a group of other recruits and suddenly, they all laughed (the key experience). He knew that they were laughing about his small penis. From that time on, he knew that he had a small penis and that this was common knowledge. Later, his wife became unable to tolerate his repeated questioning about whether he was too small for her. When she left him for another man, he knew his small penis was the reason. When seen, he lived alone, padded his underwear, and prefaced any sexual encounter with an apology to the prospective partner.

A discussion of the psychogenesis of paranoid disorder would be incomplete without mentioning Freud's analysis of the Schreber Memoirs. Daniel Schreber was 51 and President of the Court of Appeals of Saxony, when he developed 'paranoia' and was confined in hospital for the next nine years. His memoirs, written to secure his release, are a vivid personal account of this illness. Freud concluded that Schreber's paranoia was attributable to his repressed homosexual impulses towards his father. The central conflict in paranoia, for males, was the unacceptable homosexual wish to love another man. The principal forms of paranoia could be explained as contradictions of "I, a man, love him" (Freud, 1950).

Persecutory delusions. The contradiction is "I do not love him, I hate him". This by projection becomes "He hates me" and by rationalisation "I hate him".

Delusions of jealousy. The contradiction is "I do not love him, she loves him".

Delusions of love. The contradiction is "I do not love him, I love her", which by projection becomes "She loves me".

Grandiose delusions. The contradiction is "I do not love him, I love myself".

Unfortunately for this theory, the conscious profession of homosexuality is neither a remedy for, nor a prophylactic against the development of delusional disorders.

The second hypothesis that delusional disorder was attributable to a biological 'process' gained support from Kolle. He followed up cases of paranoia including those described by Kraepelin, and found that most of them developed schizophrenia. Another possibility raised by this theory was that a somatic disorder might play a role in the development of delusional disorder. Munro (1988*a*), in a review of 50 patients, found that 40% had suffered some form of brain insult. He suggested that delusional disorder might arise in individuals with a weak genetic loading for schizophrenia who had suffered a brain insult before or during adolescence.

Clinical presentation

Patients with delusional disorder rarely complain directly of their delusions. Usually, they have been coerced into seeing a psychiatrist by their family, or by some legal process. In delusional disorder an independent account of the illness from someone who knows the patient well is a necessity, particularly if the delusional content is 'culturally acceptable'.

The subject of the patient's delusions should be approached circumspectly. Patients with delusional disorder are often hostile, sarcastic and marshal many reasons against cooperating in the psychiatric assessment. Once the area of the delusional belief is touched upon it is important for the examiner to convey an attitude of open-mindedness and of sympathetic interest in the patient's concerns. This usually reduces the patient's distrust and evasiveness and leads to a disclosure of the delusional content. Although one should not agree with the patient's delusional beliefs, one should not disagree with them either, unless a challenge to the strength of the delusional formation is deemed necessary.

The rest of the mental examination should be normal, although most criteria permit occasional hallucinations. Assessing the danger that the patient poses to the subjects of the delusions is most important. In making such an assessment, the presence of anger toward the subjects of the delusions should be sought. Progression of this anger into plans for exacting revenge, or stopping the 'harmful' activities by physical means, indicates that there is a risk and preventive action is needed. Delusional disorder is usually categorised according to the delusional content. The major subtypes are:

Erotomania – this is sometimes referred to as de Clérambault's syndrome, in which the patient believes that a particular person is in love with them. This person may be a superior at work, a public figure, or a celebrity, and is less frequently someone of equivalent status. When this 'lover' denies any feelings for the patient and rejects all approaches, further delusional elaborations often occur. These provide reasons why the 'lover' cannot publicly acknowledge this love and must communicate through secret messages and signs, which the patient can interpret. For example, a patient who believed that a current rock star was in love with her interpreted his sequence of songs as having a secret message meant only for her. More women than men are seen with erotomania, but men present the major forensic problems. Legal remedies, including imprisonment, have no effect on the patients' beliefs and do little to modify their behaviour over the long term. The feelings of love, although still declared, can become mixed over time with those of hostility and jealousy. When this happens a patient may pose a significant risk to the 'lover' and those close to him or her.

Grandiose – these patients have erroneous and extravagant delusional beliefs about themselves. These beliefs may involve social status, wealth, intellectual powers and spiritual gifts.

A patient, who believed he was the only legitimate and direct heir of Charles II, attributed his considerable financial problems to machinations of the Royal Family. He knew that they had usurped his throne and were trying to discredit him.

Jealous – this is characterised by delusions that a partner, usually a spouse, has been unfaithful. It is also known, more dramatically, as the 'Othello syndrome'. Morbid jealousy is a general term for pathological jealousy, which may be a symptom of psychiatric conditions other than delusional disorder (alcoholism is probably the commonest cause). Morbid jealousy is not always delusional; for example, it can be an over-valued idea or a compulsive thought.

When jealousy is attributable to a delusional disorder it appears to develop insidiously in middle life. However, careful inquiry will sometimes reveal episodes of unjustifiable jealousy in the past. This development is sometimes associated with erectile impotence in the male and concomitant sexual dysfunction in the female. However, the psychosexual difficulties are more often an effect rather than a cause of the disorder, but they secondarily reinforce the delusion.

Sometimes the jealousy appears to be evoked by a 'key' experience, termed the 'jealous flash' by Enoch (1991) in a review.

Patients will persistently question their partner as they seek evidence to support the delusion. These partners may be spied upon, followed, traps are set for them, mail intercepted and underwear scrutinised. There will be frequent confrontations and attempts to extort a confession. Some partners worn down by these continuous demands make a false confession, with disastrous consequences. At best, further information about other lovers will be demanded. At worst, physical violence will erupt and murder results. The condition is difficult to treat and tends to recur with a new partner. It should be suspected in cases of domestic violence and if confirmed measures should be taken to protect the spouse. On occasions, the 'rival' may require protection as well.

Persecutory – the patients are usually the subject of the persecution, but occasionally it is someone close to them. The delusional system is very well organised, much better so than in other psychiatric conditions. Convinced that the evidence supporting their belief is irrefutable, and frustrated that the proper authorities will take no action, patients may attempt to expose their persecutors in a public forum; the law courts and 'letters to the editor' serve this purpose.

Somatic – delusions of physical abnormality, or of physical disorder characterise this subtype. If the delusional content is concerned with aspects of physical size or form (see case JW above) then it may be identified as delusional dysmorphophobia. The content can also be of illness, infestation, and leaking smells and secretions from body orifices, which is often referred to as monosymptomatic hypochondriacal psychosis (see also page 728).

Differential diagnosis

Paranoid, or delusional disorder is a diagnosis of exclusion. Symptoms found in the paranoid syndromes may be found in any of the other psychoses – schizophrenia, affective and organic.

Schizophrenia

Hallucinations, particularly in sensory modalities with little relationship to the content of the delusion, suggest a diagnosis of schizophrenia. Delusions of attempted control by others may be described by patients with delusional disorder. These can be readily distinguished from the superficially similar experiences reported by schizophrenic patients. This type of experience in delusional disorder is simply a delusion and nothing more. The so-called 'delusions of control' in schizophrenia are far more complex experiences. A mental activity such as thinking is experienced as not being part of the self (ego), but 'made' or alien. These 'made' thoughts usually pass between the external world and the self through the ego boundary. The delusion of attempted control provides an explanation for this strange experience. These 'made' experiences and other first-rank symptoms of schizophrenia are unusual in paranoid disorder. The presence of positive or negative formal thought disorder, affective disorganisation and affective flattening also raises the possibility of schizophrenia.

Psychotic affective disorder

Patients with delusional states often have mood disorder. The possibility that delusional symptomatology is due to depression is greater if the delusions are mood-congruent delusion-like ideas. However, the diagnosis of depression will rest largely upon the presence of neurovegetative signs. Manic delusions are grandiose in content. Mania of such severity that it gives rise to delusions will be characterised by obvious psychomotor acceleration.

Organic delusional disorder

Some patients, particularly those with a paranoid personality, may develop delusional disorder when they are affected by some physical insult to the brain. The commonest physical cause of acute delusional disorder is drug intoxication. Stimulants such as amphetamine, cocaine, and methyl-phenidate are notorious for producing a delusional disorder without evidence of impaired consciousness. Therefore, a history of drug use should always be sought in delusional disorder. Alcoholism may be a factor in the development of delusions, particularly those of morbid jealousy. Other drugs particularly associated with organic paranoid disorders are steroid hormones and dopamine agonists such as L-dopa and disulfiram.

The possibility that the delusions are secondary to a dementia should be considered in older patients. When a patient with delusional disorder continues to deteriorate, dementia and schizophrenia should be considered as possible diagnoses.

Management

The first goal in treatment is the most difficult. This is to achieve a therapeutic relationship with a patient who does not want to participate in psychiatric treatment. The patients do not see why they should enter into such a relationship, because they do not believe that they need psychiatric treatment. Also militating against this relationship which requires a large measure of trust, are the suspiciousness and distrust which are part of the illness. Patients are usually angry and hostile towards those responsible for their entry into treatment, and these feelings are immediately extended to psychiatric staff.

At this stage, the patients have come to expect that their beliefs will be met by disbelief and argument and may be sullen, resentful and evasive. The approach to eliciting the delusions has already been described and the importance of maintaining an attitude of concerned and sympathetic interest stressed. Because a patient is suspicious and distrustful, the psychiatrist should do nothing to reinforce these feelings, but try to allay them. It helps to appear open and friendly, maintain eye contact, avoid physical contact and be consistent. It does not help to argue against or agree with the delusion, attempt any type of deception, break promises or show anger.

Physical treatment can often be initiated by focusing on symptoms other than the delusion, particularly anxiety and depression. By keeping the delusion in the background, the patient may be encouraged to accept medication for these associated symptoms. At subsequent interviews to assess progress, the question of the delusion should not be raised immediately, but approached after inquiring into the progress of the other symptoms.

Physical treatment

Pimozide, a piperidine derivative, appears to be the treatment of choice for delusional disorders. Following reports of its efficacy in the treatment of monosymptomatic hypochondriasis other reports of its effectiveness in erotomania and persecutory delusions followed. Munro (1988*b*) described the development of secondary depression when delusions remit with pimozide. Following treatment with an antidepressant and withdrawal of the pimozide, the depression remits, and the delusions return. Therefore, he advocates combining pimozide with an antidepressant in those subject to depression. The efficacy of the other neuroleptics in the management of this condition is not as well established and nor is the use of carbamazepine or lithium, but all merit a trial in cases with resistant delusions.

Patients with delusional disorder may require admission to hospital, particularly if there is evidence of poor impulse control, a threat of suicide or of danger to others. Those who misuse alcohol or drugs pose a higher risk to themselves and others.

Rare delusional disorders

It is customary to include certain unusual and fascinating delusional syndromes under the heading of delusional disorders. However, the majority of them are secondary to some other cause, such as an organic brain disorder or schizophrenia.

Folie à deux, or shared delusional disorder, is the development in a second person of the delusions already entertained by someone who is a close personal contact. There is no other evidence of mental illness in the second person, who has usually been in a subordinate relationship to the first.

Case example
A patient with paranoid schizophrenia believed that he should go into space, so that he might destroy a satellite which was transmitting thought waves into his mind. His wife, who had a dependent personality and borderline intelligence, but was otherwise normal, believed in his mission and his capabilities as a 'rocket scientist'. Some time after his discharge from hospital both were apprehended by the police as they attempted to launch a three metre high, plywood and aluminium foil 'spaceship'. He was sitting in this structure, which she was attempting to ignite.

Delusions of misidentification

(1)   Capgras syndrome: a familiar person, or persons, has been replaced by an exact double.
(2)   Fregoli syndrome: an unfamiliar person, or persons is believed to be someone very familiar (usually a persecutor), even though their physical appearance is not the same.
(3)   Intermetamorphosis syndrome: similar to the Fregoli syndrome except that the stranger is believed to have both the physical and psychological characteristics of the familiar person.
(4)   Subjective doubles syndrome: other people have the same physical appearance as the patient.

References

Abrams, R. (1984) Genetic studies of the schizoaffective syndrome: a selective review. *Schizophrenia Bulletin*, **10**, 26–29.

American Psychiatric Association (1968) *Diagnostic and Statistical Manual of Mental Disorders* (2nd edn) (DSM–II). Washington, DC: APA.

——(1980) *Diagnostic and Statistical Manual of Mental Disorders* (3rd edn) (DSM–III). Washington, DC: APA.

—— (1987) *Diagnostic and Statistical Manual of Mental Disorders* (3rd edn, revised) (DSM–III–R). Washington, DC: APA.

—— (1994) *Diagnostic and Statistical Manual of Mental Disorders* (4th edn) (DSM–IV). Washington, DC: APA.

Beiser, M., Fleming, J. A. E. & Lin, T. (1988) Refining the diagnosis of schizophreniform disorder. *American Journal of Psychiatry*, **145**, 695–700.

Bergem, A. L. M., Dahl, A. A., Guldberg, C., *et al* (1990) Langfeldt's schizophreniform psychoses fifty years later. *British Journal of Psychiatry*, **157**, 351–354.

Brockington, I. F., Kendell, R. E., Kellett, J. M., *et al* (1978) Trials of lithium, chlorpromazine and amitryptiline in schizoaffective patients. *British Journal of Psychiatry*, **133**, 162–168.

—— & Leff, J. P. (1979) Schizoaffective psychosis: definitions and incidence. *Psychological Medicine*, **9**, 91–99.

—— & Meltzer, H. Y. (1983) The nosology of schizoaffective psychosis. Psychiatric Developments, 4, 317–338.

Clayton, P. J. (1982) Schizoaffective disorders. *Journal of Nervous and Mental Diseases*, **11**, 646–650.

Enoch, D. (1991) Delusional jealousy and awareness of reality. *British Journal of Psychiatry*, **159**, 52–56.

Faegerman, P. M. (1963) *Psychogenic Psychoses*. London: Butterworths.

Freud, S. (1950) Psychoanalytic notes upon an autobiographical account of a case of paranoia (dementia paranoides). In *Collected Papers, Vol 3*. London: Hogarth Press.

Gaupp, R. (1974) The scientific significance of the case of Ernst Wagner. In *Themes and Variations in European Psychiatry* (eds S. R. Hirsch & M. Shepherd), pp. 121–134. Charlottesville: University Press of Virginia.

Gjessing, L. R. (1974) A review of periodic catatonia. *Biological Psychiatry*, **8**, 23–45.

Harrow, M. & Grossman H. S. (1984) Outcome in schizoaffective disorders: a critical review of the literature. *Schizophrenia Bulletin*, **10**, 87–108.

Jaspers, K. (1963) *General Psychopathology*. Engl. translation. Manchester: Manchester University Press.

Kasanin, J. (1933) The acute schizoaffective psychoses. *American Journal of Psychiatry*, **13**, 97–126.

Kendler, K. S. (1991) Mood-incongruent psychotic affective illness. *Archives of General Psychiatry*, **48**, 362–369.

Kleist, K. (1928) Über zycloide, paranoide und epileptoid Psychosen und über die frage der Degenerationspsychosen. *Schweizer Archive für Neurologie und Psychiatrie*, **23**, 1–35.

Kraepelin, E. (1919) *Dementia Praecox and Paraphrenia* (trans. R. M. Barclay). Edinburgh: E & S Livingstone.

Kretschmer, E. (1974) The sensitive delusions of reference. In *Themes and Variations in European Psychiatry* (eds S. R. Hirsch & M. Shepherd), pp. 153–196. Charlottesville: University Press of Virginia.

Krishnan, K. R. R., Raysam, K. & Carroll, B. J. (1990) Dexamethasone suppression test in schizoaffective disorders. In *Affective and Schizoaffective Disorders* (eds A. Marneros & M. Tsuang), pp. 208–217. London: Springer-Verlag.

Langfeldt, G. (1982) Definition of schizophreniform psychoses. *American Journal of Psychiatry*, **139**, 703.

Leonhard, K. (1979) *The Classification of Endogenous Psychoses* (5th edn). New York: Irvington Publishers.

Levinson, D. F. & Levitt, M. E. M. (1987) Schizoaffective mania reconsidered. *American Journal of Psychiatry*, **144**, 415–425.

Lewis, A. (1934) Melancholia: a historical review. Journal of Mental Science, 80, 1–42.

—— (1970) Paranoia and Paranoid: a historical perspective. *Psychological Medicine*, **1**, 2–12.

Lindvall, M., Hagnell, O. & Ohman, R. (1990) Epidemiology of cycloid psychosis. *Psychopathology*, **23**, 228–232.

Maj, M. (1988) Lithium prophylaxis of schizoaffective disorders: a prospective study. *Journal of Affective Disorders*, **14**, 129–135.

—— & Perris, C. (1990) Patterns of course in patients with a cross-sectional diagnosis of schizoaffective disorder. *Journal of Affective Disorders*, **20**, 70–77.

——, Starace, F., & Pinozzi, R. (1991) A family study of schizoaffective disorder depressive type, compared with schizophrenia and psychotic and nonpsychotic major depression. *American Journal of Psychiatry*, **148**, 612–616.

Mattes, J. A. & Nayak, D. (1984) Lithium vs fluphenazine for prophylaxis in mainly schizophrenia schizoaffectives. *Biological Psychiatry*, **19**, 445–449.

Meltzer, H. Y., Arora, R. E. & Metz, J. (1984) Biological studies of schizoaffective disorders. *Schizophrenia Bulletin*, **10**, 49–70.

Mitsuda, H. (1965) The concept of "atypical psychoses" from the aspect of clinical genetics. *Acta Psychiatrica Scandinavica*, **41**, 372–377.

Moller, H. J., Schmid-Bode, W., Cording-Tommel, C., et al (1988) Psychopathological and social outcome in schizophrenia versus affective/schizoaffective psychoses and prediction of poor outcome in schizophrenia. *Acta Psychiatrica Scandinavica*, **77**, 379–389.

Munro, A. (1988a) Delusional (paranoid) disorder: etiologic and taxonomic considerations. I. The possible significance of organic brain factors in the etiology of delusional disorders. *Canadian Journal of Psychiatry*, **33**, 171–174.

——— (1988b) Delusional (paranoid) disorder: etiologic and taxonomic considerations. II. A possible relationship between delusional and affective disorders. *Canadian Journal of Psychiatry*, **33**, 175–177.

Perris, C. (1988) The concept of cycloid psychotic disorders. *Psychiatric Developments*, **1**, 37–56.

—— & Brockington, I. F. (1981) Cycloid psychoses and their relation to the major psychoses. In *Biological Psychiatry* (eds C. Perris et al), pp. 447–450. Amsterdam: Elsevier.

Pull, C. B., Pull, M. C. & Pichot, P. (1985) Comparing French and International Classification Schemes: I. Schizophrenia. In *Psychiatry the State of the Art. Vol I Clinical Psychopathology Nomenclature and Classification* (eds P. Berner, R. Wolf & K. Thau), pp. 87–92. New York: Plenum Press.

Rettersol, N. (1978) The Scandinavian concept of reactive psychosis, schizophreniform psychosis and schizophrenia. *Psychiatria Clinica*, **11**, 180–187.

—— (1986) Classification of functional psychoses with special reference to follow-up studies. *Psychopathology*, **19**, 5–15.

Schneider, K. (1959) *Clinical Psychopathology* (English translation). New York: Grune and Stratton.

Spitzer, R. L., Endicott, J. & Robins, E. (1978) *Research Diagnostic Criteria (RDC) for a Selected Group of Functional Disorders* (3rd edn). New York: New York State Psychiatric Institute.

Tsuang, M. T. (1991) Morbidity risks of schizophrenia and affective disorders among first-degree relatives of patients with schizoaffective disorder. *British Journal of Psychiatry*, **158**, 165–170.

Wahby, V. S., Ibrahim, G. A., Leechuy, I., et al (1990) Prolactin response to thyrotropin-releasing hormone in schizoaffective depressed compared to depressed and schizophrenic men and healthy controls. *Schizophrenia Research*, **3**, 227–281.

——,——, Giller, E. L., *et al* (1991) The dexamethasone suppression test in a group of research diagnostic criteria schizoaffective depressed men. *Neuropsychobiology*, **23**, 129–133.

World Health Organization (1978) *Mental Disorders: Glossary and Guide to their Classification in Accordance with the Ninth Revision of the International Classification of Diseases* (ICD–9). Geneva: WHO.

—— (1992) Mental Disorders: *The Tenth Revision of the International Classification of Diseases and Related Health Problems* (ICD–10). Geneva: WHO.

12 Suicide and deliberate self-harm

Christopher Vassilas, Gethin Morgan & John Owen

History of suicide ● Definition of suicide ● Incidence of suicide ● Aetiology of suicide ● Special groups ● Assessment ● Management of high risk individuals ● Prevention of suicide ● The aftermath of suicide ● Audit ● Non-fatal deliberate self-harm ● Aetiology ● Special groups ● Methods of DSH ● Assessment and management of DSH ● Secondary prevention of DSH ● Prognosis in DSH

Acts of suicide and non-fatal deliberate self-harm (DSH) usually have a complex aetiology. This chapter considers some theoretical issues, particularly the relevance of clinical, psychosocial and biological factors, before setting out the principles of sound clinical practice. Suicide is discussed separately from non-fatal deliberate self-harm.

History of suicide

Suicide is a phenomenon unique to human beings, and can be traced back to antiquity. Some societies sanctioned it, as in ancient Greece where the Senate would allow an individual to take hemlock if a case for suicide had been made. The Greek founder of the Stoic school of philosophy, Zenon, hanged himself at the age of 98, finding that after dislocating his big toe life was not worth living. The Stoics defended suicide in certain specific situations.

The early Christians also sometimes took their own lives in the face of persecution. St Augustine (AD 354–430), however, later declared suicide to be "a greater sin than any one might avoid by committing it"; and in England from the middle of the 16th century suicide became a criminal offence *felo de se* (literally a felony against oneself) which was equivalent to murder. Punitive attitudes were reflected in the practice of burying the body of a suicide at a crossroads with a stake through the heart and a stone over the face in order to prevent the ghost from returning to haunt the survivors. If suicides were regarded as being insane at the time of the act, they were exempt from the religious and legal punishments.

The Emperor of China would send a yellow silk scarf to a person of high rank who had lost face through breaking the law. The intention was that the scarf was used by the 'criminal' to hang himself in order to avoid criminal prosecution and disgrace.

In the 18th century fear grew that fictional portrayals of suicide might trigger imitation suicides, and as result Goethe's *The Sorrow of Young Werther* was banned in some countries (Schmidtke & Hafner, 1988). Hume, the 18th century Scottish writer, published a book arguing that an individual had a right to take his or her own life. Suicide and attempted suicide remained criminal offences in England and Wales until the Suicide Act became law in 1961, although in Scotland it had ceased to be a criminal act a century earlier, while France repealed her laws against suicide after the French Revolution. A detailed historical account is given in Morgan (1979) and Retterstol (1993).

Definition of suicide

All definitions of suicide are problematic in that each has to address the issue of intent and this can only be assessed retrospectively.

The legal definition of suicide depends on evidence (in the legal sense) being available, and this process differs from the clinical procedure by which a diagnosis is reached. Psychiatrists have argued that official figures underestimate the number of suicides. For the purposes of epidemiological research, official statistics are certainly useful (Sainsbury & Jenkins, 1982) but in individual cases there is no doubt that a coroner is far less likely to return a suicide verdict than would a clinician.

In England and Wales a coroner brings in a verdict of suicide only when there is good evidence of suicidal intent. In the case of self-inflicted death where there is insufficient evidence of intent to commit suicide, the coroner will give either an open verdict, or one of accidental death or death by misadventure (these latter two terms are synonymous in legal meaning). Holding & Barraclough (1975, 1978) examined a series of deaths where the coroner had brought in an open verdict or a verdict of accidental death. They concluded that a proportion of the open verdicts were in fact suicides. Some of the accidental deaths were also misclassified suicides but fewer than in the case of the open verdicts.

There appears to be a wide variation in the ratio of suicide to open verdicts recorded in different coroners' districts in England and Wales. Sainsbury & Jenkins (1982) suggested that because the correlation between suicide verdicts in different districts is constant over time even if the coroner changes, the idiosyncrasies of different coroners have little effect on the differences between districts. However, it may be that this apparent stability is in part due to the fact that a new coroner is often selected from the same solicitors' practice as the old coroner (Nicholson,1992). A more accurate measure for comparing coroners' districts than relying on the suicide rate alone may be to use the combined open verdict and suicide verdict rate (Renvoize & Clayden, 1990).

Incidence of suicide

Suicide accounts for approximately 1% of all deaths, and in young males it is the second commonest form of death after accidents (OPCS, 1991). Rates have varied considerably throughout this century. In common with other countries during both World Wars, the suicide rate declined in the UK when the degree of national and social cohesion rose. By contrast during the economic depression of the 1930s, a time of economic loss, rates peaked. Although poverty itself is not correlated with increased suicide risk, loss of social cohesion, possessions or personal status probably are. In the 1960s the suicide rate in England and Wales fell by about 30%, in contrast with the situation in most other European countries at that time. The extent to which this drop may have been attributable to the detoxification of domestic gas in the UK during this period has been the focus of much debate (Kreitman, 1976). Suicide rates are higher in spring and summer, a trend common to countries in both northern and southern hemispheres. Possible explanations include the idea that intrinsic annual changes in biological rhythms occur or that increased alienation is experienced by depressed individuals when communities emerge from winter.

As can be seen from Fig. 12.1 the rate of suicide in males in England and Wales is at all ages higher than in females, although this gender-related difference has gradually become less marked. The overall suicide rate in England and Wales during 1989 was 7.4/100 000 population and the rate for females was 3.7/100 000, while that for males was 11.2/100 000 (OPCS, 1991). The risk is higher in the elderly, although as Figs 12.1 and

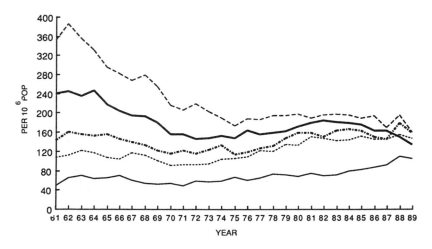

Fig 12.1 Age specific rates of male suicide per million population, in England and Wales from 1961–1989.——,15–24 years; ---- , 24–34; —·—·—, 35–44;———, 45–64; --- , 65+.

12.2 illustrate there has been a progressive fall in the last three decades in the older age group. Fig. 12.1 also shows the increase in the suicide rate among young men mentioned above. The most recent statistics indicate that suicides among men aged 15 to 44 in England and Wales rose by a third between 1980 and 1990. Most of this change was due to an increase of 78% in those aged 14 to 24 (Hawton, 1992). International comparisons of suicide rates have long been popular although their interpretation is hazardous in view of inevitable variation in methods of diagnosis and case detection from one country to another; it is generally accepted that intra-national analysis is more reliable and amenable to detailed analysis. Trends in national rates allow us to monitor changes in any given country over an extended period of time. Intra-national comparison may involve different areas of the country or various subgroups in the population selected according to criteria such as age, sex, ethnic group, and marital status or clinical variables such as the presence of physical and mental illness.

Sainsbury (1973) has indicated how suicide statistics may be used in the search for causes. For all practical epidemiological purposes, underreporting or seeking the elusive 'absolute' rate of suicide is of small consequence. What matters, and what the epidemiologist needs to establish clearly, is whether the differences he observes between the rates of particular social, clinical or other categories are valid: we discern causes by showing that certain groups of people differ in having an exceptional incidence of suicide.

A word of caution is still required. Even when a consistent association is found between social conditions and the incidence of suicide, it is

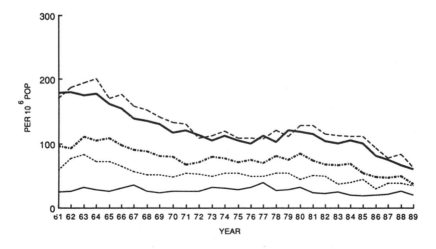

Fig 12.2 Age specific rates of female suicide per million population, in England and Wales from 1961–1989.⎯ ,15–24 years; ----, 24–34; –·–·–, 35–44; ⎯ , 45–64; – – –, 65+.

important to remember that the relationship may be indirect and is not necessarily causal. Such associations may, however, provide useful leads to other related variables such as mental disorder which might not themselves be measured easily. When dealing with small population subgroups such as different ethnic minorities, care is needed in interpreting the figures as the calculation of rates may be highly unreliable if small numbers are involved.

Marked international differences in suicide rates clearly do occur but the rate in each country shows a considerable degree of stability and consistency over time. Although they should be interpreted with caution such data can at least facilitate the study of variations in the definition and detection of suicide, as well as in the compilation of national statistics in different countries. The suicide rates in 24 European countries are shown in Table 12.1.

There has been much concern about the situation in Hungary where suicide rates have risen significantly in the last 30 years, the increase being higher in men, particularly in rural areas. The precise reasons for this rise are not clear, although it has been suggested that the rapid cultural change from an immobile semi-feudal system towards greater emphasis on the nuclear family and female employment may be relevant (Ozsváth, 1988).

The methods used to commit suicide depend to some extent on the availability of the agent used. For example, in the United States, car exhaust controls have been in force since 1968 and the proportion of carbon monoxide emitted by car exhausts has fallen massively. Suicides due to car exhaust fumes in the USA have recently levelled off and may have begun to decline, in contrast to the UK where the use of car exhaust fumes in suicide has increased dramatically. The OPCS statistics for 1989 indicate that 25% of suicides in England and Wales were carried out with the use of motor vehicle exhaust fumes. This method is particularly common in men (30% of male suicides used this method compared with only 11% of female suicides). Women tend to kill themselves using non-violent means. In 1989, 22% of suicides were due to self-poisoning, accounting for only 15% of male suicides but 42% of female suicides. The most commonly used drugs are analgesics and antidepressants. The use of barbiturates in suicides has become less frequent as their prescription has fallen. The figures for more violent means of suicide indicate a higher rate for men. Twenty-five per cent of suicides in 1989 were by hanging (28% of male suicides and 17% of female suicides). A similar pattern of male predominance occurs with other violent methods including the use of firearms, jumping from high places, jumping in front of moving objects and suicide by drowning. The most favoured methods used in suicide vary from one country to another depending upon the availability of the agent and social customs. Examples of this include firearm suicide in the USA and self-immolation in certain parts of India.

Table 12.1 Changes in the crude suicide rate per 100 000 aged 15+ years in 24 European countries, by gender (mean 1972–3 to mean 1983–4)

Country	Men			Women		
	Mean 1972–3	Mean 1983–4[1]	Change (%)	Mean 1972–3	Mean 1983–4[1]	Change (%)
Austria	43.7	50.1	+14.6	18.1	18.2	+0.6
Belgium	27.8	39.2	+41.0	12.6	19.0	+50.8
Bulgaria	20.6	28.0	+35.9	8.9	10.6	+19.1
Czechoslovakia	45.6	38.7	−15.1	16.0	12.2	−23.8
Denmark	38.8	45.7	+17.8	23.5	25.3	+7.7
Finland	50.5	51.0	+1.0	13.0	12.2	−6.2
France	30.3	41.3	+36.3	11.6	15.4	+32.8
Germany (West)	35.2	34.5	−2.0	18.2	16.1	−11.5
Greece	5.4	7.2	+33.3	2.3	2.6	+13.0
Hungary	67.4	86.9	+28.9	26.5	32.7	+23.4
Iceland	23.4	38.9	+66.2	8.4	8.0	−4.8
Ireland	6.8	15.5	+127.9	2.6	5.9	+126.9
Italy	10.9	12.9	+18.3	4.6	5.5	+19.6
Luxembourg	25.2	36.7	+45.6	11.0	14.1	+28.2
The Netherlands	13.5	18.7	+38.5	9.4	11.8	+25.5
Norway	17.3	27.2	+57.2	6.1	9.6	+57.4
Poland	26.7	29.9	+12.0	5.5	6.0	+9.1
Portugal	19.0	19.5	+2.6	5.2	7.1	+36.5
Spain	8.9	8.9	—	3.1	2.9	−6.5
Sweden	37.4	33.8	−9.6	14.6	13.8	−5.5
Switzerland	36.6	44.6	+21.9	14.0	16.9	+20.7
United Kingdom						
England & Wales	12.4	14.7	+18.5	8.0	7.0	−12.5
Northern Ireland	5.9	14.0	+137.3	4.9	7.5	+53.1
Scotland	13.5	18.0	+33.3	8.9	7.4	−16.9

1. Except for the following countries (latest years in parentheses): Ireland (1982–83), Italy (1979–80), Spain (1979–80)
Source: WHO data bank (Platt, 1988)

Aetiology of suicide

Psychiatric illness

Representative samples of suicides may be examined using the so-called 'psychological autopsy' method. This involves interviewing relatives and friends of the deceased as well as scrutinising medical records. Using this method it has been found that over 90% of suicides have been judged to have some form of psychiatric illness (Barraclough *et al*, 1974; Rich *et al*, 1986). In those few suicides which lacked evidence of such illness, it may have been present but undetected because of the unreliability of retrospective analysis. 'Rational' suicide therefore appears to be rare in Western countries.

All categories of psychiatric illness carry an increased risk of suicide. The various diagnostic groups can be ranked in decreasing order of risk:

1. Depression (all forms)
2. Schizophrenia
3. Alcoholism
4. Drug addiction
5. Organic disorder (e.g. epilepsy, brain injury, mild dementia)
6. Personality disorder (especially sociopathy)
7. Neuroses (recent studies suggest that the risk of suicide among former in-patients with primary anxiety neurosis is higher than was previously thought (Allgulander, 1994)).

Within high risk diagnostic categories attempts have been made to identify specific clinical features associated with increased risk (Table 12.2).

Psychosocial factors

Societal factors

Although psychiatric illness is an important aetiological factor, causal mechanisms leading to suicide are usually multifactorial. It is worth knowing that 85% of sufferers from depression do not kill themselves. Adverse aspects of a person's life situation should always be assessed because they often play a central role in the development of suicidal despair whatever the precise categorisation of psychiatric illness. The importance of social factors is illustrated by the fact that the incidence of suicide in pregnancy and the puerperium appears to have fallen dramatically in recent years so that now the incidence is lower than the rate expected in the general population, even though the puerperium is a time of major biological and psychological stress. Such a reduction in morbidity may be due to changes in social attitudes to pregnancy, the availability of contraception and abortion (thereby reducing the likelihood that a pregnancy will be unwanted) and the lessening of stigma attached to a unwanted pregnancy (Appleby, 1991).

Durkheim, a 19th century French sociologist, examined the suicide rates in various European countries (Durkheim, 1951) in what was the first attempt to produce a sociological theory of suicide. Finding a remarkable stability in rank order of national suicide rates over successive five year periods, he suggested that suicide results primarily from social factors. Durkheim argued that the society in which people live exerts control over them in two ways: individuals are integrated into the values and norms of their social group, and in turn society regulates their goals and aspirations. He proposed four

Table 12.2 Suicide and psychiatric disorders: high risk factors within high risk diagnoses

Diagnosis	Risk factors
Depression (Lifetime risk of suicide = 15% (Miles, 1977))	Severe illness Persistent insomnia, self-neglect, impaired memory, agitation Male, older Single/separated Socially isolated Previous DSH

Schizophrenia
(Lifetime risk of suicide =
10% (Miles, 1977))
	Younger, unemployed, socially isolated
	Previous DSH
	Depressive episode with anorexia/
	    weight loss
	More serious illness, recurrent relapse
	Fear of deterioration, especially in those
	    of high intellectual ability

Alcohol addiction (Lifetime risk of suicide = 3.4% (Murphy & Wetzel, 1990))	Male, peak age 40–60 years old High level of dependency Long history of drinking Disruption of major interpersonal relationship Depressed mood, poor physical health Poor work record in previous four years Social isolation Previous DSH

(This table should be interpreted in the light of individual correlates as shown in Box 12.1, page 522)

types of suicide: *egoistic, altruistic, anomic* and *fatalistic.* Egoistic suicide results from poor integration into society as a result of the way an individual behaves, for example, by virtue of mental illness. In altruistic suicide there is an over-integration into society. An example is the act of hara-kiri in which the customs of feudal Japanese society obliged an individual to commit suicide in certain circumstances. 'Protest' suicide which may happen, for example, as a result of political protest is not easy to categorise under Durkheim's system but presumably reflects an over-identification with a social subgroup or set of ideals. Anomic suicide occurs if the bonds between people have been loosened, as in an inner city area, and norms regulating behaviour no longer apply. In fatalistic suicide there is excessive regulation by society so that the individual has no personal freedom and no hope. An example is the suicide of a slave.

Societal attitudes to suicide may themselves be of aetiological importance. Diekstra & Kerkhoff (1989) suggest that the development of more permissive views towards taking one's life have played a part in the trend towards increased suicide rates in certain population subgroups.

Imitation

Imitation may be a precipitating factor in some cases of suicide. Such a mechanism might underlie the phenomenon of clusters of suicides which occur both in the community and in psychiatric hospitals from time to time (see later), or those suicides which follow the suicide of a well known celebrity (Schmidtke & Hafner, 1988).

Adverse life events

Adverse life stress has been shown to occur more commonly prior to suicide than in a control group (Barraclough, 1987). The relationship between mental illness, suicide and adverse life stress is complex because mental illness itself may predispose an individual to adverse life stress and vice versa.

Occupation

The profile of the incidence of suicides across all social classes forms a U-shaped curve. The upper social classes have the highest suicide mortality, while the number of deaths from suicide in unskilled workers exceeds that in skilled artisans. In men after retirement age, the rate of suicide in the lower social classes is higher than in the upper social classes and this may reflect the way in which factors such as the degree of economic security in retirement vary from one social class to another.

Certain occupations carry an increased risk of suicide with veterinary surgeons topping the list with three times the expected number of deaths; pharmacists, dentists, farmers and doctors have twice the expected mortality (Charlton *et al*, 1993) and all these professions have easy access to potentially lethal drugs. Farmers also have easy access to chemicals, drugs and firearms. Among medical practitioners younger doctors appear to be at particular risk (Richings *et al*, 1986). Medicine is clearly a stressful profession. Furthermore it involves frequent contact with death which may distort attitudes concerning the value of life and therefore reduce internal resistance to suicide. It appears that some specialities such as psychiatry and anaesthetics may carry a particular risk but further research is required before this can be confirmed.

Unemployment

High rates of suicide are positively correlated with increased unemployment (Platt, 1984). However the nature of the association is by no means clear. Psychiatric disorder may, for instance, predispose to unemployment. The stigma of unemployment has been suggested as one possible underlying mechanism in this association. Changes in the unemployment rate are not necessarily reflected in suicide rates (Charlton *et al*, 1993).

Biological factors

The role of serotonin

Disturbances in serotonin-mediated neurotransmission in the brain have been implicated as playing a part in the production of depressive illness. Some postmortem studies of suicide have reported low levels of 5-HT and 5-HIAA (metabolites of serotonin) in the brain. Such findings are only provisional because recent studies have failed to replicate them (Cheetham *et al*, 1989).

Genetic factors

The mere fact that suicide runs in families would not in itself prove that genetic mechanisms are involved, as an increased familial incidence could perhaps be due to shared psychosocial factors. However, there is evidence from adoption studies that genetic factors can probably predispose an individual towards suicide. Study of twin pairs in which one twin has committed suicide shows a higher concordance for suicide among monozygotic pairs of twins than for dizygotic pairs (Roy *et al*, 1991) indicating the involvement of a genetic factor. The inheritance of psychiatric disorders, such as depression, is not the only possible explanation for a familial increase in vulnerability to suicide. Lack of control of impulsive behaviour which has been found to correspond with low levels of CSF 5-HIAA (Roy, 1990) may be a genetically transmitted factor independent of psychiatric illness, that increases the risk of suicide. Suggestions that there might be a genetic factor responsible for suicide which is transmitted independently of psychiatric illness have not as yet been confirmed.

Individual correlates

Box 12.1 lists various sociodemographic and clinical factors which are associated with an increased risk of suicide.

Special groups

Psychiatric in-patients

The incidence of suicide among psychiatric in-patients is higher than in the general population. Given the relationship between mental illness

---

Box 12.1 Individual correlates of suicide

Elderly
Male
Divorced> widowed> single
Unemployed/retired
Living alone (socially isolated)
Physical illness (especially terminal illness,
    painful/debilitating illness
History of DSH
Family history of affective disorder/alcoholism/suicide
Bereavement in childhood
Social classes I and V
Personality traits: impulsive, aggressive, lability of mood

---

and suicide this is not altogether unexpected. In recent decades, several countries have reported an increase in the number of suicides occurring among psychiatric in-patients. It is unclear why this disturbing development has happened, although several authors have noted that such increases followed a change to an open ward system as the old Victorian style asylums were dismantled. Techniques used in caring for suicidal individuals have also come under critical scrutiny. Complex factors need to be taken into account in analysing the statistics involved. For example, a larger proportion of the psychiatric population (i.e. that part of the general population at the highest risk) is probably now admitted at some time to hospital compared with before. The number of individuals at risk far outnumbers the bed complement because of short stays and rapid patient turnover; unless this is allowed for, a spuriously low denominator leads to misleadingly high rates. There may also be changes in the type of patients admitted to hospitals. For example, those admitted with personality disorder or substance misuse represent individuals at significantly increased risk (Wolfersdorf *et al*, 1988) and they may now constitute a larger proportion of the total number of psychiatric in-patients.

Suicide in prisons

Rates of suicide in UK prisons have increased dramatically over recent years. This has particularly affected remand prisoners whose numbers have escalated with resulting gross overcrowding (Dooley, 1990). Factors associated with the increased risk of suicide in prison are listed in Box 12.2.

Box 12.2 Individual correlates of prison suicide

Past history of psychiatric contact (33%)
Previous DSH (43%)
In remand
Age > 30 years
Conviction for serious offence
Long sentence

Physical illness

Physical illness is associated with an increased risk of suicide especially among the elderly. Neoplastic disease is thought to show a particular association with suicide, although estimates of the risk vary (Whitlock, 1986). Epilepsy, especially when it affects the temporal lobe, is associated with a 25-fold risk (Barraclough, 1987). More recently there have been reports of high rates of suicide among men diagnosed as having AIDS. Such patients may account for up to 25% of suicides occurring in general hospitals in the USA (Marzuk *et al*, 1988). This is also discussed in on page 1070.

Youth suicide

Over the last two decades there has been a dramatic increase in the number of youth suicides reported in the USA and Australia. There is evidence of a similar phenomenon in the UK, particularly among young men aged 15–24 years (Burton *et al*, 1990) (see Fig. 12.1). The reasons for this are far from clear. Recent studies in the USA and Scandinavia have found that a large number of youth suicides appear to reflect involvement in substance misuse (Fowler *et al*, 1986; Runeson, 1989; Martunnen *et al*, 1991).

Suicide clusters

The problems in ascertaining whether time-space clusters of suicide occur are considerable because some clustering of suicide is bound to happen by chance alone even if suicides are essentially a random phenomenon. Gould *et al* (1990) have, however, reported this phenomenon among teenage suicides.

Assessment

Suicide risk should not be considered in isolation. A full psychiatric history and mental state examination is necessary in every patient to establish a diagnosis with regard to the associated psychiatric problem. This may pose risks other than suicide (for example aggressive behaviour related to psychotic illness) and in every patient these require assessment and management in their own right in parallel with suicide risk.

Interviewing

A skilled interview technique facilitates assessment of the severity of suicide risk and should lead to formulation of an appropriate management plan. It is vital to remember that the assessment process itself can have a significant effect on outcome.

There are a number of features in the mental state examination that are commonly associated with a suicidal state of mind. They include despair, a sense of humiliation and marked ambivalence concerning the wish to live or die. Forming an understanding, empathic relationship with the individual and promoting mutual trust are therefore essential ingredients in generating hope. Listening and allowing discussion of important issues are crucial features in establishing such rapport. Too liberal reassurance may merely confirm a person's fears that others do not understand what it means to have lost hope; such an approach can be as hazardous as not empathising at all. Suicidal individuals often declare their intent to die to a number of people prior to killing themselves, and it is a fallacy to assume that those who admit to such ideas are less likely to commit suicide. The principles relevant to good interviewing technique are shown in Box 12.3.

Questionnaires

Although suicide–risk questionnaires may be a useful adjunct to the clinical interview (Beck *et al*, 1974) they cannot replace a full psychiatric assessment. They are most effective in the long-term prediction of suicide within a population but are far less reliable in the short term, as is the case in day-to-day clinical work. In this setting, careful assessment of an individual's mental state, recent behaviour and relationships with others will provide the most important indicator of immediate risk when considered in parallel with the well established demographic factors which are heavily represented in standardised questionnaires.

Questioning about suicidal ideas

While it is essential to address the issue of suicidal thoughts openly, in practice it is advisable to lead into the topic gradually. In this way, the interviewer indicates sensitivity to the individual's distress and so makes it appear more likely that such feelings can be shared safely. Box 12.4 illustrates such an approach.

Box 12.3 How to interview a suicidal patient

Quiet uninterrupted setting
Unhurried
Initiate interview with non-directive, open questioning, allowing
    airing of issues and feelings important to the patient
Use language that is appropriate for the patient, taking account
    of variation in cultural values and religious beliefs
Build up trust and rapport quickly
Avoid brusque, challenging or judgemental approach
Listen to what the patient says
Allow repetitive discussion of issues if necessary
Take note of non-verbal behaviour that may be of significance
    regarding suicide risk
Evaluate recent events
Take a full psychiatric, medical and social history
Evaluate the mental state
Beware of hazards in assessment
Careful evaluation of suicidal motivation
Consider use of risk questionnaire

The degree of despair should be acknowledged but at the same time it is beneficial to build on positive aspects of the situation. Questions such as "When are your suicidal thoughts not so strong?" or "What other options have you considered apart from suicide?" may lead to constructive dialogue. Exploration of factors which reduce suicidal ideas, such as close support from others, is also worthwhile.

Difficulties in assessment

These are shown in Box 12.5. Suicidal patients may exhibit provocative or uncooperative behaviour. As a result, health care professionals often lose sympathy and become critical of a person at real risk of suicide, who then perceives staff as unhelpful and rejecting. Similarly, recurrent relapses of symptoms can lead to staff frustration and breakdown of the therapeutic relationship (Morgan, 1979; Morgan & Priest, 1991). Morgan has termed this process malignant alienation and has suggested that it is a common and important problem which needs to be recognised when caring for suicidal individuals.

The importance of short-lasting and therefore misleading clinical improvement prior to suicide has been highlighted by a recently reported series which found this phenomenon in 45% of psychiatric in-patient suicides (Morgan & Priest, 1991). Such improvement in symptoms may be related to a disengagement from stressful situational factors in the patient's life. Care must be taken to avoid the premature discharge of patients who have been at risk of suicide; certainly this should not happen before relevant stress factors have been effectively addressed and incorporated into a treatment plan. Lack of overt distress may also follow a final decision to commit suicide, with the resulting freedom from agonising indecision.

Management of high risk individuals

It should be remembered throughout that suicide risk is something which complicates psychiatric disorders, rather than being an illness in itself. Therefore treatment requirements for each individual must be dictated by the nature of the associated psychiatric disorder. In particular great care should be taken to observe the requirements of the 1983 Mental Health Act in the care of patients who have been admitted under any of its provisos.

Psychiatric in-patients

General principles

The hazards of delivering adequate care for in-patients at risk of suicide need to be understood fully if only because the rate of suicides among

---

Box 12.4 Interview sequence of topics in assessing suicidal motivation

Hope that things will turn out well
Get pleasure out of life
Able to face each day
Ever despair about things
Feel life is a burden
Wish self dead
Why feeling this way (e.g. be with a person who has died, life bleak, morbid guilt)
Thoughts of ending life; if so, how persistently
Thought specifically about method of suicide (means readily available)
Ever acted on them
Feel able to resist them; anything that makes them disappear
How likely to kill self
Ability to give reassurance about safety, for example until next appointment
Circumstances likely to make things worse
Willingness to turn for help if crisis occurs
Risk to others

**Box 12.5 Difficulties in the assessment and management
of suicide risk**

Variability in degree of distress (ambivalence towards suicide)
Misleading improvement (when removed from stress factors
    or calm following final decision to kill self)
Deliberate denial of suicidal ideas
Uncooperative and difficult behaviour
Anger, resentment, sometimes displaced onto staff
False assumptions made by health care professionals
– belief that suicidal ideas which are openly admitted are
    manipulative threats rather than indicative of serious risk
– fear that direct questioning about suicidal ideas will
    encourage the patient to entertain these ideas
Surveillance difficulties
Physical hazards in hospital ward/surroundings
Malignant alienation (see below)
Setting over-ambitious goals which foster sense of failure

---

such patients is significantly higher than in the general population.
Wolfersdorf *et al* (1988) quote recent figures from the United States and
Europe in the order of 50 to 600 suicides per 100 000 psychiatric in-patients
each year. These rates should be compared with those for the general
population in different European countries which are set out in Table
12.1. The current open-door policy should not mean a laissez-faire
approach to the care of the suicidal individual, and the principles of
good clinical practice must be set out clearly. These are now considered
below.

Thorough admission procedures

At or soon after admission the patient at risk of suicide is particularly
vulnerable, and inadequate admission procedures, such as the curtailment
or delay of proper assessment, present serious hazards. Clear policies
need to be understood by all staff members.

Supportive observation

The Victorian asylum, at the expense of therapeutic enlightenment, was
quite effective in preventing suicide. A style of care which utilised the
'suicide caution' card was developed for at-risk individuals. This card had
to be signed by the member of staff who had responsibility for the patient
at that time. The policy fell into disrepute because it often meant no more
than impersonal surveillance and a dehumanising denial of personal

privacy. However it would be ill-judged to assume that it can be replaced by an uncritical reliance merely on a relaxed open-door policy and good communications between ward staff. Over and above this, a clear care policy for the suicidal individual is imperative, inherent in which should be the principle that increased risk must be matched by more intensive care in terms of relationships with staff, control of physical hazards in the ward and provision of an adequate number of staff. The precise levels of supportive observation are not absolute and systems may vary between hospitals, but it is crucial that the terminology used is explicit and unambiguous: words such as close or special convey little to newcomers or to those who work in other hospital units and are a recipe for confusion. In essence the process involves intensive support for the patient rather than unwelcome intrusive surveillance. A recommended system might be as follows:

Level 3: Known place supportive observation. A designated nurse should know where the patient is. The patient may be allowed to leave the ward for short periods (10–15 minutes) but should keep the nursing staff informed about this at all times.

Level 2. 15 minute supportive observation. A designated nurse should undertake to maintain intermittent visual contact with the patient at not more than 15 minute intervals (varying 10–20 minutes). The patient should not leave the ward but is allowed to visit the toilet unaccompanied. The patient should be accompanied by a nurse when leaving the ward.

Level 1. Constant supportive observation. A designated nurse should keep the patient under constant visual supportive observation. This is appropriate in an observation area or an open psychiatric unit but care should be taken to ensure that there is only one exit, and that levels of staff are adequate at all times.

Level 1A. Constant nearby supportive observation. As in Level 1, but the designated nurse should remain physically close to the patient. This applies in the case of serious risk accompanied by impulsive behaviour. Special care may be needed to ensure the safety of staff when there is a risk of violence.

Working with the suicidal patient

Even though the precise tasks may vary with the type of illness and the nature of the situational factors, there are certain principles which apply throughout. It is necessary to move as quickly as possible towards establishing a close supportive relationship, one which may even be to some extent authoritative at times of crisis. Identifying the real suffering inherent in depression and acknowledging its painful reality is a useful early step and similarly indicating one's understanding of feelings of ambivalence and anger towards others. Isolating the suicidal drive by seeing it as part of an illness, agreeing on ways of minimising it (having identified what worsens or relieves it), explaining how depressive illness is self-limiting and that it distorts ways of thinking and the cool conveyance of fact without excessive reassurance all help to regenerate hope. Where relatives become included in morbid ideation concerning the need to die, risks to their safety should be evaluated. The importance of taking advice on trust, for example, concern over the value of treatment in spite of utter hopelessness, may have to be discussed when morbid ideation is making it difficult for a patient to accept help. Failure to respond should lead to not only a review of medication but also a search for intractable adverse life events and situations. The therapist should be consistent in what is said and done and must see the patient regularly, because even the most despairing can derive great comfort from another's willingness to sit with and listen, although loss of insight may make it seem that the patient is unable to accept support and reassurance.

When suicide risk is managed on an out-patient basis, an agreed plan for the time until the next appointment including ways of getting help in crisis must be discussed at each interview. The therapist's attitude is crucial whatever the setting, and a refusal to adopt a patient's despair and hopelessness should be a guiding principle throughout. The involvement of other key persons, by keeping them fully informed and enlisting their support, can be a crucial aspect of providing more support.

Use of medication

If medication is judged to be necessary it is important to target it correctly according to the specific symptoms which the patient presents. Barraclough *et al* (1974) demonstrated convincingly how individuals who proceed to commit suicide often receive inappropriate medication in a low ineffective dose during the last weeks or months of their lives. The addition of lithium may provide effective prophylaxis against suicide in those with an affective disorder (Modestin & Schwarzenbach, 1992). Whatever the medication prescribed, care should be taken to dispense it in a sufficient dose but in limited quantities so that patients who are at risk of suicide do not accumulate large quantities of potentially lethal medication.

Particular hazards

The ongoing management of a suicidal patient requires paying attention to the mental state and relevant psychosocial problems. In the UK approximately two-thirds of patients who commit suicide are said to have seen their GP in the month prior to death (Barraclough *et al*, 1974; Ovenstone & Kreitman, 1974). However more recently Vassilas & Morgan (1993) reported a lower figure of 36% of patients having had contact with their GP in the four weeks before death, suggesting that patterns of contact with GPs may be changing. The GP may have a key role to play in the prevention of suicide. Rutz *et al* (1989, 1992) achieved a reduction in the suicide rate following an educational programme aimed at GPs. These studies took place on a sparsely populated Swedish island and it is not clear how far the results would apply, for example, to general practice in a large city in the UK.

Whatever the specific clinical problem, certain common themes add to the complexity of assessing the risk of suicide. Occasionally the risk is very great yet a patient deceptively pretends to feel better, and this is especially likely to arise when the patient is not well known to staff as, for example, at or soon after admission. Those factors already identified as liable to confound accurate assessment (Box 12.5) may also be present: rapid fluctuation in the degree of distress, testing out and challenging behaviour, suspiciousness and reticence, aggressive outbursts, misleading clinical improvement and unusual symptoms which do not conform to the usual diagnostic categories. Any of these may test the clinical skills of staff members to the full. If alienation of staff from a patient is detected, it is wise to include it on the agenda of staff meetings in order to review why it is happening, and to encourage staff to examine their attitudes of frustration and hostility towards the patient.

Suicide clusters

A suicide which occurs in a relatively closed community such as a hospital may kindle an intensive preoccupation with suicidal ideas in other vulnerable individuals and a cluster of suicides within that hospital can follow. Intense local media publicity increases the risk of this happening. Such kindling of the suicide risk is poorly understood but is certainly a real hazard and should be taken into account by those who have clinical responsibility for in-patient services. The needs of all individuals who are at particular risk should be considered without delay whenever a patient commits suicide.

Occasionally suicide results from pacts in which two or more people form an agreement to kill themselves (Rosen, 1981). Epidemiological evidence is scarce, but it is thought approximately one in a hundred suicides in the UK occur in this way. The rate in other cultures is likely to vary substantially.

Characteristically such pacts involve two close emotionally inter-dependent partners of whom one is dominant. At least one of the couple suffers from a mental illness (Brown *et al,* 1995). The partners are frequently spouses but may also be lovers, friends or other family members. The stronger partner, who usually has the more powerful drive towards self-harm, persuades the weaker more dependant person to enter the pact. Common issues appear to be the avoidance of separation or joint guilt, such as might occur in an illicit relationship. Not infrequently one of the partners survives the suicide pact.

On rarer occasions, family or mass suicide pacts occur. These usually arise as a response to an overwhelming crisis facing the group. There are numerous historical examples of mass suicide, perhaps the most famous of which are the Jewish Zealots at Masada and the Jonestown massacre in the jungles of Guyana. These both illustrate several common themes: a charismatic leader, strong loyalties and religious beliefs under threat. Explanatory theories for such episodes have included *Folie collective* and mass hysteria, but they are difficult to study retrospectively with any degree of certainty.

Treating the unwilling patient

When the immediate risk escalates beyond a certain degree it may be necessary to treat a patient against his or her will, perhaps by preventing self-discharge and the use of physical treatment. Any such action must be strictly in compliance with the 1983 Mental Health Act. The dilemma with this approach is that it may seem an unwarranted intrusion into a patient's autonomy, yet, if carried out with scrupulous care, a patient may later be grateful to those who face up to difficult decisions during the stage of severe illness.

Discharge and leave

Decisions concerning leave and discharge need to be made carefully. Patients should be fully assessed drawing on the principles described above. The judicious use of leave under strictly controlled conditions and the anticipation of likely adverse reactions to stressful situations in the community will pave the way towards successful discharge. In the case of patients who have been detained under any section of the 1983 Mental Health Act, great care should be taken to ensure that leave arrangements are consistent with the Act's requirements in each instance. In particular it must be remembered that Section 17 of the Act directs that the relevant consultant responsible medical officer must give specific permission for any leave arrangements. Decisions should be multidisciplinary, based on the care programme approach (Kingdon,1994). Where necessary placement on the supervision risk register (Harrison & Bartlett, 1994) should be considered. Assessment of the degree of social support is vital and enlisting the help and involvement of friends and relatives is often beneficial. Discussion of how to cope until the next agreed contact and how to get help if things go wrong are both useful strategies. The period after discharge is well known as a time of high suicide risk, and arrangements which ensure continuity of care should be made explicit before the patient leaves hospital. It should be noted that in-patients who take their own discharge against medical advice are at increased risk of suicide (Flood & Seager, 1968).

There are particular difficulties in patients with depressive illnesses complicated by long-standing personality problems and current adverse life events. It may be tempting to withdraw from such a therapeutic dilemma by seeing the depressive state as reactive and understandable, with the implication that the patient is not ill and should take personal responsibility for themselves. However, such clinical problems commonly precede suicide. A decision about whether or not to invoke the Mental Health Act should be based primarily on the degree of imminent suicide risk: it is unwise to assume that physiological features of depression, such as early morning wakening or weight loss, need to be present before the risk should be taken seriously.

In the community

As the availability of in-patient facilities becomes more limited with the shift to community care, it is increasingly important to set out guidelines for the care of suicidal individuals who are not admitted to hospital. Unless this happens, there is a risk that the number of suicides in the community, which are silent in that they may not be known to mental health services and certainly not to in-patient units, will rise significantly. The principle of matching the level of supportive observation to the degree of suicide risk applies to patients in the community as much as in hospital. Strategies such as increasing the frequency of contact, deciding when to initiate day care or seek more senior help, and perhaps even admission to a hospital in-patient unit, must be set out explicitly as a code of practice by every community care service. Such decisions cannot be left entirely to the clinical judgement and possibly idiosyncratic theoretical assumptions of individual care workers.

Prevention of suicide

General principles

Murphy (1984) stated that if suicide prevention is successful:

> "The patient will live. A suicide will have been prevented. Yet to quantify this effect is impossible. It is important to realise that the absence of a suicide generates no data. Thus, we can never prove what has been accomplished. Yet we can hardly doubt that it occurs".

It is not surprising that it has proved difficult to evaluate attempts at suicide prevention. It is, however, worth discussing what potential causal factors should be addressed if prevention is to succeed. The circumstances of a person's life need as much attention as do factors within the individual.

Problems of urban living, stresses specific to young adults or to the elderly, adverse life events such as losses or alienation from others are all potentially relevant. Events must be assessed in terms of their personal meaning for the individual, bearing in mind long-standing values, attitudes and personality traits. The additive effect of such adverse events, especially if they develop rapidly, must be gauged against possible protective factors. Impulsivity and the relevance of access to lethal agents such as drugs, or structures such as bridges which may have a symbolic significance and have been used by others to commit suicide all need evaluation, in the light of an individual's previous behaviour in crisis.

The prevention of suicide is now clearly on the public health agenda in the UK with the publication of the Government's White Paper, *The Health of the Nation* (Secretary of State for Health, 1992). This sets targets that aim to reduce the suicide rate overall by at least 15% by the year 2000 and the suicide rate of severely mentally ill people by at least 33%.

Reduced access to means of suicide

As mentioned above the 30% reduction in suicides in the UK during the 1960s may well have been related to the removal of toxic coal-gas from the domestic scene at that time. In the UK as catalytic converters fitted to car exhausts are becoming more common a decline in suicides from carbon monoxide poisoning may become apparent; this has already happened in the USA (Clarke & Lester, 1987). Altering the shape of the exhaust pipe to make it harder to attach tubing might also result in a fall in deaths (Hawton, 1992). One easy way to reduce the number of deaths due to paracetamol poisoning could be to restrict sale of paracetamol to small quantities. This is the policy in France and the number of deaths due to this cause is now very small (Garnier & Bismuth, 1993).

Older tricyclic antidepressant drugs are more lethal in overdose than newer antidepressants. Some authors have suggested that by prescribing the new selective serotonin reuptake inhibitor (SSRI) antidepressants as opposed to the more familiar tricyclic antidepressants a significant reduction in the suicide rate could be achieved. Jick *et al* (1995) looked at a large cohort of people who had been prescribed a variety of antidepressants (including older tricyclics and SSRIs) over a 5 year period. Although they found that several factors correlated with the risk of suicide, choice of antidepressant was not one of them (also discussed on page 196).

In the USA, stricter gun control laws have in certain states been associated with a fall in the number of suicides using fire arms (Lester & Murrel, 1980) and there is now a convincing body of evidence that controls on gun ownership would significantly reduce suicide rates (Winokur & Black, 1992).

Specific measures are more likely to have an effect on the overall rate of suicides if they address the problem of impulsivity and the ease of access to the chosen method because the delay inherent in devising another plan may abort the suicidal crisis.

Suicide prevention agencies

Voluntary community agencies such as the Samaritans aim to reach out and make contact with vulnerable individuals. Given the problems of doing research in this area, as might be expected, proof of the Samaritans' suicide preventive role is still lacking (Jennings *et al*, 1978). In the USA suicide prevention centres (SPCs) have been set up which are usually centred around a telephone hotline operating in a similar way to the Samaritans, although they may also have a walk-in service. There is some evidence that these facilities may be beneficial to young white women (Miller *et al*, 1984). These services need to be targeted more specifically to high risk groups such as young men and the unemployed. There can, however, be no doubt that the principle of listening in a non-judgemental way is an essential part of good clinical practice, and should be supported in whatever form it is developed.

Help-seekers

A smaller proportion of men who commit suicide have been in contact with medical and psychiatric services preceding their deaths compared with women (Morgan & Priest, 1991); younger suicides in particular are less likely to have had contact with these services (Vassilas & Morgan, 1993). This contrasts strongly with elderly suicides where in the same study Vassilas & Morgan (1994) found that 68% of suicides over 65 years of age had seen their GP in the four weeks before death. The reasons for this pattern of behaviour are unclear and warrant further investigation. Any preventative measures need to be targeted at specific groups.

The role of substance misuse

Vassilas (1993) found rates of alcohol abuse to be far higher in a consecutive series of suicides in Avon than had been reported in a similar study 30 years earlier in the same area (Seager & Flood, 1965). Varnick & Wasserman (1992) have reported that the suicide rate in the USSR declined significantly between 1984 and 1988. This was the period during which perestroika was introduced in the Soviet Union: in addition strict limitations on the sale of alcohol were imposed. This latter fact may have been of importance in the reduction of suicide rates. Hawton *et al* (1993) recently reported that substance misuse was a factor particularly associated with suicide after an episode of DSH in the young. The proper assessment and management of such individuals is clearly of importance.

Media reporting

Etzersdorfer *et al* (1992) described the effect of publication of media guidelines by the Austrian Association for Suicide Prevention. Before 1987 dramatic reports on suicides in the Vienna subway appeared in the Austrian media. Following the publication of the guidelines and their adoption by the media the number of suicides in the subway system apparently declined abruptly. Barraclough *et al* (1977) called for restrictions on media reporting of suicides in the UK and recently the BBC has produced guidelines on how suicides should be reported (BBC, 1993).

Education

As suicide rates are rising in young men, one group among whom it might be thought reasonable to develop educational programmes about suicide is schoolchildren. There have been many such initiatives in the US but it is not clear how effective such measures are (Vieland *et al*, 1991) and there are suggestions that certain types of programmes may have a detrimental effect (Lester, 1992).

The aftermath of suicide

The consequences of suicide are particularly traumatic for the bereaved family because the act is self-inflicted, often unexpected and sometimes violent in nature. It can be especially difficult for relatives to resolve their grief in the face of strong conflicting feelings which may include guilt, perplexity and anger. If the deceased has been receiving psychiatric treatment, anger towards others is probably less likely to develop in those cases where the relatives felt they had previously been involved, and kept well informed during treatment.

Routine clinical practice should encompass interviewing relatives soon after a suicide has occurred in order to provide support. In the community, the GP is well placed to recognise the need for such help (Shepherd & Barraclough, 1979). If the person who committed suicide had received help from health care services, the staff may also need support as may any patients who had contact with the deceased.

Audit

Morgan & Priest (1991) in their recent study of unexpected deaths in psychiatric patients showed that it is feasible to incorporate a routine audit-type review into clinical service. Deaths from suicide can be identified, without any need for specialised research staff, by cross-checking coroner inquest data with hospital admission/discharge registers and recent mortality statistics (King, 1983). Although suicide audit procedures have never been evaluated systematically, the principles on which they should be based are clear. Within 24 hours of the suicide an initial meeting of the ward community should be held. This is not strictly for audit because the primary aim of this first meeting should be to provide support for both patients and staff. The key audit meeting should be restricted to the three or four key staff members who have been involved in the patient's care. Use of a standard check list should ensure that the review includes all relevant issues and does not avoid controversial matters which might be difficult to discuss. If such a procedure is to succeed it has to be supportive yet encourage full exchange of information. The utmost tact is required by whoever acts as chairperson. In a similar way routine suicide audit should be developed in community services. Further details are given in Morgan (1993).

Non-fatal deliberate self-harm (DSH)

History

For many years suicide and 'attempted suicide' were regarded as varieties of the same behaviour until it was pointed out that two different but overlapping populations are involved (Stengel, 1952; Stengel *et al*, 1958). Prior to the Suicide Act of 1961, behaviour which appeared to be in the nature of failed suicide was punishable under English law as a misdemeanour. Until that time, the number of reported episodes was small and it is only in the last 30 years that it has reached such a magnitude as to become a major challenge in health care.

Defining DSH

Non-fatal deliberate self-harm (DSH) is defined here as:

> "a deliberate non-fatal act, whether physical, drug overdosage or poisoning, done in the knowledge that it was potentially harmful, and in the case of drug overdosage, that the amount taken was excessive" (Morgan, 1979).

The advantage of this definition is that motivation, which is very difficult to evaluate, is not a necessary component (see below). Synonyms include parasuicide "any act deliberately undertaken by a patient which mimics the act of suicide but which does not result in a fatal outcome" (Kreitman, 1988) and attempted suicide, "an act of self-damage inflicted with the intention of self-destruction" (Stengel, 1952).

Deliberate self-harm may take the form of cutting and other types of self-mutilation. The condition is comprehensively reviewed by Hawton (1989) and Tantam & Whittaker (1992).

It is difficult to establish accurately the frequency of DSH largely because many such events occur in the community and never come to the attention of the health services. At the most, only 70% of DSH episodes may be referred to hospital (Kennedy & Kreitman, 1973). When discussing the incidence of DSH, it is important to distinguish between the number of individuals as opposed to the number of episodes during any specified time, because some individuals will harm themselves more than once. It is also useful both from a statistical and a clinical perspective to differentiate 'first timers' from those who repeat.

In the UK and the rest of the developed world, there was a marked increase in the incidence of DSH in the 1960s and '70s. The reasons for this are not fully clear, but may include social changes in attitude toward self-harm, changes in prescribing habits, particularly an increase in the use of minor tranquillisers and antidepressants, and other social changes such as increased rates of marital breakdown and patterns of alcohol intake. Over the last decade, the rate of DSH in this country has stabilised and recently there has been a slight fall, accounted for mainly by a reduction in the number of women who harm themselves.

Figure 12.3 shows in-patient admission rates for DSH in Edinburgh. With changes in hospital admission policies concerning DSH, up to a third of such patients are now discharged home directly from accident and emergency departments (Dennis *et al*, 1990; Owens *et al*, 1991). However, self-poisoning still remains the commonest cause of acute medical admissions in women, and in men is second only to ischaemic heart disease. Episodes of DSH are rare under the age of 12, they peak

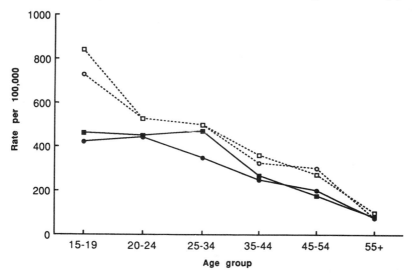

Fig. 12.3 Age and gender specific admission rates for deliberate self-harmers in Edinburgh. ——●—, males 1988; ——■—,males 1989; - - ○- - , females 1988; - -□- - , females 1989.

in the late teens and young adulthood, and then progressively decrease in frequency with increasing age (see Fig. 12.3). In non-Western countries the incidence of DSH is lower, with the gender and social class distribution varying from one country to another.

Age and gender

The ratio of female to male admissions to hospital following DSH has until recently been 1.5–2:1 but this gap is narrowing. Figure 12.3 shows that rates are higher in younger adults of either sex. DSH occurs most frequently in young women in the 15–19 year age group. In the 1990s, one in 100 girls of this age were referred to a general hospital each year following an episode of DSH, although the rate has fallen recently. The peak for men occurs later, between 25–34 years and this rate for men has increased since the 1970s. Reasons for the female predominance in DSH are not firmly established but may be due to differences in the types of problem faced by men and women, the adoption of alternative coping mechanisms, variation in the social acceptability of such behaviour, and the differential prescription of psychotropic drugs.

Self-cutters tend to be young and epidemiologically based studies suggest a roughly equal male to female sex ratio (Weissman, 1975), although females more commonly present for treatment.

Socio-economic status

DSH rates among those in social class V are seven times higher than those in social class I (Holding *et al*, 1977) and are higher in areas of overcrowding and relative social deprivation (Morgan *et al*, 1975*b*). The exact relationship between DSH and unemployment is difficult to disentangle because of the many intervening variables. However it does appear that the long-term unemployed are more at risk of DSH (Platt, 1986). Demographic and social correlates of DSH in individuals are shown in Box 12.6.

Aetiology

Psychiatric illness

Symptoms

When patients are interviewed shortly after the episode of DSH nearly two-thirds are found to be suffering from significant psychological symptoms which subside rapidly over the next few months. Actual psychiatric illness is found in 30% of patients at the time of the act, reducing to 8% at 3 months, and in most instances the disorder is depressive in type (Newson-Smith & Hirsch, 1979*b*). Repeated overdosing and self-cutting

---

Box 12.6 Correlates of deliberate self-harm

Female
Social class V
Divorced
Age under 25
Overcrowded accommodation
Current unemployment
Significant debts
At present address less than one year

---

have also been found among women suffering from bulimia nervosa (Lacey, 1993).

Personality

Longstanding difficulties in psychological adjustment may occur in up to a third of cases of deliberate self-harm (Morgan *et al*, 1975*a*). In those who present with self-cutting there is often evidence of an associated personality disorder with its origins sometimes in an earlier disruptive, abusive or broken home (Tantam & Whittaker, 1992). Self-cutting is associated with dissocial personality disorder and borderline personality disorder but it should be noted that self-mutilation is one of the diagnostic criteria for borderline personality disorder.

Alcohol misuse

Alcohol is taken by 55% of men within 6 hours of the act and by 25% of women (Morgan *et al*, 1975*a*). The problem is even greater in Scotland (Holding *et al*, 1977).

Psychosocial factors

Motivation

Stengel *et al* (1958) were the first to point out that it is a mistake to regard 'attempted suicide' as being merely a failure to destroy the self. Each episode has a social meaning that has to be addressed in order to understand the reasons for the act. In support of their approach they noted that people who attempted suicide commonly remain in contact with others, and there is often an element of warning, or appeal, with a marked 'Janus faced' ambivalence. The precise causes of an act of DSH are notoriously difficult to assess and often they are not clear to the patient. Bancroft *et al* (1979), in a retrospective study, found that only about half of such patients, when interviewed on the day after the episode, stated that they had, at the time, wished to die. Psychiatrists, who evaluated the interviews in this study, considered hostility to others as an important and common theme. Morgan *et al* (1975*a*) found that 65% of DSH patients had acted impulsively, although during the previous month half had considered the idea of harming themselves.

Hopelessness

Hopelessness and pessimism about the future may be key cognitions preceding suicide. Suicidal intent among DSH patients has been reported as having a close correlation with an attitude of hopelessness (Dyer & Kreitman, 1984).

Life events

DSH patients frequently experience adverse life events prior to the act of self-harm. Paykel (1980) compared the number and type of recent life events experienced prior to deliberate self-harm with those before the onset of depressive illness, and a first episode of schizophrenia. He measured the relative risk, which is an epidemiological measure of the degree to which being exposed to an aetiological factor increases the risk of developing an illness as compared to not being exposed to that factor. Relative risks were calculated for the six months following a life event and were highest for DSH. The figures for the three groups were: 3.0 for schizophrenia; 5.4 for depression; and 6.7 for deliberate self-harm indicating that DSH was the most 'life event sensitive' condition. In the month following a life event the relative risk of DSH is raised to ten times that of the general population indicating a strong and immediate relationship. Serious arguments with a spouse comprise the single event most commonly reported by the DSH group, most of whom reported interpersonal arguments.

Communication

Kreitman *et al* (1970) found that patients in any locality who have committed an act of DSH know one another more often than would be expected by chance, and hypothesised that DSH might in certain individuals represent a form of communication.

Imitation

As with suicide an imitation effect may occur in DSH and produce, in a similar way, clusters of non-fatal DSH. It is difficult to obtain clear epidemiological evidence to support this hypothesis (Platt, 1989) but those involved in psychiatric in-patient units should proceed with caution when several vulnerable individuals are present at one time. Social influences probably explain the phenomena of epidemics of self-mutilation which occasionally spread through a hospital ward (Walsh & Rosen, 1985).

Prescription of psychotropic drugs

It is salutary to note that the rise in numbers of young women admitted to hospital because of DSH has coincided with an increase in prescription of psychotropic drugs, particularly in young women. Interpretation of these findings is complicated by the fact that, during the same period of time, the number of DSH episodes involving non-prescribed analgesics also rose.

Physical illness

Among those admitted for DSH there is a higher than expected incidence of physical illness and recent admission to hospital (Bancroft *et al*, 1975). Increased rates of self-mutilation have been observed among those who have experienced surgery or hospital treatment before the age of five (Rosenthal *et al*, 1972).

Biological factors

Psychiatric patients with a history of DSH (particularly if this is associated with violence), have lower levels of CSF 5-HIAA (a metabolite of serotonin) than those with no history of DSH (Roy, 1990). Replication of this finding would have implications regarding the relevance of disordered serotonin metabolism and affective disorder in certain types of DSH. There is one very rare form of self-mutilation, the Lesch Nyhan syndrome, which may have a definite biochemical basis resulting from an underlying inherited disorder of uric acid metabolism.

Special groups

Adolescents

The majority of adolescent DSH patients are female. They comprise 70% of 12–20-year-olds admitted to hospitals in Oxford following deliberate self-harm (Sellar *et al*, 1990). It has already been noted that nearly 1% of all young women aged 15–19 years are referred to hospital because of DSH each year. Interpersonal problems, particularly relationships with parents, friends and at school are commonly reported. DSH has a positive association with broken homes, family psychiatric illness and sexual abuse in children (Hawton & Catalan, 1987).

Ethnic minorities

In the UK, the rate of DSH in the Asian community has in the past been regarded as lower than in the host community, but recent evidence suggests that the incidence of DSH among Asian women may be higher than in white females. Asian patients are younger, more likely to be married and less likely to be diagnosed as psychiatrically ill or suffering from a personality disorder, when compared to UK born white DSH patients (Merrill & Owens, 1986).

Mothers and children

Hawton *et al* (1985) found that the risk of committing child abuse among mothers who are deliberate self-harmers was nearly 30% above that of a control group and it is important to bear this in mind when assessing DSH in a young mother.

Methods of DSH

Approximately 90% of episodes of non-fatal DSH in the UK involve a drug overdose. In Edinburgh analgesics account for a third of the total (particularly paracetamol which poses the specific hazard of liver damage), followed by minor tranquillisers/sedatives in 15% of cases, and antidepressants in approximately 10%. Two-thirds of the drugs used originate from medical prescriptions and the agent used reflects prescribing habits. Barbiturate overdoses, for example, have fallen in frequency since the 1960s when this group of drugs was prescribed more commonly. In both Edinburgh and Oxford there has also been a recent fall in benzodiazepine overdoses which may relate to greater discrimination in the way they are prescribed.

The second most common method used in DSH is laceration, usually of the wrist or arm. Some 8–15% of those referred to A & E departments with deliberate self-harm have self-mutilated. Robinson & Duffey (1989) give a figure of 8.2% for those referred to the Edinburgh Regional Poisoning Treatment Centre. Weissman (1975) gave a corresponding figure of 11.7% in the USA. A more thorough Canadian study of DSH occurring in general practices, nursing homes, jails and hospital found that self-cutting accounted for 17.5% of all episodes (Johnson *et al*, 1975). Other methods include falls, jumping in front of vehicles, and non-fatal self-asphyxiation. Violent methods are more frequent in men.

Hawton (1989) provides a classification for those presenting with self-cutting:

    (a) superficial self-cutting with little or no suicidal intent
    (b) deep cutting sometimes involving major blood vessels, nerves and tendons. Sometimes (though not necessarily) associated with serious suicidal intent, but usually associated with severe psychiatric disorder
    (c) self-mutilation, as occurs in psychotics.

Individuals who produce superficial cuts appear to form a characteristic subgroup of self-harmers. They tend to be young with personality traits which include impulsive or aggressive behaviour and unstable moods. They typically have problems with low self-esteem, sexual identity, interpersonal relationships and alcohol or drug misuse. The cuts themselves are often multiple and appear to bring relief from feelings of increasing tension and irritability. People who harm themselves in this way sometimes report a state of detachment in which no pain is perceived at the time of the lacerations. In the female prison population, at a London reception centre, a previous history of self-mutilation was found in 7.5% of the cases. A subgroup showed strong association with severe personality disorder and multiple disorders of impulse (Wilkins & Coid, 1991).

In Favazza's (1987) series of 240 subjects presenting with self-cutting to hospital, the cutting occurred on the wrists in 74% of cases, legs 44%, abdomen 45%, head and neck 23%, chest 18% and the genitalia in 8%. Almost any kind of implement was used to inflict the damage. Razor blades, knives, broken glass, broken metal and cigarette burns were the methods most frequently employed. Self-wounding typically continued for about five to ten years thereafter.

Psychotic self-mutilation is a rare phenomenon, most commonly affecting the eyes, tongue or genitalia. Enucleation of the eye is extremely rare and probably only occurs in subjects with schizophrenia. Greilsheimer & Groves (1979) reviewed 53 case reports of male self-castration published between 1901 to 1977 which summarised all the then known published case reports. Most were single men between 20 and 40-years-old and the majority were patients with schizophrenia. The castration sometimes occurred in response to command hallucinations which sought to exorcise demons. In other cases there were psychotic transvestite or transsexual impulses. In a third group there were a few transsexuals who had either been refused surgery or who had elected to conduct the surgery on themselves. In a few instances the act was carried out in a state of acute mania, and in others there was evidence of alcoholism combined with schizophrenia, where the disinhibition due to alcohol may have played a role. Eighty-seven per cent of reported cases were thought to have been psychotic at the time of self-castration but only one patient in this series committed suicide.

Assessment and management of DSH

Initial interview

During the initial interview the doctor should pay particular attention to difficulties in interpersonal relationships, the exploration of unresolved adverse life events, as well as assessing the severity of suicidal ideation and its degree of persistence. It is important to note that the severity of physical dangerousness does not correlate closely with degree of suicide intent. Traditional clinical practice has involved the admission of patients for at least an overnight in-patient stay following an episode of deliberate self-harm. This recommendation has become increasingly difficult to observe as in-patient resources have become more scarce. In some areas, as many as 31% of DSH patients are discharged home directly from the A & E department, possibly without major adverse sequelae (Owens *et al*, 1991), although adolescents may receive inadequate assessment (O'Dwyer *et al*, 1991). This situation needs further evaluation.

Management

Hawton & Catalan (1987) have outlined an approach to the management of patients who have been admitted to hospital following DSH, the principles of which may be listed as follows:

(a) assessment of the problems associated with the overdose
(b) problem solving:
    (i) clarify the problems to be tackled
    (ii) Establish goals which are realistic and specific
    (iii) Define what steps need to be carried out to obtain these goals
    (iv) Agree what the patient has to do before the next session
    (v) Review progress. Explore in detail any difficulties encountered
(c) preventative measures. Prepare for future crises by exploring alternative approaches and enhancing coping skills
(d) minimise potential problems of terminating the therapeutic relationship by providing ample warning and preparation. A follow-up appointment 1–2 months later can facilitate this process.

There are no specific management techniques for self-mutilation *per se*, and indeed focusing on the act itself may heighten its importance and may worsen the situation (particularly among those with personality disorder) or increase the frequency of self-mutilation. A comprehensive account of both the psychotherapy and pharmacological management of the personality disorders is given in Chapter 19.

Who should assess self-harmers?

The Hill Report on the hospital treatment of acute poisoning (Central Health Services Council, 1968), recommended the provision of special poisoning treatment centres and participation of psychiatrists in the assessment of all cases. In practice, however, it was not always feasible to follow this advice and the potential clinical role of other professionals in the assessment and management of DSH patients has now become clearer. In 1984, the DHSS issued revised guidelines which advised that apart from psychiatrists other professionals such as specialist social workers, nurses and junior physicians might, under certain circumstances, undertake the psychosocial assessment and aftercare of DSH patients. This approach is supported by a substantial body of research evidence (Gardner *et al*, 1977; Newson-Smith & Hirsch, 1979*a*; Catalan *et al*, 1980; Waterhouse & Platt, 1990). The DHSS guidelines indicate that when responsibility for assessment of DSH is delegated by psychiatrists to other professionals, thorough preliminary training as well as good regular and continuing clinical supervision should be the rule (Department of Health and Social Security, 1984).

Secondary prevention of DSH

It has been difficult to establish any effective intervention in reducing repetition of DSH. Greer & Bagley (1971) examined retrospectively a group of self-harmers and found that those who attended psychiatric follow-up repeated less often than those who had no further contact. It is not clear, however, whether the psychiatric support itself reduced the rate or whether those patients willing to accept help were a self-selected lower risk group. Kennedy (1972) suggested that those admitted to a regional poisons unit fared better than those who were not. Gibbons *et al* (1978) compared the influence of a social work service with that of normal management. Repetition rates in the two groups were the same, although the social work group eventually had fewer social problems. Chowdhury *et al* (1973) and Hawton *et al* (1981) found that domiciliary outreach teams do not reduce repetition rates. Wulliemier *et al* (1977) suggested that pre-arranged contacts at regular intervals following DSH might reduce rates although this strategy requires further evaluation. Salkovskis *et al* (1990) examined the effect of a series of five hour-long sessions of cognitive–behavioural problem-solving therapy and found improvements in ratings of hopelessness, despair and suicide intent after one year, but again repetition rates were not reduced.

Patients suffering from borderline personality disorder who repeatedly deliberately self-harm are particularly difficult to treat. Linehan et al (1991) looked at the effect of a variant of cognitive–behavioural therapy on this group of patients. Patients were randomly assigned to either a treatment group, which received a package consisting of weekly one hour individual therapy sessions and group therapy of two-and-a-half hours a week, or to a control group. The treatment continued for one year. Although only 44 subjects were involved in the study, those in the treatment group were significantly less likely to have deliberately self-harmed and to have spent fewer days hospitalised in a psychiatric ward over the one year study period.

Some researchers have evaluated the effect of medication. Hirsch *et al* (1982) concluded that mianserin improved mental state more than a placebo, but did not affect the number of repeat self-harm episodes. The use of flupenthixol decanoate has been reported to reduce repetition rates in chronic repeaters when compared with placebo, but the numbers of patients were small and this finding requires replication (Montgomery *et al*, 1979).

Hitherto, attempts to demonstrate effective secondary prevention of DSH have been disappointing. New initiatives are greatly needed, both in hospital and community practice. Non-compliance in attending out-patient appointments may reach as high as 40%, and ways of reducing this need to be considered (O'Brien & Hurren, 1987). Possible lines of approach include the recognition that specific subgroups of DSH patients, such as first timers or chronic repeaters, may need different therapeutic strategies. Ways of making help available at times of crisis are likely to be more effective than a more rigid approach which depends entirely on fixed out-patient appointments. Morgan *et al* (1993) suggest one way forward in a study in which those presenting with DSH for the first time were given a card which had a contact telephone number they could phone if they felt they were at risk of further episodes of DSH. At one year follow-up there was a significant reduction of actual or seriously threatened DSH in the experimental group. Practices of prescribing minor psychotropic drugs for persons distressed because of social problems also need scrutiny.

Prognosis in DSH

Repetition

Kreitman & Foster (1991) have recently reported the development of scales predicting DSH repetition. Factors found to be important in increasing risk include previous DSH, personality disorder, previous psychiatric treatment, unemployment, social class V, alcohol and drug misuse, criminal record, involvement in violence, age 25–54 years and being single, divorced or separated.

Suicide

Studies have shown consistently that the risk of suicide following DSH is far larger than would be expected in the general population (Hawton & Fagg, 1988). The period of greatest risk for suicide appears to be in the first 3 years, particularly in the first 6 months following DSH. After an episode of DSH about 1% of patients kill themselves in the next year; this is about 100 times the expected rate for the general population. Box 12.7 shows the main correlates of increased suicide risk following an episode of DSH (Hawton & Fagg, 1988). It is self-evident that all the problems identified earlier as relevant to suicide risk, particularly those of social

---

Box 12.7 Risk factors for suicide in patients admitted to hospital following DSH

Male
Advancing age (women only)
Psychiatric disorder
Long-term use of hypnotics
Poor physical health
Repeated attempts

---

isolation and conflict with others, contribute to the overall risk and should be taken into clinical consideration. About 15% of patients who have self-mutilated eventually kill themselves (Nelson & Grunebaum, 1971).

Social and family outcome

An act of DSH often has dramatic impact upon relationships with others, sometimes ending the relationship, in others introducing tension and perhaps, in some, generating support which previously was not forthcoming.

References

Allgulander, C. (1994) Suicide and mortality patterns in anxiety neurosis and depressive neurosis. *Archives of General Psychiatry*, **51**, 708–712.

Appleby, L. (1991) Suicide during pregnancy and in the first postnatal year. *British Medical Journal*, **302**, 137–140.

Bancroft, J., Hawton, K., Simkin, S., *et al* (1979) The reasons people give for taking overdoses, a further inquiry. *British Journal of Medical Psychology*, **52**, 353–365.

——, Reynolds, F., Simkins, S., *et al* (1975) Self poisoning and self-injury in the Oxford area. *British Journal of Preventative and Social Medicine*, **29**, 170–177.

Barraclough, B.M. (1987) The suicide rate of epilepsy. *Acta Psychiatrica Scandinavica*, **76**, 339–345.

——, Bunch, J., Nelson, B., *et al* (1974) A hundred cases of suicide: clinical aspects. *British Journal of Psychiatry*, **125**, 355–373.

——, Shepherd, D.M. & Jennings, C. (1977) Do newspaper reports of coroners'inquests incite people to commit suicide? *British Journal of Psychiatry*, **150**, 528–532,

BBC (1993) Suicide. In *Producers Guidelines*. London: BBC Publications.

Beck, A.T., Schuyler, D. & Herman, J. (1974) Development of suicidal intent scales. In *The Prediction of Suicide* (eds A.T. Beck, H. L. P. Resnick & A. J. Lettieri), pp. 45–56. Bowie: Charles Press Publishers.

Brown, M., King, E. & Barraclough, B. (1995) Nine suicide pacts. A clinical study of a consecutive series 1974–93. *British Journal of Psychiatry*, **167**, 448–451.

Burton, P., Lowry, A. & Briggs, A. (1990) Increasing suicide rates among young men in England & Wales. *British Medical Journal*, **330**, 1695–1696.

Catalan, J., Marsack, P., Hawton, K. E., *et al* (1980) Comparison of doctors and nurses in the assessment of deliberate self poisoning patients. *Psychological Medicine*, **10**, 483–491.

Charlton, J., Kelly, S., Dunnell, K., *et al* (1993) Suicide deaths in England and Wales: trends factors associated with suicide deaths. *Population Trends*, **70**, 34–42.

Cheetham, S. C., Crompton, M., Czudek, C., *et al* (1989) Serotonin concentrations and turnover in brains of depressed suicides. *Brain Research*, **502**, 332–339.

Chowdhury, N., Hicks, R. & Kreitman, N. (1973) Evaluation of an aftercare service of parasuicide ('attempted suicide') patients. *Social Psychiatry*, **8**, 67–81.

Clarke, R. U. & Lester, D. (1987) Toxicity of car exhausts and opportunity for suicide. *Social Science and Medicine*, **441**, 114–120.

Dennis, M., Owens, D. & Jones, S. (1990) Epidemiology of deliberate self poisoning: trends in hospital attendances. *Health Trends*, **22**, 125–126.

Department of Health and Social Security (1984) *The Management of Deliberate Self Harm*. Health Notice HN(84)25. London: DHSS.

Diekstra, R. F. W. & Kerkhoff, A. J. F. M. (1989) Attitudes towards suicide. The development of a suicide attitude questionnaire. In *Suicide and its Prevention* (eds R. F. W. Diekstra, R. Maris, S. Platt, *et al*), pp. 91–108. Leiden: E. J. Brill.

Dooley, E. (1990) Prison suicide in England and Wales (1972–1987). *British Journal of Psychiatry*, **156**, 40–45.

Durkheim, E. (1951) *Suicide: A Study in Sociology* (transl. J. A. Spaudling & G. Simpson). Illinois: Glencoe.

Dyer, J. & Kreitman, N. (1984) Hopelessness, depression and suicidal intent in parasuicide. *British Journal of Psychiatry*, **144**, 127–133.

Etzersdorfer, E., Sonneck, G. & Nagel-Kuess, S. (1992) Newspaper reports and suicide. *The New England Journal of Medicine*, **327**, 502–503.

Favazza, A. R. (1987) *Bodies under Siege*. Baltimore: Johns Hopkins University Press.

Flood, R. A. & Seager, C. P. (1968) A retrospective examination of psychiatric case records of patients who subsequently committed suicide. *British Journal of Psychiatry*, **114**, 443–450.

Fowler, R. C., Rich, C. L. & Young, D. (1986) San Diego Suicide Study II. Substance abuse in young cases. *Archives of General Psychiatry*, **43**, 962–965.

Gardner, R., Hanka, R., O'Brien, V. C., *et al* (1977) Psychological and social evaluation in cases of deliberate self-poisoning admitted to a general hospital. *British Medical Journal*, **ii**, 1567–1570.

Garnier, R. & Bismuth, C. (1993) Liver failure induced by paracetamol. *British Medical Journal*, **306**, 718.

Gibbons, J., Butler, J., Urwin, P., *et al* (1978) Evaluation of a social work service for self poisoning patients. *British Journal of Psychiatry*, **133**, 111–118.

Gould, M. S., Wallenstein, S. & Kleinman, M. (1990) Time–space clustering of teenage suicide. *American Journal of Epidemiology*, **131**, 71–78.

Greer, S. & Bagley, C. (1971) Effect of psychiatric intervention in attempted suicide: a controlled study. *British Medical Journal*, **i**, 310–312.

Greilsheimer, H. & Groves, J. E. (1979) Male genital self mutilation. *Archives of General Psychiatry*, **36**, 441–446.

Harrison, G. & Bartlett, P. (1994) Supervision registers for mentally ill people. *British Medical Journal*, **309**, 551–552.

Hawton, K. (1989) Self-cutting: Can it be prevented. In *Dilemmas and Difficulties in the Management of Psychiatric Patients* (eds K. Hawton & P. Cowen), pp. 91–104. Oxford: Oxford Medical Publications.

—— (1992) By their own young hand. *British Medical Journal,* **304,**1000.

——, Bancroft, J., Catalan, J., *et al* (1981) Domiciliary and out-patient treatment by self poisoning patients by medical and non-medical staff. *Psychological Medicine,* **11,** 169–177.

——, Roberts, J. & Goodwin, G. (1985) The risk of child abuse among mothers who attempt suicide. *British Journal of Psychiatry,* **146,** 486–489.

—— & Catalan, J. (1987) *Attempted Suicide. A Practical Guide to its Nature and Management* (2nd edn). Oxford: Oxford University Press.

—— & Fagg, J. (1988) Suicide and other causes of death following attempted suicide. *British Journal of Psychiatry,* **152,** 359–366

——, ——, Platt, S. & Hawkins, M. (1993) Factors associated with suicide after parasuicide in young people. *British Medical Journal,* **306,**1641–1644.

Central Health Services Council (1968) *Hospital Treatment of Acute Poisoning.* Report of the Joint Subcommittee of the Standing Medical Advisory Committee. HMSO: London.

Hirsch, S. R., Walsh, C. & Draper, R. (1982) Parasuicide. A review of treatment interventions. *Journal of Affective Disorders,* **4,** 299–311.

Holding, T. A. & Barraclough, B. M. (1975) Psychiatric morbidity in a sample of a London coroner's open verdicts. *British Journal of Psychiatry,* **127,**133–143.

——, Bluglass, D., Duffy, J. C., *et al* (1977) Parasuicide in Edinburgh. A seven year review, 1968–74. *British Journal of Psychiatry,* **146,** 481–485.

—— & Barraclough, B. M. (1978) Undetermined deaths, suicide or accident? *British Journal of Psychiatry,* **133,** 542–549.

Jennings, C., Barraclough, B. M. & Moss, J. R. (1978) Have the Samaritans lowered the suicide rate? A controlled study. *Psychological Medicine,* **8,** 413–422.

Jick, S. S., Dean, A. D. & Jick, H. (1995) Antidepressants and suicide. *British Medical Journal,* **310,** 215–218.

Johnson, F., Frankel, B., Ferrence, R., *et al* (1975) Self-injury in London, Canada: a prospective study. *Canadian Journal of Public Health,* **66,** 307–316.

Kennedy, P. F. (1972) Efficacy of a regional poisoning treatment centre in preventing further suicidal behaviour. *British Medical Journal,* **iv,** 255–257.

—— & Kreitman, N. (1973) An epidemiological survey of parasuicide ('attempted suicide') in general practice. *British Journal of Psychiatry,* **123,** 23–34.

King, E. (1983) Identifying out-patients and ex-patients who have died suddenly. *Bulletin of the Royal College of Psychiatrists,* **7,** 4–7.

Kingdon, D. (1994) Care programme approach. *Psychiatric Bulletin,* **18,** 68–70.

Kreitman, N. (1976) The Coal Gas Story. *British Journal of Preventative & Social Medicine,* **30,** 86–93.

—— (1988) Suicide and Parasuicide. In *Companion to Psychiatric Studies (4th edn)* (eds R. E. Kendell & A. K. Zealley), pp. 459–475. Edinburgh: Churchill Livingstone.

——, Smith, P. & Eng Seong Tan (1970) Attempted suicide as language. An empirical study. *British Journal of Psychiatry,* **116,** 465–473.

—— & Foster, J. (1991) The construction and selection of predictive scales with particular referral to parasuicide. *British Journal of Psychiatry,* **159,** 185–192.

Lacey, J. H. (1993) Self-damaging and addictive behaviour in bulimia nervosa. *British Journal of Psychiatry*, **163**, 190–194.

Lester, D. (1992) State initiatives in addressing youth suicide: evidence for their effectiveness. *Social Psychiatry and Psychiatric Epidemiology*, **27**, 75–77.

—— & Murrell, M. E. (1980) The influence of gun control laws on suicidal behaviour. *American Journal of Psychiatry*, **137**, 121.

Lineham, M. M., Armstrong, H. E., Suarez, A., *et al* (1991) Cognitive–behavioural treatment of chronically parasuicidal borderline patients. *Archives of General Psychiatry*, **48**, 1060–1064.

Miller, H. L., Coombs, D. W., Leeper, J. D., *et al* (1984) An analysis of the effects of suicide prevention facilities on suicide rates in the United States. *American Journal of Public Health*, **74**, 340–343.

Martunnen, M. J., Aro, H. M., Henriksson, M. M., *et al* (1991) Mental disorders in adolescent suicide. *Archives of General Psychiatry*, **48**, 834–839.

Marzuk, P. M., Tierney, H., Tardiff, K., *et al* (1988) Increased risk of suicide in persons with AIDS. *Journal of the American Medical Association*, **259**, 1333–1337.

Merrill, J. & Owens, J. (1986) Ethnic differences in self-poisoning. A comparison of Asian and White groups. *British Journal of Psychiatry*, **148**, 708–712.

Miles, C. P. (1977) Conditions predisposing to suicide: a review. *Journal of Nervous and Mental Disease*, **164**, 231–246.

Modestin, J. & Schwarzenbach, F. (1992) Effect of psychopharmacotherapy on suicide risk on discharged psychiatric inpatients. *Acta Psychiatrica Scandinavica*, **85**, 173–175.

Montgomery, S. A., Montgomery, D. B., Rani, S. J., *et al* (1979) Maintenance therapy in repeat suicidal behaviour – A placebo controlled trial. *Proceedings of the 19th International Congress of Suicide Prevention and Crisis Intervention*, pp. 227–229. Ottawa.

Morgan, H. G. (1979) *Death Wishes? The Understanding and Management of Deliberate Self Harm*. Chichester: Wiley.

—— (1993) Suicide prevention and the 'Health of the Nation'. *Psychiatric Bulletin*, **17**, 135–136.

——, Burns-Cox, C. J., Pocock, H., *et al* (1975a) Deliberate self-harm. Clinical and socio-economic characteristics of 368 patients. *British Journal of Psychiatry*, **126**, 564–574.

——, Pocock, H. & Pottle, S. (1975b) The urban distribution of non-fatal deliberate self-harm. *British Journal of Psychiatry*, **126**, 319–328.

—— & Priest, P. (1991) Suicide and other unexpected deaths among psychiatric in-patients. *British Journal of Psychiatry*, **158**, 368–374.

——, Jones, E. M. & Owen, J. H. (1993) Secondary prevention of non-fatal deliberate self-harm. The green card study. *British Journal of Psychiatry*, **163**,111–112.

Murphy, G. E. (1984) The prediction of suicide: why is it so difficult? *American Journal of Psychotherapy*, **38**, 341–349.

—— & Wetzel, R. D. (1990) The lifetime risk of suicide in alcoholism. *Archives of General Psychiatry*, **47**, 383–392.

Nelson, S. & Grunebaum, H. (1971) A follow-up study of wrist slashers. *American Journal of Psychiatry*, **127**, 1345–1349.

Newson-Smith, J. G. B. & Hirsch, S. R. (1979a) A comparison of social workers and psychiatrists in evaluating parasuicide. *British Journal of Psychiatry*, **134**, 335–342.

—— & —— (1979*b*) Psychiatric symptoms in self-poisoning patients. *Psychological Medicine*, **9**, 493–500.

Nicholson, S. D. (1992) Suicide in North Devon. Epidemic or problem of classification? *Health Trends*, **24**, 95–97.

O'Brien, G. A. & Hurren, K. (1987) Deliberate self-harm and out-patient attendance. *British Journal of Psychiatry*, **150**, 246–247.

O'Dwyer, F. G., Dalton, A. & Pearce, J. B. (1991) Audit in practice: adolescent self-harm patients – audit of assessment in an accident and emergency department. *British Medical Journal*, **303**, 629–630.

Office of Population Censuses and Surveys 1989 (1991) *Mortality Statistics: Cause*. London: HMSO.

Ovenstone, M. K. & Kreitman, N. (1974) Two syndromes of suicide. *British Journal of Psychiatry*, **124**, 336–345.

Owens, D., Dennis, M., Jones, S., *et al* (1991) Self-poisoning patients discharged from accident and emergency: Risk factors and outcome. *Journal of the Royal College of Physicians*, **25**, 218–222.

Ozsváth, K. (1988) Epidemiology of suicide event in a Hungarian country. In *Current Issues of Suicidology* (eds H. J. Möller, A. Schmidtke & R. Welz), pp. 38–45. Berlin: Springer-Verlag.

Paykel, E. S. (1980) Recent life events and attempted suicide. *In The Suicide Syndrome* (eds R. Farmer & S. Hirsch), pp. 105–115. London: Croom Helm.

Platt, S. (1984) Unemployment and suicidal behaviour – a review of the literature. *Social Science and Medicine*, **19**, 93–115.

—— (1986) Parasuicide and unemployment. *British Journal of Psychiatry*, **149**, 401–405.

—— (1988) Suicide trends in 24 European countries 1972–1984. In *Current Issues in Suicidology* (eds H. J. Möller, A. Schmidtke & A. Velz), pp. 3–13. Berlin: Springer-Verlag.

—— (1989) The consequence of a televised soap opera drug overdose. Is there a mass media imitation effect? In *Suicide and its Prevention* (eds R. F. W. Diekstra, R. Maris, S. Platt, *et al*), pp. 341–359. Leiden: E. J. Brill.

Renvoize, E. & Clayden, D. (1990) Can the suicide rate be used as a performance indicator in mental illness? *Health Trends*, **22**, 16–20.

Retterstol, N. (1993) *Suicide: a European Perspective*. Cambridge: Cambridge University Press.

Runeson, B. (1989) Mental disorder in youth suicide. *Acta Psychiatrica Scandinavica*, **79**, 490–497.

Rich, C. L., Young, D. & Fowler, R. C. (1986) The San Diego suicide study : 1. Young vs old cases. *Archives of General Psychiatry*, **43**, 577–582.

Richings, J. C., Khara, G. S. & McDowell, M. (1986) Suicide in young doctors. *British Journal of Psychiatry*, **149**, 475–478.

Robinson, A. & Duffy, J. (1989) A comparison of self-injury and self-poisoning from the Regional Poisoning Treatment Centre, Edinburgh. *Acta Psychiatrica Scandinavica*, **80**, 272–279.

Rosenthall, R. J., Rinzler, C., Walsh, R., *et al* (1972) Wrist-cutting syndrome: the meaning of a gesture. *American Journal of Psychiatry*, **128**, 1363–1368.

Roy, A. (1990) Possible biologic determinants of suicide. In *Current Concepts of Suicide* (ed D. Lester), pp. 40–56. Philadelphia: The Charles Press.

——, Segal, N. L., Centerwall, B. S., *et al* (1991) Suicide in Twins. *Archives of General Psychiatry*, **48**, 29–32.

Rosen, B. K. (1981) Suicide pacts: a review. *Psychological Medicine*, 11, 525–533.

Rutz, W., Von Knorring, L. & Walinder, L. (1989) Frequency of suicide on Gotland after systematic postgraduate education of general practitioners. *Acta Psychiatrica Scandinavica*, **80**, 151–154.

——, —— & —— (1992) Long-term effects of an educational program for general practitioners given by the Swedish Committee for the Prevention and Treatment of Depression. *Acta Psychiatrica Scandinavica*, **85**, 83–88.

Sainsbury, P. (1973) Suicide opinions and facts. *Proceedings of the Royal Society of Medicine*, **66**, 579–587.

—— & Jenkins, J. S. (1982) The accuracy of officially reported suicide statistics for purposes of epidemiological research. *Journal of Epidemiology and Community Health*, **36**, 43–48.

Salkovskis, P. M., Atha, C. & Storer, D. (1990) Cognitive–behavioural problem solving in the treatment of patients who repeatedly attempt suicide. *British Journal of Psychiatry*, **157**, 871–876.

Schmidtke, A. & Hafner, H. (1988) The 'Werther' effect after television: new evidence for an old hypothesis. *Psychological Medicine*, **18**, 665–667.

Seager, C. P. & Flood, R. A. (1965) Suicide in Bristol. *British Journal of Psychiatry*, **111**, 919–932.

Secretary of State for Health (1992) *The Health of the Nation. A strategy for health in England*. London: HMSO.

Sellar, C., Hawton. K. & Goldacre, M. J. (1990) Self-poisoning in adolescents. Hospital admissions and death in the Oxford region 1980–1985. *British Journal of Psychiatry*, **156**, 866–870.

Shepherd, D. M. & Barraclough, B. M. (1979) Help for those bereaved by suicide. *British Journal of Social Work*, **9**, 69–74.

Stengel, E. (1952) Enquiries into attempted suicide. *Proceedings of the Royal Society of Medicine*, **45**, 613–620.

——, Cook, N. G. & Kreeger, I. S. (1958) *Attempted Suicide; Its Social Significance and Effects*. Maudsley Monograph No 4. London: Chapman & Hall.

Tantam, D. & Whittaker, J. (1992) Personality disorder and self-wounding. *British Journal of Psychiatry*, **161**, 451–464.

Varnik, A. & Wasserman, D. (1992) Suicides in the former Soviet republics. *Acta Psychiatrica Scandinavica*, **86**, 76–78.

Vassilas, C. A. (1993) *Pathways to Suicide: Health Care Use in Persons who Commit Suicide*. MD thesis. University of Bristol.

—— & Morgan, H. G. (1993) General practitioners' contact with victims of suicide. *British Medical Journal*, **307**, 300–301.

—— & —— (1994) Elderly suicides. Contact with their general practitioners before death. *International Journal of Geriatric Psychiatry*, **9**, 1008–1009.

Vieland, V., Whittle, B., Garland, A., *et al* (1991) The impact of curriculum based suicide prevention programs for teenagers: an 18 month follow-up. *Journal of the American Academy of Child and Adolescent Psychiatry*, **30**, 811–815.

Walsh, P. & Rosen, P. M. (1985) Self-mutilation and contagion, an empirical test. *American Journal of Psychiatry*, **141**, 119–120.

Waterhouse, J. & Platt, S. (1990) General hospital admission in the management of parasuicide. *British Journal of Psychiatry*, **156**, 236–242.

Weissman, M. M. (1975) Wrist-cutting: relationship between clinical observations and epidemiological findings. *Archives of General Psychiatry*, **32**, 1166–1171.

Whitlock, F. A. (1986) Suicide and physical illness. In *Suicide* (ed. A. Roy), pp. 151–170. Baltimore: Williams & Wilkins.

Winokur, G. & Black, D. W. (1992) Suicide – what can be done. *The New England Journal of Medicine*, **327**, 190–191.

Wilkins, J. & Coid, J. (1991) Self-mutilation in female remanded prisoners. An indicator of severe psychopathology. *Criminal Behaviour and Mental Health*, **1**, 247–267.

Wolfersdorf, M. G., Vogel, R. & Hole, G. (1988) Suicide in psychiatric hospitals. In *Current Issues of Suicidology* (eds H. J. Möller, A. Schmidtke & R. Welz), pp. 83–100. Berlin: Springer-Verlag.

Wulliemier, F., Kremer, P. & Bovet, J. (1977) Comparison study of two intervention modes on suicide attempters hospitalised in general hospital. *Proceedings of the 9th International Congress of Suicide Prevention and Crisis Intervention*, pp. 81–87. Helsinki.

13 Anxiety disorders

George Stein

---

*History • Classification today • Generalised anxiety disorder • Panic
disorder • Post-traumatic stress disorder • Adjustment disorder •
Epidemiology • Aetiology theories • Treatment • Appendix*

History

The category of neurosis has been in use for more than a century to
describe the anxieties, phobias, obsessions, hysteria, hypochondriasis and
a few other non-psychotic conditions, but it has now finally been
abandoned as an official category in both the ICD–10 and DSM–IV. The
word neurosis is derived from the Greek root meaning nerve, and was
first introduced into the English language by Lovell in 1661, as a 'neurotick'
which was a herbal medicine made from rose syrup or vegetables, claimed
to have a bracing effect on the nervous system (Oxford English Dictionary,
1989). Cullen, the leading Scottish physician of the eighteenth century
was the first to apply the term neurosis to a class of illnesses in *First Lines
in the Practice of Physic* (1784; quoted in Hunter & MacAlpine, 1963):

> In a certain view, almost the whole of the diseases of the human
> body might be called nervous ... in this place I propose to
> comprehend the title neurosis to all those preternatural affections
> of sense and motion which are without pyrexia as part of the primary
> disease and which do not depend on a topical affection of the
> organs but upon a more general affectation of the nervous system.

Cullen distinguished 'local diseases' from 'general diseases' and the
neuroses were general disorders which lacked fever. Pinel (1801)
translated Cullen's work, but at the same time criticised his view that the
neuroses were physical disorders and in *Treatise on Mental Alienation*
wrote that the neuroses were disorders of sense and movement without
any neuropathological basis and put forward an explanation of moral or
sympathetic causes. The moral element was explained in terms of the
'passions' or 'affections of the soul' while 'the sympathetic cause' described
influences arising from the stomach, the reproductive organs or other
parts of the body and their effect on the brain. Georget (1840) further
developed Pinel's ideas and was the first to formulate the modern concept
of neurosis as non-fatal, non-psychotic disorders and he included hysteria,
asthma, nervous palpitations, gastralgia with or without vomiting and the

neuralgias among the neuroses. In England a more mechanistic view prevailed and the terms spinal irritation and reflex functional nervous disease came into use.

Two American physicians made further important contributions. During the American Civil War, Da Costa (1871) described cases of severe chest pain and panic in otherwise healthy young men who suffered from a condition he called the irritable heart. This was caused by:

> ... quick long marches producing the affection or even slight exertion in those whose constitution had been impaired by insufficient or indigestible food ... It seems to me most likely that the heart has become irritable from its overactive and frequent excitement and disordered innervation keeps it so.

During the First World War, Da Costa's syndrome once more assumed importance and the British Army had an official category known as 'disordered action of the heart' which was diagnosed in over 60 000 British soldiers. In peacetime this was renamed as the 'effort syndrome' by Sir Thomas Lewis, a cardiologist from UCH.

The second American contribution came from George Beard (1869) who proposed the term 'neurasthaenia' to describe a group of patients who suffered from severe fatigue and mood disorders, which seem to defy other explanations. Beard considered it to be mainly an hereditary disorder, and it became a fashionable diagnosis in the latter part of the nineteenth century but then fell into disrepute, but has recently experienced a revival and is included in ICD–10.

A variant of neurasthaenia, which combined features of Beard's neurasthaenia, together with those of Da Costa's irritable heart, neurocirculatory asthaenia, was described by Oppenheimer (Oppenheimer & Rothschild, 1918), a pupil of Lewis. This disorder comprised cardiovascular symptoms combined with anxiety, and most cases would now be diagnosed as panic disorder.

No historical overview would be complete without mentioning the work of I. P. Pavlov, the Russian physiologist who described the conditioned reflex. His ideas were later taken up and extensively modified by Skinner, and later by Wolpe, Marks and others. Although the idea of simple conditioned reflexes and faulty learning as the cause of neuroses has long since been discarded, the notion that the treatment of neurotic disorders should involve new learning, and take place in the here and now rather than through exploration of the distant past, has been widely influential.

The distinction from psychosis

The separation of the neurosis from the psychosis is attributed to Huxley in 1871 (Oxford English Dictionary, 1989) but this distinction had until recently assumed rather more importance than the facts warranted.

According to ICD–9 (WHO, 1978) the neuroses were disorders characterised by unimpaired reality testing with preservation of insight and an absence of any demonstrable organic basis. By contrast subjects with psychoses lacked insight and mental function was so impaired that contact with reality was lost and even the ordinary demands of life could not be met. Thus the psychotics are extremely ill but fail to recognise it, while neurotic patients are much less ill, but realise only too well how ill they are (Tyrer, 1989). This old, somewhat arbitrary, distinction has little validity in clinical practice because the majority of those who suffer from psychoses are all too painfully aware of their disabilities. Also many neurotic patients have a severe and life-long incapacity, and may not be particularly insightful, for example patients with severe hypochondriasis. Insight is a difficult attribute to define or assess with any degree of reliability and so its presence or absence is not a particularly useful diagnostic pointer.

The demise of neurosis as a category

The final nail in the coffin of the concept of neurosis came with the advent of DSM–III and this is well described by Bayer & Spitzer (1985). The American Psychiatric Association (APA) had delegated the DSM–III task force to base the new classification scheme exclusively on scientific evidence. Spitzer who led the task force soon came to the conclusion that "there was no group of disorders which together comprise the neuroses". He suggested that the term 'neurosis' should be dropped altogether but this provoked a furious backlash from the American psychoanalytic profession who argued that a symptom-based diagnostic scheme which precluded any psychodynamic insight into why patients fell ill at the time they did, could only be a second-rate diagnosis. More pertinently the analysts were concerned that if the term neurosis were dropped from the new official glossary, then the insurance companies might cease to pay for the treatment of neurosis and so jeopardise their income.

In 1979 a solution was reached within the APA and the term neurosis was dropped as a main category for the forthcoming DSM–III, but it was to be placed in parenthesis after each disorder, thus dysthymia became 'dysthymic disorder (depressive neurosis)', hypochodriasis became 'hypochondriacal disorder (hypochondrical neurosis)'. This system was continued in DSM–III–R (APA, 1987) but the DSM–IV (APA, 1994) has dropped the pretence altogether and the word neurosis does not appear anywhere in either the text or the index, and dysthmia is now 'dysthymic disorder' only.

Classification today

Disorders previously classified in the ICD–9 (WHO, 1978) as neurosis were reassigned; thus depressive neurosis became dysthymia and was grouped with the mood disorders, while hypochondriasis was placed in the section on somatisation.

The ICD–10 (WHO, 1992) has also almost completely dropped the term neurosis and also makes no distinction between neurosis and psychosis. It states, however, that the term 'neurotic' is still retained for occasional use and as the heading of a major group of disorders called 'neurotic, stress related, and somatoform disorders'. Within this general grouping are two sections, the phobic anxiety disorders (F.40) and other anxiety disorders (F.41). DSM–IV includes a slightly different group of disorders in its chapter on anxiety. Thus obsessional disorder and the stress disorders, acute stress reaction, and post-traumatic stress disorder are grouped with the anxiety disorders in DSM–IV, but in ICD–10 are accorded a separate category. A minor difference between the two schemes is the inclusion of anxiety depression in ICD–10 but not in DSM–IV where it is only included in the section 'anxiety disorders not otherwise specified'. The main categories of anxiety in the two schemes are shown in Table 13.1.

Patterns of anxiety disorders

The anxiety disorders are much less clear cut than the depressive disorders and therefore several different definitions and concepts of anxiety are described in this account. Lewis (1970) considered the word to be somewhat ambiguous and outlined what he believed were the main features of anxiety (Box 13.1). Lewis also traced the origins of the word anxiety back to its Indo-European root *angh*, which gave rise to the Greek word *anxo* (meaning to squeeze or throttle), the Latin *anxietas* (literally painful mind) and the German word *angst* (anguish or dread).

These are all fairly specific concepts. Psychotherapists use the word anxiety in a wider sense to denote a state of emotional dysharmony which may appear in a variety of other psychological and somatic disorders.

A more recent definition is given by Barlow (1991) who considers that anxiety can best be characterised as a diffuse cognitive–affective structure. At the heart of this structure is high negative affect, composed of various levels and combinations of activation or arousal, perceptions of lack of control over future events, and shifts in attention to self-evaluative concerns. This structure is described as diffuse because it can be associated with any number of situations or events and may be expressed somewhat differently from one individual to another or even within a given individual across time.

Anxiety is an ubiquitous and normal phenomenon. The biological function of fear and anxiety is adaptive; to alert the organism to threats to its survival, so that appropriate action may be taken. In more primitive animals it manifests as the 'fight and flight reaction' as described by the American physiologist W. B. Cannon. Hoehn-Saric & McLeod (1986) considers anxiety to become abnormal when it is excessively intense or disproportionate to the stimulus, or continues beyond the exposure to

Table 13.1 Classification of anxiety disorders

ICD–10	DSM–IV
Anxiety disorders	*Anxiety disorders*
Panic disorder	Panic disorder with/without agoraphobia
Generalised anxiety	Generalised anxiety disorder
Mixed anxiety and depressive	Agoraphobia without history of panic
disorder	Social phobia
Other mixed anxiety disorders	Specific phobia (formerly simple phobia)
Anxiety disorder unspecified	Obsessive–compulsive disorder
	Post-traumatic stress disorder
Phobic disorders	Acute stress disorder
Agoraphobia, with or without panic	Anxiety disorder due to a general
disorder	medical condition
Social phobia	Substance-induced anxiety disorder
Specific phobia (isolated phobias)	Anxiety disorder not otherwise specified

danger, or when it is triggered by situations known to be harmless, or occurs without cause. For many psychiatric disorders, particularly those which blur into normality, the distinction between a pathological symptom and normality is made on the grounds of 'a significant impairment of function'. In the case of anxiety the relationship between functional performance and anxiety levels has the shape of an inverted U and this is known as the Yerkes-Dodson Law. Thus, mild degrees of anxiety improve function, but high levels of anxiety can have an inhibiting effect.

> A student begins to worry a few months before his finals and the anxiety serves him well to motivate him to open his textbook and study, but in the week immediately before the exam he becomes so paralysed with anxiety that he can no longer concentrate or take in any of the material.

The symptoms of anxiety

The symptoms of anxiety are numerous and are both psychological and somatic (Box 13.2). It is important to note that several of these symptoms should be present before a clinical anxiety state should be diagnosed.

The mood of anxiety is one of fearful apprehension that some calamity is about to occur. Sometimes the person can name the feared event but often the apprehension cannot be attributed to any particular event. Thoughts are dominated by the possibility of mishap or failure. Typically the thoughts centre upon the possibility of failure to cope with some eventuality, appearing foolish or incompetent, or there are themes of serious illness or death to oneself or others. Piotrowsky (1957) in an

---

Box 13.1 Lewis' concept of anxiety

An emotional state with the subjective experience of fear
An unpleasant emotion which may be accompanied by a
    feeling of impending death
Anxiety is directed to the future, with the feeling of some
    kind of threat
There may be no recognisable threat or one which, by
    reasonable standards, is insufficient to provoke the
    degree of anxiety
There may be subjective bodily discomfort and manifest
    bodily disturbance

---

attempt to analyse the subjective experience of anxiety observed at least
five separate components: awareness of one's own powerlessness in the
face of threat; a feeling of impending danger; a state of tense alertness;
apprehensive self-absorption; and doubts as to the effectiveness of action
to counter the threat. Increased levels of arousal lead to restless behaviour
and if this is combined with muscular tension there may be futile attempts
to divert anxiety-laden thoughts into some trivial activity. Others develop
avoidant behaviour and make strenuous attempts to avoid situations
known to trigger anxiety. In extreme cases, there may be little evidence
of the original 'anxiety disorder', for example, a socially phobic person
may have developed a completely hermit-like existence as a result of
avoidant behaviour and display little of the earlier anxiety disorder.

Excessive worrying is central to anxiety and the Present State
Examination (PSE; Wing *et al*, 1974) defines it as "a round of painful,
unpleasant or uncomfortable thoughts which cannot be stopped
voluntarily and are out of proportion to the subject worried about". These
should be distinguished from obsessions where the thought is more
repetitive and there is a tendency to resist. Complaints of nervous tension
also occur and these include worrying as well as feelings of being keyed
up or on edge.

One common manifestion of anxiety is a sense of retro-sternal
constriction, often accompanied by a feeling that sufficient air cannot be
breathed in. This leads to an increase in the respiratory rate with
consequent hyperventilation. If this is at a chronic low-grade level,
hypocapnia and hypocalcaemia may result leading to feelings of faintness,
parasthaesia, and in extreme cases, the characteristic carpo-pedal spasms
of tetany. Palpitations, as well as an excessive awareness of the normal
heartbeat are also common, and tachycardia occurs during panic attacks.
However, the presence of tachycardia should also alert the clinician to
the possibility of an organic cause.

Box 13.2 Manifestations of anxiety

Increased arousal
    Wakefulness
    Restlessness
    Increased startle response
Mood
    Fearfulness
    Apprehension
Thoughts
    Unrealistic appraisal of danger or illness to self or others
    Belief in personal inability to cope with stress
Behaviour
    Constriction of purposeful activity
    Restless purposeless activity
    Avoidance of situations which increase feelings of insecurity
Somatic
    Sense of retrosternal constriction
    Hyperventilation:
        faintness, paraesthesia, carpo-pedal spasm
    Muscular tension:
        fatigue, pain, stiffness, tremor
    Autonomic nervous system overactivity:
        tachycardia, hot and cold flushes, dryness of mouth,
        diarrhoea, frequency of micturition, sweating
Associated symptoms
    Depersonalisation, secondary demoralisation, irritability

---

Muscle tension can occur together with worrying and the subject describes an unpleasant feeling of tension in one or more groups of muscles. If the muscle tension is severe there may be muscle pain, most commonly sited retro-sternally, in the neck, shoulders and back. Tension pains in the head should be carefully distinguished from other causes of headache, such as migraine. In some cases the muscle tension, if severe, leads to fidgeting, restlessness and pacing. Two types of tremor occur, a rather gross irregular tremor and a fine tremor resembling the tremor of thyrotoxicosis.

Some of the somatic manifestations of temporal lobe epilepsy also may occur in acute anxiety states, even when no organic basis can be found: these include sensations of epigastric nausea, and the experience of some movement starting from the stomach, which subjects describe as warmth or a feeling of a swelling, rising up through the body. This particular symptom is the basis of the ancient theory of migration of the womb as the cause of hysteria and also of the term 'globus hystericus'. Almost any combination of symptoms can occur in a given individual. Some patients appear to have predominantly muscular tension, a second group have mainly cardio-respiratory symptoms, a third group present with trembling in their hands, dry mouths, upper abdominal sensations, nausea, or have increased frequency of urination, while a fourth group develop panic attacks, and have panic disorder. Some or all of the above symptoms may occur together and these groupings are not rigid, but there is a tendency for an individual to display the same or a characteristic stereotyped pattern in different episodes, even when the external stressors vary.

Sleep disturbance is a common feature of anxiety and there is typically initial insomnia (difficulty in getting off to sleep), intermittent waking in the night and early morning wakening at around 4 am. Dreaming is frequent with the dreams having a threatening quality often with themes of disaster and in more severe cases there may be nightmares. Appetite is usually decreased but a few subjects take comfort in over-eating, while interest in sex is generally diminished. A variety of other symptoms also may sometimes accompany anxiety. These include depersonalisation (page 15), exhaustion (page 733) and irritability which is discussed later in this chapter.

Generalised anxiety disorder (GAD)

This disorder is undoubtedly very common. High rates of anxiety have been reported in community surveys, for example Dean *et al* (1983) gave a figure of 7%, and even higher rates are reported among general practice attenders and among general medical out-patients. The more restricted DSM–III diagnosis is probably less common and may have a lifetime prevalence of around 3.8%. However in clinic populations a rather different picture emerges. Thus in specialised anxiety disorder clinics only 11% of the new patients had GAD compared with 50% who had panic disorder. This suggests that most 'chronic worriers' with GAD do not seek medical advice, or if they do, are not referred on by their general practitioner (GP), while panic disorder appears to elicit treatment-seeking behaviour more readily.

Generalised anxiety disorder was originally a residual category, describing those patients with an anxiety disorder who did not have panic attacks. Panic disorder had been separated off from the other anxiety disorders by virtue of its response to small doses of imipramine. The first definition of GAD given in DSM–III (1980) comprised feelings of anxiety combined with three out of four categories of symptoms: motor tension, autonomic hyperactivity, apprehensive expectation, and vigilance or scanning. The text specified that symptoms should have been present for at least a month. Unfortunately this definition was shown to be unreliable with a low interrater reliability (Cohen's Kappa = 0.47; Barlow, 1988). The definition was therefore modified in the DSM–III–R and again in DSM–IV in three important ways. First, the new definition specified that the worry and concern should focus on a number of different areas to show that the anxiety was 'generalised'; second, the duration was increased from one month to at least six months (though not necessarily continuously); and third, there should be at least three out of six symptoms (Box 13.3).

ICD–10 also includes GAD but has a rather less restrictive definition:

> The essential feature is anxiety which is generalised and persistent but not restricted to or even strongly predominating in any particular environmental circumstance (i.e. it is free-floating). As in the other anxiety disorders the dominant symptoms are highly variable but complaints of continuous feelings of nervousness, trembling, muscular tension, sweating, lightheadedness, palpitations, dizziness and epigastric discomfort are common.

The symptoms should have been present usually for several months and symptoms of apprehension, motor tension, and autonomic overactivity should be present, but the text does not state how many or for how long symptoms are required for the diagnosis, nor are exclusion criteria given.

Because anxiety is so common, Sanderson & Barlow (1990) made an attempt to formulate GAD as a more positive syndrome rather than merely a residual category. They identified 22 subjects attending their anxiety disorders clinic who fulfilled criteria for a primary diagnosis of DSM–III–R (1987) GAD. The mean duration of the symptoms prior to presentation was five years four months, indicating that the condition elicits only weak treatment-seeking behaviour and also there is tendency to chronicity. Around two-thirds of the subjects were female, and 85% of their subjects spent more than half of their day in a state of anxiety or worry. Excessive

---

Box 13.3 DSM–IV generalised anxiety disorder

Excessive anxiety or worry occurring on more days than not for at least six months about a number of events or activities
Difficult to control the worry
Three or more of the following symptoms:
  restlessness
  easily fatigued
  difficulty concentrating or mind going blank
  irritability
  muscle tension
  sleep disorder
The focus of the worry is not some other Axis I disorder
Significant distress or impairment of function
Not drug induced or due to a general medical condition

Adapted with permission from DSM–IV. Copyright 1994 American Psychiatric Association.

or unrealistic worries focused around four main areas: family concerns, money, work and illness, in decreasing frequency. Almost all of their cases (91%) were comorbid for at least one other psychiatric diagnosis with social phobia being the most frequent but 25% also had panic disorder as a secondary diagnosis, while simple phobia, obsessive–compulsive disorder, dysthymia and major depression also occurred. These authors concluded that the core features of GAD were a sense of apprehensive expectation and chronic worrying.

Case example

> A 36-year-old geophysicist presented with symptoms of anxiety and worries mainly focused around his work. His job was to lead a team of computer programmers for an oil exploration company, and the task of the team was to analyse sonic explosive data used to best guess the site of possible oil deposits. The work was anxiety provoking because mistakes (e.g. drilling in the wrong place) could be very costly, and there were penalty clauses attached to delays in the data analysis, and in addition there were some aspects of the computer programme he did not understand. The illness started with aerophagy which always occurred before any important business meetings although once in the meeting he functioned well. Later he developed headaches which he described as "tensing of the muscles, sometimes in the front and sometimes at the back of the head which feel like muscle cramps and seem to come on even when the original reasons have passed". He also developed sweating, palpitations and difficulties in concentrating which ... "bring the fog down over my thought patterns. When I get home from work I just sit down and watch a TV programme, and I couldn't tell you what it was about because all these worries just whizz around my head but when it cleared it was like the curtains being pulled away". Symptoms were worse in crowded shops or in traffic jams and were particularly bad when he was driving to work down the motorway. Once he arrived at work the headache tended to diminish. "If I get the headache, I have not got the anxiety, they are sort of mutually exclusive. When I focus on the work, I seem to get anxious." Symptoms cleared completely at weekends or on holiday and were obviously work related. There was no evidence of any depression or panic attacks. At first he showed little response to relaxation or anxiety management techniques, but after some hesitancy agreed to take amitriptyline. Dosage was slowly titrated up to 120 mg (over four months) and his symptoms were greatly reduced. He then found that the relaxation tapes were helpful.

The distinction between panic disorder and generalised anxiety is blurred and may also be artificial. Thus in the series of Sanderson & Barlow (1990) 25% also concurrently suffered from panic disorder as a secondary diagnosis, but more significantly 73% had previously experienced at least one panic attack during the previous year. Life charts of those with panic disorder suggest that the onset of panic disorder is often preceded by a prolonged period of generalised anxiety disorder (Uhde *et al*, 1985). Breier *et al* (1985) have commented on the lack of any temporal separation for panic disorder and GAD and suggest that the separation may be artificial and that GAD may be "a prodromal, incomplete, or residual manifestation of other psychiatric disorders". GAD may be continuous or episodic and interspersed with periods of remission.

Panic disorder

The essential features of panic disorder are recurrent attacks of very severe anxiety or panics which do not occur in any particular situation and are largely unpredictable. The roots of the experience of panic are to be found in Greek mythology. Pan, the god of nature, had a habit of sleeping in a small cave near the road, but when disturbed from his sleep by a passer by, would let out a blood curdling scream so intense that many a terrified traveller died. This sudden overwhelming terror or fright came to be known as 'panic' and Pan would use his unique talent to vanquish his foes and even frighten the other gods (after Barlow, 1988).

The delineation of panic disorder owes much to an observation made by Klein (1964) who found that small doses of imipramine led to a complete resolution of the symptoms of non-situational panic attacks but had little effect on anticipatory anxiety or more generalised anxiety. The significance of this finding was not immediately obvious, and Klein recounts how, when he described his findings to Sergeant (a prominent British expert on physical treatments), that the latter commented that "he had probably missed cases of depression". Gradually, however, it became clear that subjects with panic attacks were not suffering from depression but had had a very severe and disabling type of anxiety. The presence of reasonably clear cut phenomenology and specific therapy led to its inclusion as a separate disorder initially in the Feighner Criteria and later in the DSM–III, DSM–IV and the ICD–10, although in ICD–10 it is also called episodic paroxysmal anxiety.

Clinical features

The PSE defines panic attacks as discrete episodes of autonomic anxiety which the subject tries to terminate by taking some drastic avoiding action. For example, a subject who cannot get his or her breath may rush outside for air, the subject who is anxious when left alone may telephone her husband, or the subject with a phobia of travelling may have to leave the bus. The DSM–IV definition of a panic is shown in Box 13.4.

A rather more detailed description of an individual panic attack is given by Hoehn-Saric & McLeod (1988) and when listening to patients describe their panic attacks it is helpful to compare their accounts with the description given below. Panic attacks usually start with paroxysms of intense fear and apprehension which strike suddenly, without warning and usually with no apparent reason. The physical symptoms are predominantly cardio-respiratory, combined with shakiness but frequently include feelings of lightheadedness and depersonalisation. Along with feelings of intense terror and fear patients may complain of rapid heartbeat, palpitations, discomfort in the chest, rapid or difficult breathing, sweating, hot and cold spells, urgency to urinate or to defaecate, trembling, nausea, dizziness and feelings of faintness. The symptoms may last from a few minutes to half an hour but rarely for longer, after which they gradually fade. Afterwards subjects still continue to feel tense, shaky or exhausted for several hours to come. During the early phases of the panic attack patients may believe they are about to die, are having a heart attack or a stroke or that they are going insane. Even among those with many previous attacks, who know they are going to survive the present episode, there are strong feelings of dread and fear because the experience itself is so unpleasant. Sometimes those with severe panic attacks may also get minor panics which are similar but briefer and less severe.

There is some variation in the number of episodes required to meet diagnostic criteria, e.g. DSM–III–R (APA, 1987) requires four attacks over four weeks, DSM–IV (Box 13.5) specifies at least two attacks and ICD–10 (Box 13.5) requires 'several episodes' over the previous month.

Box 13.4 DSM–IV criteria for a panic attack

A discrete period of intense fear or discomfort in which four (or more) of the following symptoms developed abruptly and reached a peak within 10 minutes:
palpitations
sweating
trembling
sensation of shortness of breath
feeling of choking
chest pain or discomfort
nausea or abdominal distress
dizzy or faint
derealisation or depersonalisation
fear of loosing control or going crazy
fear of dying
paraesthesias
chills or hot flushes

Adapted with permission from DSM–IV. Copyright 1994 American Psychiatric Association.

Studies of college undergraduates have shown that panic attacks are also common among young people in the community. Thus, Norton *et al* (1985) found that 35% of young adults reported at least one panic attack in the previous year, while 17% described experiencing a panic attack in the last three weeks. Non-clinical panickers had fewer associated symptoms and reported getting the panics out of the blue. Interestingly, these subjects also reported a high frequency of panic attacks in their first-degree relatives (Norton *et al*, 1986).

During a panic attack there is often a rise in resting heart rate. Hyperventilation usually accompanies panic attacks but subjects with panic disorder have a lower pCO_2 even before their panic attacks, suggesting that they may be chronic hyperventilators. In some cases, the hyperventilation itself may precede and cause the panic attacks, but in most instances the panic precedes the hyperventilation (Bass & Gardner, 1985).

There is a strong association with agorophobia, and DSM–IV describes panic disorder as being either associated or not associated with agoraphobia. A spontaneous attack of severe anxiety may lead to avoidance of the situation where it occurred and anticipatory anxiety is common among panic disorder subjects. However, this is unlikely to be the whole explanation of the association between agoraphobia and panic attacks because agoraphobia consists of more complex fears, such as fears of being alone, fears of travel, fears of crowds, etc., rather than

---

Box 13.5 Panic disorder in DSM–IV and ICD–10

DSM–IV
Both (1) and (2)
1. Recurrent unexpected panic attacks
2. Attacks followed by one month or more of one of the following:
   (a) concern about having more attacks
   (b) worry about implications of the attack (going crazy, having a heart attack)
   (c) change in behaviour due to the attacks
3. Panic attacks not due to a general medical condition, a substance or another anxiety disorder
4. Panic disorder may occur with or without agoraphobia

ICD–10
1. Panics occur where there is no objective danger
2. Not occurring in predictable situations
3. Freedom from anxiety between attacks (though anticipatory anxiety is common)

Adapted with permission from DSM–IV. Copyright 1994 American Psychiatric Association.

---

simply the avoidance of more panic attacks (agoraphobia is further discussed in Chapter 14).

The natural history of panic disorder is typically episodic with the panic attacks clustering for a few weeks or months at a time and then followed by phases of spontaneous remission, with recurrences occurring later following new stresses. Regular cycles, as sometimes occurs in bipolar disorder, have not been observed, but the course of panic disorder may extend over many years.

Stress reaction and adjustment disorder

ICD–10 includes categories for the classification of understandable anxiety, that is anxiety in relation to situations and particular circumstances. In these categories the anxiety would be accepted by anyone, as a normal reaction. Even so, the experience of anxiety is, to most people, unusual and alarming; the manifestations of anxiety are easily misattributed to some other cause, usually somatic illness; the clinician must therefore be clear about what are the manifestations of anxiety only, how these differ from (or become added to) the symptoms of an organic disease and be able to explain all this to the patient in clear terms. Such explanations alone often constitute the major part of the treatment of stress reactions. The clinician must also be clear about what constitutes a stressful event and how this may vary from one person to another, taking into account the background and life experience of the individual as well as constititutional predisposition. For instance, an episode of chest pain resulting from muscular strain may be shrugged off as 'normal' by an individual who has experienced it frequently before or by someone who is aware that violent and unaccustomed exertion may lead to transient pain. Another person, perhaps a young man whose father or friend has recently died from a myocardial infarction, may interpret the pain in a more sinister light and the fear will add to the muscular tension and so increase the pain. Acute stress reactions and adjustment disorder are relatively common in community and general practice settings, but only rarely reach the attention of the specialist.

Acute stress reaction

> A transient disorder of significant severity which develops in an individual without any other apparent mental disorder in response to exceptional physical and/or mental stress and which usually subsides within hours or days ... Individual variation and coping capacity play a role in the occurrence and severity of acute stress reactions ... The symptoms show great variability but typically include an intial state of 'daze' with some constriction of the field of consciousness and narrowing of attention, inability to

comprehend stimuli and disorientation ... The state may be followed either by further withdrawal from the surrounding situation, or by agitation and overactivity. Autonomic signs such as tachycardia, sweating or flushing are commonly present ... Partial or complete amnesia for the episode may be present. (ICD–10, 1992)

Previous personality factors may play a role, and the diagnosis should not be made if the symptoms are no more than an exacerbation of a previous mental disorder. DSM–IV (1994) describes a similar condition but highlights the presence of dissociative symptoms including dissociative amnesia, depersonalisation, derealisation, being in a daze and subjective numbing.

Post-traumatic stress disorder (PTSD)

Kraepelin described the schreck-neurosis (German, *schreck* = terror), a nervous disorder that occurred after shocks or accidents, while English authors wrote of a condition called 'railway spine' caused by concussion of the spine following railway collisions. Shell shock, battle fatigue and combat neuroses were all terms used in First World War and the early history of PTSD is reviewed by Trimble (1981). The modern concept of PTSD was first formulated by Kardiner (1941), who considered it to be a physio-neurosis, a mental disorder with both physiological and psychological components. He described the five principal features of PTSD: (1) the persistence of the startle response and irritability; (2) a tendency to explosive outbursts of aggression; (3) fixation on the trauma; (4) constriction of the general level of the personality functioning, and (5) typical dream life. More recently the Vietnam War, with around half a million psychiatric casualties, brought the disorder into prominence, and led American psychiatrists to press for its inclusion in the DSM–III (1980).

Clinical features of PTSD

The re-experiencing of the trauma in the form of intrusive or unwanted memories is the most characteristic symptom of PTSD. Intrusive memories may be triggered by relatively minor stimuli, for example for some Vietnam veterans a rainy day (the monsoon lasts for months in Vietnam), the noise of a helicopter or any loud discharge could evoke the traumatic wartime memories. Intrusive memories tend to be of short duration and the subject remains in touch with reality. Sometimes there are flashbacks when the person feels they are reliving the events and in severe cases there may be dissociated states and the subject acts as if the original trauma is occurring in the present time. Intrusive memories may be troublesome for many years after the original trauma, or as one Vietnam veteran put it, "It was bad enough that I had to go to Vietnam in the first place, but to live through it over and over again is just too much" (Southwick *et al,* 1994, p. 258).

Sufferers complain of difficulties in sleeping, usually initial insomnia associated with a fear of disturbing dreams and nightmares during which the trauma is often vividly recalled in detail. There may be recurrent dreams of specific traumatic episodes such as being shot, running away or witnessing the death of friends in battles among the military cases. The dream content tends to be repetitious and is all too easily recalled in contrast to the variable pattern found in normal dreaming when recall is more remote or absent. Sometimes alcohol is used to treat the insomnia, or other symptoms, and this may complicate the picture.

Avoidance behaviour is also a core symptom of PTSD and is particularly marked among those with strong re-experiencing symptoms as they try to escape from troublesome memories and dreams. Horowitz (1986) describes an avoidance/denial phase of the disorder with a tendency to either deny or play down any connection between the traumatic event in the past and present psychological problems. There may be excessive pointless activity or the use of fantasy to avoid reality, and accompanying this denial there may be a general lack of emotional responsiveness, and a constriction of thinking and affect which results in a lack of experience of either pleasure or pain causing detachment from friends and family and ultimately isolation. Titchener (1985) considered this to be the most malignant feature of PTSD because it may explain the severe social and psychiatric decline sometimes seen in PTSD. Depression is often associated with this anhedonia.

An increased startle response may be characteristic, with flinching, grimacing or even shouting when stimuli reminiscent of the original trauma occur and may have the appearance of an over-reaction. Hypervigilance is shown by excessive alertness, preparation of flight or other forms of self-protection in situations which most would consider innocuous but the individual views as dangerous. Occasionally hypervigilance may approach the bizarre. After the Buffalo Creek flood in West Virginia, Titchener & Kapp (1976, p. 297) wrote:

> The community leader and his wife never slept at the same times so that at least one of them could always remain alert. On rainy nights he would be deluged with phone call rumours that another dam might break. He would then spend the night sitting on the dam with a rifle. Other community members stayed on shore nearby in order to protect him from attack.

A variety of symptoms may be associated with PTSD and these depend on the particular nature of the trauma, the individual and the circumstance. Among war veterans survivor guilt is common (Why did I survive when other more worthy people did not?). Paramedics who witnessed many deaths were particularly susceptible to survivor guilt and for years afterwards would castigate themselves for being responsible for the deaths of their fellow soldiers, because they were either too slow or incompetent.

Victims of assault or rape may be prone to feelings of anger or rage, fears of loss of control, uncontrollable crying, and feelings of shame. Recurrent nightmares of the attack occur, sometimes with the patient waking up immediately before the attack while in other cases during the dream the victim masters the assailant and fights off the attack. Some women become depressed later. A few women develop a 'silent rape reaction' where the most recent episode serves to reawaken a long history of earlier childhood sexual molestation. Following natural disasters, fears of the elements are common, for example, after the Buffalo Creek disaster many people developed obsessions and phobias about water and rain and other reminders of the disaster.

Measurement

A variety of interviews and rating scales are available for the measurement of PTSD, mainly for use in research. The structured interview for PTSD (Davidson *et al*, 1989) and the PTSD module of the SCID will yield a DSM–III–R diagnosis. The most widely used scale is the Impact of Events Scale (Horowitz *et al*, 1979) which has 15 items and two subscales which measure the symptoms of intrusion and avoidance. There are also PTSD subscales in the MMPI and the SCL–90. The Mississippi Scale for Combat Related PTSD (Keane *et al*, 1989) is a 35-item scale which gives a numerical score and has been modified for use in cases of civilian trauma.

Differential diagnosis

Adjustment disorder may be associated with a stressor of any severity (usually less severe), is of shorter duration and is a less severe condition with a different symptom pattern. Acute stress reaction should have resolved within a four-week period while PTSD is a more prolonged condition. Recurrent intrusive thoughts are also a feature of obsessive–compulsive disorder. In the latter condition the thoughts are felt to be inappropriate, may be resisted and even if the obsessions started after some life event the content of the thought is usually unrelated to the trauma. Flashbacks may occur in dissociative disorders or occasionally in brief psychosis. Malingering should always be excluded if financial gain is a possibility or when forensic considerations are present.

Comorbidity

A distressing condition such as PTSD, which impairs functioning, might itself cause additional psychiatric problems but these are generally non-psychotic. The Centres for Disease Control study (1988) of a non-clinic population of Vietnam veterans with PTSD gave comorbid rates for major depression as 34%, GAD 45%, alcohol misuse 70%, and drug misuse 25%. Among Israeli veterans with PTSD, alcohol and drug misuse were very uncommon, possibly because public attitudes to the veterans are more positive, but also because base rates for alcohol and drug misuse are much lower in Israel.

Following a natural disaster the pattern is also different, possibly because different age groups and social strata are exposed. Thus, after the Mt St Helens volcano eruption, PTSD was more strongly associated with anxiety, 76% had GAD, 51% depression, 27% alcohol misuse, and only 8% drug misuse (Shore *et al*, 1986). A comorbid disorder such as alcohol misuse or major depression may initially dominate the clinical picture and require treatment first before the PTSD itself can be dealt with.

Classification

Ramsay (1990) points out how the American DSM system has waxed and waned in its enthusiasm for incorporating PTSD according to whether the US is at war or not. DSM–I (1952) was published soon after the Second World War, and included a category of 'gross stress reaction', but DSM–II (1968) formulated during peacetime dropped this category. The catastrophic effect of the Vietnam War led to the first inclusion of PTSD in the DSM–III (1980) and later DSM–III–R (1987), but as there have only been a few military casualties since then, the DSM–IV (1994) has switched its emphasis back to civilian and childhood trauma, although the conditon of PTSD has been retained.

ICD–10, DSM–III and DSM–III–R give as their main criteria that "the trauma should be of an exceptionally threatening or catastrophic nature which is likely to cause pervasive distress in anyone" (ICD–10, 1992). The DSM–III–R added a clause "that the stress should be outside the range of the usual human experience". The DSM–IV has a different approach and provides a symptom-based definition (Table 13.2) only requiring that the subject "should have experienced, witnessed or confronted life-threatening events and the patients response involved intense fear, helplessness or horror". The reason for this change, and the removal of the phrase "the stress should be outside the range of the usual human experiences" was because in the DSM–IV field trials, stresses of this type proved to be quite common and difficult to define, and proved to be an unreliable item.

The types of possible trauma listed in ICD–10 include natural or man-made disasters, combat, serious accidents, witnessing the violent death of others, or being the victim or witness of torture, terrorism, rape, or other crime. DSM–IV has a rather broader concept, and in addition to the above includes traumas that others close to the subject have experienced, and the subject has learnt about. For children, it also includes

---

Box 13.6 DSM–IV criteria for post-traumatic stress disorder

A. i. The person experienced, witnessed, or was confronted with an event that involved actual or threatened death or serious injury, or a threat to the physical integrity of the self or others and
ii. The person's response involves intense fear, helplessness or horror

B. Re-experiencing symptoms (one of the following):
recurrent intrusive recollections
recurrent distressing dreams
acting or feeling as if the event was still occurring
distress on exposure to cues that recall the event
physiological reactivity on exposure to cues

C. Persistent avoidance of stimuli associated with the trauma (three or more of the following):
efforts to avoid, thoughts, feelings or conversations
associated with the trauma
avoid activity or places associated with the trauma
diminished interest or participation in activities
detachment or estrangement from others
restricted range of affects (e.g. unable to have loving feelings)
sense of a foreshortened future

D. Symptoms of increased arousal (not present before the trauma, at least two of the following):
insomnia
increased anger
poor concentration
hypervigilance
exaggerted startle response

E. Criteria B, C, D last more than one month

F. Clinically significant distress or impairment of function

DSM–IV recognises an acute type of PTSD when the duration of symptoms is less than three months, a chronic type when the symptoms last for more than three months, and a type with delayed onset starting at least six months after the trauma. Separate but broadly similar criteria are given for children.

---

inappropriate sexual experiences (without threatened or actual violence). Cases with a period of six months or more separating the onset of symptoms from the original trauma are classified in the DSM–IV as 'with delayed onset'. ICD–10 specifies the onset should be within six months of the trauma; cases with a later onset should be given a diagnosis of probable PTSD and the more chronic cases should be classified under the category enduring personality change (see page 795).

Aetiology

The nature of the trauma is generally seen as one of the prime aetiological factors. Figley (1985) suggests that the trauma should be sudden so there is no time for psychological preparation, dangerous with a life-threatening potential, and overwhelming, leaving the survivor with at least a temporary sense of helplessness and being out of control.

Among Vietnam veterans the intensity and length of contact exposure were critical variables in the development of PTSD. Kulka *et al* (1990) found that 38.5% of those with high war zone exposure developed PTSD compared with 8.5% who had low battle exposure; higher rates were also found among Black and Hispanic soldiers.

The severity of the trauma is also a factor in the aetiology of PTSD during peacetime, for example, following crime. Kilpatrick & Resnick (1993) in a large follow-up study of the victims of crime found the following rates for DSM–III PTSD: rape 57%, physical assault 37%, other sexual assault 16–33%, robbery 18–28%. The risk for PTSD among victims where there was a threat to life was 35%, if physical injury occurred 43%, and if both were present the rate rose to 59%. The inference from these figures is that both objective injury and subjective fear may contribute to PTSD.

A neurobiological basis to PTSD is suggested on the basis of studies of three different animal models (for review see Friedman, 1994). These include the learned helpless model which arises if there is inescapable stress. This model involves the limbic system and locus coerulus and so may possibly involve noradrenergic, dopaminergic, GABA and opioid systems. The fear-potentiated startle model of PTSD suggests the activity of the central nucleus of the amygdala with its projections to the brain stem. This system may also involve noradrenergic, GABA and opioid systems. Finally the kindling/long-term potentiation model postulates sensitisation of the limbic nuclei which are involved in emotional arousal, memory and other behaviours. Kindling is associated with increased benzodiazepine receptor binding and sensitivity of catecholaminergic neurones and suggests a possible role for anticonvulsants such as carbamazepine in treatment.

As with most other psychiatric disorders aetiology is multi-factorial (for review see Ramsay, 1990) and in addition to the trauma, genetic and premorbid personality traits and a disturbed early environment also contribute.

A recent large twin study of Vietnam veterans found hereditabilities of 0.13–0.30 for the re-experiencing cluster (painful memories, nightmares), 0.30 for the avoidant cluster and 0.30 for the arousal cluster (insomnia, irritability, easily startled) (True *et al*, 1993). Family studies have also shown high rates of alcoholism among siblings. Introversion and extroversion were associated with the development of PTSD among fire fighters exposed to the Australian bush fire, a disturbed child environment, poor parent–child relationships, high rates of parental separation, and history of alcohol misuse were associated with PTSD in the veterans from Vietnam. Public attitudes to war can also be important. The soldiers returning from the Second World War in America were welcomed home as war heroes but those returning from Vietnam, an unpopular war, were sometimes subjected to abuse and so the rates for PTSD were higher.

Assessing the relevance of the background features in an individual patient is helpful in planning treatment as well as in medico-legal cases because for some patients the pre-existing psychopathology may be sufficient to explain the whole clinical picture with the trauma serving only as a trigger, while in other cases, the trauma may be the primary cause.

PTSD and the law

An increasing number of patients with PTSD are claiming damages for personal emotional injury through the courts. This comes under tort law, which roughly translated means an injury. Tort law provides monetary compensation for wrongs inflicted on one party by another and it is quite separate from criminal law. Keenan (1989) defines the legal essence of a tort:

> The fact that a person has suffered damage does not necessarily entitle him to maintain an action in tort. Before an action can succeed the harm suffered must be caused by an act which is a violation of a right which the law vests in the plaintiff or injured party. The law of torts is concerned with the effects of injurious contact rather than the motives. It makes little difference whether the motive is intentional, malicious or innocent or due to negligence.

To establish a tort in a case of personal injury, courts are required to establish fault, causation, and the assessment of damages. The question of fault does not usually concern the psychiatrist but the court will seek a psychiatrist's opinion on the issue of causation and, to some extent, on the assessment of damages.

For causation the law looks to proximate causes, that is the logical and timely connection between the actions of one party and their effects on another party. No such simple type of causation exists in psychiatry and the notion of multi-factorial causation is unfamiliar to judges, lawyers, and the lay public. The psychiatrist should still attempt to assess the nature and strength of the link betwen the trauma and the subsequent psychiatric disorder. Other factors that may have contributed to the symptoms should be listed although it may not be possible to quantify to what extent the psychiatric disorder is due to the trauma and how much of it is due to the other factors. Cases of delayed onset of PTSD may be particularly difficult to explain to the court. If the trauma is trivial and lies within the realm of normal experience the Court is unlikely to accept a causal link, and this may even arouse a suspicion of malingering.

Keenan (1989) suggests that damages should be assessed under three headings: (1) pain and suffering; (2) loss of enjoyment of life or amenity; and (3) loss of earnings, both actual and prospective; and the premorbid function in these three areas should always be addressed in the report. Courts are likely to be less generous when the trauma has only served to reactivate some pre-existing problem, rather than when the only episode of psychiatric disorder followed the trauma.

Outcome

The naural history of PTSD has yet to be clarified but most individuals recover from the acute effects of trauma. A series of studies on the effect of rape (Rothbaum & Foa, 1993) showed a fairly rapid attentuation of symptom severity in the first few months. Thus, at two weeks 94% of the victims fulfilled criteria for PTSD, this figure fell to 65% at four weeks and continued falling to 40% at 12 months, but other studies have shown that even 15 years later around 15% of subjects still have symptoms. A recrudescence of symptoms can sometimes occur, for example after the Enniskillen bombing most survivors were thought to have recovered after six months but then experienced renewed symptoms at one year at the anniversary of the event.

Traumas due to interpersonal violence or of human design (for example, torture) are generally more potent causes than the stress caused by natural disasters, and long-term follow-up studies have shown that extremely severe stress may have a lifelong damaging effect. Thus among American prisoners of war (POWs) the degree of maltreatment by their captors appeared to determine subsquent rates of PTSD; 11% of those incarcerated in Europe after the Second World War developed PTSD, while 28% of those in Japanese camps developed PTSD (Langer, 1987). However, a long-term follow-up study of the POW survivors of the Korean War (where the prisoners had been subjected to a particularly cruel regime, including mock executions, brain-washing, exposure to the elements for months on end, etc.) found that 86% of subjects still fulfilled criteria for PTSD or another DSM–III anxiety disorder 30 years after their release, and they continued to be suspicious, confused, isolated and guilt-ridden (Sulker *et al*, 1991).

Treatment

The earliest treatments for PTSD included abreaction with or without drugs. Group methods were used during the Second World War and again proved successful in the treatment of Vietnam veterans. Possibly soldiers feel more comfortable sharing their experiences with others who have also gone through equally horrific experiences. Horowitz (1986) recommends brief psychotherapy with a mainly dynamic orientation which aims to help the subject integrate their memories in a more controlled fashion with less painful affects. The victim is encouraged to realise that he is basically a healthy individual but the pressure that cracked him would have cracked anyone. A wide variety of different approaches are used to achieve this, and the particular method adopted will depend on whether the patient is in the 'arousal phase' or the 'denial numbing phase' of the disorder (Table 13.2). A more recent and comprehensive account of treatment is given in Williams & Sommer (1994).

Drug treatments

There is no drug of choice in the treatment of PTSD but a common finding of the few available controlled studies is that only the 'arousal symptoms' and not the 'denial-numbing' features of the disorder respond to medication (for review see Friedman, 1994). Tricyclic antidepressants improve PTSD symptoms although, as might be expected, improvement is greater in the presence of comorbid depression. Monoamine oxidase inhibitors may also help some cases of PTSD. Because the intrusive phenomena show some resemblance to obsessive–compulsive symptoms serotonergic drugs may have a place and a recent open study of fluoxetine (20–80 mg daily) showed benefits for both intrusive and even for some avoidant symptoms (McDougle *et al*, 1990). Anti-kindling drugs such as valproate and carbamazepine may help and there are a few reports suggesting lithium may help some patients. Benzodiazeines decrease anxiety levels but have little effect on the core PTSD symptoms, and benzodiazepine withdrawal has been associated with severe exacerbations of the original PTSD symptoms. Neuroleptics are best reserved for patients with aggressive outbursts due to flashbacks, paranoia or other types of behavioural dyscontrol. Medication should only be used as part of combined psychological and treatment programme, and drug selection should be empirically based.

Adjustment disorders

The concept of adjustment disorder is that of a rather more prolonged disturbance than a stress reaction. However, the stressor is usually much less severe than in cases of PTSD. Adjustment disorders are states of subjective distress and emotional disturbance which may interfere with social functioning and arise during the period of adaptation to a life change or life event. Individual predisposition or vulnerability plays an important role in this disorder. Symptoms usually include depressed mood, anxiety, a feeling of inability to cope, plan ahead or continue in the

Table 13.2 Treatment for PTSD according to presenting symptoms

Denial numbing phase	*Intrusive repetitive phase*
1. Reduce controls by: (a) encouraging recollection of the trauma (b) interpret defences and attitudes that make controls necessary	1. Supply structure to patients frightening world: (a) organise information (b) reduce external demands (c) reduce stimuli, particularly reminders (d) provide an identification model. Permit dependency, over-idealisation and offer support
2. Encourage abreaction: by (a) verbal description (b) free association (c) use of images in recollection rather than solely relying on words (d) creative OT therapies, such as art therapy, role play, etc. (e) recreate the scene of the original trauma, e.g. visit the battle field, fly in a helicopter	2. Work through and reorganise painful experiences: (a) differentiate reality from fantasy (b) past from current schemata (c) self-attribute from object attributes (d) teach patient to switch off from stress-related information
3. Explore emotional aspects of relationships: (a) relationship with self and others at the time of the trauma (b) support and encourage current social relationships which help to counteract numbness	3 (a) Suppress emotion with anti-anxiety agents (see below) (b) teach patient desensitisation and relaxation techniques

Adapted from Horowitz (1986). Published with kind permission of Jason Aronson Inc.

present situation as well as some interference with the performance of the daily routine. Some individuals may feel liable to dramatic behaviour, or outbursts of violence, although this is rare. Among adolescents with conduct disorder for example, aggressive or antisocial behaviour may occur. The ICD–10 specifies that the onset should be within one month of the stressful event, and DSM–IV specifies within three months of the event and the duration should not exceed six months, nor should the symptoms be sufficiently severe to justify any other more specific diagnosis. The diagnosis should only be made in the presence of a relatively strong stressor, and then only if the symptoms would not have occurred without the stressor. Personality disorder or immature personality may predispose to adjustment disorders.

The DSM–IV describes a broadly similar condition (Box 13.7), and also regards adjustment disorder as a residual category for those reactions to stress which do not meet criteria for other (generally more severe) psychiatric disorders. It specifically excludes bereavement which should be classified separately. The severity of the reaction bears little relationship to the severity of the stressor. Specifiers of adjustment disorder are described according to their most prominent symptoms: depressed mood, anxiety, mixed anxiety depression, disturbances of conduct, and with mixed disturbance of emotions and conduct. Adjustment disorders are common in the community and among general practice attenders but are less frequent among those presenting to psychiatric clinics.

Mixed anxiety and depression

The ICD–10 proposes this as a new category. It is important to note that this category refers to patients who have relatively mild symptoms of anxiety and depression, which are not severe enough to justify a separate diagnosis for either major depression or one of the anxiety disorders. This category should be considered if there is mild depression, some anxiety and perhaps a few autonomic symptoms such as tremor or palpitations. Individuals with this condition are commonly found in the community and may sometimes visit their GPs but rarely reach specialist attention. If these milder symptoms are associated with a stressful event, a diagnosis of adjustment disorder should be made, while if the symptoms are prolonged, a diagnosis of dysthymia is better. The DSM–IV (1994) does not have a special section for this type of disorder but mentions it in the section "Anxiety disorder not otherwise specified".

Irritability

The state of irritability is not an anxiety disorder although it is convenient to consider it here. The recognition of irritability as a form of emotional disorder has been long neglected, and as described here, it is the manifestation of purposeless, ill-directed verbal or physical expressions of irascibility. The actual expression may be suppressed but the subjects sense, as do those close to them, an uncomfortable lack of control over angry expression. A definition is provided by Snaith & Taylor (1985):

> Irritability is a feeling state characterised by reduced control over temper which results in irascible verbal or behavioural outbursts, although irritable mood may be present without observed manifestation. It may be experienced as brief episodes in particular circumstances or it may be prolonged and generalised. The experience of irritability is always unpleasant for the individual and overt manifestation lacks the cathartic effect of justified outbursts of anger.

Box 13.7 DSM–IV criteria for adjustment disorder

Emotional or behavioural symptoms occurring within three months of an identifiable stressor

Symptoms or behaviours are clinically significant as evidenced by:

Distress is greater than what would be expected by exposure to the stressor

Impairment of social, occupational or academic function

Does not meet criteria for another Axis I disorder or an exacerbation of a pre-existing Axis I or Axis II disorder

Symptoms not due to bereavement

Once the stressor has terminated, symptoms do not last for more than six months

Specify whether acute (symptoms for less than six months) or chronic (more than six months)

Adapted with permission from DSM–IV. Copyright 1994 American Psychiatric Association.

This definition recognises that irritability is primarily a mood which may be expressed as behaviour. Irritability may be directed outwardly or turned inwardly so that the person feels angry with himself. The outwardly directed irritability concept is probably a mixture of a general impulse towards behaviour, suicidal impulses combined with personal dissatisfaction with one's own performance as well as that of others. The outward irritability construct is best understood (and differentiated from the states of aggression and hostility which are more interpersonally directed) by consideration of the items of the Outward Irritability subscale of the Irritability Depression Anxiety Scale (Snaith *et al*, 1978).

(1) I lose my temper and shout or snap at others.
(2) I feel I might lose control and hit or hurt someone.
(3) I am impatient with other people.
(4) People upset me so that I feel like slamming doors or banging about.

Irritability has many associations: it may be an aspect of personality, it is prominent in both premenstrual tension and postnatal depression (Pitt, 1968). It may be an expression of discomfort in intimate relationships. Weissman & Paykel (1974) noted a 'continuum of intimacy', that is the closer the personal relationship the more likely irritability would be expressed. Pharmacological factors, such as the 'paradoxical' effect of the benzodiazepine drugs may increase irritability (Editorial, 1975), and it may also be a troublesome after-effect among those with head injuries (Brooks & McKinlay, 1983).

Differential diagnosis

The differential diagnoses of the anxiety disorders, but particularly generalised anxiety and panic disorder, are essentially similar and represent one of the most important differential diagnoses in medicine. Anxiety is an ubiquitous symptom and may be a presenting feature of many physical and psychiatric conditions. The clinician must always entertain alternative diagnoses apart from simple anxiety (or any of the anxiety disorders), but in the vast majority of cases a few additional questions, a physical examination, or simple laboratory test will soon clarify the diagnosis. Cardiac, endocrine and neurological diseases figure prominently but almost any organ system may be involved. Although a few patients may present with the complete list of anxiety symptoms which render a psychiatric diagnosis more likely, the majority present with only a few anxiety symptoms, generally confined to one organ system only. Thus, a symptom-based approach to differential diagnosis may be more helpful and the account that follows is drawn largely from the work of Jacob & Rapport (1984).

Cardiovascular symptoms are perhaps the most frequent, and the more organic cardiac disorders tend to be more common with increasing age, whereas the anxiety disorders occur more often in younger age groups. The presence of palpitations should suggest the possibility of supraventricular tachycardias, extrasystoles and other arrythmias. Dyspnoea and hyperventilation indicate the possibility of congestive heart failure, mitral valve disease, chest infections and chronic lung disease. In asthma, common among young people, the breathing difficulty is greater during expiration than during inspiration. The distinction from asthma is particularly important because some of the drugs used to treat panic disorder such as propranolol may worsen asthma. Over-breathing may also be a feature of alcohol withdrawal states. Among the middle-aged, chest pain is a cardinal feature of myocardial infarction and angina pectoris. Retrosternal pain also occurs in anxiety but in these cases the patient usually looks physically well. In pleuritic conditions, the pain is confined to coughing and expiration. Chest pain of psychological origin may resemble costal chondritis which may also have retrosternal tenderness.

The symptoms of tremor and sweating should alert the clinician to the possibility of hypoglycaemia which may be reactive due to diabetes, or oral hypoglycaemics and very rarely an insulinoma. Dizziness is commonly due to orthostatic hypotension and occurs in anaemia, but in psychiatric patients is most commonly the result of drug side-effects, such as those of the tricyclics or sedative antipsychotics. Sometimes subjects with Menière's disease, who are also anxious, complain of dizziness but closer questioning reveals the rotational component of the vertigo which is not a feature of the anxiety disorders. Depersonalisation and feelings of unreality, particularly if intermittent, should suggest temporal lobe epilepsy. Complaints of weakness may indicate neurological disorder such as multiple sclerosis, transient ischaemic attacks and myasthenia gravis. Some patients report feelings of being hot and cold, which is also common during the menopause when patients complain of hot flushes but the same symptom may also occur in the rare carcinoid syndrome.

A number of other conditions, mainly endocrine or metabolic disorders may mimic the complete picture of DSM–IV generalised anxiety disorder. The most important of these is thyrotoxicosis, which is readily excluded if considered. The anxious subject usually sweats and has a cold clammy hand in contrast to the warm sweaty palm of the thyrotoxic patient. Less commonly hypothyroidism may present with anxiety although the mood is more characteristically one of lethargy and depression. Both hypo- and hyperparathyroidism and other disorders causing hypocalcaemia can present with anxiety and tetany which confusingly may be worsened by hyperventilation. Episodic attacks of fear sometimes associated with headache and sweating may be a presenting feature of the rare phaeochromocytoma and a variety of drugs can precipitate attacks of anxiety in porphyria. Caffeinism due to drinking excess tea or coffee may also present with anxiety symptoms and this is described more extensively on page 1130. Finally, a picture resembling panic disorder can occur in cases of alcohol and substance misuse, particularly during phases of withdrawal from alcohol, amphetamines or opiates.

Assessment of anxiety

Anxiety is mainly a subjective experience, and therefore self-rating is commonly used. One of the earliest and most widely used scales was the Hamilton Anxiety Scale (Hamilton, 1959) composed of 14 items each of which is rated on a five point scale. The scale is quite long and heavily biased toward somatic symptoms making it unreliable in the presence of physical illness. A derivative of the Hamilton Scale which is shorter and places less emphasis on somatic symptomatology is the Clinical Anxiety Scale (Snaith *et al*, 1982). Comprehensive interviews such as the Present State Examination and the Comprehensive Psychopathological Rating Scale, the Structured Clinical interview for the DSM–III and the Diagnostic Interview Schedule (DIS) all include subsections which measure anxiety and these interviews and references are described in Chapter 25. Finally the Anxiety Disorders Interview Schedule (Dinardo *et al*, 1983) is a comprehensive interview which gives a DSM–III diagnosis for the anxiety disorders as well as scores on the Hamilton Depression and Anxiety Scales.

The Spielberger State–Trait Anxiety Inventory (Spielberger *et al*, 1970) provides two measures of anxiety: the present state which has 20 items and refers to the past three days;, and in the second part the underlying proneness to anxiety is measured in which subjects respond to the questions in the light of their feelings over the past year. The Hospital

Anxiety and Depression Scale (Zigmond & Snaith, 1983) distinguishes between the concepts of depression and anxiety, with little emphasis on somatic symptoms. The scale is brief, making it a practical instrument for use in general hospital settings, primary care and community work. Two rating scales based on adjective check-lists are the Multiple Affect Adjective Checklist (Zuckerman, 1960) and the Profile of Mood States (McNair *et al*, 1987) which cover a variety of different anxiety-related dimensions and can be used repeatedly, for example on a daily basis.

The advent of behavioural therapy, and more recently cognitive therapy, has led to the development of several new instruments which help monitor progress in treatment. The Fear Questionnaire (Marks & Mathews, 1979) is perhaps the best known and yields factor analytic subscales for measuring agoraphobia, blood injury and social phobia as well as a total phobia score. A variety of other tests and interviews for monitoring therapy are reviewed by Snaith & Turpin (1990). Physiological measures such as heart rate, the galvanic skin response, blood pressure and electromyography which may correlate with anxiety are mainly used in research.

Epidemiology

Anxiety disorders are common in the community, presenting more frequently to GPs and medical out-patient departments than psychiatric clinics. The Epidemiological Catchment Area (ECA) data suggest that around one in 20 people suffer from an anxiety disorder, with the phobias being the most common disorder (Robius & Regier, 1991). The six-month prevalence for all phobias was around 6%, with agoraphobia and simple phobia accounting for roughly equal proportions although there was considerable variation between the different sites in the ECA. The six-month prevalence of panic disorder in the five ECA sites was found to be a little under 1% with a lifetime prevalence of around 1.5%. The prevalence of GAD (DSM–III criteria) was 2.4% for men, 4.95% for women and 3.8% overall. The lifetime prevalence of agoraphobia was around 5% with a six-month prevalence of 4%. The lifetime prevalence for PTSD was 1.2%

An epidemiological study in the UK which used the PSE to give ICD–8 and RDC diagnoses found essentially similar figures: 2.9% for all anxiety disorders and 7% for anxiety symptoms. Agoraphobic symptoms were present in 17.4% but were severe in only 0.2%, and panic disorder was present in 0.7% (Dean *et al*, 1983). Differences between the British and American studies probably reflect the different methods employed for diagnostic assessment.

Almost all epidemiological studies show a female preponderance of around 2:1 for both generalised anxiety disorder and panic disorder, but this gender difference only applies for younger people. Thus for those

over 30, the prevalence of panic disorder is the same in males and females
(Wittchen, *et al* 1986). Panic disorder is more common among the younger
age groups, for example Bland *et al* (1988) reported a prevalence of 2.1%
in the 25–34 age group but for those over 65 the rate was only 0.3%, while
rates for phobias are equally distributed across all ages. ECA data suggest
that rates for panic disorder are increased among the separated and
divorced, but there is conflicting information on the relevance of race,
level of education, and urban/rural differences.

Aetiological theories

The symptoms of anxiety represent the end point of several different multifactorial processes; genetics, neurophysiology, psychodynamics and social
factors all influence clinical anxiety syndromes and the contribution of
these items is reviewed below.

Genetic aspects

Twin studies

Evidence from twin and family studies points to a significant genetic
contribution to the anxiety disorders but this is probably more in the
form of the inheritance of a personality trait such as neuroticism rather
than the transmission of specific DSM–IV symptom disorders. A large
Swedish study of 13 000 twin pairs who were given the short form of the
EPQ (Eysenck, 1959) found the heritability of neuroticism was 0.50 for
men and 0.58 for women, and for extraversion the scores were 0.54 and
0.66 respectively (Floderns-Myrhed *et al*, 1980). More recently the
inheritance of the symptoms of anxiety and depression was examined in
a large Australian twin study and heritability of 0.34–0.46 was reported
(Kendler *et al*, 1986).

Further analysis of the Australian twin data by Jardine *et al* (1984)
showed a high genetic correlation between the EPQ scores for neuroticism
with measures of the symptoms of anxiety and depression indicating that
they were probably measuring the same underlying factor. On this basis,
Kendler (1986) suggested that at least in the case of anxiety the distinction
between personality traits and symptoms was not clear-cut. Several earlier
studies have shown that current psychiatric disorder, particularly
depression may have large effects on the 'N' score of the EPI (Ingham,
1966).

For the clinical anxiety disorders, the twin series of Slater & Shields
(1969) and Torgersen (1983) are comparable because both are based on
probands who were hospitalised and diagnosed with ICD–9 criteria. Slater

& Shields found that seven (47%) of 17 monozygotic twins (MZs) were concordant as compared to only five (18%) of 28 concordant dizygotic twins (DZs). With the application of stricter diagnostic criteria, that is the presence of only anxiety disorder in the co-twin the MZ:DZ ratio increased to 41:4. In Torgerson's rather smaller series there was a concordance ratio of 36% for MZs and only 13% for DZs, also suggesting a significant genetic component. On the other hand, a more recent community-based interview study in Australia which applied DSM–III criteria found no difference between MZ and DZ concordance rates (Andrews *et al*, 1990). The most likely explanation for the discrepancy between the community-based twin study and the previous hospital-based studies may relate to how the probands are identified. Thus Torgerson (1983), in a twin study on neurosis, showed that if probands were selected from hospitalised cases, the MZ:DZ ratio was around two indicating a genetic contribution, but when probands were selected from out-patient samples there were negligible MZ:DZ differences (no genetic effect), and this would presumably also apply to community-based samples as well.

Family studies

Noyes *et al* (1978) compared the first-degree relatives of probands with anxiety disorders with surgical controls, and found a much higher rate (18 *v*. 3%) of anxiety disorders among the relatives of the anxiety probands. Female relatives had an even higher risk for the anxiety disorders possibly because the prevalence of anxiety is greater among women. An additive effect for genetic loading was observed in this study. Thus, if only the proband and no other family member had an anxiety disorder then the risk for the siblings was 9%; if one parent as well as the proband had anxiety disorder this risk rose to 26%, but if both parents and the proband had an anxiety disorder this risk to rose 44% (Noyes *et al*, 1978).

Panic disorder appears to be the most strongly genetically determined subtype of anxiety. Thus, Crowe *et al* (1983) selected 21 subjects with panic disorder from the original study of Noyes *et al* (1978) and found that 31% of their first-degree relatives also had panic disorder compared with only 4% of the control relatives. High rates of alcoholism (15 *v*. 4% in controls) were also present in the relatives of panic disorder probands. Panic disorder is often comorbid with depression and there has been much debate as to whether panic disorder represents a more extreme form of either anxiety or depression or whether panic disorder is phenomenologically and genetically distinct from depression. In a recent elegant study utilising three groups of probands, those with pure panic disorder, pure major depression, and those with combined panic disorder and major depression, Weissman *et al* (1993) showed that the first-degree relatives of panic disordered subjects had a 20-fold greater risk for panic disorder but had little or no increased risk for major depression. Relatives of probands with major depression had only a threefold increased risk for panic disorder, but a sixfold increased risk for major depression while relatives of probands with combined disorders had increased risks for both disorders. These results support the hypothesis that panic disorder is genetically distinct from major depression, even though panic attacks respond well to standard antidepressant treatment.

Generalised anxiety disorder is a less distinct condition than panic disorder, but recently Noyes *et al* (1987) has reported a rate of 19.5% for GAD among first-degree relatives of probands with GAD which is considerably elevated over population base rates. In another study, although the prevalence of GAD was only 3.8% among the first degree relatives, 3.8% also had major depression, 15% had alcoholism and 11% had other disorders giving a total of 34% of the first-degree relatives who had some type of psychiatric disorder (Davidson *et al*, 1985). These authors suggested that GAD was probably one manifestation of some underlying diathesis which could present with a variety of different symptom disorders.

Neuroanatomical and physiological aspects

The role of a neuronal system or 'circuit' subserving the experience of emotion was put foward by Papez in 1937. Gray (1981, 1982), basing his views on animal studies, has stressed the importance of the septohippo-campal function. He suggests that the hippocampus acts as a comparator, that is a mechanism which compares actual to expected stimuli (see also page 660). The system also has links with the Papez circuit and with a structure on the floor of the fourth ventricle, the locus coeruleus, from which descending pathways affect the sympathetic division of the autonomic nervous system and which therefore probably has an important role in generating the experience of anxiety. Using positron emission tomography (PET) Reimann (1990) has demonstrated the involvement of the temporal poles of the brain in pathological and normal forms of human anxiety.

Panic attacks are one of the few (and perhaps only) psychiatric disorders that can be regularly induced in the laboratory. Pitts & McClure (1967) observed that infusion of sodium lactate provoked anxiety in susceptible subjects. Approximately three-quarters of patients with panic disorder or agoraphobia with panic disorder developed panic during the lactate infusions compared with none among the normal controls (Liebowitz *et al*, 1984). The mechanism remains uncertain; it is not due to hypocal-caemia, nor is it the result of a metabolic disturbance (see review by Nutt & Lawson, 1992).

Catecholamines (adrenaline and noradrenaline) induce sensations with a quality similar to anxiety. Isoprenaline, a selective beta-agonist, induced panic attacks in five out of eight panic disorder subjects, but only in one out of nine controls, although lactate was found to be more likely to induce panic attacks in the same subjects (Freedman *et al*, 1984). Infusions of sympathomimetics such as isoprenaline may act via beta adrenergic receptors in the autonomic nervous system, as well as in the CNS. Yohimbine is an α_2-adrenoceptor antagonist which may precipitate panic attacks and it is thought to act centrally at the locus coerulus. There are extensive noradrenergic projections from the locus coerulus to the cortex and the noradrenaline is thought to serve more of a neuromodulatory than a neurotransmitter function (Charney, 1990). By blocking α_2-adrenoceptors, the neural release of noradrenaline from the locus coeruleus projections may be enhanced. Both diazepam and clonidine block yohimbine-induced anxiety (Charney *et al*, 1984*a*).

No doubt clinically the most important substance to provoke anxiety is caffeine. Charney *et al* (1984*b*) gave 10 mg/per kg body weight by mouth to 21 patients, 15 reported panic attacks which resembled their own panics, while the healthy controls reported only increased anxiety but no panic. Caffeine interacts weakly with the benzodiazepine receptor but its central effect is probably via the adenosine receptor site (Boulenger *et al*, 1982). Large doses produce symptoms of an anxiety state including insomnia, headache, tremor, nausea and diarrhoea. Instant coffee contains 80–100 mg caffeine per cup and percolated, filtered or boiled coffee rather higher concentrations. Tea contains rather lower concentrations and caffeine is a constituent of certain carbonated drinks such as Coca Cola. An estimate of caffeine consumption is important in all people presenting with anxiety states and a consumption of over 600 mg a day may contribute to the state, and the condition is further discussed on page 1170.

Anxiety may occur in states of abnormal brain function, especially in temporal lobe epilepsy. Jackson (1881) remarked: "There are other kinds of psychic states in connection with epileptic paroxyms. It is not uncommon for a patient to have an emotion of terror and to look terrified at the onset of the seizures. When this is so there is usually the epigastric sensation with it". Williams (1956), a neurologist, observed that temporal lobe epilepsy could also present with a variety of different emotional disturbances, but anxiety attacks seemed to be preferentially associated with lesions in the anterior portions of the temporal lobes. The relationship between CNS disorders and anxiety is reviewed by Strian & Ploog (1988).

Psychoanalytic theories

Psychoanalytic theories of anxiety are of two main types. Earlier Freudian theories highlighted the role of sexual drives and instinctual forces while later analysts, particuarly Sullivan, Horney and Bowlby, stressed the interpersonal realm rather than the instinctual drives. Only Freud's writing on anxiety neurosis corresponds to the modern DSM–IV concept of generalised anxiety and panic disorders. Other analysts have tended to use the word 'anxiety' to cover a much wider range of non-psychotic disorder.

Freud's toxic theory of anxiety and signal anxiety

In 1895 Freud proposed his first theory of anxiety, the toxic theory. He suggested anxiety resulted from the transformation of ungratified or undischarged sexual impulses, and these arose from prolonged sexual deprivation, frustration or unnatural sexual practices such as coitus interruptus. In this model, the undischarged impulses would build up into a state of excessive excitation and this in turn would result in anxiety. Freud called this an 'aktual neurosis'. In other cases, such as in hysteria, there was a strangulation of affect and the excessive libidinal excitation was transformed by mental processes into symptoms such as hysteria and these were called 'the psychoneurosis'. Before long the term 'aktual neurosis' was dropped and psychoneurosis was applied to all neurotic disorders. The rather mechanistic overtone of the toxic theory of anxiety is best understood as a product of its time, for its description coincided with the discovery of bacteria and their toxins as well as the invention of the motor car. As a way of explaining human emotion it proved untenable and was soon discarded.

In his *New Introductory Lectures* Freud (1933) proposed a rather more subtle concept, signal anxiety. In a situation of danger, the ego generates a small amount of anxiety which serves as a signal to alert the organism to the threat. While this type of anxiety appears to bear a superficial resemblance to W. B. Cannon's fight and flight reaction in which the threat is an external one, in signal anxiety the threat arises internally from intra-psychic conflicts. Any instinctual wish or impulse that had previously been associated with disappointment or punishment could elicit signal anxiety. As the pleasure principle rules that anxiety and psychic pain are to be avoided, signal anxiety serves to mobilise defences, such as repression to ward off any anxiety provoking thoughts or impulses, and so prevent them from reaching consciousness. Different types of threat, such as object loss or castration anxiety, may elicit signal anxiety, and Freud believed that signal anxiety played a role in the causation of phobias.

Sullivan

Sullivan rejected the drive instinct model of anxiety and shifted the focus of both the theory and the practice of psychotherapy to the arena of human relationships. According to Sullivan (1953) anxiety played a central role in life "... anybody and everybody devotes much of his lifetime, a great deal of energy and a good part of his effort in dealing with others to avoid anxiety and if possible to get rid of anxiety". He tried to link adult anxiety to disturbances in the mother–infant interaction. Central to the relationship between mother and infant is the quality of empathy linkage which Sullivan defined as "the peculiar emotional linkage that sustains the relationship of the infant with other significant people – the mother or the nurse". In an over-simplified model he suggests that early pleasurable experiences with the mother become transformed into a self-image of 'the good me' and the painful experiences into a notion of 'bad me', while unintegrated realms of experience become a 'not me' view of the self. These images become stored cognitions within the child and later in the adult and he wrote "a person's character is his or her history". In the presence of danger, the self institutes security operations (which are analagous to Freud's defences) and the earlier self-images are brought into play. The security operations also result in rigid patterns of interpersonal behaviour and any information which threatens to arouse anxiety is shut out. In Sullivan's scheme therapy will involve disruption of the security operations, which entails personality change and will inevitably meet with resistance, as well as the experiencing of anxiety.

Karen Horney

Karen Horney's views on anxiety are in many ways similar to Sullivan's, also emphasising the importance of the interpersonal realm (Horney, 1937). Writing in the 1930s during the run up to the Second World War, she saw that human aggression and hostility were far more serious threats to existence and causes of anxiety than simple undischarged libido. Such ideas were deemed heretical at the time and she was expelled from the Freudian New York Psychiatric Institute and went on to found the American Institute of Psychoanalysis, becoming its Dean until her death in 1952.

She described a condition of basic anxiety " ... as feelings of being isolated and helpless in a world conceived as potentially hostile". Such basic anxiety could arise from many different kinds of adversity in childhood: indifference, lack of warmth, over-protectiveness, misuse, injustice, etc. In Horney's system there were four means of escaping from the basic anxiety: rationalisation or denial; narcosis with sedatives and alcohol; avoidance; and developing a neurotic pattern. This pattern is originally developed as a way of surviving in disturbing circumstances but gradually it becomes the organising principle governing a person's life (Aveline, 1991). The individual needs to suppress hostile feelings because they are usually directed towards loved ones or those who are close, and in these instances "it is unbearable to be aware that one is hostile". In Horney's scheme self-realisation (a theme that was later taken up by Maslow) was just as important as the instinctual drives as a force for motivation. Rejection and hostility in the parents would impair self-actualisation, a basic need present in every child, as well as in all adults and this could later result in anxiety "... the child does not develop a feeling of we but instead a profound sense of insecurity and apprehensiveness". Formulated more than 50 years ago the views of Sullivan, Horney and others now may appear to be oversimplistic, but at the time represented a significant advance from the early Freudian instinctual theories and notions of undischarged libido and set the scene for Bowlby's theory of attachment.

Bowlby

Bowlby's theory of attachment draws heavily from ethology and animal work. In his scheme anxiety is viewed as a direct innately based response to separation or threat of separation from the caretaker. Holmes (1993) in a lucid account has recently considered the implications of attachment theory for psychotherapy.

(1) Bowlby postulates that there is a primary attachment relationship (Bowlby, 1969). This appears in the human infant at around seven months and its original main function was protection from predators. Animal work by Lorenz in ducks, and Harlow in monkeys, has shown that attachment and bonding behaviours are of central importance and are separate from feeding behaviours. Attachment is also fundamental to all types of psychotherapy. The universality of attachment may possibly explain the paradox why all types of psychotherapy are equally efficacious despite wide differences in underlying philosophies and methods of treatment (Frank, 1971).

(2) Attachment is characterised by proximity-seeking behaviour, which is activated in young children by separation from the carer. There is initially increased anxiety and a protest reaction such as a temper tantrum or crying: this is an adaptive response, termed separation anxiety, and its aim is to reunite the infant with the caregiver. Darwin observed that primates may also show separation anxiety, while Freud believed that anxiety in children represented the feeling of loss for the person they love. In later life, threats of separation, losses, illnesses and other catastrophies may trigger this earlier separation anxiety.

(3) Attachment results in the secure base phenomenon. When an infant feels securely attached and physically close to his attachment figure, he feels safe and engages in exploratory behaviour. An analogy is made with attachment in psychotherapy in which one aim is to help the patient explore new and better ways of coping with the environment as well as their own internal affects. To facilitate this, the therapist needs to provide a secure environment which is consistent, predictable and has warmth – all of which are also clearly the requirements for good mothering. In the absence of secure feelings, anxious attachments may develop, manifested by a pattern of clinging dependent behaviour, little in the way of exploratory behaviour, as well as a constant fear of separation and a proneness to separation anxiety. Bowlby (1969) suggested that school phobia might at least in part be explained as a result of anxious attachments and separation anxiety.

(4) The individual carries within him an internal working model, or a map which represents the relationship patterns that exist between himself and his attachment figures. The 'map' consists of self-images, core affective states and cognitive schemata which describe the expectations the subject has of both himself and the external world. Analysts have tended to focus on the unconscious schemata. More recently cognitive therapists have shown the value of exploring the patient's conscious schemata in psychotherapy.

(5) The attachment dynamic is essential for physical and mental wellbeing and protection in childhood but it continues throughout life. The same attachment dynamic is found in all later psychosocial relationships, such as work or marriage and also provides the dynamic for attachment in psychotherapy.

Bowlby's theory of attachment has derived some support from the experimental work of Mary Ainsworth (1969), a colleague of Bowlby. She devised the Strange Situation Test, a reliable rating for measuring the security of a one-year-old's attachment to his parent. In this test the parent leaves the room, while the infant remains alone with the investigator. Around 65% of one-year-old infants display a secure pattern, where they make an initial protest but are easily pacified, 20% show an 'insecure avoidant pattern', where there is little protest on the initial separation but on the parents' return the infant hovers warily nearby unable to play freely, 15% have an 'insecure ambivalent pattern' where they protest at the separation, and cannot be pacified and they cling tenaciously to the mother on her return, and around 4% of infants seem to just freeze and are described as 'insecure disorganised'. These patterns appear to be both innate and persistent. Thus an avoidant pattern shown at one year is also found when the child is five, and again at 10 years of age. Although Bowlby's theory of attachment has stimulated much research Rutter (1972) has criticised it on the grounds that it fails to take account of the numerous studies pointing to the role of genetic factors, as well as current stress as causes of anxiety.

Psychological models of anxiety

Individual vulnerability to external stresses and anxiety symptoms are linked together, but their interaction is complex. The additive model is simplest and proposes two independent variables, the personal vulnerability and the external stress. Too much stress in a vulnerable subject results in symptoms or breakdown, while a similar stress in a more robust individual has little effect. Apart from being rather mechanistic, this model ignores cognitive and interactive processes. People do not react passively to situations, but are constantly weighing up and interpreting events or working out the meaning events have for themselves, and sometimes intervene or try to master situations and so alter the course of events. Coping ability decreases an individual's vulnerability. Lazarus & Faulkmann (1984) define coping as "constantly changing cognitive and behavioural efforts to manage specific external, and/or internal demands that are appraised as taxing or exceeding the resources of the person". A host of factors contribute to coping ability including: people's beliefs, for example whether they have a stoical nature, their state of general health, energy levels, problem-solving ability, their social skills, and so forth. Endler & Magnusson (1976) propose an interactive model for anxiety which is the result of several process variables including personal vulnerability and coping ability, rather than anxiety simply being the result of genetically endowed anxiety traits.

In another, rather different model Barlow (1991) proposed that anxiety (and depressive) disorders are the product of tightly organised basic emotions which are stored in the memory and are then fired inappropriately. Vulnerable individuals may find these emotions difficult to cope with, and so eventually these emotions also become the focus of anxiety.

The model of Andrews (1991) proposes three separate components to explain clinical anxiety: a general vulnerability to anxiety (trait anxiety), comorbidity with other psychiatric disorders, and treatment-seeking behaviour. In this model, external stress acts as a trigger for symptom formation particularly for those with high trait anxiety, and if symptoms become chronic they eventually become transformed into irrational beliefs or despair. The ability to cope or otherwise may modify this response. The model is of interest because Duncan Jones (1987) has tried to estimate how much of the variance in anxiety symptoms could be explained by each item in subjects in the community. Only 5% of the variance of anxiety symptoms could be accounted for by external life events, and most of the explained variance (around 44%) could be attributed to a high trait anxiety as measured by the neuroticism score on the EPQ.

The addition of a second personality variable, locus of control, increased the explained variance of the symptoms up to 60%. An internal locus of control refers to a person's perception that stressful events relate to one's own behaviour or character, whereas an external locus of control refers to the belief that the stressful event is due to luck, fate or the influence of powerful others (Rotter, 1966). Internals tend to seek out and use more information and employ coping strategies such as humour whereas externals may become tense if confronted with feelings of failure. A life events study showed a correlation between symptoms and negative life events held true only for externals, but not for internals who presumably had better coping mechanisms (Johnson & Sarason, 1978).

The third factor in the model of Andrews (1991) is comorbidity and this appears to be critically important for initiating treatment-seeking behaviour. Isolated feelings of anxiety and panic are common in the community but this on its own does not elicit treatment-seeking behaviour. Those who seek help usually have other psychiatric disorders as well as anxiety and it is the combination of disorders which leads patients to seek help.

Stress and anxiety

In any discussion of anxiety, stress should be mentioned because anxiety and stress reflect the two opposite faces of the same coin. Anxiety is a description of a subjective state of specific symptoms while stress is the explanation made by an external observer of what he sees happening to a person who reports feeling anxious (Snaith, 1991). The concept of stress was originally borrowed from physics where the term 'stress' was used to describe the actions of a force on a body. Selye (1956) popularised its use in the biological sciences in his description of the general adaption syndrome, as a response to external stress, with its characteristic adreno-corticol response. Most significant stressors imply some degree of threat to the organism.

Spielberger (1976) makes an important distinction between threat as defined in terms of the objective properties of a situation (e.g. a life threatening situation) and threat as defined in terms of the individual's perception of the situation. Lazarus & Launier (1978) suggest that stress should not be defined in terms of either the situation or the person and his vulnerability, but rather as a transaction between the two: " ... stress is a particular relationship between the person and the environment that is appraised by the person as taxing his or her resources and endangering his or her well being".

Social factors

The role of life events and other social factors in the anxiety disorders has been less extensively investigated than for depression, possibly because the link is not so strong. In a community study, Finlay-Jones & Brown (1981) found that depressive symptoms tended to be linked with loss events, while the symptoms of anxiety were associated with events that implied some threat or harm in the future, for example hearing of a diagnosis of cancer in a close relative. Mixed pictures of anxiety and depression were associated with both types of events.

In the study of Prudo *et al* (1984) in the Outer Hebrides, where family life is relatively stable, the type of severe disruptive life events commonly found in inner city populations are relatively uncommon and so depression was less frequent. However rates for phobias and anxiety were high and symptoms were often chronic. Life events, particularly bereveavement (in 64% of the cases), tended to be associated with the onset of disorders, but there was little evidence that life events played any maintenance role.

Among clinical populations the evidence for an association between the onset of anxiety disorders and life events is stronger. Sheehan *et al*

(1981) found that 91% of a group of patients with anxiety disorders experienced either a major life event or physical illness in the six months prior to the onset of their anxiety disorder. Last *et al* (1984) reported the onset of anxiety in around one-third of their subjects started following either childbirth, miscarriage or hysterectomy, and in another third of cases it followed the death of a close relative. Panic disorder appears to be more specifically associated with medically related life events, serious illness in the subject, or serious illness and/or death in a close relative, and in most subjects the life events occurred in the month immediately prior to the onset of the panics (Faravelli, 1985).

Mortality

The suicide literature has tended to regard suicide as almost always stemming from depressive disorders with a consequent neglect of the anxiety disorders, but there is good evidence that anxiety, particularly panic disorder, has a raised mortality. Brill & Beebe (1955) followed a large cohort of US veterans diagnosed as having 'psychoneuroses' in 1944 and nine years later found a threefold increased risk of suicide. Sims (1973) traced 157 subjects admitted to hospital with a diagnosis of a neurosis, and some 12 years later found that 20 had died. There were eight possible and three definite suicides while the expected number was only six. However, in Barraclough's series of 100 completed suicides only three subjects had a primary diagnosis of an anxiety disorder (phobic neurosis) although anxiety symptoms were common in the weeks before the suicide: thus 60% looked anxious, 31% complained of anxiety, 34% were restless, and 24% were trembling (Barraclough *et al*, 1974).

Panic disorder appears to carry a raised mortality and probably accounts for most if not all of the raised mortality due to anxiety disorders. Thus Coryell *et al* (1982) traced the death certificates of 117 subjects who were admitted between 1925 and 1955 with panic disorder. Suicide was responsible for the death of around 20% of those with panic disorder, and 16% of those with major depression and the group as a whole had an increased mortality mainly due to cardiovascular disease. More recently Lepine *et al* (1993) found that 42% of the series of 100 consecutive out-patients with panic disorder had made a suicide attempt, and this was most common at around the time of onset of the panic disorder. Rates were higher (52%) for those who were also comorbid for other psychiatric disorders (mainly alcoholism, major depression and personality disorder) whereas only 17% of those with pure panic disorder had made suicide attempts.

Comorbidity

Anxiety disorders are the most common psychiatric disorders in the community (Robins, 1991) and they also appear frequently in clinical populations. Comorbidity with other disorders is the rule, rather than the exception, for example in the ECA, 60% of those with anxiety had more than one diagnosis. Wittchen *et al* (1986) found that 69% of a community sample and 95% of a clinical sample of subjects with an anxiety disorder had more than one diagnosis. Anxiety is the main motivating force for treatment-seeking behaviour for other disorders and this explains the high comorbidity rates.

Comorbidity with depression

Anxiety and depressive disorders are inextricably entangled. The word 'depression' covers a wide variety of states of misery: it describes a state of grief at loss; disappointment at failed aspiration; a pessimistic attitude of hopelessness and helplessness; a persisting trait of low self-esteem; demoralisation in the face of persistent adversity or chronic illness, as well as depressive illness. While the old 'endogenous–reactive' distinction has now been largely discarded, the so-called reactive depressions were thought to have more in the way of anxiety symptoms. More recently, at least in the American literature, the term 'atypical depressive disorder' has reappeared, and reactivity of mood, anxiety and other symptoms are said to characterise this disorder. Klein (1974) proposed that failure of the pleasure response, anhedonia, is one of the best clinical markers for depression disorder. Anxiety may be an accompanying feature of all these states, and may occur as a consequence of the depressed state. Conversely, depression (in the sense of demoralisation, helplessness and low self-esteem) may follow from any persisting anxiety disorder, but this will generally resolve if the anxiety disorder is successfully treated. Also both anxiety and depression may have a common origin in psychosocial, interpersonal or neurophysiological mechanisms. These comorbid associations of severe disorders should be distinguished from the milder ICD–10 category of 'mixed anxiety depression' as described previously (page 578).

Depressive states and anxiety states in the same individual may be separated in time. For example, anxiety symptoms may precede the onset of a depression and the anxiety may then subside as the depression intensifies; or anxiety states may commence in the setting of a depressive disorder and then persist as the depression resolves.

There is now some evidence that panic disorder and major depressive illness are related (Breier *et al*, 1985; Stavrakaki & Vargo, 1986), and one state may precede the other by many years or the two states may occur together. The Collaborative Study on Depression (Coryell *et al*, 1988) found that 22% of subjects with major depression also had panic disorder. Patients with the combined disorders had more severe ratings for most depressive symptoms, and there were increased rates for the agitated, endogenous, and melancholic subtypes. Family history data showed that the panic disorder was probably primary in 3.5% of the cases, as these subjects had positive family histories for anxiety disorders, with the depression being secondary. Patients with combined disorders were also less likely to have recovered from the index admission at one year, were more symptomatic at follow-up and had worse ratings of social function indicating that the combined condition was probably more severe than pure depression. Making the diagnosis of the combined disorder is clinically important because these patients will require more in the way of antidepressant treatment and psychotherapy.

Comorbidity with alcoholism

The notion that alcohol may help reduce anxiety dates back to antiquity. Hippocrates' (1886) wrote: "wine, drunk with an equal quantity of water puts away anxiety and terrors". Alcoholism and anxiety are both common disorders, and so some degree of comorbidity is to be expected, but the rates found in practice are considerably higher than those expected by chance. Prevalence studies indicate that around 40% of alcoholics display anxious or mixed anxiety/depressive symptoms (Weissman *et al*, 1985). Thus in a clinical sample of 102 hospitalised alcoholics 32% were phobic, 17% had agoraphobia and 24% had social phobia (Mullaney & Trippett, 1979). In another study 11 subjects (23%) had generalised anxiety disorder and 10 subjects (21%) had panic disorder and of these in six subjects the panic disorder preceded their alcoholism, but in four it developed following the alcoholism (Bowen *et al*, 1984). High rates of alcoholism are found in cohorts of subjects with agoraphobia and panic disorder; for example, Bibb & Chambless (1986) using the Michigan Alcohol Screening Test found 21% of their subjects were alcoholic. Men were more likely to have both diagnoses. Family studies with probands who have anxiety disorders, agoraphobia and panic also reveal increased rates of alcoholism among first-degree relatives.

Alcohol is used to decrease social tension and is widely used as an anxiolytic, and in clinical practice it may be important to try and work out whether alcoholism is the primary problem or alcohol is being used as an anxiolytic (or antidepressant), although this is not always possible. Schuckit & Monteiro (1988) suggested that the chronology of symptoms, that is which disorder came first, as well as the symptom pattern during periods of abstinence may provide useful clues. Kushnir *et al* (1990) suggests that if the anxiety disorder is either agoraphobia or social phobia, then the alcohol is probably a form of self-medication, while panic disorder or generalised anxiety disorder are more likely to follow on from pathological drinking. In either case both the drinking and anxiety disorder may require independent treatment. George *et al* (1990) point out that alcohol withdrawal and panic disorder have a common clinical picture (sweating, non-directed fear, palpitations, tremor, etc.) and a similar neurobiological mechanism involving the hippocampus in susceptible individuals and this may explain both the comorbidity and recurrent nature of the two disorders.

Comorbidity with personality disorders

At one time it was thought that the neurotic disorders and personality disorders were closely related and indeed Schneider made no distinction between the two (Mulder *et al*, 1991). In keeping with this, Roth *et al* (1972) described increased rates of dependency, immaturity and sensitivity to criticism, neuroticism and other personality traits among those with anxiety disorders as compared with depressed subjects. More recently, Tyrer (1989) has argued in favour of a combined 'general neurotic syndrome' which incorporates both the anxiety symptoms and certain personality traits.

However, the modern trend, particularly in the DSM–IV, has been to separate Axis I and Axis II disorders. Both should be diagnosed when they occur together, but the separation gives the opportunity for only one condition to be recorded if they occur separately. Although there is now a substantial literature, mainly on out-patient samples, applying DSM–III criteria for personality disorder to out-patients presenting with anxiety disorders the range of published figures, from 12% (Klass *et al*, 1989) up to 83% (Alnaes & Torgersen, 1990), is so wide as to make these figures almost meaningless.

In treating any anxiety disorder, it is useful to note whether there is any associated personality disorder because its presence may make therapy more difficult and may worsen the outcome (Tyrer *et al*, 1993). However, some recent studies have shown that both abnormal personality traits and personality disorders can improve following the successful treatment of a comorbid anxiety disorder, particularly obsessional disorder and agoraphobia (Baer *et al*, 1992).

Treatment

Patients with anxiety symptoms usually present with a wide spectrum of problems including relationship difficulties, and these may require separate attention. However, this section will focus more on describing methods that can help patients overcome their anxiety symptoms using specific anxiety management techniques. They are applicable to all the anxiety disorders.

There are many different types of psychological therapy for anxiety which have quite different theoretical bases, but all recognise that the interaction between the patient and the therapist is crucial. Jerome Frank (1971) noted that there were certain 'common therapeutic factors' on which a successful outcome of any psychotherapeutic technique depends and these were:

(1) An intense, emotionally charged confiding relationship with a helping person, often with the participation of a group.
(2) A rationale for the therapy which is compatible with the prevailing cultural view.
(3) Provision of new information concerning the nature of the patient's problems and ways for dealing with them.
(4) Faith in the therapist.
(5) Provision of success experiences which enhance the sense of self-mastery.
(6) The facilitation of emotional arousal, thereby learning to cope with strong emotion be it anxiety and/or depression.

As well as incorporating all the above elements most modern anxiety management techniques have four separate elements:

(1) Education on the nature of the problem and the proposed method of treatment.
(2) Eliciting negative thoughts, and then modifying the destructive patterns of thinking through cognitive restructuring. The lifestyle itself may need modifying as well.
(3) Introduction to techniques of self-mastery, e.g. relaxation, breathing exercises, distraction, specific anxiety control techniques, such as the rehearsal of cue words or images associated with control over anxiety.
(4) Exposure to the original anxiety where the newly acquired techniques can be practised and so enabling the anxiety to be mastered.

Making lifestyle changes

Although some patients with anxiety will describe obvious symptom-generating behaviours during their initial diagnostic interviews, in other cases these may only become apparent when the daily diary has been examined. The housewife who drinks endless cups of coffee may be unaware of the effect of caffeinism, similarly the financial dealer who panics each morning before the screen may have failed to make any connection between his panic attacks and his nightly drinking sessions. Another example is the worried executive who presents a diary showing a time-pressured and work-filled schedule in which every moment of the week and weekend is taken up with work or some work-related activity. Such anxious concerns may result in giving up hobbies or simple leisure and social activities such as gardening or playing a game of cards with friends. Often these apparently trivial activities, which had once given pleasure, may also have made subtle yet important contributions to a person's sense of worth and feelings of control over their environment as well as their sanity; restoration of these once pleasurable and other non-pressurised activities may be helpful.

Education

Anxiety forms a major part of the adaptive response to stress and anxious subjects are generally very receptive to new information, particularly with regard to anything which may help explain or reduce their anxiety levels. Education packages usually contain descriptions of the symptoms, their probable causes as well as details of the proposed treatment programmes. Anxiety management should be regarded as a skill which the therapist hopes to teach the patient rather than as a treatment which merely soothes the symptoms or as an explanation or interpretation which provides only an intellectual understanding of the complaint. As with any other skill it needs to be broken down into a number of simpler components, each of which can be easily learnt, and there should be practice between sessions (homework) so that gains made during the sessions may be consolidated. In some clinics, the education on the nature of the symptoms is given as a lecture to a group of patients or as a handout. However, it may be more helpful if the education is ongoing, with the relevant information being imparted during therapy as and when particular issues arise. Group methods are particularly useful in anxiety management because groups help decrease the sense of isolation which is common among anxious subjects. Also, the more assertive subjects may voice concerns that reticent members are reluctant to make.

Earlier anxiety management methods

One of the earliest specifically behavioural techniques was Wolpe's (1958) reciprocal inhibition of anxiety by systematic desensitisation. The subject is required to imagine a hierarchy of increasingly anxiety-provoking situations and to manage the anxiety that this generates by progressive muscular relaxation or light hypnosis. Suinn & Richardson (1971) developed an anxiety management programme in which subjects were taught to visualise a scene which aroused anxiety, a scene which reintegrated competency or success, and a scene which was associated with feelings of relaxation. They were then given a tape with instructions on it to switch between the three different types of scene. The technique has been modified and further developed as an anxiety control treatment (Snaith, 1991).

Frankl (1960)was probably the first to describe the method of parodoxical intention when the subject is deliberately encouraged to produce and even exaggerate his symptoms and so confront the anxiety. A medical student who had listened to Frankl's lecture would tremble every time the anatomy instructor entered the room. She said to herself before the anatomy lecture, "Oh, here is the instructor – now I will really show him what a good trembler I am". She said this thought to herself repeatedly so that when the lecturer finally entered the room she was quite unable to tremble. Malleson (1959) treated a student with severe examination nerves by instructing him to try and imagine that he was sitting the exam in the university examination hall and staring at the exam paper. He was then asked to try and experience as much anxiety as he possibly could, and not to push this anxiety away and repeat this exercise as often as possible. When it came to the day of the actual examination there were no anxiety symptoms.

While most of the early methods depended on the use of imagination, research studies have demonstrated that exposure to the anxiety *in vivo* is a rather more effective method of treatment. In recent years this has been combined with cognitive therapy, and present-day anxiety management programmes usually incorporate both cognitive and behavioural methods combined with exposure (Clarke, 1989).

Cognitive approaches

> Men are disturbed not by things but by the view that they take of them.   (Epictetus (Stoic philosopher) quoted in Ellis, 1962)

Eliciting the destructive thought patterns

The primary task is to work out in as much detail as possible precisely what the patient's belief system (negative thoughts) is concerning their anxiety. These congitions differ according to the underlying disorder. In panic disorder they are characterised by catastrophic misinterpretations of bodily sensations and cognitive therapy focuses specifically on these conditions. Generalised anxiety disorder is characterised by a rather wider range of anxiety-based cognitions.

A useful way to elicit negative thoughts is to engage in a detailed discussion of a recent emotional experience, or of a panic attack, and to ask the patient to recall these experiences (see also Chapter 6 for a description of cognitive therapy). For a panic attack questioning should focus on the particular sensations experienced at the time, as well as the thoughts accompanying the sensations. "Going over the panic attack, what was your worst moment?"; "What went through your mind at that point?"; "What did you think would happen to you?". During the calm of the session a patient might explain, "I had palpitations and sweating and I thought I was going to have a heart attack". The therapist tries to separate the sensations the patient experiences, from their interpretation of these feelings. Thus palpitations are a physical sensation, while the thought that these symptoms signify an imminent heart attack is but one of several possible (and incorrect) interpretations of these sensations. Although it would be fruitless to argue with the patient about the physical sensations the patient will usually be more prepared to discuss the interpretation placed upon these sensations. Another useful method to elicit a more detailed understanding of the negative thoughts is the use of the daily diary. An example is shown in Table 13.3, and this also shows how the strength of belief and anxiety levels may be rated.

Sometimes during a session the therapist may observe a sudden shift of mood when a particular topic is discussed. At this point it is sometimes helpful to ask the patient, "What passed through your mind just then?", to elicit the key morbid thought processes. More active techniques, such as role play or asking the patient to imagine an anxious scene may also help elicit automatic negative thoughts.

Rapee & Barlow (1991) suggest that anxious individuals tend to make two types of logical errors, they over-estimate the likelihood that an adverse event will occur, particularly to themselves, and, having decided that such an event will probably occur, they tend to overdramatise or catastrophise the consequences. Focusing on these two types of logical error is useful in cognitive restructuring.

Cognitive restructuring and modifying the negative thoughts

Rapee & Barlow (1991) highlight the importance of explaining at the outset what cognitive restructuring is to their patients and they offer the following explanation:

> the way we interpret and think about eventful situations determines our emotional reaction to it. Thus altering these interpretations or thoughts can change the resulting emotion. Cognitive restructuring is not the same as positive thinking. Positive thinking encourages us to look at life through rose coloured glasses and may be unrealistic. Cognitive restructuring encourages us to look at life in a realistic and rational manner. Sadness and anxiety are realistic emotions but they may not have to happen as frequently or intensely as you are currently experiencing them ...

Once the negative and automatic thoughts have been elicited, it is the therapist's task to engage the patient in a debate, and the skill of the therapist lies in the ability to somehow help the patient modify these negative thought patterns, and place a less catastrophic interpretation on their thoughts and feelings.

Clarke (1989) also lists 10 questions which can be used as opening strategies to engage anxious subjects in a debate on their negative thoughts.

(1) What is the evidence that I have for this thought? Is there any alternative way of looking at this situation? Is there an alternative

explanation? A patient expressed a fear of fainting during her panic attacks. Direct questioning revealed that she had never actually fainted but she interpreted the feeling of dizziness as the precursor to an inevitable fainting episode. A detailed discussion of all the symptoms and physiological changes that occur during a panic attack proved helpful to her.

(2) How would someone else think about the situation? Sometimes another person is able to reassure the patient that the situation is not as dangerous as they perceive it. The patient can be asked how they might counsel a friend who was experiencing a similar situation.

(3) Are your judgments based more on how you felt rather than what you actually did? Anxious subjects often believe they cannot cope with situations but direct questioning usually shows they cope extremely well and behave entirely appropriately.

(4) Aren't you setting yourself an unrealistic or unobtainable standard? Many anxious subjects tend to be perfectionists. Themes of over-control may underly such thoughts.

(5) Are you focusing on irrelevant items? Subjects with anxiety have a tendency to worry about trivia.

(6) Are you thinking in all or nothing terms? "If I cannot do a job perfectly it is not worth doing at all". "If people do not show they like me, then they dislike me". A useful strategy to counter such thinking is to introduce the concept of a dimension by producing

Table 13.3 Monitoring and practice form for cognitive modification

For each panic attack or anxious event this week, please describe your beliefs

Actual event (trigger)	Initial thought	Probability (0–100)	Consequence	Anxiety level (0–8)
Riding on a bus	I cannot get off	50	My heart will pound	6
	My heart will pound	80	I will have a heart attack	2
	I will have a heart attack	0		
Difficult examination	I will fail	10	I will be expelled	4
	I will be expelled	1	I will never have a job	2
	I will never have a job	0		

After Rapee & Barlow (1991)

a linear analogue scale with the patient's extreme positions at either end and asking the patient to place his belief somewhere on the continuum of the line. The assumptions are then gently probed and in later sessions the strength of the patient's beliefs are once more tested on the scale.

(7) Am I over-estimating how responsible I am for the way things work out? Am I over-estimating how much control I have over events? Some anxious subjects see themselves as responsible for all the ills that befall themselves or their families. Analysts use the word 'omnipotence' to describe this phenomenon, but the concept is also helpful in other types of treatment.

(8) What if it does happen, what would be so bad about that? Clarke (1989) recommends pushing subjects to think about the worst possible consequences of the specific events they dread so much, and imagine the worse possible scenario.

(9) How will things be in x months/years time? Asking patients to imagine the future is sometimes helpful when they are faced with some immediate situational crisis or anticipated loss or imminent breakup of a relationship. Things may not be quite as catastrophic as the patient makes out and life usually just carries on. However, if there is any associated depression, or despair, this may need to be addressed separately.

(10) Are you over-estimating how likely an event is to occur? As previously noted anxious patients believe that an adverse event is highly likely, for example a patient who was frightened of flying believed that if other people flew, there was only a remote chance of a crash, but if they themselves were on the aeroplane, a crash was a near certainty.

Behavioural experiments

Inducing panic attacks

Hyperventilation will cause panic or panic-like sensations in around 60% of susceptible subjects. Once patients are able to make the connection between symptoms induced by voluntary hyperventilation and their panic attacks they find it easier to discard their catastrophic interpretation of having a heart attack, suffocating or going insane. If during a therapy session, hyperventilation does lead on to a panic attack, the remainder of the session should be devoted to teaching breathing control. In this way a sense of control is restored to patients as they learn how to switch their symptoms on and off by the simple physiological manoeuvres of overbreathing and then breathing slowly.

Some patients are unable to adequately hyperventilate and in these cases the therapist hyperventilates together with the patient, or alternatively uses a tape which has instructions to breathe in and out every two seconds.

The technique of inducing panic attacks by hyperventilation is perhaps best reserved for younger patients and younger therapists, and is contra-indicated among those with chest or heart disease, epilepsy or during pregnancy. After a session of voluntary hyperventilation patients and therapists should not drive for at least 30 minutes.

Avoiding avoidance

Three types of avoidance behaviour occur in general anxiety. Most patients are anxious about social evaluative situations, such as talking in public, or eating or drinking in public. Around 20% have an agora-phobic type pattern, such as avoiding crowds, shopping or travelling on public transport, while a further 20% avoid activities which bring on the feared situation, such as exercise. Avoidance strategies are commonplace, such as clutching on to the wall to avoid fainting, or taking a pram when going out walking, etc. In all cases it is essential to try and get the patient to confront avoidant behaviour to and prevent it from becoming entrenched, but a certain amount of ingenuity may be required to devise ways to help the patient confront their own particular avoidance strategy.

Role play

Some patients describe a type of anxiety that occurs in a particular situation that can be re-enacted during the session.

> Francis was a 17-year-old student who was studying for her 'A' levels. She was very anxious when she came home from school and developed panic attacks. This was quite clearly related to her mother questioning her about her day at school, and criticising her if she obtained low marks, and this would make her anxious and reduce her to silence. At other times the mother would nag her or her father. After a few exploratory sessions, when a good rapport had developed, the therapist assumed the role of the mother and asked Francis to reply to any criticisms as vociferously as possible. In another session Francis, herself, had to play her hypercritical mother, while the therapist assumed the role of the patient. After three sessions Francis was able to laugh at both the therapist's impression of her mother and herself, as well as see the pointlessness of her distress at her mother's temperamental difficulties. Anxiety and panic attacks disappeared, although her mother's behaviour remained unchanged, her reaction to it was much diminished.

Role play is used particularly in the treatment of social anxiety and social phobia (see Chapter 14).

Prediction testing

Many patients with anxiety believe that frightening or humiliating things are likely to happen to them in everyday situations. It can be helpful for these patients to plan situations in which they can test out their prediction of impending disaster. For these patients, there may be no evidence of avoidance, and so a purely artificial situation may have to be devised to carry out the behavioural experiment.

Case example

> Raymond was a 25-year-old clerk whose anxiety symptoms were particularly bad if he thought people were looking at him. He did not avoid social situations and was a regular churchgoer. He was asked to imagine the most frightening situation for him, and replied that this would be to stand up at a meeting and talk, or stand on stage and address an audience. Underneath this fear about talking in public was the fear that he would stumble over his words and that the audience would then laugh at him. After some discussion it was agreed that a suitable target for him to aim for was to read the lesson in church. As an intermediate step he agreed to read to the smaller weekly bible reading class before attempting to read to the full church congregation. Both tasks were successfully accomplished and prediction testing in this way served to show him that the consequences of his worst fear did not happen.

Strategies to decrease the anxiety

Breathing exercises. The aim of breathing exercises is to produce slow smooth deep breathing and so prevent hyperventilation and excessive blowing off of carbon dioxide. This can be done by asking the patient to place their hand on the abdomen. Subjects should feel their abdomen going out during inspiration and in during expiration. If this is not the case diaphragmatic breathing is not being used and practice will be required to achieve it. Once diaphragmatic breathing is achieved the patient is taught to breathe more slowly by the therapist, e.g. five seconds to breathe in and five seconds to breathe out. This can also be done with a tape which has pacing instructions. An alternative method is to ask patients to breath in slowly through their nose keeping their mouth shut, and then to expire only through their mouth. Acquiring this skill is helpful because most patients learn that even such a simple manoeuvre as placing their hand on their abdomen may have a calming effect in the presence of prodromal panic symptoms. Once hyperventilation has occurred, rebreathing from a paper bag will rapidly help restore blood pCO_2 and reduce anxiety.

Relaxation training. Edmond Jacobson, the originator of progressive muscular relaxation, developed his methods over 40 years, and most present-day relaxation techniques are derived from his earlier methods. Although relaxation therapy is probably insufficient as a sole treatment for an anxiety disorder it may be usefully combined with other therapies. Acquiring the skill to relax may be particularly helpful for those with a lifelong tendency to anxiety.

The essential component of progressive muscular relaxation is for the subject to cultivate an ability to make sensitive observations on their own internal sensory world and recognise a subtle state of tension. To achieve control, the subject contrasts this state of tension with the state of eliminating tension – and this is the state of relaxation. A key point in Jacobson's method is that the subject does not actively try and relax, the process is rather more one of discontinuing tensing the muscles – perhaps analgous to switching the power off. Each muscle group is systematically contracted so that the learner can identify the unique tension sensation (the control signal) for that particular muscle group and then this tension is released to achieve the state of relaxation. The patient is taught to tense and relax each muscle group in turn and a full course of training in Jacobsen's day would have lasted 90 days. Jacobson (1938) soon observed the anxiety-reducing effect of muscular relaxation as his subjects were unable to engage in any mental processes or be at all emotional while simultaneously relaxing. Today much briefer schedules are used, but relaxation training may still take 8–12 sessions. These procedures are commonly taught to patients by occupational therapists often in groups, or by nursing staff with a particular interest in anxiety control techniques (for details see Clarke, 1989) and one set of instructions for progressive muscular relaxation is given in Appendix 1.

Flashcards. Some patients find that reading flashcards during a spell of anxiety or a panic attack can be helpful. Statements which the patient finds particularly reassuring should be elicited and they should be devised jointly with the therapist. One patient found the examples given below helpful:

(1) Anxiety is very unpleasant but if I wait it will pass.
(2) Breathing too fast worsens my symptoms.
(3) All my symptoms are typical of anxiety.

Distraction techniques

These are described by Fennell (1989) and are probably more useful in mild depression and anxiety than in the more severe states, and they depend on the subject having at least a modicum of concentration. Some patients are able to distract themselves by doing crosswords, playing sport, hobbies or getting absorbed in a TV programme or video. Housewives may sometimes report that certain activities which are not too demanding or complex such as ironing have a soothing effect, and should therefore be encouraged.

More contrived distraction techniques include trying to focus on an object, for example during a panic attack and then describing its shape, size and colour in one's mind. Another technique is teaching patients increased sensory awareness and instructing them to focus on their surroundings rather than their anxious preoccupations. This may entail thinking about the decor of the room, the shape of the furniture, the feel of their clothes, extraneous noises, and so forth. A few subjects are able to engage in mental exercises such as subtracting seven from 1000 repeatedly or thinking of animal names beginning with the first letter of the alphabet. Imagining pleasant situations may also help to distract, for example, imagining a nice holiday or winning the national lottery, but subjects who are too depressed may have difficulty recalling pleasant cognitions. A demonstration during a treatment session that distraction can modify or reduce anxiety can help to restore patients' sense of mastery over their anxiety as well as show the rapid effectiveness of simple psychological measures.

Drug treatments

Alcohol and opiates were the traditional remedies for anxiety for many hundreds of years, later to be replaced by the almost equally harmful bromides and barbiturates and more recently by the benzodiazepines. Almost all anxiolytic drugs have invariably also become substances of misuse and addiction as well.

Although the benzodiazepines are no longer recommended for the treatment of anxiety, epidemiological studies show they are still widely used. The 1979 National Household Survey in America showed that 11% of the adult population had taken an anxiolytic in the previous year, but a repeat survey in 1990 showed this figure had fallen to 1.3% (Juergens, 1993).

The benzodiazepines

The primary pharmacological effects of the benzodiazepines are related to their ability to potentiate γ-aminobutyric acid (GABA) and the $GABA_A$ receptors. GABA is widely distributed in the CNS and is an inhibitory neurotransmitter. GABA receptors are present in 30% of brain synapses and GABA probably influences a variety of systems via pre-synaptic inhibition at nerve terminals decreasing the release of neurotransmitters. There are probably specific benzodiazepine receptors in the CNS and, once activated, they increase the affinity of the GABA receptor for its ligand GABA. This, in turn, permits an increased flux of negative chloride ions through the cell membrane and results in hyperpolarisation of the cell and so inhibits its function.

Pharmacokinetics. Most benzodiazepines are rapidly absorbed, and diazepam is the most rapidly absorbed so it may have effects within minutes. They are rather more erratically absorbed when given by intramuscular injection. Benzodiazepines are mainly protein bound (to albumen) in plasma and they also have high lipid solubility and are therefore stored in brain and adipose tissue. The duration of the anxiolytic effect and the elimination half-life depends on the rate of release from adipose tissue back into plasma. Elimination is mainly via hepatic metabolism usually by acetyletion or conjugation, and it is of interest that slow acetylators may have an increased benzodiazepine elimination half-life. Renal excretion of unchanged drugs is negligible. Some metabolites, for example desmethyldiazepam, are clinically active and have a very long half-life. The elimination half-life depends partly on hepatic function but also on age, for example for diazepam this may be 20 hours in young adults but rises to over 40 hours for those over 65, and there is also very wide individual variation. Using a regular dose schedule, a steady state concentration may take 4–10 days to achieve. Differences in efficacy between the different benzodiazpenes depends on their lipid solubility, and breakdown metabolism. The different properties of the more commonly used benzodiazepines are shown in Table 13.4.

Effects and side-effects. The main clinical effects are as anxiolytics, sedatives or hypnotic drugs, and they are also anticonvulsants. Their principal side-effects relate to these actions and are sedation and psychomotor impairment, resulting in impaired driving skills or the ability to operate machinery safely. Less common side-effects include dry mouth, blurred vision, gastrointestinal upset, ataxia, headache and low blood pressure, restlessness and rashes. A more subtle effect on memory, particularly on the recall and recognition of items, has also been described, and the risks of their use in pregnancy are discussed in Chapter 21.

In comparison with most other drugs the benzodiazepines are relatively safe and there are few recorded fatalities of overdose of benzodiazepines when taken on their own. However, they interact with alcohol, possibly as alcohol competes for the same metabolic pathways in the liver, and the majority of recorded fatalities have been associated with the concomitant use of either alcohol or other CNS depressants. Much has been written about the ability of benzodiazepines to trigger rage reactions (Editorial, 1975) and these undoubtedly occur particularly among those with personality disorders; however, a recent review of the larger controlled epidemiological studies of the phenomenon showed that violent episodes were equally common (at around 1%) in control non-drug-taking populations (Deitch & Jennings, 1988).

Table 13.4 Pharmacokinetic characteristics of commonly used benzodiazepines

Benzodiazepine	Approximate dose clinically equivalent to diazepam 10 mg (mg)	Mean to peak concentration after oral administration (hours)	Mean elimination half-life (hours)
Chloridazepoxide	20	1.5	40–60
Diazepam	10	0.9	40–60
Oxazepam	20	2.3	8.5
Clorazepate	15	1.2	60
Lorazepam	1	1.9	14
Temazepam	15	2.5	15
Alprazolam	1	1–2	11

There is a wide range, particularly for the eliminiation half-life between individuals, and these figures are only an approximate guide.

Dependence.   The most serious adverse effects of the benzodiazepines are dependence and substance misuse. Tolerance, which is defined as the need to use increasing doses of a drug to achieve the same clinical effect, is common to all the benzodiazepines. It can occur after a single dose but normally takes a few days or two to three weeks to develop. Cross-tolerance occurs with alcohol, between the benzodiazepines and the barbiturates, as well as between different benzodiazepines. The adaptive changes that take place during the development of tolerance mean that if the drug is abruptly withdrawn, these adaptive changes act unopposed and this unopposed action causes the withdrawal syndrome. In this way drugs which cause tolerance may result in dependency, addiction and substance misuse.

Benzodiazepene withdrawal states.   For many years it was thought that the symptoms that followed on when a benzodiazepine was stopped reflected no more than a return of the patient's original anxiety. More recently it has become clear that there is a specific benzodiazepine withdrawal syndrome, and Petursson & Lader (1981) showed that withdrawal symptoms could occur after taking the drug for as little as six weeks. The withdrawal symptoms are of two types, more general anxiety symptoms and some more specific sensory symptoms (Box 13.8). The onset is usually 1–10 days after stopping the drug or dosage reduction and the withdrawal state usually lasts 5–25 days but may last up to 12 weeks. More severe withdrawal states occur with drugs that have shorter half-lives, such as lorazepam and triazolam.

Management.   The management of withdrawal states usually entails switching from a drug with a short half-life to one with a longer half-life, such as switching from lorazepam to diazepam, and this is accomplished slowly over a period of weeks and then the diazepam is gradually tapered off. During the period of withdrawal there should be adequate psychological support and the withdrawal should always be supervised because sometimes a severe depression may supervene. Some patients find anxiety management or group support helpful during drug withdrawal. There are reports that clonidine, propranolol, carbamazepine and tricyclic antidepressants may reduce the severity of withdrawal symptoms, but in practice experience with these drugs is often disappointing. Most patients who have decided to come off one drug are a little wary of starting another one.

The use of benzodiazepines in the anxiety disorders. The high rates of drug dependence as well as recent legal actions directed against the drug companies which manufactured the benzodiazepines has led to a sharp decline in their use. These drugs should be prescribed only under special circumstances. The Committee of Safety of Medicine, and the Royal College of Psychiatrists (Priest & Montgomery, 1988) have issued guidelines, which essentially recommend that benzodiazepines should only be used in the treatment of anxiety for short periods, e.g. for no more than 2–4 weeks at a time, and then only for severe anxiety. At one time, even relatively mild anxiety states associated with the problems of everyday living were treated with benzodiazepines (usually diazepam or chordiazepoxide) and up to three million people in the UK were taking one or another drug of this group. Even now a large numbers of patients continue to take benzodiazepines, but how many take them for anxiety and how many are simply addicted is unknown.

Recent placebo-controlled studies have shown that benzodiazepines are effective in the more severe anxiety disorders such as GAD (DSM–III–R criteria). Rickels *et al* (1993) showed that 66% of those treated with diazepam (26 mg daily) responded compared with only 47% in the placebo group. Diazepam was the most effective drug in the first two weeks of the trial. It should be noted, however, that in the same trial imipramine 150 mg led to a response rate of 73%. Barlow (1988), reviewing a series of older studies, concluded that benzodiazepines had a relatively small effect in anxiety states and reduced scores on the Hamilton Anxiety Scale by only 3.7 units or about 10%, and their use is virtually precluded because of the risks of dependence as the anxiety disorders are chronic illnesses.

Tricyclic antidepressants

Tricyclic antidepressants are probably the drug of choice for both panic disorder and GAD. Although much of the earlier literature, for example Klein (1964), focused on the specific effect of small doses of imipramine

---

Box 13.8 Specific and non-specific symptoms of benzo-diazepine withdrawal syndromes

Specific symptoms (but uncommon)
Increased intensity of sensations
Hyperacusis, tinnitus
Photophobia
Blurred vision
Abnormal perception of motion
Muscle twitching
Hyperreflexia
Depression
Confusion
Psychosis
Seizures
Delirium

Non-specific symptoms (common)
Anxiety
Insomnia
Irritability
Nausea
Palpitations
Headache and muscle tension
Tremor

(30 mg) in panic disorder, more recent studies have shown that GAD responds quite well at doses of 75–150 mg imipramine. Almost all studies have shown that tricyclics are superior to placebo. The antipanic effect normally only appears in the third week, and the main reasons for failure are premature cessation and inadequate dosage, and patients who have no antipanic effects in the lower dose ranges should have their dosage increased to 150–200 mg daily.

A recent large scale and longitudinal study of panic disorder which compared alprazolam (mean dosage 5.7 mg), imipramine (mean dosage 175 mg daily), and placebo showed that alprazolam and imipramine were equally effective in producing a panic-free state (Schweiger *et al*, 1993). During a six-month maintenance phase in this study, there was no tendency to increase drug dosage for either drug, nor was there any other evidence of tolerance. However, during the drug taper phase a withdrawal syndrome occurred in almost all the patients on alprazolam but only in a few subjects on imipramine, and around one-third of the alprazolam-treated group were unable to come off medication. One year later 85% of the subjects were free of panic attacks although 55% were still taking medication.

Some patients, particularly those with pure panic disorder (those without depression) are very sensitive to even low doses of tricyclic antidepressants and because of this it is best to start with imipramine 10 mg nocte and then slowly titrate the dose upwards. Caetano (1985) suggests that panic disorder patients are particularly sensitive to clomipramine and in his study the mean dosage of clomipramine was only 26.4 mg. Patients with generalised anxiety disorder appear to require higher doses (in the 100–150 mg range). A small number of patients, around 15%, seem to get worse on imipramine. They develop insomnia and increased agitation and tolerate tricyclics poorly and they should be switched to other medications. Antidepressants may also be helpful when the predominant disorder is one of mixed anxiety/depression.

Selective serotonin reuptake inhibitors

There are few published studies of the SSRIs in the anxiety disorders, but they are probably effective and almost certainly are widely used. A recent trial by Black *et al* (1993) showed that fluvoxamine was an effective treatment for panic disorder. In this study, 57% of patients receiving fluvoxamine were rated as improved, compared with only 40% of those treated with cognitive therapy, and 22% on placebo. A comparison of paroxetine 20–60 mg with placebo in patients with panic disorder, in which both treatment groups received standard cognitive–behavioural therapy, showed a definite advantage for paroxetine. Thus a reduction to one or zero panics was achieved in 36% of the paroxetine-treated group, but only 16% among the placebo group, although the beneficial effect of treatments were only statistically significant after 12 weeks (Oehrberg *et al*, 1995).

Beta-blockers

Propranolol was introduced as a non-addictive alternative to the benzodiazepines in the management of anxiety. Granville-Grossman & Turner (1966) showed that in doses of up to 80 mg daily, it was an effective treatment for the autonomic but not for the psychological symptoms of anxiety. Other controlled studies have confirmed these findings but propranolol is probably less effective than the benzodiazepines. Noyes *et al* (1984) studied patients with panic disorder and agoraphobia and compared diazepam 30 mg with propranolol 240 mg daily, and found that 86% of the diazepam-treated group improved compared with only 33% of those receiving propranolol. Propanolol is ineffective in lactate-induced panic (Gorman *et al*, 1983). Although propranolol has been widely advocated, its efficacy in the more severe DSM–IV disorders such as GAD and panic disorder is questionable. Stern & Drummond (1991) suggest that beta-blockers may be particularly helpful for the somatic symptoms of tremor, palpitations and diarrhoea. There is also a suggestion that it may be helpful in performance anxiety of the stage fright type, for example for performing musicians (James *et al,* 1977), but it is uncertain whether this relates to its anxiolytic or anti-tremor actions.

Beta-blockers must be used with caution in patients with congestive heart failure, asthma and in diabetics on oral hypoglycaemics or others prone to hypoglycaemia, as they inhibit gluconeogenesis. At low doses they tend not to cause bradycardia, but if higher doses are used, pulse and blood pressure should be monitored for bradycardia and hypotension. Beta-blockers should be tapered off slowly to prevent rebound anxiety or if the drop is from high doses to prevent rebound hypertension. Their main side-effects are gastro-intestinal, including nausea, abdominal distension, diarrhoea, and constipation. CNS side-effects include dizziness, insomnia, fatigue, and if beta-blockers are used in very high doses (2000 mg daily) delirium has been reported. Their most troublesome side-effect is depressed mood and this appears to be common.

Buspirone

Buspirone is a relatively new drug and is an azaspirodecanedione and therefore not a benzodiazepene. It has no anticonvulsant, sedative, muscle relaxant or alcohol interactive properties, and acts as an agonist to $5HT_1$ receptors. These receptors are found among the serotonergic neurones of the raphe nuclei and stimulation of these receptors reduces the firing rate for the serotonergic neurones. Its action is delayed, often taking up to three weeks to appear but it may be effective in some patients with GAD.

Monoamine oxidase inhibitors.

At one time these drugs were extensively used in the treatment of phobias, particularly agoraphobia, as well as in syndromes of the mixed anxiety/depressive type, such as atypical depressive disorder, and they are described in Chapter 4. The advent of the selective serotonin reuptake inhibitors, which do not have any dietary restrictions, has largely displaced the use of these drugs, in anxiety as well as depression.

Combined drug and psychological approaches

Most patients presenting with an anxiety disorder require a combination of treatment approaches, usually with the doctor managing the pharmacotherapy and a psychologist, occupational therapist or nurse undertaking the cognitive therapy or anxiety management. There are few comparative studies of the relative merits of the different treatments. Johnstone *et al* (1980) examined a heterogenous group of out-patients with anxiety and milder depression and found that most patients improved, and only the tricyclic proved to be marginally superior to placebo. Tyrer *et al* (1988) conducted a randomised control trial of cognitive therapy, dothiepin, diazepam and a self-help group, among patients with DSM–III–R GAD, panic disorder and dysthymia and found little difference between the three treatments, although diazepam was marginally worse than the other treatments.

Anxiety management techniques should be taught to all patients but many indivdiuals cannot sustain a course of behavioural therapy, or lack the fortitude to expose themselves to feared situations. Drugs may be particularly helpful in panic disorder where up to 85% of patients respond (Klein, 1985) whereas cognitive–behavioural psychotherapy for panic disorder is not an easy treatment to conduct. A recent study has shown that the majority (93%) of patients with anxiety disorders eventually end up on medication (Evans *et al*, 1988).

Aveline (1991), a psychotherapist, remarks that the psychiatrist should not neglect speedy biological remedies when they are indicated, but the overall aim should always be to help the patient manage his life better without recourse to medication.

Appendix 1: Progressive muscular relaxation training

The procedure begins with an explanation to the patient of the value of relaxation and it is helpful if the relaxation training takes place in a quiet room. In some cases the patient is asked to sit in a comfortable chair with armrests and a headrest and foot stool, but in many departments the patient lies on the floor on a mattress. After a brief introduction the relaxation instructions begin:

"Settle back in the chair as comfortably as you can and we shall start with relaxation of your arms ... This begins with a contraction of the right biceps muscle. Hold the contraction of the biceps for a few moments now until I tell you to stop (about seven seconds). Now relax the biceps by gradually straightening out your arm and resting it on the armrest of the chair ... Now focus on the feelings of relaxation in that muscle ... Try to think of your right biceps and nothing else for the moment (about fifteen seconds). Next I want you to contract your forearm muscles. Do this by making a fist with your right hand and holding it until I tell you to stop (about seven seconds). Now let your fingers gradually straighten out and rest your hand over the armrest of the chair ... Focus now on the feeling of relaxation on your forearm and hand (about 15 seconds). Now I am going to repeat these exercises in the same way for the other arm so that both arms become completely relaxed (repeat as above for the left arm)".

The therapist then asks the patient to alternately tense and relax the scalp muscles, eye lids, jaw muscles, muscles at the back of their neck, their chest and abdomen (tummy muscles), thighs, calves, etc. The session usually ends with asking the patient to relax their whole body

"... I am going to assist you in this. I am going to name each of the parts we have just relaxed but instead of contracting them just make sure you are not contracting them and relax them. Now check that you are taking nice slow easy breaths and that your abdomen is completely relaxed. Now check that the muscles at the top of your leg are relaxed, your right calf, etc."

At the end of the instructions the patient is told the training exercises are over and they are instructed to remain relaxed for a further five minutes. Patients often report they feel sleepy but it is not the aim of relaxation therapy to induce sleep unless it is being used as a treatment for insomnia. At the end of the session the patient is given a tape recording of the session that they have attended and is then asked to play it at home each day for two weeks to practice relaxation before attending for their next appointment (after Stern & Drummond, 1991).

References

Ainsworth, M. (1969) Object relations dependency and attachment. A theoretical review of the mother infant relationship. *Child Development*, **40**, 969–1025.

Alnaes, R. & Torgersen, S. (1990) DSM–III personality disorders among patients with major depression, anxiety disorders and mixed conditions. *Journal of Nervous and Mental Disease*, **178**, 693–698.

American Psychiatric Association (1952) *Diagnostic and Statistical Manual of Mental Disorders* (1st edn) (DSM–I). Washington, DC: APA.

—— (1968) *Diagnositc and Statistical Manual of Mental Disorders* (2nd edn) (DSM–II). Washington, DC: APA.

—— (1980) *Diagnostic and Statistical Manual of Mental Disorders* (3rd edn) (DSM–III). Washington, DC: APA.

—— (1987) *Diagnostic and Statistical Manual of Mental Disorders* (3rd edn, revised) (DSM–III–R). Washington, DC: APA.

—— (1994) *Diagnositc and Statistical Manual of Mental Disorders* (4th edn) (DSM–IV). Washington, DC: APA.

Andrews, G. (1991) Anxiety, personality and anxiety disorders. *International Review of Psychiatry*, **3**, 293–302.

——, Stewart, G. W., Allen, R., *et al* (1990) The genetics of six neurotic disorders: a twin study. *Journal of Affective Disorders*, **19**, 23–29.

Aveline, M. (1991) Anxiety and stress related disorders. In *Textbook of Psychotherapy in Psychiatric Practice* (ed. J. Holmes), pp. 239–264. Edinburgh: Churchill Livingstone.

Baer, L., Jenike, M. A., Black, D. W., *et al* (1992) Effect of axis II diagnoses in treatment outcomes with clomipramine in 55 patients with obsessive compulsive disorder. *Archives of General Psychiatry*, **49**, 862–866.

Barlow, D. H. (1988) Generalised anxiety disorder. In *Anxiety and its Disorders* (ed. D.H. Barlow), pp. 566–597. New York: Guilford Press.

—— (1991) Disorders of emotion. *Psychological Inquiry*, **2**, 58–105.

Barraclough, B., Bunch, J., Nelson, B., *et al* (1974) A hundred cases of suicide: clinical aspects. *British Journal of Psychiatry*, **125**, 355–373.

Bass, C. & Gardner, W. (1985) Emotional influences on breathing and breathlessness. *Journal of Psychosomatic Research*, **29**, 599–609.

Bayer, R. & Spitzer, R. L. (1985) Neurosis, psychodynamics and DSM–III; a history of the controversy. *Archives of General Psychiatry*, **42**, 187–196.

Beard, G. (1869) Neurasthenia or nervous exhaustion. *Boston Medical and Surgical Journal*, **80**, 217–221.

Bibb, J. L. & Chambless, D. L. (1986) Alcohol use and abuse among diagnosed agoraphobics. *Behaviour Research and Therapy*, **24**, 49–58.

Black, D. W., Wesher, R., Bowers, W., *et al* (1993) A comparison of fluvoxamine, cognitive therapy and placebo in the treatment of panic disorder. *Archives of General Psychiatry*, **50**, 44–50.

Bland, R. C., Newman, S. C. & Orn, H. (1988) Period prevalence of psychiatric disorders. *Acta Psychiatrica Scandanavica*, **77** (suppl. 338), 43–49.

Boulenger, J. P., Patel, J. & Marangos, P. J. (1982) Effects of caffeine and theophylline on adenosine and benzodiazepine receptors in human brain. *Neuroscience Letters*, **30**, 161–166.

Bowen, R. C., Cipwayk, C. N., D'Arcy, C., *et al* (1984) Alcoholism, anxiety disorders and agoraphobia. *Alcoholism: Clinical and Experimental Research*, **8**, 48–50.

Bowlby, J. (1969) Attachment. In *Attachment and Loss*, Vol. 1. London: Hogarth Press.

Breier, A., Charney, D. & Heninger, G. R. (1985) The diagnostic validity of anxiety disorders and their relationship to depressive illness. *American Journal of Psychiatry*, **142**, 787–797.

Brill, N. & Beebe, G. (1955) *A Follow-Up Study of War Neurosis*. Veterans Administration Medical Monograph. Washington, DC:Veterans Administration.

Brooks, D. N. & McKinlay, W. (1983) Personality behavioural change after severe blunt head injury, a relative's view. *Journal of Neurology, Neurosurgery and Psychiatry*, **46**, 336–344.

Caetano, D. (1985) Treatment for panic disorders with clomipramine (Anafranil): An open study of 22 cases. Ciba-Geigy reprint. *Journal Brasileiro de Psiquiatria*, **34**, 125–132.

Centres For Disease Control (1988) Health status of Vietnam veterans psychosocial characteristics. *Journal of the American Medical Association*, **249**, 2701–2707.

Charney, D.S., Heninger, G.R. & Breier, A. (1984*a*) Noradrenergic function in panic anxiety: Effects of yohimbine in healthy subjects and patients with agoraphobia and panic disorder. *Archives of General Psychiatry*, **41**, 751–763.

——, Galloway, M. P. & Heninger, G. R. (1984*b*) The effects of caffeine on plasma MHPG, subjective anxiety, autonomic symptoms and blood pressure in healthy humans. *Life Sciences*, **35**, 135–144.

——, Woods, S. W., Price, L. H., *et al* (1990) Noradrenergic dysregulation in panic disorder. In *Neurobiology of Panic Disorder* (ed. J. C. Ballenger). New York: Wiley.

Clarke, D. (1989) Anxiety States. In *Cognitive Behaviour Therapy for Psychiatric Problems* (eds K. Hawton, P. Salkovskis, J. Kirk, *et al*), pp. 52–96. Oxford: Oxford University Press.

Coryell, W., Endicott, J., Andreasen, N. C., *et al* (1988) Depression and panic attacks: The significance of overlap as reflected in follow-up and family study data. *American Journal of Psychiatry*, **145**, 293–300.

——, Noyes, R. & Clancy, J. (1982) Excess mortality in panic disorder: a comparison with primary unipolar depression. *Archives of General Psychiatry*, **39**, 701–703.

Crowe, R. R., Noyes, R., Pauls, D., *et al* (1983) A family study of panic disorder. *Archives of General Psychiatry*, **40**, 1065–1069.

Cullen, W. (1784) *First Lines in the Practice of Physic*. Edinburgh: Elliott.

Da Costa, J. M. (1871) On irritable heart: a clinical study of a functional cardiac disorder and its consequences. *American Journal of Medical Science*, **61**, 17–52.

Davidson, J., Schwartz, M., Storck, M., *et al* (1985) A diagnostic and family study of posttraumatic stress disorder. *American Journal of Psychiatry*, **142**, 90–93.

Davidson, J. R. T., Smith, K. D. & Kadler, H. S. (1989) Validity and reliability of the DSM–III criteria for posttraumatic stress disorder. Experiences with a structural interview. *Journal of Nervous and Mental Disorders*, **177**, 336–341.

Dean, C., Surtees, P. G. & Sashidharan, S. P. (1983) Comparison of research diagnostic systems in an Edinburgh community sample. *British Journal of Psychiatry*, **142**, 247–256.

Deitch, J. T. & Jennings, R. K. (1988) Aggressive dyscontrol in patients treated with benzodiazepines. *Journal of Clinical Psychiatry*, **49**, 184–188.

Dinardo, P. A., O'Brien, G. T., Barlow, D. H., *et al* (1983) Reliability of DSM–III anxiety disorder categories using a new structured interview. *Archives of General Psychiatry*, **40**, 1070–1075.

Duncan-Jones, P. (1987) Modelling the aetiology of neurosis: Long-term and short-term factors. In *Psychiatric Epidemiology: Progress and Prospects* (ed. B. Cooper). London: Croom Helm.

Editorial (1975) Tranquillizers causing aggression. *British Medical Journal*, *i*, 113–114.

Ellis, A. (1962) *Reason and Emotion in Psychotherapy*. New York: Lyle Stuart.

Endler, N. S. & Magnusson, D. (1976) Towards an interactional psychology of personality. *Psychological Bulletin*, **83**, 956–974.

Evans, L., Opie, T. P. S. & Hoey, H. (1988) Prescribing patterns in agoraphobia with panic attacks. *Medical Journal of Australia*, **148**, 74–77.

Eysenck, H. J. (1959) *The Maudsley Personality Inventory*. London: University of London Press.

Faravelli, C. (1985) Life events preceding the onset of panic disorder. *Journal of Affective Disorders*, **9**, 103–105.

Fennell, M. (1989) Depression. In *Cognitive Behaviour Therapy for Psychiatric Problems* (eds K. Hawton, P. Salkowskis, J. Kirk, *et al*), pp. 169–234. Oxford: Oxford University Press.

Figley, C. R. (1985) Traumatic stress: the role of the family and social support system. In *Trauma and its Wake. The Study of Post-Traumatic Stress Disorder* (ed. C. R. Figley), pp. 39–56. New York: Brunner/Mazel.

Finlay-Jones, R. & Brown, G. W. (1981) Types of stressful life event and the onset of anxiety and depressive disorders. *Psychological Medicine*, **11**, 803–815.

Floderns-Myrhed, B., Pederson, N. & Rasmuson, I. (1980) Assessment of heritability for personality. Based on a short form of the Eysenck Personality Inventory: A study of 12,898 twin pairs. *Behaviour Genetics*, **10**, 153–162.

Frank, J. D. (1971) Therapeutic factors in psychotherapy. *American Journal of Psychotherapy*, **25**, 350–361.

Frankl, V. E. (1960) Paradoxical intention: a logotherapeutic technique. *American Journal of Psychotherapy*, **4**, 520–535.

Freedman, R. R., Ianni, P., Ettedgui, E., *et al* (1984) Psychophysiological factors in panic disorder. *Psychopathology*, **17** (suppl. 1), 66–73.

Freud, S. (1895) On the grounds for detaching a particular syndrome from neurasthenia as anxiety neurosis. In *Complete Psychological Works*, Vol. 3 (trans. J. Strachey). London: Hogarth Press (1962).

—— (1933) *New Introductory Lectures on Psychoanalysis*. New York: Norton.

Friedman., M. J. (1994) Biological and pharmacological aspects of the treatment of PTSD. In *Handbook of Post-traumatic Stress Disorder Therapy* (eds. M. Williams, M. Sommer, M. Westport), pp. 495–509. West Port, CT: Greenwood Press.

George, D. T., Nutt, D. J., Dwyer, B. A., *et al* (1990) Alcoholism and panic disorder: is the comorbidity more than coincidence? *Acta Psychiatrica Scandinavica*, **81**, 97–107.

Georget, E. J. (1840) Neuroses. In *Dictionnaire de Medicine*, Vol. XXV, pp. 27–41. Paris: Bechet.

Gorman, J. M., Leroy, S. F., Liebowitz, M. R., *et al* (1983) Effect of acute beta-adrenergic blockade on lactate induced panic. *Archives of General Psychiatry*, **40**, 1079–1082.

Granville-Grossman, K. L. & Turner, P. (1966) The effect of propranolol on anxiety. *Lancet*, *i*, 788–790.

Gray, J. A. (1981) Anxiety as a paradigm case of emotion. *British Medical Bulletin*, **37**, 193–197.

—— (1982) The neuropsychology of anxiety: an enquiry into the functions of the septohippocampal system. Oxford: Oxford University Press.

Hamilton, M. (1959) The assessment of anxiety states by rating scale. *British Journal of Medical Psychology*, **32**, 50–55.

Hippocrates (1886) Aphorisms. Vii, 56. In *The Works of Hippocrates*. New York: William Word.

Hoehn-Saric, R. & McLeod, D. R. (1988) Panic and generalised anxiety disorders. In *Handbook of Anxiety Disorders* (eds C.G. Last & M. Hersen), pp. 109–127. New York: Pergammon Press.

Holmes, J. (1993) Attachment theory: a biological basis for psychotherapy. *British Journal of Psychiatry*, **163**, 430–438.

Horowitz, M. J. (1986) General treatment principles. In *Stress Response Syndrome* (2nd edn), pp. 111–146. Northvale, NY: Jason Aronson.

——, Wilmer, N. & Alvarez, W. (1979) Impact of events scale: A measure of subjective stress. *Psychosomatic Stress*, **41**, 209–218.

Horney, K. (1937) *The Neurotic Personality of Our Time*. New York: Norton.

Hunter, R. & Macalpine, I. (eds) (1963) William Cullen. In *Three Hundred Years of Psychiatry 1535–1860*, pp. 473–479. London: Oxford University Press.

Ingham, J. G. (1966) Changes in MPI scores of neurotic patients: a three year follow up. *British Journal of Psychiatry*, **112**, 931–939.

Jackson, J. H. (1881) On right or left-sided spasms at the onset of epileptic paroxysms and on crude sensation warnings and elaborate mental states. *Brain*, **3**, 192–197.

Jacob, R. G. & Rapport, M. D. (1984) Panic disorder. In *Behavioural Theories and Treatment of Anxiety* (ed. S. M. Turner). New York: Plenum.

Jacobson, E. (1938) *Progressive Relaxation*. Chicago: University of Chicago Press.

James, I. M., Pearson, R. M., Griffith, D. N. W., *et al* (1977) Effect of oxprenolol on stage fright in musicians. *Lancet, ii,* 952–954.

Jardine, R., Martin, N. G. & Henderson, A. S. (1984) Genetic covariation between neuroticism and the symptoms of anxiety and depression. *Genetic Epidemiology,* 1, 89–107.

Johnson, J. H. & Sarason, I. G. (1978) Life stress, depression and anxiety: Internal–external control as a moderator variable. *Journal of Psychosomatic Research,* 22, 205–208.

Johnstone, E. C., Owens, D. G. C., Frith, C. D., *et al* (1980) Neurotic illness and its response to anxiolytic and antidepressant treatment. *Psychological Medicine,* 10, 321–328.

Juergens, S. M. (1993) Benzodiazepines and addiction. *Psychiatric Clinics of North America,* 16, 75–86.

Kardiner, A. (1941) The traumatic neurosis of war. *Psychological Medicine Monograph* (I–II). Washington, DC: National Research Council.

Keane, T. M. Fairbank, J. M., Cadell, R. T., *et al* (1989) Clinical evaluation of a measure to assess combat exposure. *Journal of Consulting and Clinical Psychology,* 1, 53–55.

Keenan, D. (1989) The Law of Torts. In *Smith and Keenan's English Law* (9th edn) (ed. D. Keenan), pp. 340–420. London: Pitman.

Kendler, K. S., Heath, A., Martin, N. G., *et al* (1986) Symptoms of anxiety and depression in a volunteer twin population: The aetiologic role of genetic and environmental factors. *Archives of General Psychiatry,* 43, 213–221.

Kilpatrick, D. G. & Resnick, H. S. (1993) Post-traumatic stress disorder associated with exposure to criminal victimization in a clinical and a community population. In *Post-traumatic Stress Disorder Dsm–IV and Beyond* (eds J. Davidson & E. B. Foa), pp. 113–146. Washington, DC: American Psychiatric Association.

Klass, E. T., Dinardo, P. A. & Barlow, D. H. (1989) DSM–III–R personality diagnoses in anxiety disorder patients. *Comprehensive Psychiatry,* 30, 251–258.

Klein, D. F. (1964) Delineation of two drug responsive anxiety syndromes. *Psychopharmacologia,* 5, 397–408.

—— (1974) Endeogenomorphic depression. *Archives of General Psychiatry,* 31, 447–454.

Kulka, R. A., Schlenger, W. E., Fairbank, R. L., *et al* (1990) *Trauma and the Vietnam War Generation: Report of findings from the National Vietnam Veterans Readjustment Study.* New York: Brunner Mazel.

Kushnir, M. G., Sher, K. J. & Beitman, B. D. (1990) The relation between alcohol problems and the anxiety disorders. *American Journal of Psychiatry,* 147, 685–695.

Langer, R. (1987) Post-traumatic stress disorder in former POWs. In *Post-traumatic Stress Disorders: A Handbook for Clinicians* (ed. T. Williams), pp. 35–51. Cincinnati, OH: Disabled American Veterans.

Last, C. G., Barlow, D. H. & O'Brien, G. T. (1984) Precipitants of agoraphobia: role of stressful life events. *Psychological Reports,* 54, 567–570.

Lazarus, R. S. & Launier, R. (1978) Stress related transactions between person and environment. In *Perspectives in Interactional Psychology* (eds L. A. Pervin & M. Lewis), pp. 287–327. New York: Plenum.

—— & Faulkmann, S. (1984) *Stress, Appraisal and Coping*. New York: Springer.

Lepine, J. P., Chignon, J. M. & Teherani, M. (1993) Suicide attempts in patients with panic disorder. *Archives of General Psychiatry*, **50**, 144–149.

Lewis, A. (1970) The ambiguous word 'anxiety'. *International Journal of Psychiatry*, **9**, 62–79.

Liebowitz, M. R., Fyer, A. J., Gorman, J. M., *et al* (1984) Lactate provocation of panic attacks. I: Clinical and behavioural findings. *Archives of General Psychiatry*, **41**, 764–770.

McDougle, C. S., Southwick, R., St James, S., *et al* (1990) An open trial of fluoxetine. *PTSD Research Quarterly*, **1**, 7.

McNair, D., Law, M. & Droppleman, L. (1987) *The Profile of Mood States*. Windsor: NFER–Nelson.

Malleson, N. (1959) Panic and phobia. *Lancet*, *i*, 225–227.

Marks, I. & Matthews, A. M. (1979) Brief standard self-rating for phobic patients. *Behaviour Research and Therapy*, **17**, 263–267.

Mulder, R. T., Sellman, J. D. & Joyce, P. R. (1991) The comorbidity of anxiety disorders with depressive alcohol and drug disorders. *International Review of Psychiatry*, **3**, 253–263.

Mullaney, J. A. & Trippett, C. J. (1979) Alcohol dependance and phobias: Clinical description. *British Journal of Psychiatry*, **135**, 565–573.

Norton, G. R., Harrison, B., Hauch, J., *et al* (1985) Characteristics of people with infrequent panic attacks. *Journal of Abnormal Psychology*, **94**, 216–221.

——, Dorward, J. & Cox, B. J. (1986) Factors associated with panic attacks in non-clinical subjects. *Behaviour Therapy*, **17**, 239–252.

Noyes, H. V., Clancy, J., Crowe, R., *et al* (1978) The familial prevalence of anxiety neurosis. *Archives of General Psychiatry*, **35**, 1057–1074.

Noyes, R., Jr., Anderson, D. J., Clancy, J., *et al* (1984) Diazepam and propranolol in panic disorder and agoraphobia. *Archives of General Psychiatry*, **41**, 287–292.

——, Clarkson, C. R., Crowe, R. R., *et al* (1987) A family study of generalized anxiety disorder. *Archives of General Psychiatry*, **43**, 227–232.

Nutt, D. J. & Lawson, C. (1992) Panic attacks. A neurochemical overview of models and mechanisms. *British Journal of Psychiatry*, **160**, 165–178.

Oehrberg, S., Christiansen, P., Behtkek, *et al* (1995) Paroxetine in the treatment of panic disorder. A randomised double blind controlled study. *British Journal of Psychiatry*, **167**, 374–379.

Oppenheimer, B. S. & Rothschild, M. A. (1918) The psychoneurotic factor in the "irritable heart" of soldiers. *British Medical Journal*, *ii*, 29–31.

Oxford English Dictionary (1989) Second Edition. Oxford: Clarendon Press.

Papez, J. W. (1937) A proposed mechanism of emotion. *Annals of Neurology and Psychiatry*, **38**, 725–743.

Petursson, H. & Lader, M. H. (1981) Benzodiazepine dependence. *British Journal of Addiction*, **76**, 133–145.

Piotrowski, Z. (1957) Quoted in *Psychiatric Dictionary* (5th edn) (ed. R. J. Campbell). London: Oxford University Press.

Pinel, P. (1801) *A Treatise on Insanity* (trans. D. D. Davis, 1962). New York: Hagner.

Pitt, B. (1968) Atypical depression following childbirth. *British Journal of Psychiatry*, **114**, 1325–1335.

Pitts, F. N. & McClure, J. N. (1967) Lactate metabolism in anxiety neurosis. *New England Journal of Medicine*, **277**, 1329–1336.

Priest, R. G. & Montgomery, S. A. (1988) Benzodiazepines and dependence. A College statement. *Psychiatric Bulletin*, **12**, 107–108.

Prudo, R., Harris, T. & Brown, G. W. (1984) Psychiatric disorder in a rural and an urban population: 3. Social integration and the morphology of affective disorder. *Psychological Medicine*, **14**, 327–345.

Ramsay, R. (1990) Post-traumatic stress disorder: a new clinical entity? *Journal of Psychomatic Research*, **34**, 355–365.

Rapee, R. M. & Barlow, D. H. (1991) The cognitive–behavioural treatment of panic attacks and agoraphobic avoidance. In *Panic Disorder and Agoraphobic Avoidance* (eds J. R. Walker, G. R. Norton & C. A. Ross), pp. 252–305. Pacific Grove, CA: Brookes Cole.

Reiman, E. M. (1990) Pet, panic disorder and normal anticipatory anxiety. In *Neurobiology of Panic Disorder* (ed. J. C. Ballenger), pp. 245–270. New York: Wiley.

Rickels, K., Schweizer, E., Weiss, S., *et al* (1993) Maintenance drug treatment for panic disorder. II: Short and long term outcome after drug taper. *Archives of General Psychiatry*, **50**, 61–66.

Robius, L. N. & Regier, D. A. (1991) *Psychiatric Disorders in North America: The Epidemiologic Catchment Area Study*. New York: Free Press.

Roth, M., Gurney, C., Garside, R. F., *et al* (1972) Studies in the classification of affective disorders. The relationship between anxiety states and depressive illness. I. *British Journal of Psychiatry*, **121**, 147–161.

Rothbaum, B. O. & Foa, E. B. (1993) Subtypes of post-traumatic stress disorder and duration of symptoms. In *Post-traumatic Stress Disorder: DSM–IV and Beyond*, pp. 23–36. Washington, DC: American Psychiatric Assocation.

Rotter, J. B. (1966) Generalized expectancies for internal versus external control of reinforcement. *Psychological Monographs*, **80** (1, No. 609).

Rutter, M. (1972) *Maternal Deprivation Reassessed*. Harmondsworth: Penguin.

Sanderson, W. C. & Barlow, D. H. (1990) A description of patients diagnosed with DSM–III–R generalised anxiety disorder. *Journal of Nervous and Mental Diseases*, **178**, 588–591.

Schuckit, M. A. & Monteiro, M. G. (1988) Alcoholism, anxiety and depression. *British Journal of Addiction*, **83**, 1373–1380.

Schweiger, E., Richeb, K., Weiss, R. N., *et al* (1993) Maintenance drug treatment of panic disorder. I: Results of a prospective placebo controlled comparison of alprazolam and imipramine. *Archives of General Psychiatry*, **50**, 51–60.

Seyle, H. (1956) *The Stress of Life*. New York: McGraw Hill.

Sheehan, D. V., Sheehan, K. E. & Minichiello, W. E. (1981) Age of onset of phobic disorders: A re-evaluation. *Comprehensive Psychiatry*, **22**, 544–553.

Shore, J. H., Tatum, E. L. & Volmer, W. M. (1986) Psychiatric reaction to disaster. The Mt St Helens experience. *American Journal of Psychiatry*, **143**, 590–595.

Sims, A. (1973) Mortality in neurosis. *Lancet*, **ii**, 1072–1076.

Slater, E. & Shields, J. (1969) Genetical aspects of anxiety. In *Studies of Anxiety* (ed. M. H. Lader), pp. 62–71. Kent: Headley Bros.

Snaith, R. P. (1991) *Clinical Neurosis* (2nd edn). Oxford: Oxford Medical.

——, Constantopoulos, A. A., Jardine, M. Y., *et al* (1978) A clinical scale for the self-assessment of irritability. *British Journal of Psychiatry*, **132**, 164–171.

——, Baugh, S. J., Clayden, A. D., *et al* (1982) The Clinical Anxiety Scale: an instrument derived from the Hamilton Anxiety Scale. *British Journal of Psychiatry*, **141**, 518–523.

—— & Taylor, C. M. (1985) Irritability: definition, assessment and associated factors. *British Journal of Psychiatry*, **147**, 127–136.

—— & Turpin, G. (1990) Clinical anxiety states. In *Measuring Human Problems* (eds D. Peck & C. Shapiro), pp. 67–89. Chichester: Wiley.

Southwick, S. M., Bremner, D., Krystal, J. H., *et al* (1994) Psychobiological research in post-traumatic stress disorder. *Psychiatric Clinics of North America*, **17**, 251–264.

Spielberger, C. D. (1976) The nature and measurement of anxiety. In *Cross Cultural Anxiety* (eds C. D. Spielberger & R. Diaz-Guerro), pp. 3–12. Washington, DC: Hemisphere.

——, Gorsuch, R. R. & Lushene, R. E. (1970) *State-Trait Anxiety Inventory Test Manual.* Palo Alto, CA: Consulting Psychologists Press.

Stavrakaki, C. & Vargo, B. (1986) The relationship of anxiety and depression: a review of the literature. *British Journal of Psychiatry*, **149**, 7–16.

Stern, R. S. & Drummond, L. (1991) *The Practice of Behavioural and Cognitive Psychotherapy.* Cambridge: Cambridge University Press.

Strian, F. & Ploog, D. (1988) Anxiety related to central nervous system dysfunction. In *Handbook of Anxiety*, Vol. 2. (eds R. Noyes, M. Roth & G. D. Burows), pp. 431–476. Amsterdam: Elsevier Science.

Suinn, R. M. & Richardson, F. (1971) Anxiety management training: A nonspecific behaviour therapy programme for anxiety control. *Behaviour Therapy*, **2**, 510–698.

Sullivan, H. S. (1953) *The Interpersonal Theory of Psychiatry.* New York: Norton.

Sulker, P. B., Winstead, D. K., Galine, Z. H., *et al* (1991) Cognitive deficit and pscyhopathology among former prisoners of war and combat veterans of the Korean conflict. *American Journal of Psychiatry*, **148**, 67–72.

Titchener, J. L. (1985) Post-traumatic decline: A consequence of unresolved destructive drives. In *Trauma and its Wake, Traumatic Stress Theory Research and Intervention*, Vol. 2 (ed. C. R. Figley), pp. 5–19. New York: Brunner/Mazel.

—— & Kapp, F. (1976) Family and character change at Buffalo Creek. *American Journal of Psychiatry*, **153**, 295–299.

Torgersen, S. (1983) Genetic factors in anxiety disorders. *Archives of General Psychiatry*, **40**, 1085–1089.

Trimble (1981) *Post-Traumatic Neurosis.* Wiley: Chichester.

True, W. R., Rice, J., Eisen, S. A., *et al* (1993) A twin study of genetic and environmental contributions to liability for post-traumatic stress symptoms. *Archives of General Psychiatry*, **50**, 257–264.

Tyrer, P. (1989) *Classification of Neurosis.* Wiley: Chichester.

——, Seivewright, N. & Murphy, S., et al (1988) The Nottingham study of neurotic disorder. Comparison of drug and psychological treatments. *Lancet*, *ii*, 235–240.

Uhde, T. W., Boulenger, J. P., Roy-Byrne, P. P., *et al* (1985) Longitudinal course of panic disorder: Clinical and biological considerations. *Progress in Neuro-Pharmacology and Biological Psychiatry*, **9**, 39–51.

Weissman, M. M., Leaf, P. J., Holzer, C. E., *et al* (1985) Epidemiology of anxiety disorders. *Psychopharmacology Bulletin*, **21**, 538–541.

Weissman, M. M., Wichramanaratne, P., Adams, P. B., *et al* (1993) The relationship between panic disorder and major depression. *Archives of General Psychiatry*, **50**, 767–780.

—— & Paykel, E.S. (1974). *The Depressed Women: A Study of Social Relationships.* Chicago, IL: University of Chicago Press.

Williams, D. (1956) The structure of emotions reflected in epileptic experience. *Brain,* **79**, 29–67.

Williams, M. B. & Sommer, M. (1994) *Handbook of Post-traumatic Stress Disorder Therapy.* West Port, CT: Greenwood Press.

Wing, J. K. Cooper, J. E. & Sartorius, N. (1974) *The Measurement and Classification of Psychiatric Symptoms.* Cambridge: Cambridge University Press.

Wittchen, H. U., Semler, G. & Von Zerssen, D. (1986) Diagnostic reliability of anxiety disorders. In *Panic and Phobias,* Vol. 1 (eds I. Hand & U. Wittchen). Heidelberg: Springer.

Wolpe, J. (1958) *Psychotherapy by Reciprocal Inhibition.* Standford, CA: Stanford University Press.

World Health Organization (1978) *Mental Disorders: Glossary and Guide to their Classification in Accordance with the Ninth Revision of the International Classification of Diseases* (ICD–9). Geneva: WHO.

—— (1992) *The Tenth Revision of the International Classification of Diseases and Related Health Problems* (ICD–10). Geneva: WHO.

Zigmond, A. & Snaith, R. P. (1983) The Hospital Anxiety and Depression Scale. *Acta Psychiatrica Scandanavica,* **67**, 361–370.

Zuckerman, M. (1960) The development of an affect adjective checklist for the measurement of anxiety. *Journal of Consulting and Clinical Psychology,* **24**, 457–462.

14 Phobic disorders

Richard Stern

Agoraphobia ● Social phobia ● Differential diagnosis of phobic disorders ● Other specific phobias ● Natural history ● Epidemiology ● Psychological theories ● Treatment ● The role of medication

---

A phobia is defined as an irrational fear leading to avoidance of a particular situation or object. In this definition it is important to recognise that although patients themselves recognise that the fear is irrational, they cannot face the feared situation without discomfort, or in an extreme emergency.

Agoraphobia

Agoraphobia, the main phobic disorder, was vividly described by Westphal more than a century ago:

> "Agony was much increased at those hours when the particular streets dreaded were deserted and the shops closed. The subjects experienced great comfort from the companionship of men or even an inanimate object, such as a vehicle or cane. The use of beer or wine also allowed the patient to pass through the feared locality with comparative comfort. One man even sought, without immoral motives, the companionship of a prostitute as far as his own door ... some localities are more difficult of access than others; the patient walked far in order not to traverse the dreaded spaces... in one instance the open country was less feared than sparsely housed streets in town. One case also had a dislike for crossing a certain bridge. He feared he would fall into the water. In this case, there also was apprehension of impending insanity."
> (Westphal, 1871)

Clinical features

Agoraphobia is also known as the "housebound housewife syndrome", and this characterisation is a useful starting point since the majority of sufferers are married women. The term implies that the main fear is of the outside world (*agora* means an assembly place or market place, and *phobos* fear in Greek). Patients with agoraphobia fear and avoid large open spaces, as well as crowded places, and the means to travel to them if it involves public transport, although driving a car is often possible.

If patients try to venture out they are likely to experience a variety of anxiety symptoms: sweating, palpitations, dizziness in the head, weakness in the legs, and breathing problems (either a sensation that it is difficult to catch their breath, or, more commonly, breathing too rapidly, which is known as hyperventilation). There may be attacks of such anxiety lasting from a few minutes to several hours; these are known as panic attacks (see also page 564).

Patients have various underlying fears about what might happen to them during these episodes. A common fear is that they will faint, or make a fool of themselves in some way, or that they might go mad.

Following on from the attacks of panic, phobic avoidance develops. For example, a patient who describes an attack occurring in a supermarket may afterwards show total avoidance of returning to the supermarket. The next stage might be having a panic attack at the small corner shop, and then avoiding that as well. If the patient then has an attack just outside her home she may stop going out altogether.

Underlying fears, together with the actual anxiety symptoms, lead to phobic avoidance. There are also subtle kinds of avoidance that patients develop, such as total concentration on a book or newspaper to the extent that the external stimuli do not impinge on them. Other patients strike up endless conversation with strangers on public transport with the same reason in mind. Other classical counterphobic activities include wearing dark glasses, sucking strong-tasting sweets, going out in the rain or in the dark, sticking to small alleyways and avoiding crossing roads, and holding onto something such as a shopping basket on wheels, a dog on a leash or a pram (with or without a baby inside). Such patients may also carry bottles of tablets, or flasks of a favourite alcoholic beverage, but usually do not actually consume these substances. Another strategy is to carry a card with the name, address and telephone number of the sufferer "in case of emergency". These counterphobic items are called 'soteria', and are usually idiosyncratic to particular patients.

In addition to the anxiety which patients experience when facing the phobic situation, they also describe "fear of the fear", phobophobia, or anticipatory anxiety. For example, a patient who fears bus travel may cope if the bus comes along straight away, but if there is a delay, fear builds up and the patient may give up and retreat home.

Case example 1
Wendy, a 35-year-old woman, was travelling to work by bus, a journey of some 20 minutes, when a panic attack occurred in the middle of her journey. She got off the bus at the next stop and hailed a passing taxi to take her home. The following day she had anticipatory anxiety about going to work, and pleaded with her husband to take her there by car although it was inconvenient for

him to do so. Being a caring and concerned man, he drove her in to work the rest of the week. After that she prevailed upon a friend to give her a lift in her car, and avoided any need for travelling by bus until she gave up work to have children. She now organised her husband to drive her to the supermarket to avoid catching the bus there. Her husband usually dropped her off at the supermarket entrance, and picked her up at a pre-arranged time. One day when he came to meet her she was trembling with anxiety, after having a panic attack in the supermarket. She would not return to the supermarket and instead went to the local corner shop. In spite of the extra expense involved, her husband readily agreed to this idea as he found the regular chauffeuring of his wife had become tedious. She bought herself a shopping basket on wheels, and felt more confident gripping its handle. She soon noticed that she never went out without it, even if she was only buying one or two items. She later found that she lacked the confidence to go out except on dark or rainy days, and when she did venture out she always followed a particular route along small back streets, although it would have been quicker to walk beside the main road.

This case illustrates many of the classical features of agoraphobia. Wendy's gradual deterioration led to her increasing isolation and dependence on others, especially her husband. She developed a lack of confidence in social situations, and avoided them.

Patients with agoraphobia often avoid travel by plane or train, which limits their ability to go on holiday. They may also avoid elevators, tunnels, and any closed-in spaces as well as open ones. Rarely, patients feel insecure in their own home, either at night or if they feel shut in. It is most common for home to represent the one safe place they prefer never to leave.

Social phobia

According to ICD–10 (WHO, 1992), social phobias are centred around a fear of scrutiny by other people in comparatively small groups (as opposed to crowds), leading to avoidance of social situations. The fears may be discrete (e.g. eating in public, speaking in public, or encounters with the opposite sex) or they may be diffuse, involving almost all social situations outside the family. A fear of vomiting in public may be important. Common symptoms include low self-esteem, fear of criticism, blushing, hand tremors, nausea and urgency of micturition. Avoidance is often marked, and in extreme cases may result in almost complete isolation.

Although patients with agoraphobia often have social difficulties, patients with social phobia differ from them in a number of ways (see Table 14.1).

Table 14.1 Differences between social phobia and agoraphobia

Feature	Social phobia	Agoraphobia
Situations avoided	Parties, social gatherings, work meetings, seeing friends or acquaintances	Crowds, supermarkets, public transport, being alone
Activity avoided	Speaking, eating, writing in public	Travel, shopping
Anticipatory thoughts	What if I stutter? Will I blush?	What if I faint, die, go insane, lose control?
Response	Blushing, tremor, stammering	Panic, dyspnoea, tachycardia, faintness

After Solyom *et al* (1986).

Social phobia is more common in men than women. For example, in a study of patients selected for social skills training, 77% were men (Stravynski *et al*, 1982). Most of these patients feel worse in crowded restaurants, and some are afraid to go out to dinner, or to invite others to dine with them at home. They often avoid writing in public or handling money in front of others for fear that their hands will shake. The fear may be worse in front of the opposite sex, although patients usually have no specific sexual problems.

As with agoraphobia, the fears lead to avoidance and have major implications for how patients live. They avoid talking in public, eating in public, walking past bus queues, sitting opposite others on a train or a bus, going to parties, or swimming in a public swimming pool. They sometimes start to use alcohol or minor tranquillisers to help them to cope with social situations, with the added risks of dependency on these substances.

The underlying fears of these patients include the thought that they are blushing and that people are looking at them. This fear of others increases the anxiety, so that any blushing that was present becomes worse. They may also fear that their hands will tremble or shake when performing some action such as drinking a cup of tea, and the *fear* of trembling is usually quite out of proportion to the actual minor tremor the patients have. Sufferers may also have an underlying fear of vomiting, without ever having vomited. The fear of vomiting may be made worse by being in the presence of others who might vomit. This led to one patient avoiding public houses or being with young children, because there was the increased possibility of witnessing vomiting in these situations.

Case example 2
Jeffrey was hiding behind a newspaper in the waiting room, and when called for his appointment kept his eyes firmly fixed on the floor. During the interview he did not look at the therapist, and his voice was barely audible. In muted tones Jeffrey described how he had always been shy, even at school, in spite of having a close, warm relationship with his parents. When he went to university his shyness had prevented him from joining in with social activities, and he spent his holidays with his parents or other family members. He trained as a librarian and enjoyed his job, except when it brought him into contact with the public. His shyness in this situation was threatening to hold up his promotion. He always ate lunch alone in order to avoid dining with colleagues. His social life was poor as he feared going out into social situations, and so he had become a recluse, with his main spare time activities restricted to watching television or playing chess with a computer. The most fearful situation for Jeffrey was talking to a young woman. At these times he would become lost for words and feared blushing.

Differential diagnosis of phobic disorders

Physical disorders such as hypoglycaemia, phaeochromocytoma and thyrotoxicosis must be excluded.

Substance-induced conditions should also be considered, including the common over-indulgence in tea or coffee or other caffeine-rich drinks leading to caffeine-induced symptoms. Other stimulants such as amphetamines may cause symptoms, and so may withdrawal from substances such as barbiturates and benzodiazepines.

Depressive illness may be associated with panic attacks, and phobias may result from depression if a patient avoids a situation because it is overwhelming. *Somatisation disorder* and *generalised anxiety disorder* should also be considered in the differential diagnosis.

In a *psychotic disorder with persecutory features,* patients may avoid situations that they believe will make them vulnerable to attack.

In the diagnosis of social phobia, it is important to recognise that the normal fear of giving a speech in public does not amount to a social phobia. *Avoidant personality disorder* also leads to anxiety and avoidance of many social situations. Panic disorder and specific phobias can often coexist with social phobia.

Other specific phobias

The possible list of phobic situations or objects is limitless, but common ones are phobias of heights, elevators or other enclosed spaces, as well as of thunderstorms and lightning. Patients with the latter problem will often avoid listening to the weather forecast, and will not go outside if the weather looks overcast or dark, in case it becomes stormy.

There are also isolated phobias of certain animals, for example, domestic animals such as dogs and cats, and others such as birds, moths, bees, wasps and spiders. These phobias generally start in early childhood, although they commonly present in adult life. They are associated with fewer other psychiatric symptoms than agoraphobia or social phobia, and tend to run a steady, rather than a fluctuating, course.

Some patients have a phobia of dental treatment or having an injection, which can lead to their avoiding medical or dental treatment. A rare syndrome is "space phobia" described in four patients by Marks & Bebbington (1976), in which intense fear is evoked by spatial cues, when standing without support close by. It differs from agoraphobia in that the key feature of agoraphobia is a fear not of open spaces, but of public places, although a mild fear of open spaces sometimes occurs.

So-called "illness phobia" is no longer classified as a phobic disorder, since although patients have a fear of disease which persists in spite of medical reassurance, their need for this reassurance is closer to obsessive–compulsive disorder. Illness phobia is best categorised as hypochondriasis (DSM–IV) and is described on page 712.

> *Case example 3*
> Bill had a vague memory that he had always disliked spiders. He said that as a child he would run in from the garden crying if he saw a spider, but he only presented for treatment of his spider phobia at the age of 17. At interview he looked an unlikely candidate for an anxiety disorder of any kind: he was a large man dressed in motorcyclists' clothing. He described his long-standing fear of spiders, and how it prevented him from putting his motorcycle away in the garden shed, because he knew it was frequented by spiders. Bill's motorcycle was his pride and joy, and he was unhappy to leave it in front of his house instead of in the garden shed.

This case illustrates the very discrete nature of the disability of a patient with a discrete phobia, as well as the feature common to all the phobias, avoidance.

In many adults the origins of phobias are unclear. In children the common animal fears subside rapidly without any apparent reason, or because the patient has been exposed to gradual relearning situations. It is not known why a small percentage of these phobias continue after puberty.

Natural history

Phobic disorders pursue a course of remissions and relapses of varying durations. At the start of the phobia a short episode may resolve completely within a few days or weeks, but in cases seen by psychiatrists where severe phobias have been present for a year or more, a partial rather than total remission seems to be the usual outcome without treatment until patients reach later life (Buglass *et al*, 1977). In one sample only 20% of cases reported periods of complete remission after the initial onset of their phobia (Marks & Herst, 1970).

Epidemiology

Agoraphobia accounts for 60% of phobias (Marks, 1987). At least two-thirds of patients are women, usually aged between 15 and 35 years. When the condition has been present for more than a year it runs a fluctuating course with minor remissions and relapses over many years.

The prevalence of phobic disorders varies across different studies and depends on the setting, with general practice, general hospital and psychiatric out-patient studies showing different rates.

A major community survey was carried out in Vermont (Agras *et al*, 1969). In a sample of 325 subjects, the current prevalence of phobic disorder was 7.7%, including a prevalence of illness/injury phobias of 3.1%, agoraphobia 0.6%, and severe phobias 0.2%. Therefore agoraphobia accounted for only 8% of all phobic cases, but 50% of patients with a phobia who had been treated, showing how the frequency of a condition in psychiatric practice is not a good indicator of its prevalence in the community.

Phobic disorder has also been investigated as part of the Epidemiological Catchment Area (ECA) study, looking at the rates and risks for psychiatric disorders in a sample of over 18 000 adults in five communities in the USA (Markowitz *et al*, 1989). In three communities (*n*=11 506), the pooled six-month prevalence rate was 0.8% for panic (60% more in women), 3.8% for agoraphobia (300% more in women),1.7% for social phobia (50% more in women), and 7.0% for specific phobias (100% more in women). Rates were highest between ages 25 and 44, and lowest above age 64 (Weissman *et al*, 1985).

Genetic factors

Of all the phobic disorders, agoraphobia has been most systematically studied from the genetic point of view. Harris *et al* (1983) found that relatives of patients with agoraphobia were at increased risk not only for agoraphobia, but also for panic disorder and for other phobias, while relatives of patients with panic disorder had only a raised risk of panic disorder. Moran & Andrews (1985) studied the familial risk of agoraphobia by questionnaire and interview, and found that probands tended to have either a parent or a sibling affected, but not both; the risk to parents was not less than that to children, contrary to what would be expected with transmission from a single recessive gene. The familial prevalence of agoraphobia is unlikely to result from modelling by family members, as most of the probands had never met a sufferer. Of the probands, 85% came from a family in which neither parent was reported to have agoraphobia.

A high rate of phobic disorders has been found among mothers (31%), along with an increase in other neuroses among both parents (55% of mothers, 24% of fathers; Solyom *et al*, 1974), and a higher than expected rate of school phobia among the children (14% for ages 11 to 15; Berg, 1976).

In a family study of agoraphobia, panic disorder and non-anxious controls (20 probands per group), the morbidity risk for all anxiety disorders among first-degree relatives was respectively 32%, 33%, and 15%, the risk for relatives of controls being significantly lower (Harris *et al*, 1983).

Why agoraphobia runs in families, and especially among female relatives, is still unclear. Among twins with panic disorder or agoraphobia, anxiety disorders were more than five times as frequent in monozygotic (MZ) as dizygotic (DZ) co-twins (Torgerson, 1983). Carey (1982) studied 21 twin probands with phobic disorders, and of these, seven of the eight MZ co-twins had either a phobic disorder or phobic features, compared with only five of the 13 DZ co-twins. This is likely to be a genetic rather than a modelling effect, as even twins raised apart were concordant. Also, in at least two of the concordant MZ pairs the type of phobia present in one twin was unknown to the other.

A remarkable fact has emerged about one of the specific phobias, a phobia of blood and of having injections: 68% of patients had biological relatives with the same condition. This rate is 3–6 times higher than the frequency of corresponding phobias among the relatives of patients with agoraphobia or social phobia (Marks, 1969). It has been suggested that the strong family history might mean that blood-injury phobia originates in a genetically-determined extreme autonomic response. This group is also unusual in that the response to the phobic stimulus is bradycardia rather than the more usual tachycardia. The tendency to bradycardia leads patients to faint readily, and this may give a predisposition to the phobia.

Comorbid factors

Depression

Many agoraphobic patients complain of the common symptoms of depression: irritability, difficulty in sleeping, lack of energy and feelings of hopelessness. In clinical practice, if patients have the symptoms of both depression and agoraphobia, the depression should be treated in its own right. In most cases of agoraphobia the phobic symptoms will persist. However, in patients prone to both conditions, agoraphobia may be aggravated during a depressive episode.

Depersonalisation

Depersonalisation (feeling unreal and disembodied) and derealisation (feeling that the surroundings are unreal) can occur in agoraphobia (see also page 15). Roth (1959) has proposed a distinct syndrome, the "phobic anxiety depersonalisation syndrome", in which 80% of his cases had agoraphobia. There were also other symptoms said to indicate a temporal lobe abnormality. It has not been substantiated that patients with agoraphobia and depersonalisation also have temporal lobe dysfunction, and this particular syndrome is no longer diagnosed.

Generalised anxiety and panic attacks

Generalised anxiety is common in agoraphobia and may be constant or variable. Panic attacks can be very dramatic and are often the reason precipitating the consultation. There is great variability in the frequency of general anxiety and panic attacks: 33% to 70% of patients did not complain of these symptoms in various studies (Weissman *et al*, 1985). DSM–IV (APA, 1994) distinguishes between agoraphobia with panic attacks, and those cases without panic attacks.

Psychological theories

Psychoanalysts have stressed the importance of symbolism in the generation of phobic disorders. In the classic case of little Hans, described by Freud, Hans developed a phobia of horses after the experience of witnessing an accident involving a horse while out walking with his father. Freud proposed that the horse symbolised a feared retaliation from his father:

> "If an individual no longer feels threatened by his father but by a horse, he can avoid hating his father; here the distortion was a way out of the conflict of ambivalence. The father, who had been hated and loved simultaneously, is loved only, and the hatred is displaced onto the bad horse. Freud also brings to our attention that a boy is forced to associate with his father every day, whereas the threatening horse can be avoided by simply not going outdoors."
> (Fenichel, 1944*a*)

In a later theoretical framework, Freud viewed phobic disorders as resulting from conflicts centred on unresolved childhood oedipal situations.

In adults, because the sex drive had oedipal associations, its arousal caused anxiety that was characteristically a fear of castration. The anxiety alerts the ego to exert repression to keep the drive away from consciousness. Freud gives an example of a patient with a phobia of boats which he attributed to sexual feelings towards her father in childhood:

> "From these observations, it was clear that, through the mechanism of displacement and because of their association with the sexual activity that had initially aroused her anxiety, boats had come to be the symbol of the patient's sexual conflict, which was manifested clinically as a simple phobia."(Fenichel, 1944*b*)

One variant of the theme of unconscious motivation, held more recently, is that patients with agoraphobia are really suffering from something wrong with their marriage (Milton & Hafner, 1979). The phobic behaviour is seen as a means of expressing or coping with aspects of an unsatisfactory marital relationship. A more likely explanation, however, is that anxiety caused by marital conflict may increase the probability of panic attacks, and high neuroticism may lead both to conflict in marriage and a poor response to treatment. Marital factors should not be disregarded in treatment: the author has seen a case in which the husband has sabotaged treatment for agoraphobia because he did not want his wife to go out shopping without him. Clearly marital assessment is important before individual treatment of a phobia is embarked upon.

In the 1920s, psychologists in the USA turned to conditioned reflex theories to explain the origin of phobias. John B. Watson described the famous case of Little Albert, an 11-month-old baby who was systematically exposed to a battery of objects such as rats, rabbits, dogs, and a variety of masks, and showed no concern about them (Watson & Rayner, 1920). However, when Albert was shown a white rat and simultaneously an iron bar was struck loudly behind him, Albert withdrew from the rat.

Seven days later, when Albert was shown the rat unaccompanied by the noise, he showed a fear response that the experimenters claimed to be a *conditioned response*. Seventeen days later the response had waned, but it was strengthened by a further banging of the bar in the presence of the rat. One month later, Albert had a strong fear response to rats, dogs, fur coats and a mask of Santa Claus with a long beard. No follow-up of Albert's progress was reported, but as a result of this case claims were made indicating the conditioned reflex theory of phobias.

Both these theories have now been supplanted. Studies have failed to confirm the idea that boys desire to replace their fathers as their mothers' lovers (Fisher & Greenberg, 1977). Watson's conditioned reflex experiments have been repeated, but the early results were *not* replicated. This promoted a search for theories to explain both the origin and the maintenance of phobic disorders.

Since the 1950s, theories derived from the psychology of learning have underpinned advances in behavioural treatments. It is worth emphasising that there is no *one* theory of learning; there are a number of different theories which have developed over the years. Some proved of more influence at first, until they were replaced by another theory, and so on. For this reason it makes no sense to talk of behavioural therapy as "behaviourist", because there are many theories behind behavioural therapy, not just that of behaviourism, which derives from the theories of J. B. Watson and states that much human behaviour, including the development of phobias, is based on the principles of classical conditioning.

It is doubtful that this model can explain why phobias *persist*. After fear has been classically conditioned in the laboratory by pairing a tone with a shock a few times, extinction will occur rapidly if the tone is presented without the shock. Within 10 or 20 presentations of tone without shock, fear will always disappear. Even when the shock is extremely painful, fear of the tone will extinguish in no more than 40 trials (Annau & Kamin, 1961). On the other hand, phobias resist extinction often for years, or even a lifetime. The classical conditioning model cannot explain their persistence.

Theories of avoidance and escape conditioning may help with this problem. In laboratory experiments, a rat is put in a box where it has previously received electric shocks. A fear-evoking tone that has been paired with shocks comes on, but no shock is presented. The rat can do nothing to escape the tone and is exposed to the fact that the tone no longer predicts a shock. In this situation fear does extinguish rapidly (Baum, 1969).

Phobic patients rarely test the reality of their fears, but characteristically avoid the phobic situation, as in the case examples in this chapter. In the laboratory, using rats in an avoidance conditioning experiment, a cage has a platform on to which the rats can jump and escape from the shock. A tone comes on, and at the end of ten seconds a shock occurs. If the rat jumps on to the platform before the ten seconds are up, the tone will go off and the shock will not occur. In this situation the rat will learn to jump up, and does so in less than two seconds on every trial. When extinction trials start, the shock is disconnected: this is analogous to the clinical situation where the phobic situation no longer signals trauma. The rat now undergoes 100 trials in which it jumps up within two seconds of tone, the tone goes off quickly, and shock never occurs. If the rat's fear of the two-second tone is measured, it is seen that the fear has extinguished. The crucial test now is to see if the rat fears the ten-second tone. It must be born in mind that the rat has not tested reality: it has not remained on the grid floor for ten seconds and has not found out that the shock is no longer delivered. When the rat is exposed to the full ten-second tone, it does indeed show great fear. Escaping the tone and avoidance of shock has protected the fear of the signal from extinction.

The avoidance conditioning model of fear acquisition allows tests to be carried out on procedures that might help fear extinction. Lederhendler &

Baum (1970) devised an apparatus to force a rat to walk about and explore a feared grid floor, and showed how it was possible to help the rat overcome avoidance in a way that is similar to modern behavioural therapy with patients today.

In the clinical situation, patients avoid and escape the phobic situation, preventing the fear of the phobic situation from being extinguished. Some learning theories can help explain the persistence of phobic disorders, and also make predictions that procedures which extinguish fear in the laboratory situation should also be therapeutic in the treatment of phobic disorders.

Treatment

Behavioural treatment begins with a behavioural formulation, which is a hypothesis about a disorder, behaviour or symptom attempting to identify any possible predisposing, precipitating and perpetuating factors. It is not carved in tablets of stone, and may alter as treatment progresses and other factors come to light. Sharing the behavioural formulation with the patients allows them to see that their problems, which may have seemed insurmountable, can be summarised in a few short sentences and so appear more manageable. Such a discussion also ensures that the therapist has understood the problem fully, as well as helping the patients to feel that the therapist has taken note of them.

Measures and rating scales

Measurement of the problem is an important part of behavioural and cognitive treatments, in which patients may be considered as their own single-case experiment. There are several advantages to this approach. In the initial stages it can encourage patients to express their

---

Box 14.1 Psychological theories

Psychoanalytical theories are now mainly considered of historic interest. However, theories derived from the psychology of learning have underpinned advances in modern behavioural and cognitive treatments. The most commonly used and proven treatment is that of graduated exposure, where the exposure should be for a reasonably long period of time and in real life rather than in imagination. Self-exposure homework task and self-help manuals also play an important role in treatment.

own targets and goals of treatment, which may prevent a therapist fruitlessly pursuing a course which does not interest the patient. Also, measurement allows the patient and the therapist to monitor progress and to ensure the treatment programme is working. Failure to progress can be recognised early, and the treatment redirected.

> *Case example 4*
> A trainee psychiatrist was treating a patient with agoraphobic and social phobic problems. Progress was slow, in spite of the trainee spending 2–3 hours in the supermarket with the patient twice a week. Further questioning by the trainee's supervisor revealed that the programme had been almost entirely suggested by the trainee, with little input from the patient. Also the trainee had taken no measurements as he felt they were superfluous. The supervisor instructed the trainee to have another session with the patient in which she completed a full list of measures. This revealed that the patient had little interest in being able to travel to a supermarket, as she was quite happy for her sister to do the shopping! As a result she had never performed any of the self-exposure homework tasks suggested by the trainee. Her only target of treatment was to be able to travel on a bus to visit her elderly parents who lived some miles away. Changing the treatment programme to tackle this goal allowed the patient to achieve her target.

In this example, if the trainee had monitored his patient properly, he would have realised sooner that she was failing to make progress, and could have saved himself several fruitless hours standing in a supermarket. He would have been able to question the patient and discover her failure to comply with homework tasks and her lack of interest in the target of treatment. Examples of useful measures and rating scales that can be used in phobic disorders are given in Stern & Drummond (1991).

Treatment using graduated exposure

The most effective exposure has been shown to be: (a) of prolonged rather than short duration (Stern & Marks, 1973); (b) real life rather than fantasy exposure (Emmelkamp & Wessels, 1975); and (c) regularly practised with self-exposure homework tasks (McDonald *et al*, 1978).

Although the flooding versus desensitisation debate has sunk into oblivion, there is some confusion in clinical practice about the optimal speed of exposure programmes. Taking a highly anxious patient who has not been out of the house for 20 years on a train to the January sales may be effective in dealing with her agoraphobia, but any therapist who adopts such tactics is likely to have problems with compliance with treatment. Also, painstakingly working through a very structured hierarchy with a patient who experiences little or no anxiety at each step is likely to lead to boredom in the patient, and frustration in the therapist about the slow rate of improvement after many hours of treatment. It is best to tailor the speed of treatment to the needs of the individual patient. Some patients are highly anxious and need hours of exposure before they arrive at their treatment goals, while others require little more than an explanation of the rationale of exposure to enable them to tackle their most feared situations.

Example of treatment of agoraphobia using graduated exposure

June, a 22-year-old married woman, was brought to the clinic by her husband. She had married one year previously, and since that time had been unable to go to work due to her fear of travelling alone. June had a panic attack when her husband Barry was at work, and had called her general practitioner as she believed she was going to die.

She avoided travelling on buses or trains for fear that she might faint. Immediately prior to her marriage, she had passed her driving test, but was unable to drive unaccompanied as she feared fainting at the wheel.

She had attempted to get to work on the first day after moving to a flat after her wedding, but had panicked at the bus stop and returned home. Since that time she had remained off work.

The therapist established a working hypothesis for the origin and maintenance of June's symptoms, explaining:

"Although you have always been a shy and nervous person, it seems that your problems really began after you fainted at school. This was an unpleasant experience, which you learned to associate with being away from your family. Following this episode, you avoided going anywhere alone, and this strengthened the belief. You never allowed yourself to discover whether or not you could be alone without fainting."

It was next necessary to educate June and Barry about anxiety. Firstly, the possible physical and emotional symptoms of anxiety were explained to them. Then it was described how avoidance of feared situations leads to further avoidance:

"Currently, whenever you are in danger of being alone, you take precautions to prevent this. When you went to the bus stop to go to work, you were tense because of your expectation that something dreadful might happen. Due to your tense state, you began to notice the physical symptoms of your anxiety, such as your heart pounding, and believed this was evidence that something terrible was about to happen and that you might die."

To help them remember all this information it was summarised as "three golden rules" for exposure treatment:

(1) Anxiety is unpleasant but it does no harm (i.e. I will not die, go mad or lose control).
(2) Anxiety does eventually reduce (i.e. it cannot continue indefinitely if I continue to face up to the situation).
(3) Practice makes perfect (i.e. the more a particular exposure exercise is repeated, the easier it becomes).

Following this explanation, June was asked to identify five specific tasks which she would like to be able to perform by the end of treatment, and which would demonstrate to both herself and her therapist that she had improved:

(1) To drive alone on the motorway to visit an old school friend in Camberley.
(2) To travel to work alone on the bus during the rush hour.
(3) To travel to work alone on the train during the rush hour.
(4) To travel alone by bus and underground train into the centre of London, and to visit the main shopping areas.
(5) To remain in the flat alone overnight while Barry is on a night shift.

June decided that it would be easiest for her to start by tackling her problem of walking alone. Barry agreed to be involved in the treatment, and to act as her co-therapist. Every evening, when Barry returned from work, they were to go out for a walk. June was to leave first and to go along a predetermined route, while Barry was to wait for five minutes and then follow in her footsteps. They were to take care that the exposure time was long enough for June's anxiety to reduce (habituation), which usually took between 1–2 hours. June was to record the details of the exposure exercises in a diary, and to note down her anxiety levels at the beginning, middle and towards the end of the exposure task. To introduce some consistency into the anxiety ratings, she was asked to record the level of anxiety using a 0–8 scale, where 0 meant no anxiety and 8 indicated extreme anxiety or panic. If June found her anxiety levels reducing during the week, she was to go out for a long walk alone with Barry remaining in the house.

At the second session the following week, June and Barry were pleased with her progress. June had not only managed to go for a walk alone, but had even visited the local shops and done some shopping while Barry remained at home. The therapist praised her for this progress and suggested that with her consent, they could use the session to start tackling bus travel. At first, June asked if Barry could sit next to her, but eventually she agreed to sit at the front of the bus, while Barry and the therapist sat at the back. After a few minutes, June became very anxious and came to the therapist complaining of symptoms of panic. The therapist gently reminded her that this feeling, although unpleasant, would eventually pass, while, if she gave up now, her anxiety might be even worse next time. She returned to her seat and after a further 45 minutes looked more relaxed and cheerful. At the prearranged stop, June, Barry and the therapist left the bus. The therapist praised June saying: "You have done extremely well. Although you felt panicky you have managed to face up to your fear, and have learned that these frightening and nasty symptoms do eventually reduce."

In this case, it became clear to the patient that her anxiety levels were reducing, which gave her confidence to proceed. The therapist's comment that she had done well acted as a reinforcer, but the fact that the therapist was a sympathetic humane person is probably also important.

On the return journey, June sat alone upstairs on the bus while her husband and the therapist sat downstairs. Again, she coped well, and agreed to continue this practice with Barry during the following week. She was to start using driver-only buses once her confidence increased, and also to tackle bus travel alone while Barry remained at home.

June and Barry gradually increased the homework exposure, so that June practised travelling alone to her place of work by bus and train, and was able to return to work before the end of the fifth week. During this time, June began working on her fear of remaining alone in the house overnight. Initially, she stayed alone in the house during the day and evening, and then progressed to remaining alone overnight when she knew that her sister was at home. She was pleased and surprised with herself when she did not feel the need to telephone her sister, and felt able to try being alone without taking these precautions. Throughout this time the therapist monitored her progress, praised her for her success, and suggested tasks which she should attempt.

By session six, June had achieved most treatment targets except driving alone, which proved more difficult. Barry was concerned that she might become very anxious when driving and "do something silly". As June found it easier to drive on quiet roads, the therapist and Barry sat in the car while June drove from the clinic into the country. Again, she found this easier than she had anticipated and agreed that, after 45 minutes of driving, she would stop at a station and leave the therapist and Barry to catch a train while she drove herself back to the clinic. This demonstration proved to both June and Barry that she was able to drive sensibly and safely. Afer this session, June continued to practise driving over the next three weeks. At first she continued to go on quiet roads, and then on increasingly busy roads in town. Driving in lines of traffic when she was in the right-hand lane and felt unable to "escape" was particularly difficult for her, and so she devised some routes which involved doing this. Her confidence increased as she practised, and she began travelling on motorways. Once again, she began by driving on motorways at relatively quiet times, and then progressed to busier times.

Session seven was used to reiterate the principles of treatment, which June had successfully applied; she had achieved all her targets of treatment. The therapist warned her that she would still need to continue practising over the following months. Everyone has good and bad days, weeks or months and the important thing would be for June to continue to face up to difficult situations even during these 'bad' times.

The use of modelling

Modelling is a procedure often used to facilitate exposure therapy. In this technique, the therapist models an activity that the patient is afraid to perform and asks the patient to follow suit.

Example of treatment of a specific dog phobia using modelling

In the first treatment session, Julie eventually agreed to remain in the same room as a small dog, but only if the dog was on a leash and never closer to her than four metres. The therapist sat on a chair next to the dog and petted and stroked it while talking to Julie. After about 20 minutes, Julie approached the dog and was able to imitate the therapist's stroking action along the dog's back. In the first session, she could not be persuaded to touch the head of the dog and would only touch its body if the therapist kept it on a leash.

Julie required four more sessions in which the emphasis was on modelling to facilitate exposure to the dog. The therapist modelled touching the dog's head, even putting a hand into the dog's mouth. Eventually Julie was able to copy the therapist, even when the dog was unleashed.

Part of the treatment involved 'homework' exercises in which Julie had to visit a friend with a large dog. By the end of treatment she could remain alone with the dog in the friend's room. At follow-up one year later, she was able to visit public parks and had no fears of encountering dogs off the leash.

Self-exposure

The early exposure techniques often carried implicit instructions to patients that it would be therapeutic for them to practise going out into a feared situation between therapy sessions. In retrospect, this variable may have explained the apparent effectiveness of weak exposure techniques like systematic desensitisation (e.g. Gelder *et al*, 1967). When later work showed imaginal exposure could also be effective (Johnston *et al*, 1976), the role of self-exposure was investigated and 'homework' tasks shown to be vital for successful treatment (McDonald *et al*, 1978).

The efficacy of this form of self-treatment led to the development of self-help books, such as *Mastering Phobias* (Stern, 1995). The success of self-exposure methods, with their obvious advantage of increased cost effectiveness, may lead some to wonder if there is any need to train mental health care workers in the behavioural treatments. However, the reality is often more complicated than just giving a patient a book to read. There are several reasons why therapists need to gain experience of exposure treatment. Although some patients seem to be able to read a treatment manual and apply it to themselves without any further intervention, a substantial number cannot without the motivation of regularly reporting their progress to a therapist. In addition, therapists should not only understand and be familiar with the contents of the self-help manual, but may also need to explain the exposure principle in alternative language, troubleshoot specific problems, and be aware of potential pitfalls.

Treatment of social phobia

This will be illustrated by the case of the socially phobic young man (Jeffrey) who was described above in case example 2. Jeffrey had a poor opinion of himself and thought that he would fail in certain situations even before he tried. This expectation of failure had become self-fulfilling, as he now avoided feared situations, and had become a recluse, which made him think even more badly of himself.

Treatment followed four stages:

(1) a description of new behaviour to be learnt
(2) learning a new behaviour through guidance and demonstration
(3) practice of the new behaviour with feedback
(4) transfer of the new behaviour to the natural environment.

(1) *Description of new behaviour to be learnt*

The therapist asked Jeffrey in what ways he thought he should change his behaviour: "Tell me, Jeffrey, what would you like to do that you find too difficult or painful at the moment?"

He responded:

"I suppose I ought to be able to look you in the face. Then I'd like to be able to talk to people without blushing. I would like to be able to eat in front of other people, especially at work."

Finally he admitted in a whisper:

"It would be great if I could chat to women like other blokes do."

These four statements were taken as behavioural targets.

(2) *Learning new behaviour through guidance and demonstration*

The therapist used techniques to deal with the problem of gaze aversion. Firstly a co-therapist and therapist demonstrated how they looked at each other during a conversation, and Jeffrey was asked to watch. When the therapist asked him to copy the behaviour, however, he reverted to his habitual gaze aversion. He then received direct training in looking the therapist in the face.

Therapist: "I am going to look *you* in the face and I want you to stare directly back at me, no matter how hard it is, do not look away."

After staring at each other for two minutes, the therapist asked Jeffrey how he felt, and he said "Most uncomfortable. I wish the earth would open and swallow me up. I feel hot and red, and very embarrassed."

In spite of these feelings, it was possible to encourage Jeffrey to carry out brief periods of mutual gazing. Jeffrey gradually increased the time he spent looking until he could tolerate it for five seconds.

Next the time spent looking was increased, first with the therapist speaking while he listened, and finally reversing roles with the therapist listening. At the end of six sessions along these lines, Jeffrey no longer felt hot and uncomfortable.

This method encouraged direct exposure to the feared situation. Staring is itself not usually socially appropriate, and the therapist spent some time discussing with the patient the rules of eye-contact. Brief contact with the eyes is made on first meeting someone, and it is useful to make brief eye-contact again when making a point, but direct eye-contact is broken and intermittent during normal conversation. It is also usual to make brief eye-contact on parting.

After repeated practice Jeffrey gradually became less worried about looking the therapist in the face for prolonged periods, and in his homework tasks he practised looking at other people such as his landlady while engaging them in conversation, and obeying the rules of eye-contact.

(3) *Practice of the new behaviour with feedback*

The therapist next made a videotape of an interview between Jeffrey and a friendly female medical student. The student was a socially skilled, attractive young woman who asked Jeffrey all about his work in the library. When the videotape was played back, Jeffrey could see that he made good eye-contact and received praise for this. In general it is best to begin by emphasising positive behaviour before going on to make any criticisms. On the negative side, it was immediately clear that Jeffrey's conversational skills were poor, he never initiated conversation, and he spoke in a soft, barely audible voice.

They now focused on his problem with voice production. The therapist encouraged him to practise each of the following techniques after watching them modelled in the session:

(a) using an expressive tone
(b) speaking fluently
(c) speaking faster
(d) using powerful speech.

Jeffrey carried a card into the next session with these four instructions written on it. He soon began to use a more expressive tone, but had to guard against developing a high-pitched voice. Fluency likewise increased with practice, especially when he had formulated his thoughts in advance. As his confidence increased he was able to talk more rapidly and his speech became more powerful with practice and exposure to the situation. The therapist gave him a few rules to help this, such as avoiding the use of prefatory remarks such as "I think", "I guess", "I mean", "sort of" and "you know", and to avoid expressing uncertainty by making statements that sound like questions.

Whenever he used a good expressive tone, spoke fluently, and spoke faster or more powerfully, the therapist pointed out the achievement and praised him.

(4) *Transfer of the new behaviour to the natural environment*

Jeffrey's social skills deficit was partially responsible for this self-perpetuating situation. One possibility for change, however, was on his weekly visit to the launderette.

Jeffrey: "I dread having to speak to someone, so I usually take a book."

Therapist: "Leave the book behind and initiate a planned conversation with a young woman along the lines of 'could you show me how to work this machine?'"

This was successful, as the young woman then talked to him in a non-threatening way about the neighbourhood, and he was able to practise his new-found voice production and conversational skills.

Variations on the basic training

In some cases therapy is not as straightforward as described above, and more complicated techniques may be necessary.

Role play and role reversal

In this technique the patient plays the role of someone he fears encountering. In Jeffrey's case he could have pretended to be a young woman, and the therapist could have taken the role of Jeffrey. In this way the therapist would have acted as a competent model so that the patient could be exposed to a useful learning situation. In the next stage the patient plays himself again and the therapist plays the young woman.

Use of an ear-microphone

This is a useful device for a patient who is totally lost for words, to receive prompting from the therapist who watches the session through a one-way screen.

Use of a script

Again, for a patient who becomes speechless in certain situations a script can be useful. The therapist encourages the patient to write the script as a homework exercise, and they discuss and edit it together. Reading from the script in practice sessions is gradually faded out until the patient no longer requires it. The patient then carries out real-life practice.

Outcome studies of behavioural treatment

One of the longest follow-up studies of agoraphobic therapy has shown that 65 out of 66 patients maintained improvement for 5–9 years, and there was no symptom substitution (Munby & Johnston, 1980). Hand & Wittchen (1986) had similar results in agoraphobia 5–8 years after exposure therapy. Reviewing two to five-year follow-up studies of phobic disorders, Marks (1987) found that treatment gains were generally maintained and no new problems developed.

There are many studies to show the reduction in social phobia with exposure (e.g. Butler *et al*, 1984). There are also studies demonstrating that social skills training is effective in samples with varying mixtures of social phobia and dysfunction (Marks, 1987). The long-term effectiveness of exposure was compared with social skills training by Wlazlo *et al* (1990). Patients with a diagnosis of primary phobia seemed to get the same benefit from either treatment and showed slightly better gains (in all treatment modalities) than patients with skills deficits at 2.5 year follow-up.

Cognitive therapy

As exposure therapy is effective in most cases of phobic disorder, there is usually no need to use the more time-consuming cognitive approaches.

Beck's cognitive therapy draws the following model: it is not events themselves but people's expectations and interpretations of events which cause anxiety. Individuals overestimate the danger in a situation and start responding in a way that was originally meant to protect us from harm, such as flight or aggression.

Within Beck's model, two levels of disturbed thinking have been described: automatic thoughts and thinking errors.

Clark (1988) has further refined the cognitive model of panic, stating that individuals experience panic attacks because of a tendency to interpret a range of bodily sensations in a catastrophic fashion. This interpretation leads to a further increase in bodily sensations and a vicious circle ensues. Salkovskis & Clark (1990), in an experiment using volunteer subjects, showed that hyperventilation played an important role in panic attacks *only* if the subject interpreted the effect of the hyperventilation in a catastrophic way (see also page 602).

Once the vicious circle is established, two further factors make the situation worse. Firstly, hypervigilance makes patients repeatedly scan their bodies, so they notice more symptoms. Secondly, avoidance of certain activities maintains the negative thoughts. For example, thinking that exercise will bring on a heart attack can lead to avoidance of exercise, leading to the patient never testing himself out in a situation in which exercise is necessary.

The role of medication

Exposure therapy and benzodiazepines

It was common in the 1960s for benzodiazepines such as chlordiazepoxide, diazepam, and lorazepam to be prescribed for phobic disorders. In the 1980s it was increasingly recognised that, although it was easy to start treatment with a benzodiazepine, it was difficult to stop it due to the dependence it produced, and at the same time controlled studies showed the efficacy of behavioural therapy.

Wardle (1990) discusses the outcome of combining behaviour therapy and benzodiazepines. They may be mutually beneficial, inducing the ideal conditions for maximal habituation or extinction by reducing the patient's arousal levels. They might also help by reducing the unpleasantness of exposure therapy. On the other hand, there may be harmful effects which could operate by the mechanism of state-dependent learning effects, and this could prevent generalisation of new learning from the drug state to the non-drug state. State-dependent learning occurs when learning has taken place under the influence of one of a number of drugs, including alcohol, and the learning does not transfer to the non-drug state. Gray (1987) has suggested that benzodiazepines might impair the effectiveness of behaviour therapy by attenuating the development of behavioural tolerance of stress.

Giving medication to patients can have many effects apart from purely pharmacological ones. The so-called "attribution effect" may be important. This occurs when patients carry out an exposure exercise after taking a particular drug, saying that they can do so because of the medication. The effect of the drug may have been to boost a patient's confidence through a psychological mechanism, although the patients will attribute their success to a pharmacological mechanism. Other truly pharmacological effects of benzodiazepines are tolerance and withdrawal. Tolerance means that larger amounts of medication have to be given to produce the same effect, and is a very real danger with the benzodiazepine group of drugs. Withdrawal refers to the pharmacological effects of stopping the drug. One of the most important factors is that a panic attack may occur, making the patient worse than they were before treatment.

The studies combining behaviour therapy and benzodiazepines show contradictory findings, but there is tentative evidence that behavioural treatment is associated with lower levels of anxiety during exposure in patients taking anxiolytics.

In a controlled study of 60 patients with panic disorder or agoraphobia with panic attacks, patients were given alprazolam in a four-month combined drug and behavioural group treatment programme. One of the major findings was that the efficacy of alprazolam and behavioural therapy in the short-term treatment of panic appeared to be maintained during long-term alprazolam maintenance. Also, sustained clinical improvements were observed in many patients who decreased or discontinued alprazolam (Nagy *et al*, 1989).

Diazepam given in moderate doses just before exposure made no difference to the outcome, but given in regular doses was better than propranolol (Noyes *et al*, 1984). Therapists have suggested that failure to habituate to exposure often seems related to ingestion of large amounts of benzodiazepines or alcohol (Marks & O'Sullivan, 1988). In spite of this finding, clinical experience suggests that some patients are helped to overcome their avoidance by taking a small dose of diazepam. The crucial factor is that a patient has only a small supply of the drug (e.g. diazepam 5 mg) and is clearly instructed to take a tablet immediately before confronting the phobic situation. The patient receives the medication as part of a behavioural package, which includes self-exposure or therapist-assisted exposure as already described. The patient would eventually be expected to face the phobic situation without this pharmacological support.

Exposure therapy and tricyclic medication

As far back as 1964, the New York psychiatrist Klein suggested that imipramine might lower anticipatory anxiety in agoraphobia. Zitrin *et al* (1980) reported that imipramine was superior to placebo in both agoraphobic and "mixed phobic" groups, although not in "simple phobics". They also found that the combination of supportive psychotherapy and imipramine was slightly superior to the combination of desensitisation in fantasy and imipramine. However, we now consider desensitisation in fantasy to be a weak treatment. There have been ten subsequent studies of imipramine, making it the most widely studied drug, and in eight of them imipramine was superior to placebo in agoraphobia/panic disorder. Marks & O'Sullivan (1988) concluded that imipramine usually yields a non-specific short-term reduction in many agoraphobic symptoms. The size of the drug effect is uncertain, but has a delayed onset as expected. Exposure therapy facilitates the effect of imipramine, but it could also be that imipramine facilitates the effect of exposure.

In order to pursue this question, Telch *et al* (1985) randomly assigned 37 severely disabled agoraphobic patients to: (1) a group receiving imipramine and no exposure (*n*=12); (2) a group receiving imipramine plus exposure (*n*=13); and (3) a placebo plus exposure group(*n*=12). To provide a more stringent test of the pharmacological effects of imipramine independent of exposure, patients in group 1 received anti-exposure instructions during the first eight weeks of therapy. The assessments included the Fear Questionnaire (Marks & Mathews, 1979), the Beck Depression Inventory (Beck, 1978), and a specifically designed behavioural approach test in which patients had to walk unaccompanied on a predetermined route in a shopping centre as far as they could without stopping, and this point was measured, as well as subjective anxiety and heart rate. Panic attacks were recorded in detail, both via a questionnaire and in diary form. Assessments were made before therapy, and at 8 and 26 weeks follow-up.

At eight weeks the group receiving imipramine combined with exposure therapy showed more improvement than the other two groups, and was the only group to show a reduction in panic attacks. The results lend support for the combined use of imipramine and exposure in the treatment of agoraphobia. Of great interest was the finding that the combined treatment was the only condition to show a further reduction in dysphoric mood at 26 weeks. This favourable response to the combined use of imipramine and exposure is consistent with the findings of Zitrin *et al* (1980), but discrepant with those of Marks *et al* (1983) who found no synergistic effect. The controversy over how imipramine exerts its effect still remains: Telch *et al* (1985) proposed that the alteration in mood brought about by the drug affects the exposure therapy by (a) making it more likely that patients will engage in self-exposure homework; or (b) correcting any depressive undervaluation of gains made, so increasing the efficacy of behavioural therapy.

In clinical practice there is probably a role for combining exposure therapy with imipramine for patients who lack the confidence to venture into the feared situation and suffer from panic attacks, remembering that a substantial number of patients are fearful of medication, and many cannot tolerate the drug's anticholinergic side-effects, even in a low dose.

Exposure therapy and other antidepressants

Some controlled studies show beneficial effects from other antidepressants. Tyrer *et al* (1973) studied 40 out-patients with either social phobia or agoraphobia, and showed the superiority of phenelzine to placebo. Each group was matched for type of phobia, duration of phobia, depression, sex and overall severity. A flexible dose regime was used, all patients starting on one tablet (15 mg) daily and increasing up to 45 mg daily after one week. As patients were encouraged to test themselves in the phobic situations, this could have improved the overall results.

Due to the dangers of food and drug interactions with this class of drug, they are now prescribed less often, especially following the advent of the 5-HT uptake inhibitor class of drug. These seem to be free of these dangers, and do not have the anticholinergic and cardiotoxic side-effects of the tricyclics. However, controlled trials in phobic disorders are still awaited with the 5-HT uptake inhibitor class.

Exposure therapy and β-blockers

There are conflicting studies on the research in this area. For instance, Ullrich *et al* (1975) found that β-blockers were superior to placebo when given along with exposure therapy, but Noyes *et al* (1984) found them to be inferior to diazepam. In moderate doses, β-blockers have no central effects on the nervous system, so the mode of action depends on peripheral blockade of the sympathetically mediated mechanisms underlying the symptom. Bodily symptoms may reinforce anxiety, and a vicious cycle can be set up. Therefore, in patients in whom tremor, palpitations or diarrhoea are the major symptoms, β-blockers can have an important role in combination with the cognitive therapy of anxiety states. As with all

---

Box 14.2 The role of medication

Benzodiazepines can be useful in a few cases if they facilitate exposure treatment but are not advised if given alone. Tricyclic medication may also have a definite advantage when combined with behavioural treatments in some patients. Controlled trials are awaited for the effects of the SSRIs, but beta-blockers may help with certain specific anxiety symptoms.

medication, the benefits of treatment must be weighed against the side-effects, which are relatively few but in some patients can include faintness which may be unbearable. The dose of medication should be tailored to the individual patient; for example, propranolol is often started at 10 mg increasing gradually to 120 mg daily.

References

Agras, S., Sylvester, D. & Oliveau, D. (1969) The epidemiology of common fears and phobias. *Comprehensive Psychiatry*, **10**, 151–156.

Annau, Z. & Kamin, L. J. (1961) The conditional emotional response as a function of intensity of the US. *Journal of Comparative and Physiological Psychology*, **54**, 428–432.

Baum, M. (1969) Extinction of an avoidance response following response prevention. *Canadian Journal of Psychology*, **23**, 1–10.

Beck, A. T. (1978) *Depression Inventory*. Philadelphia, PA: Center for Cognitive Therapy.

Berg, I. (1976) School phobia in children of agoraphobic women. *British Journal of Psychiatry*, **128**, 86–89.

Buglass, D., Clarke, J., Henderson, A. S., *et al* (1977) A study of agoraphobic housewives. *Psychological Medicine*, **7**, 73–86.

Butler, G., Cullington, A., Munby, M., *et al* (1984) Exposure and anxiety management in the treatment of social phobia. *Journal of Consulting and Clinical Psychology*, **52**, 642–650.

Carey, G. (1982) Genetic influences on anxiety neurosis and agoraphobia . In *The Biology of Anxiety* (ed. R. J. Mathew), pp. 37–50. New York: Brunner/Mazel.

Clark, D. M. (1988) A cognitive model of panic attacks. In *Panic: Psychological Perspectives* (eds S. J. Rachman & J. Maser). Hillsdale, NJ: Erlbaum.

Emmelkamp, P. M. G. & Wessels, H. (1975) Flooding in imagination v. flooding in vivo in agoraphobics. *Behaviour Research and Therapy*, **13**, 7.

Fenichel, O. (1944a) *The Psychoanalytic Theory of Neurosis*. London: Rouledge, Kegan and Paul.

—— (1944b) Remarks on the common phobias. *Psychoanalytic Quarterly*, **13**, 313–326.

Fisher, S. & Greenberg, R. P. (1977) *The Scientific Credibility of Freud's Theories and Therapy*. New York: Basic Books.

Gelder, M. G., Marks, I. M. & Wolff, H. H. (1967) Desensitisation and psychotherapy in the treatment of phobic states: a controlled enquiry. *British Journal of Psychiatry*, **113**, 53–73.

Gray, J. A. (1987) Interaction between drugs and behaviour therapy. In *Theoretical Foundations of Behaviour Therapy* (eds H. J. Eysenck & I. Martin). New York: Plenum.

Hand, I. & Wittchen, H. U. (1986) *Panic and Phobias*. New York: Springer.

Harris, E. L., Noyes, R., Crowe, R. R., *et al* (1983) A family study of agoraphobia: a pilot study. *Archives of General Psychiatry*, **40**, 1061–1064.

Johnston, D., Lancashire, M., Mathews, A. M., *et al* (1976) Imaginal flooding and exposure to real phobic situations: changes during treatment. *British Journal of Psychiatry*, **129**, 372–377.

Lederhendler, I. & Baum, M. (1970) Mechanical facilitation of the action of response prevention (flooding) in rats. *Behaviour Research and Therapy*, **8**, 43–48.

Markowitz, J. S., Weissman, M. M., Ouellette, R., *et al* (1989) Quality of life in panic disorder. *Archives of General Psychiatry*, **46**, 984–992.

Marks, I. M. (1969) *Fears and Phobias*. New York: Academic Press.

—— (1987) *Fears, Phobias and Rituals*. Oxford: Oxford University Press.

—— & Herst, E. (1970) A survey of 1200 agoraphobics in Britain. *Social Psychiatry*, **5**, 16–24.

—— & Bebbington, P. (1976) Space phobia: syndrome or agoraphobic variant? *British Medical Journal*, **2**, 345–347.

—— & Mathews, A. M. (1979) Brief standard self-rating for phobic patients. *Behaviour Research and Therapy*, **17**, 263–267.

——, Gray, S., Cohen, D., *et al* (1983) Imipramine and brief therapist-aided exposure in agoraphobics having self-exposure homework. *Archives of General Psychiatry*, **40**, 153–162.

——, Lelliot, P., Basoglu, M., *et al* (1988) Clomipramine, self-exposure and therapist-aided exposure for obsessive–compulsive rituals. *British Journal of Psychiatry*, **152**, 522–534.

—— & O'Sullivan, G. (1988) Drugs and psychological treatments for agoraphobia/panic and obsessive–compulsive disorders: a review. *British Journal of Psychiatry*, **153**, 650–658.

McDonald, R., Sartory, G., Grey, S. J., *et al* (1978) Effects of self-exposure instructions on agoraphobic outpatients. *Behaviour Research and Therapy*, **17**, 83–85.

Milton, F. & Hafner, J. (1979) The outcome of behaviour therapy for agoraphobia in relation to marital adjustment. *Archives of General Psychiatry*, **36**, 807–811.

Moran, C. & Andrews, G. (1985) The familial occurence of agoraphobia. *British Journal of Psychiatry*, **146**, 262–267.

Munby, M. & Johnston, D. W. (1980) Agoraphobia: the long-term follow-up of behavioural treatment. *British Journal of Psychiatry*, **137**, 418–427.

Nagy, L. M., Krystal, J. H., Woods, S. W., *et al* (1989) Clinical and medication outcome after short term alprazolam and behavioral group treatment in panic disorder. *Archives of General Psychiatry*, **46**, 993–999.

Noyes, R., Anderson, D. J., Clancy, J., *et al* (1984) Diazepam and propranolol in panic disorder and agoraphobia. *Archives of General Psychiatry*, **41**, 287–292.

Roth, M. (1959) The phobic-anxiety-depersonalisation syndrome. *Proceedings of the Royal Society of Medicine*, **52**, 587.

Salkovskis, P. M. & Clark, D. M. (1990) Affective responses to hyperventilation: a test of the cognitive model of panic. *Behaviour Research and Therapy*, **28**, 51–61.

Solyom, L., Beck, P., Solyom, C., *et al* (1974) Some aetiological factors in phobic neurosis. *Journal of the Canadian Psychiatric Association*, **19**, 69–78.

——, Ledwidge, B. & Solyom, C. (1986) Delineating social phobia. *British Journal of Psychiatry*, **149**, 464–470.

Stern, R. S. (1995) *Mastering Phobias*. London: Penguin.

—— & Marks, I. M. (1973) Brief and prolonged flooding: A comparison in agoraphobic patients. *Archives of General Psychiatry*, **28**, 270–276.

—— & Drummond, L. M. (1991) *The Practice of Behavioural and Cognitive Psychotherapy*. Cambridge: Cambridge University Press.

Stravynski, A., Marks, I. M. & Yule, W. (1982) Social skills problems in neurotic outpatients. *Archives of General Psychiatry*, **39**, 1378–1385.

Telch, M. J., Agras, W. S., Taylor, C. B., *et al* (1985) Combined pharmacological and behavioral treatment for agoraphobia. *Behaviour Research and Therapy*, **23**, 325–334.

Torgersen, S. (1983) Genetics of neurosis: the effects of sampling variation upon the twin concordance ratio. *British Journal of Psychiatry*, **142**, 126–132.

Tyrer, P., Candy J. & Kelly, D. (1973) Phenelzine in phobic anxiety: a controlled trial. *Psychological Medicine*, **3**, 120–124.

Ullrich, R., Ullrich, G., Crombach, G., *et al* (1975) Three flooding procedures for agoraphobia. In *Progress in Behaviour Therapy* (ed. J. C. Brengelmann), pp. 59–67. New-York: Springer-Verlag.

Wardle, J. (1990) Behaviour therapy and benzodiazepines: allies or antagonists? *British Journal of Psychiatry*, **156**, 163–168.

Watson, J. B. & Rayner, R. (1920) Conditioned emotional reactions. *Journal of Experimental Psychology*, **3**, 1–14.

Weissman, M. M., Leaf, P. J., Holzer, C. E., *et al* (1985) Epidemiology of anxiety disorders. *Psychopharmacological Bulletin*, **26**, 543–545.

Westphal, C. (1871) Die Agoraphobie: eine neuropathische erscheinung. *Archiv fur Psychiatrie und Nervenkrankheiten*, **3**, 138–171.

Wlazlo, Z., Schroeder-Hartwig., Hand, I., *et al* (1990) Exposure in vivo vs social skills training for social phobia: long term outcome and differential effects. *Behaviour Research and Therapy*, **28**, 181–193.

World Health Organization (1992) *The Tenth Revision of the International Classification of Diseases and Related Health Problems (ICD–10)*. Geneva: WHO.

Zitrin, C. M., Klein, D. F. & Woerner, M. G. (1980) Treatment of agoraphobia with group exposure in-vivo and imipramine. *Archives of General Psychiatry*, **37**, 63–72.

15 Obsessive–compulsive disorder

Lynne M. Drummond

Clinical features ● *Comorbidity* ● *Epidemiology* ● *Aetiology* ●
Treatment

Both ICD–10 (World Health Organization, 1992) and DSM–IV (American Psychiatric Association, 1994) have similar definitions of obsessive–compulsive disorder, and state that the essential features of the disorder are obsessions and compulsions, for which broadly similar definitions are given. DSM–IV approaches the definition of obsessive–compulsive disorder by dividing it into obsessions and compulsions. *Obsessions* are intrusive and unwanted thoughts, images or impulses which the patient tries, at least in the early stages of the illness, to resist. Attempts not to have the thoughts lead to an increase in their frequency and intensity. Patients recognise the thoughts as being a product of their own mind, but they are seen as contrary to their wishes or personality and often distressing.

Examples of obsessions include a parent thinking of harming a loved child, or a religious person having blasphemous thoughts. The 17th century writer, John Bunyan, was tortured by the recurrent obsession that he would sell the body of Christ in the way that Judas was said to have done. When he had the obsessional thought, "sell him", he would also have the urge to resist and neutralise the thought by using a covert ritual or compulsion: "I will not, I will not, I will not, I will not, no, not for thousands, thousands of worlds".

Compulsions may be either overt actions or covert 'neutralising' thoughts. They are activities designed to reduce the anxiety caused by the obsessional thought or to "put the thought right" in some way. For example, a person with an obsessional thought of being contaminated by disease may compulsively wash to 'undo' the contamination; the minister plagued by blasphemous obsessions may have the covert compulsion of thinking a stereotyped prayer to 'undo' or neutralise the obsessional thought. The activities, however, are either not in reality linked with the fear, or they may be clearly excessive. For example, a man with the obsessional thought that his home will be burgled may check that he has locked the front door 25 times.

Clinical features

One of the first full descriptive accounts of obsessive–compulsive disorder (OCD) was by Sir Aubrey Lewis (1935). He emphasised the importance of unwanted thoughts which came into a patient's mind and were actively resisted by the patient. A later description by Schneider (1959) also emphasised the patient's perception that these unwanted thoughts or obsessions were senseless.

According to contemporary views, obsessions distress the patient and cause extreme anxiety. Urges are experienced to perform a neutralising or anxiety-reducing activity. Performance of the compulsion or ritual reduces the anxiety, which can be seen as a reward serving to strengthen the association between the obsessional thought and performance of the anxiety-reducing compulsion. However, a ritual is an inefficient way of decreasing anxiety, as it only reduces it by a small amount and the effect tends to be short-lived. A sufferer from OCD therefore remains in a state of high anxiety for much of the time, with only brief periods of comparative relief following the performance of the anxiety-reducing rituals.

Case example
A woman had the obsessional thought that she may cause an epidemic of tuberculosis. The thought arose after she had been in contact with an aunt who had had tuberculosis in infancy. She recognised the thought as irrational and knew she neither had nor could spread the bacillus. This insight, however, did not stop the obsessional thought being extremely anxiety-provoking. To counteract her anxiety, she would perform a set routine of compulsive activities or decontaminating rituals. These consisted of wearing newly washed clothes if she was likely to come into contact with other people, washing from head to foot prior to any social contact, repeated handwashing after touching her mouth or face, and a cognitive ritual of going through in her mind all the reasons why it was impossible for her to spread tuberculosis.
Performance of a ritual reduced her anxiety briefly, but she soon experienced the urge to repeat the ritual.

Obsessions without compulsions have also been described and are usually called obsessional ruminations. Analysis of patients complaining of intrusive and distressing thoughts has shown that most of these patients, after they experience the rumination, attempt to suppress or neutralise their distress by performing a covert compulsion or cognitive ritual (Salkovskis, 1985). Therefore, most of the patients can be shown on close examination to have both obsessions and compulsions.

Case example
A 40-year-old man presented with a 20-year history of incapacitating ruminations concerning his sexuality. He spent an average of ten hours a day ruminating, and was unable to work or socialise because of his problem. Although he was initially reluctant to discuss the ruminations, eventually he admitted that he worried he might have touched mens' bottoms if he had been near them. As a result he worried that he was homosexual in spite of being married for 15

years and having no homosexual fantasies or experience. When he was near another man he would suddenly have the thought that he might have touched him on the bottom. He then felt very anxious. He would have the urge to try and relive in his mind every movement he had made since first seeing the man to check that he had not touched the man's bottom. Although this checking reduced his anxiety a little, he would soon doubt his recall and repeat the checking activity several times.

From this example it can be seen that the obsessional thought was "I have touched his bottom", which would be followed by repeated covert checking rituals or compulsions. Because these checking rituals took the form of mentally visualising his own actions, they might easily have been overlooked if the patient had not been asked to report exactly what went through his mind.

Not all obsessional thoughts are expressed verbally, and they may take the form of obsessional images. For example, a person may have the mental image of performing an action. In the case described above the patient might have an image of touching a man's bottom.

Compulsions without obsessions have also been described. Many of these patients have had chronic problems with OCD for several decades. It appears that the original obsessional thought or reason for performing the compulsions has been lost in the mists of time but the compulsions have persisted as a type of habit. Rachman (1976) reported a group of patients with pure compulsive activity but no history of obsessions, who have a form of *compulsive slowness* (sometimes erroneously called obsessional slowness). These patients may take several hours to get up, have a bath and dress. However, they deny any clear obsessional thoughts which might lead to this extreme difficulty.

Case example
A 24-year-old man had a 10-year history of compulsive slowness. Washing and shaving in the morning took him between two and five hours to complete. This led to him feeling unable to attempt to get up and get dressed. Direct observation of his behaviour revealed that initially he would spend up to an hour going over in his mind the activities he was going to perform. Before doing anything he would set out the objects he was going to use. For example, he would put his razor on the shelf and then stand and stare at it for several minutes before picking it up and putting it down again. This sequence of moving and staring at objects could continue for as much as an hour. Once he had completed it, he methodically performed the actions of shaving and washing in a similar way, with each individual action being followed by close scrutiny, prolonged periods of thought and repetition.

Compulsive slowness is, however, extremely rare. Although these patients deny having any obsessional thoughts, the motivation for their slowness is usually an effort to ensure that everything they do is performed perfectly.

By aiming at perfection they constantly fail, and so have to try harder which takes increasingly longer. It seems likely that at least some of these patients may have obsessions about being perfect.

Patients with OCD frequently experience *obsessional doubts*. These refer to the subjective feeling of doubt that a person has performed an action even though he or she has done it. An example would be a man with obsessional fears that harm may occur to his house by fire or flood. On leaving home he checks all the electrical switches and gas taps. Immediately afterwards he experiences doubt that he has checked everything properly and therefore repeats the checks. He may repeat the compulsive activity many times. On one level he knows that he has checked everything, yet he still feels he cannot trust his memory about the checks. We can understand the phenomenon in terms of the temporary anxiety-reducing effect of carrying out a compulsive ritual.

Differential diagnosis

The main diagnosis which may be confused with OCD is phobic disorder (see Chapter 14). Important similarities and differences between the two conditions are given in Table 15.1.

An example may help to demonstrate the differences. The previous chapter includes the case history of Bill (page 628) who had a fear of spiders. His fear is an example of a specific animal phobia as it related to the presence of spiders in his vicinity. Contrast this with a case of OCD.

> *Case example*
> Eleanor had a 10-year history of fear of contamination by household dirt. She was anxious that she might catch a disease which could then be passed on to others. As a result she would feel responsible for causing a plague. She viewed spiders as evidence that a place was dusty and "unclean". Even if she saw a spider through the window in her garden, she would feel anxious and resort to cleaning rituals. These involved taking off all her clothes which she considered

Table 14.1 Obsessive–compulsive disorder (OCD) compared with phobias

Similarities	Differences
1. *Anxiety* accompanies the obsessional thought or ritual	1. In OCD the fear is not of the situation itself but of its *consequences*
2. *Avoidance* of situations which provoke thoughts, anxiety or rituals	2. In OCD, elaborate *belief systems* develop around the rituals

were contaminated and washing them. She then bathed following a set pattern and would repeat the ritual washing in multiples of four which she believed to be a good number. Eleanor's anxiety also led her to avoid any situation where she had seen spiders in the past.

In Bill's case he had a simple spider phobia which caused him to avoid spiders or any situations which reminded him of them. However, Eleanor's problem is different. She does not fear spiders themselves but the *consequences* which she worries may result from having contact with spiders and dust. Unlike Bill, whose anxiety was relieved by escaping from a spider, Eleanor would still remain anxious after the spider had left until she had performed her washing rituals to her satisfaction. Her case history also illustrates the development of an elaborate *belief system* according to which she performed the stereotyped washing rituals in multiples of four. Such belief systems only partly explain the situation, as people with OCD generally realise that their fears are irrational and their ritualistic patterns of behaviour unrealistic.

Anankastic or obsessional personality disorder

A colleague of the author once decided to examine the residual personality attributes and symptoms of patients successfully treated with behavioural psychotherapy for obsessive–compulsive disorder. He then made a serious mistake. For the control group he used medical and psychology students. This control group had more obsessional personalities and more florid obsessive–compulsive symptoms than the patient group.

On reflection, such a finding is not surprising. Anankastic or obsessional personality disorder is described in ICD–10 as leading to excessive conscientiousness, checking, stubbornness and caution, combined with perfectionism and meticulous accuracy. These personality traits may clearly be advantageous in certain careers, and people with obsessional personality disorders are frequently high achievers, entering professions such as medicine, law, accountancy and insurance as well as the media. They are also common in the history of premorbid personality in patients suffering from OCD (Black, 1974).

Obsessional personality traits lie on a spectrum from normal healthy caution to severe incapacity. The more extreme examples are likely to handicap patients themselves, or interfere with the lives of other people with whom they come into contact. When the desire for orderliness, cleanliness or perfection becomes an end in itself, rather than simply assisting in the performance of other tasks, a diagnosis of anankastic personality can be made. In more severe cases the traits are out of an individual's control, leading to distressing and persistent obsessional thoughts and compulsive rituals, and impaired functioning at home or work. In these cases a diagnosis of obsessive–compulsive disorder is made.

Anankastic personality disorder itself does not alter in response to behavioural psychotherapy, drugs or other treatment. Past sufferers of OCD are likely to remain careful, meticulous and conscientious people, which may be reassuring to a patient about to embark on therapy.

There has been evidence of anankastic personality disorder or florid OCD in a number of historical and contemporary personalities, including John Bunyan, Samuel Johnson, Hans Christian Andersen, Howard Hughes and Woody Allen (Toates, 1990). Howard Hughes is perhaps the best known contemporary example. He was a famous film producer, aircraft manufacturer and playboy. Later, obsessions about his health and fear of death led him to live the life of a recluse, living in a bare room with no clothes and hardly eating. Ironically, his obsessional personality had at first contributed to his success in the film and engineering worlds, but when these tendencies got out of hand, the more severe symptoms led to his ultimate demise.

Comorbidity

Depression

A strong association between depression and OCD has been noted for many years (e.g. Lewis, 1934; Kendell and DiScipio, 1970; Beech, 1971; Cammer, 1973; Rachman, 1976). There are three ways in which these two conditions may interact:

(1) Some patients suffering from depressive disorder have persistent and distressing worrying thoughts or ruminations. For example, Kendell & DiScipio (1970) found obsessive–compulsive symptoms and traits in over 20% of in-patients with depression. The obsessional thoughts are commonly associated with thoughts of harming others. Depressed patients may also exhibit compulsive activity. In these cases the diagnosis is usually clear since the onset of the compulsive activity occurred at the same time or after the onset of depression. Treatment of the depression improves the compulsions.

(2) OCD is a severely disabling disorder which restricts an individual's home, work and social life. It is not surprising that patients with the condition are not happy, and in many this dysphoria is severe enough to be diagnosed as neurotic depression. Treatment of the obsessive–compulsive disorder leads to an improvement in the depression as well.

(3) Severe OCD, although relatively rare, can be chronic. Depression, on the other hand, is a common disorder. They may coexist in the same patient. In these cases the patient requires treatment for both depression and OCD.

Schizophrenia and other psychoses

The bizarre nature of many obsessive–compulsive symptoms can occasionally mislead clinicians into making a diagnosis of schizophrenia.

However, no matter how bizarre the content of a patient's obsessional thoughts or how strange the compulsions, reality is maintained and patients are usually only too aware of the absurdity of their behaviour. Confusion arises when patients have difficulty in admitting to a professional that their worries are senseless and without basis, as the example below illustrates.

> *Case example*
> A 45-year-old man presented with a 20-year history of fear that he might have sexually abused children. This led to his avoidance of leaving home in case he might abuse them in the street. There was no evidence of his ever having abused a child and, indeed, the times when he was most worried about abuse were generally in a public situation where it would have proved difficult. He was, however, reluctant to admit that those thoughts were senseless, as another of his fears was that his memory might not be accurate for past events.

A small number of patients presenting with OCD later develop schizophrenia (Black, 1974). In the author's experience, such patients are usually young with more isolated lifestyles and frequently extremely bizarre obsessions. It may also be difficult to assess how strongly the patient believes that the obsessions are rational.

Foa (1979) examined a series of patients with OCD who did not respond to behavioural psychotherapy. One group who failed in treatment were individuals with overvalued ideas that their obsessions were rational. The clinical descriptions suggest that in at least some of these patients, the overvalued ideas bordered on the delusional. (The disorder could be classified as monosymptomatic psychosis.) Innovative but as yet uncontrolled work with this subgroup indicated that initial treatment with cognitive therapy to reduce the strength of belief in the obsession makes the patient more amenable to subsequent behavioural treatment (Salkovskis & Warwick, 1985).

Anorexia nervosa

The link between obsessive–compulsive symptomatology and anorexia nervosa has been recognised for many years (Palmer & Jones, 1939; Dubois, 1949). A review of this subject by Steinhousen & Glanville (1983) showed that obsessive–compulsive traits or symptoms had been reported as existing in between 3–83% of anorexic patients and it is thus difficult to gauge the extent of overlap between the conditions. Clearly many anorectics have obsessional thoughts and compulsions about their weight and food intake but it has also been shown that many have obsessions and compulsions unrelated to food.

Gilles de la Tourette's syndrome

OCD has been reported to occur more frequently in sufferers of Gilles de la Tourette's syndrome (Montgomery *et al*, 1982). It can sometimes be difficult to distinguish between compulsive rituals and true tics. Close questioning about the reasons why the movements are performed is required. Compulsive rituals are carried out to try to reduce the anxiety associated with an obsessional idea, while tics usually occur in response to discomfort or tension which may be worsened by stress and anxiety. The families of sufferers of Gilles de la Tourette's syndrome have a raised incidence of the syndrome itself, tics, OCD and agoraphobia (Montgomery *et al*, 1982); Gilles de la Tourette's syndrome is further discussed on page 1078.

Stammering and stuttering

Diagnostic confusion may arise with patients who have obsessive–compulsive symptoms and who perform rituals in the form of disordered speech patterns, which can be difficult to distinguish from a pure stammer. Examples include patients who need to check that every word they say is completely accurate, and patients who count the number of words in a sentence or letters in a word before speaking. Careful and sometimes prolonged assessment will usually reveal the problem if patients are asked about reasons for their speech difficulty.

Brain damage and learning disabilities

OCD was reported following encephalitis lethargica in the years after the First World War (e.g. Schilder, 1938). Many of these patients had Parkinsonism and other evidence of abnormalities of the basal ganglia.

Occasionally OCD develops after a head injury (Hillbom, 1960). The injury may have been very minor (McKeon *et al*, 1984*a*; Drummond & Gravestock, 1988).

There is also an association between OCD and birth injury (Capstick & Seldrup, 1977) and temporal lobe epilepsy (Kettl & Marks, 1986).

Epidemiology

Although it has previously been suggested that OCD is a rare condition affecting 0.05% of the population (Nemiah, 1985), recent large-scale epidemiological surveys in the US have shown a higher prevalence of the condition, with a six-month prevalence of 1.3–2% (Myers *et al*, 1984) and a life-time prevalence of 1.9–3.3% (Karno *et al*, 1988). These surprisingly high prevalence rates could be due to the fact that many sufferers of OCD do not seek medical help, preferring to battle alone in the community. Alternatively, high rates in community surveys may be obtained if normal people with obsessional symptoms are included, as well as those with the full-blown syndrome. For example, if standing near the edge on top of a tall building, many people may have a sudden thought that they will jump. Although this is not sufficient evidence to make a diagnosis, a researcher could mistakenly record all such episodes as indicating the presence of OCD.

Most epidemiological studies have found an equal sex ratio in the incidence of OCD (reviewed by Marks, 1987). Women more commonly suffer from compulsive washing and avoidance, while more men have checking rituals (Noshirvani *et al*, 1991).

Onset of OCD is usually in early adult life at a mean age of 22 years (Marks, 1987). The condition is rare in childhood (Berman, 1947) in spite of rituals being a normal developmental feature of children aged 7–8. Age of onset is younger in men than women, which may be related to individuals with washing rituals having a later onset (Noshirvani *et al*, 1991). Sufferers usually present for treatment many years after onset of the disorder in early middle age.

Approximately half of all obsessive–compulsive patients who present for treatment are unmarried. In the series of obsessive–compulsive patients treated by Noshirvani *et al* (1991), two-thirds of the men and a third of the women were not married.

There is some suggestion from a series of obsessive–compulsive in-patients at the Maudsley Hospital of an association with high intelligence and social class (Rachman & Hodgson, 1980). However, caution is needed in interpreting these findings as a selection bias due to more effective treatment-seeking behaviour may be in operation.

OCD occurs in a variety of cultures including Indian (Khanna *et al*, 1986), Hong Kong Chinese (Lo, 1967) and Western societies. It is not known if there are any differences in the form the disorder takes in different cultures. It has been suggested that religion may play a part in the development of some cases of OCD. It appears more common in people who have had a rigid, strictly religious upbringing rather than being related to any particular denomination (Rasmussen & Tsuang, 1986).

Aetiology

There are a number of theories about the aetiology of OCD. Most are not mutually exclusive, and a multifactorial aetiology is likely. The theories will be described under the subheadings of biological, psychological and sociological theories.

Biological theories

Genetic

The evidence for a genetic component to the neurotic disorders is harder to interpret than in the studies on schizophrenia.

There is a high rate of psychiatric illness in the relatives of patients with OCD, with 40–50% of parents, 19–39% of siblings and 16% of children having psychiatric problems (McGuffin & Reich, 1984). Higher rates of OCD in the relatives of patients compared with the general population have been reported by McGuffin & Reich (1984), although Hoover & Insel (1984) found a high rate of obsessional personality but not OCD in the relatives.

Twin studies are also not conclusive. Carey (1982) reported that monozygotic twins were more likely to be concordant for OCD or obsessional personality traits (87%) than dizygotic twins (47%). However, there are no studies of twins reared apart which could help to unravel the part played by environmental factors.

Neurotransmitters

The evidence for an abnormality in the functioning of neurotransmitters in patients with OCD comes from drug studies, which have shown a differential response when patients are treated with agents acting on different neurotransmitter functions.

In the 1970s there were several case reports which suggested that clomipramine had beneficial effects in patients with OCD. Clomipramine is a tricyclic antidepressant which reduces the uptake of 5-HT (serotonin) into the neurones after its release from the presynaptic vesicles. It only has a weak action on noradrenergic neurones, although one of its metabolites is anti-noradrenergic. The suggestion that clomipramine reduced obsessive–compulsive symptomatology led to many trials comparing it with placebo and with other tricyclic drugs. For example, clomipramine has been shown to be more effective than desipramine (Zohar & Insel, 1987) and nortriptyline (Thoren *et al*, 1980). Other studies have demonstrated that clomipramine is effective in relieving depressed or anxious mood, but not obsessive–compulsive symptoms (Marks *et al*, 1980, 1988; Mavissakalian *et al*, 1985). Overall, clomipramine appears more efficacious than other tricyclics in OCD, reducing symptoms in approximately 50% of patients (McDougle & Goodman, 1990).

Since the development of clomipramine, other more specific 5-HT reuptake inhibitors have been used in patients with OCD. The outcome of treatment with these has been variable, although fluvoxamine (Goodman *et al*, 1990) and fluoxetine (Jenicke *et al*, 1990*a*) seem to reduce symptoms in some patients. A beneficial effect with sertraline is more doubtful (Jenicke *et al*, 1990*b*).

The suggestion that OCD was the result of a dysfunction in the 5-HT system led to studies in which patients were given a 5-HT agonist to see if their symptoms got worse. Oral administration of m-chlorophenylpiperazine (MCPP) worsened obsessive–compulsive symptoms in some patients (Hollander *et al*, 1988), but other studies failed to show such an effect (Charney *et al*, 1988).

The variable findings of the effects of agents acting on the 5-HT system in patients with OCD suggest that the disorder is pathophysiologically heterogeneous. McDougle & Goodman (1991) have argued that OCD is mediated by the 5-HT neurones in most cases, but that for some patients there is an additional upset in the dopaminergic system. Evidence for this view comes from studies of combination drug treatments as well as recent neuroimaging work.

Gross brain pathology

OCD can be a rare complication of severe head injury (Lishman, 1968), and for some patients even a minor head injury seems to be the precipitating factor (McKeon *et al*, 1984a; Drummond & Gravestock, 1988).

As with the other anxiety neuroses, many previous theories about the brain pathology which might cause OCD have focused on the limbic system and its frontal connections. This followed from studies which found that stimulation of certain parts of the limbic system led to fear in animals, and that epilepsy arising in these areas resulted in a subjective experience of fear in the patient.

There is also some evidence from particular accidents. A famous example is the case of Phineas Gage. He was a conscientious, hardworking and capable foreman, with perhaps a mildly obsessional personality. In 1848 he was employed in building a railway when an explosion occurred which drove an iron bar through both his frontal lobes. Surprisingly he survived the accident, but his personality changed. He became unreliable, impulsive and childlike.

Belief that obsessive–compulsive symptoms arise due to abnormalities in the limbic system led to the development of limbic leucotomy as a treatment for severe resistant OCD (Kelly *et al*, 1973). Symptoms may arise as an abnormality independent of fear (Kelly, 1980).

Difficulties in understanding the repetitive nature of obsessive–compulsive symptoms have led to models of the disorder in which a feedback mechanism is proposed. Obsessive–compulsive symptoms are seen as developing when normal cessation of a particular behaviour fails to occur due to a disorder in the feedback system. In other words, hand-washing does not stop after a reasonable length of time because the feedback mechanism in the brain does not perceive that the goal of cleanliness has been achieved.

The septohippocampal system may also function by comparing sensory input with the input the organism is expecting. In Gray's (1982) model the septohippocampal system functions as a checking system to filter stimuli that are either new, aversive or non-rewarding. If stimuli are perceived as a major threat, the septohippocampal system causes cessation of activity, and increased arousal and attention (Gray, 1971). According to this model, OCD arises if the septohippocampal system becomes oversensitive and reacts to too many stimuli. This results in persistent searching or checking.

For example, a person may become oversensitive to stimuli connected with dirt. The slightest stimulus suggestive of dirt causes the septohippocampal system to go into checking mode. However, hypersensitivity to dirt signals means that this mode will not be switched off when normal cleanliness is achieved, which leads to excessive washing behaviour. This model explains the repetitive nature of obsessive–compulsive symptoms and is consistent with the hypothesis that obsessive–compulsive symptoms arise in the limbic system.

Modern brain-imaging techniques in OCD indicate an abnormality in the frontal lobe/basal ganglia system (McDougle & Goodman, 1990). Drawing on recent neuroimaging studies, Rapoport & Wise (1988) suggested that there is an innate stimulus recognition and behavioural releasing mechanism in the basal ganglia. Sensory information may be relayed from the sensory apparatus to the cortex and then the striatum. If the sensory stimulus matches a stored representation in the striatum, then a normal response to the sensory input occurs. However, if the sensory input originates from the anterior cingulate cortex, which might be able to generate behavioural responses in the absence of an appropriate sensory stimulus, compulsive behaviour will occur. Support for this hypothesis comes from neuroimaging studies and also neuropharmacological studies, as there are 5-HT and dopamine inputs from the midbrain to the striatum.

Psychological theories

Psychoanalytic theories

Freud (1907, 1908) proposed that the symptoms of OCD arose as a compromise between conflicting forces in the mind. He suggested that there was a constitutional predisposition to overvalue anal eroticism and a corresponding weakness in the capacity to confront and integrate the anxieties and realities of the Oedipus complex.

Freud thought that unlike patients with hysteria, obsessional neurotic patients could only incompletely repress forbidden sexual impulses, and their symptoms were both a *reaction formation* and a disguised gratification of these wishes. Reaction formation means that habitual behaviour often contradicts underlying impulses. For example a mother who has unconscious violent thoughts towards her children may be unable to discipline them. He explained the tendency of obsessional rituals and prohibitions to multiply in terms of the inefficiency of these defences and the continuing threat or temptation posed by contemporary provocations.

In a later discussion of the subject, Freud (1926) drew attention to the diphasic form of many obsessional rituals and introduced the notion of *undoing*. This is negative magic which seeks by motor activity to "blow away" not merely the consequences of an event, but the event itself. For example, a man with guilt about masturbation would repeatedly wash himself and his bedding after masturbating in order to try to change himself and his environment as if the behaviour had never occurred. Undoing relates to the notion of the omnipotence of thought or magical thinking in which the thought is as dangerous as and equivalent to the action.

Isolation is a term Freud coined to describe another mental mechanism characteristic of obsessive–compulsive people. It refers to the way in which an event or thought which is significant to the neurosis is not forgotten although it is stripped of its associative links and emotional resonance.

Along with his structural theory of the mind, Freud opened the way to the development of an object-relations theory of the mind and described OCD in terms of a relationship between an over-severe superego and an ego struggling to balance the demands of id, reality and superego. In OCD, reality can only weakly counteract powerful unconscious fantasies or repressed instinctual wishes. This accounts for the transient value of perception of reality as a reassurance.

Klein (1932) developed Freud's theory that there are conflicting instinctual forces in the mind: libidinal and destructive. Through her work with severely ill children, she concluded that obsessional symptoms developed in relation to both paranoid and depressive anxieties, which arose from destructive impulses and their confusion with libidinal ones. She regarded the recognition and resolution of paranoid anxieties, which threaten the survival of the self, as important in effecting a lasting cure, although she recognised that puberty, with the tremendous upsurge in the strength of libidinal impulses, could be a time of renewed symptoms.

Bion (1977), in his theory of thinking (and attacks on linking), has further developed the theory concerning the defence of isolation, relating it to psychotic patterns of thought.

Behavioural and cognitive theories

Obsessions can be viewed as learned responses to specific situations. For example, a 42-year-old man had a five-year history of blasphemous thoughts which were provoked by the sight of churches, crosses or clergymen. The thoughts started following the death of his mother. It could be argued that the death of his mother led him to be in an agitated and aroused state. At this time, previously neutral stimuli such as churches caused him to have aversive blasphemous thoughts. Instead of ignoring the thoughts, which would have allowed his anxiety to habituate, he tried to suppress the thoughts and avoided situations which might provoke them. Anxiety is an aversive experience, so anything reducing it can be viewed as a positive reinforcer. The man's behaviour in avoiding situations and trying to suppress his anxiety-provoking thoughts was reinforced. This reinforcement would strengthen the association between the previously neutral stimuli, the thoughts and his avoidance behaviour.

Compulsive behaviours or rituals may be introduced as an anxiety-reducing activity. However, they are an inefficient way of reducing anxiety as they only produce a small amount of temporary relief before the anxiety increases again leading to a repetition of the ritual. For example, a 30-year-old secretary had a 10-year history of fear that she might contaminate her children with toxicara from dog faeces. If she had been outside, on her return home she would remove her clothes and engage in washing rituals. By reducing her anxiety the activities were reinforced. Every time she performed the washing rituals she strengthened the association between the thoughts and the washing rituals. However, once she had completed a washing ritual, she had doubts about whether or not she had performed the ritual correctly. She would then start the washing ritual again. This sequence of anxiety followed by washing occurred 20 to 30 times before she gave up in a state of exhaustion and continued anxiety. It can be seen that most of the time she had high levels of anxiety, and gained only partial temporary relief from her rituals, which in turn increased the problem by not allowing her anxiety to habituate.

It is worth noting that the themes of obsessional thoughts are often remarkably similar. Most obsessions can be put into one of the following categories:

(1) fear of contamination (harm to self)
(2) fear of contamination (harm to others)
(3) acts of omission (harm to self)
(4) acts of omission (harm to others)
(5) acts of commission (harm to self)
(6) acts of commission (harm to others)
(7) loss of objects
(8) perfectionism.

To a limited extent obsessional symptoms can be advantageous. If as a species we were not particular about hygiene, we might have become extinct many years ago. Obsessionality may therefore have been selectively maintained within our genetic makeup. According to the theory of prepotency (Marks, 1969), members of a species are more likely to respond to stimuli of evolutionary significance than other stimuli. This may explain why it is relatively easy for a child to learn to have a fear of spiders, while fear of trees is much rarer and normally preceded by an obvious aversive event associated with a tree. Most obsessional fears occur around situations which might be prepotent to our species.

In the past, obsessional ruminations caused confusion as they were viewed purely as worrying thoughts. In such cases there is usually a clear aversive obsessional thought, but it seems difficult to understand why an individual would not habituate to the thought in time. However, careful analysis of the content of the thought will generally reveal that there is an anxiety-provoking obsession followed by an anxiety-reducing ritualistic thought, acting in the same way as covert rituals in temporarily reducing the anxiety.

Patients with OCD also use reassurance in an attempt to reduce anxiety (Warwick & Salkovskis, 1985). For example, a man with a fear that he might cause an inferno by leaving on the gas or electricity in his house when he left in the morning would perform elaborate checking rituals. After this he would repeatedly seek reassurance from his wife that everything had been switched off. His reassurance seeking was similar to performing a ritual, as it initially reduced his anxiety although the effect was only short-lived.

Sociological theories

There are difficulties in separating the effects of genetics and the environment. It is perhaps surprising that the majority of children who have a parent with OCD grow up normally. A minority exhibit obsessive–compulsive symptoms which may be similar or completely different to those of the parent. In such cases the role of genetics versus social learning (or *modelling,* to use a behavioural term) is unclear.

Although the onset of OCD may be insidious or sudden, McKeon *et al* (1984*b*) found that individuals with OCD report more life events in the year preceding onset than do matched controls. In this study the life events included bereavement, redundancy and head injury, as well as events which appeared more positive. The finding agrees with both the more biological theories as well as the behavioural theories on the aetiology of OCD. Life events might be expected to increase arousal which, if aversive, could be linked with a previously neutral stimulus such as electrical plugs. In a classical conditioning model the patient would become conditioned to respond with fear and high arousal to electrical plugs. The repetitive checking could then be explained by Gray's model of the septohippocampal system, so that the individual constantly checks for the danger of electrical plugs to ensure they are safe. Such a theory has been put forward to explain the onset of OCD in a woman following benzodiazepine withdrawal (Drummond & Matthews, 1988).

Treatment

Biological treatments

Drug therapy

Studies demonstrating the efficacy of clomipramine in the treatment of OCD have been discussed earlier in this chapter. Recently, more specific 5-HT reuptake inhibitors have been used. There have been several controlled trials using fluvoxamine and fluoxetine, but none as yet reported with sertraline.

The observation that 40–60% of patients do not benefit from a 5-HT reuptake inhibitor given alone has led to the investigation of combination therapies (McDougle & Goodman, 1991). Most of the trials have been open studies and are therefore difficult to evaluate fully. Examples include the combination of fluoxetine with buspirone (Markovitz *et al*, 1990) and fluvoxamine with a neuroleptic (McDougle *et al*, 1990).

One of the problems with treatment using clomipramine is the high incidence of side-effects. In a controlled trial of clomipramine in OCD, 70% of previously sexually active patients became anorgasmic at therapeutic levels of the drug (Monteiro *et al*, 1987). There have been no reports of major side-effects with the newer 5-HT reuptake inhibitors, although some patients complain of nausea.

Another disadvantage with drug treatment for OCD is that a large percentage of patients seem to relapse on stopping medication (see review by Marks, 1987).

Many clinicians have attempted a combined approach of using drugs and behavioural psychotherapy. A study by Marks *et al* (1980) suggested that clomipramine had an additional beneficial effect when combined with behavioural psychotherapy. However, further analysis of the data indicated that this benefit only occurred with patients who were clinically depressed. In another study, after depressed patients were excluded, combined treatment with clomipramine had no additional benefit over behavioural psychotherapy alone (Marks *et al*, 1988). Such a view of clomipramine acting solely as an antidepressant remains controversial (see McDougle & Goodman, 1991).

Psychosurgery

Although psychosurgery was used extensively in the 1950s, it is rarely advocated now. However, in a tiny percentage of patients with severe OCD who have failed to respond to all other forms of treatment, modern stereotactic surgery is sometimes recommended. After stereotactic limbic leucotomy, 84% of patients with OCD were reported to have improved (Mitchell-Heggs *et al*, 1976). There have been no controlled trials to evaluate the significance of these results. It is difficult to assess the specific effect of the brain lesions compared with the placebo effect of undergoing brain surgery.

Behavioural psychotherapy

For patients with obsessions and overt rituals, the treatment involves prolonged, graduated *exposure* in real life to the feared situation, together with *self-imposed response prevention*. The following case history demonstrates these techniques in practice.

Example of behavioural treatment for OCD

Flora, a 52-year-old lady, reported "I have always been meticulous, but recently things have got completely out of hand". Five years before she had begun to pay excessive detail to everything she did. She dreaded attempting household chores such as washing and ironing as they had become so time-consuming due to her attention to detail. She developed particular ways of doing things. Other rituals centred around dressing and personal hygiene. For example, when hanging up a dress, she had to shake it out six times and then examine it from every corner, which meant this task took at least 30 minutes. In addition, if she had touched anything that she considered "dirty" such as a rubbish bin, or "smelly" such as an onion, she became anxious and felt compelled to wash her hands for at least 40 minutes. "These rituals are ridiculous; they take up all my time and make life a misery".

Flora's husband explained how the rituals had gradually taken over her life in the last two or three years. He was keen to help in any way he could with her treatment, but Flora said she would be too embarrassed to let her husband assist in her treatment. Although the involvement of relatives is usually regarded as essential, in this case the therapist decided to respect her wishes so long as the husband's lack of involvement did not impede treatment. He understood he should not reassure her that she was not contaminated or participate in any way in the rituals.

Behavioural formulation

The behavioural assessment produced models for the aetiology and maintenance of Flora's symptoms (see Figs 15.1a and b and Box 15.1). From these model hypotheses, the therapist was able to suggest a behavioural formulation as shown in the figures. In summary, Flora had always been a meticulous, careful and obsessional person, but this had not previously caused her any real difficulties. After her two grown-up children left home, she felt abandoned and had more time on her hands. Their departure coincided with her husband starting to work with an attractive female colleague. Flora began to worry about how attractive she was to him. Her anxiety increased as she began to consider that she would shortly be menopausal. She began to try to ensure that she was as attractive as possible when her husband returned from work. Her mild depression and consequent low self-esteem led to her worrying about being dirty and smelling, and her obsessive–compulsive symptoms began to emerge. Once she had developed these symptoms they were maintained by her avoidance, rituals and reassurance-seeking, which meant that she was never able to test the validity of her fears or expose herself to the feared situations for long enough for habituation to occur.

The therapist explained the formulation to Flora. Part of the conversation is given below:

Therapist: "What happens if you touch something dirty or smelly?"

Flora: "I get very anxious, even though I realise there is no logical reason for it."

Therapist: "And then washing makes you less anxious, and that causes washing to become rewarding behaviour, which is increasingly likely to recur, because each time you wash you reward yourself again."

Flora: "You mean its like a habit, a kind of ingrained behaviour pattern?"

Therapist: "That's right! The more you wash, the more likely you are to wash again. This is why treatment is going to involve you touching something smelly and *not washing.*"

Treatment

After discussing the formulation of her case, Flora learnt about anxiety and how an exposure programme would help her to overcome her fears. The therapist asked her to record some baseline measures to estimate the extent and severity of her problems. She received an anxiety rating scale and learnt that this scale would be used as a form of short-hand for her to communicate how she felt to the therapist, and to allow the two of them to monitor her progress. The therapist asked her to rate her anxiety on a 9-point scale, with 0 meaning no anxiety, 2 mild anxiety, 4 moderate anxiety, 6 severe anxiety, and 8 meaning panic.

The therapist then asked Flora to think of tasks which she needed or would like to be able to do. She was asked to rate the anxiety each one would cause her if she did not perform a ritual or ask for reassurance. This list was arranged into a hierarchy of tasks. The therapist asked Flora which task she felt most able to attempt. The task chosen should be one that would cause her some anxiety but would not be impossible to do without carrying out a ritual or seeking reassurance.

Inexperienced behavioural psychotherapists are often concerned about how to prevent a patient from ritualising or, in other words, to perform self-imposed response prevention. However, this is rarely a problem. If patients have been educated about the effect of the temporary relief of anxiety by performing a ritual, they will usually realise from their own experience that such activity is counterproductive. It is hard to break a long-established pattern of behaviour, and many patients find themselves reverting to rituals from time to time. It is worth explaining this to patients in advance and telling them that if they do perform a ritual, they should try to re-expose themselves to the same situation immediately but this time without performing the ritual.

Flora found it difficult to think of any situation she would be able to expose herself to without performing a ritual. The therapist suggested she might cut up an onion without washing her hands afterwards. "You must be crazy, Doctor, no one would do that" was her first reaction. However, when she came to see how this could break her "ingrained behaviour pattern" by allowing her to habituate, that is become less anxious, she agreed to try. In the first session her anxiety after cutting the onion was rated 8 (maximal), but after 45 minutes had reduced to 4 (moderate).

After two more similar sessions she was able to cut up an onion with an anxiety level of 4 at the start and 1 (minimal) after 45 minutes. She commented "The more I can do something without carrying out a ritual, the easier it becomes. Now I think I can see how this idea could be used to solve my difficulty hanging up my dresses".

Flora herself suggested hanging up the dresses without shaking them out first, "but I know I am going to find this will make me very anxious". The therapist told her this was a good approach, and that although it would make her very anxious at first, her level of anxiety would decline as it had done with the first behavioural task. This is exactly what happened. Flora dealt with her other rituals in a similar way and with similar success.

At this point it is worth comparing exposure methods used for OCD with those described in Chapter 14 on phobic disorders. Modelling is used in both cases, and careful judgement on how fast to proceed is important. It is also crucial to try to guide the patient on to the next step rather than using domination or cajoling.

Recently there has been a move away from intensive therapist-aided exposure treatment towards more self-help exposure work (Ghosh *et al,*

(a)

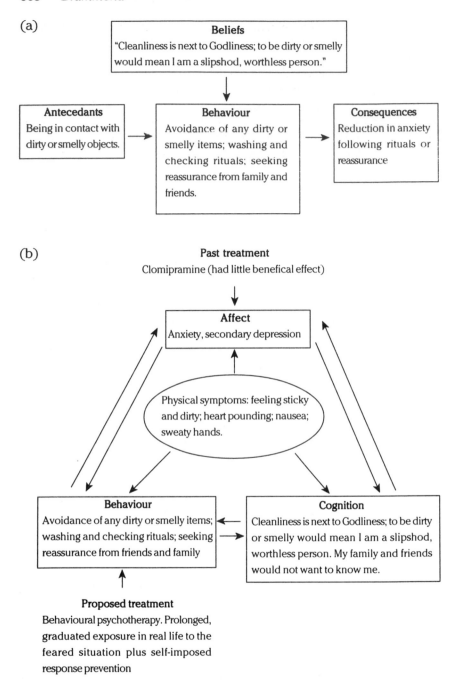

Fig. 15.1 Models for the aetiology (a) and maintenance (b) of Flora's symptoms, derived from behavioural assessment.

1988). Although this can be helpful for some patients, even with the help of a relative acting as co-therapist it can be too anxiety-provoking for patients with high anxiety levels.

In the past patients with pure obsessional ruminations were considered difficult to treat. This could be a problem if the therapist failed to analyse the thoughts into anxiety-provoking obsessions and anxiety-reducing rituals as discussed earlier. The cornerstone of treatment is exposure to the anxiety-provoking part of the ritual, but without performing the anxiety-relieving covert ritual. This may be attempted using a technique known as *satiation*.

Example illustrating satiation

Bill was a 20-year-old man with ruminations about the size of his nose. He could not stop thinking about how ugly his nose was and this thought upset him. It affected his social life and prevented him from developing a relationship with a girlfriend. It also prevented him carrying out his studies at university. When he last attempted a written examination he could not do anything because thoughts about his nose kept intruding into his consciousness. The diagnosis was OCD rather than dysmorphophobia, as Bill knew that there was nothing really wrong with his nose.

Treatment began with the therapist asking him to imagine that as he sat in the examination hall his nose grew to enormous proportions. The therapist encouraged him to let his imagination run riot and to describe in an exaggerated way the worst

---

Box 15.1   Predisposing, precipitatinig and perpetuating factors in Flora's obsessional behaviour

Predisposing factors
Parents insisted on scrupulous standards of self-care. Mother house-proud and often said that cleanliness was next to godliness. Strict religious upbringing. Marked premorbid obsessional traits.

Precipitating factors
Children leaving home had resulted in her having more time to worry about herself. Mild depressive episode following children leaving. Husband had started working with an attractive female colleague leading to Flora worrying about his fidelity.

Perpetuating factors
Washing and checking rituals prevented Flora from facing up to her fears and testing their validity. Husband and others offered frequent reassurance which also prevented her facing fears. Avoidance of dirty and smelly items when possible also reinforced her fears.

possible consequences of this happening. Bill's words provide a good illustration of the technique:

"I'm sitting there biting the end of my pencil trying to think how to answer the first question when the shadow of my nose starts to fall on the paper. I then find it has grown so big I can't see the paper at all. The other candidates turn round to look at me and I feel very foolish and embarrassed. The invigilator comes up to my desk and says 'You will have to leave. We can't have freaks like you sitting this examination'. When I try to leave the weight of my nose makes it difficult to lift up my head. It has grown so large I can hardly squeeze it through the exit. Outside I give up all hope of walking home because of the weight of my nose, and hail a taxi. The taxi driver refuses to take me because I look so revolting. I'm left standing in the street while people jeer at me. Eventually the police are called but they can't get me into the back of the van as my nose is so large. They have to improvise a kind of trolley to put my nose on as I'm marched along the street. I end my days in a kind of side-show for freaks."

Bill built up this monologue over three sessions. He then recorded it on a portable tape-recorder and played it to himself every day for three weeks. At the end of this time satiation had occurred and he no longer felt preoccupied with thoughts about his nose.

Example of habituation using a personal stereo

A novel technique in the treatment of ruminations involves a personal stereo. The aim is to use an audiotape to prolong exposure without allowing the patient time to perform any cognitive rituals. There are several case histories illustrating this treatment (Salkovskis, 1983; Headland & McDonald, 1987).

Cecil, a 42-year-old unmarried ex-schoolteacher, had a 15-year history of distressing obsessional ruminations which occupied 10–12 hours a day and had led to his early retirement from work. Whenever he saw anyone he would have the thought, "I would like to have sex with him or her". The thought was repugnant to him as he worried he might be a "pervert".

In order to reduce his anxiety, he had developed the habit of repeating the Lord's prayer and following this by saying "Jesus, forgive me" seven times. If he was interrupted by any sound or movement in his environment he would have to repeat the ritual until he had performed it perfectly. Due to the ruminations he became a recluse and had even stopped attending church. He had contemplated suicide to rid himself of them, but believed this would be an even greater sin.

Initially treatment involved graduated prolonged exposure to situations he had been avoiding. However, he made only limited progress as he could not stop himself automatically starting his 'praying ritual' which would help to maintain his anxiety.

Cecil needed to experience prolonged exposure to his anxiety-provoking thoughts without ritualising. The therapist achieved this by asking him to record the thoughts (viz. "I want to have sex with her. I want to have sex with him") in his own voice onto a continuous loop tape such as those used for telephone answer machines. After recording his thoughts, Cecil played the tape to himself via a personal stereo with headphones for at least one hour three to four times a day while in the company of other people (for example, on a bus).

At first Cecil found the treatment so aversive that he had difficulty in complying. The therapist advised him to start with the volume turned down low and to increase the volume as he became more confident.

The procedure worked well, and within two weeks of starting to use the tape Cecil reported that he had little anxiety and was able to go out at other times, have the thoughts and not ritualise. After two months he returned to work as a supply teacher and remained asymptomatic.

Two important issues, if this technique is to be successful, are that the tape should be recorded in the patient's own voice and then played through the headphones of a personal stereo. It will then be almost impossible for the patient to ignore the sound of the recording or to ritualise at the same time.

Outcome of behavioural–cognitive treatments

A behavioural approach to the treatment of OCD using graduated exposure and self-imposed response prevention has been shown by controlled trials to be effective in most patients undergoing treatment. Success rates range from 75% (Marks *et al*, 1975) to 85% of patients (Foa & Goldstein, 1978). In a series of studies, Emmelkamp (1982) demonstrated that therapist modelling did not significantly alter the response to treatment, although involvement of the family in the treatment could be helpful. There is no evidence of symptom substitution in patients with OCD treated in this way and the gains made in therapy may be maintained for at least four years (see Marks, 1981).

A minority of patients relapse and may require booster sessions of behavioural psychotherapy. After a course of treatment patients should be followed up to ensure that gains are maintained, and if signs of relapse develop they can be dealt with promptly before the person reverts to a pre-treatment level of disability. Usual practice is to see patients 1, 3, 6 and 12 months after treatment ends.

The outcome of behavioural psychotherapy for patients with obsessional ruminations appears less favourable (Emmelkamp & Kwee, 1977). The outcome of audiotaped habituation has yet to be fully evaluated by controlled trial.

Other psychotherapies

There is little evidence that cognitive therapy has any advantage over behavioural psychotherapy in the treatment of OCD. Indeed, it may make patients worse as the process of looking for evidence to confirm or refute the obsessions can become incorporated into rituals. In addition, cognitive therapy is less cost-efficient as it requires more training and supervision for the therapist and usually takes more time in therapy. A pragmatic approach is to consider using cognitive therapy for patients who failed to improve with behavioural treatment. Salkovskis & Warwick (1985) described the successful treatment of a group of patients who failed to improve with standard behavioural treatment due to the strength of belief in their obsessions.

Although some psychoanalysts still recommend psychodynamic psychotherapy for patients with OCD, most would agree with Cawley's (1974) view that "there is no evidence to support or refute the proposition that formal psychotherapy helps patients with obsessional disorders".

Acknowledgements

I am grateful to Cambridge University Press for allowing me to reproduce some of the material and case histories from *The Practice of Behavioural and Cognitive Psychotherapy* by R. S. Stern & L. M. Drummond, Cambridge University Press, 1991.

I am also grateful to Dr Sue Davison who advised and contributed to the section on psychodynamic theory.

References

American Psychiatric Association (1994) *Diagnostic and Statistical Manual for Psychiatric Disorders* (4th edn) (DSM–IV). Washington, DC: APA.

Beech, H. R. (1971) Ritualistic activity in obsessional patients. *Journal of Psychosomatic Research*, **15**, 417–422.

Berman, L. (1947) Obsessive–compulsive neurosis in children. *Journal of Nervous and Mental Disorders*, **95**, 26–39.

Bion, W. R. (1977) *Second Thoughts*. London: Karnac.

Black, A. (1974) The natural history of neurosis. In *Obsessional States* (ed. H. R. Beech), pp. 19–54. London: Methuen.

Cammer, L. (1973) Antidepressants as prophylaxis against depression in the obsessive–compulsive person. *Psychosomatics*, **14**, 201–206.

Capstick, N. & Seldrup, J. (1977) Birth abnormalities and subsequent development of obsessional symptoms. *Acta Psychiatrica Scandinavica*, **56**, 427–431.

Carey, G. (1982) Genetic influences on anxiety neurosis and agoraphobia. In *The Biology of Anxiety* (ed. R. J. Mathew), pp. 37–50. New York: Brunner/Mazel.

Cawley, R. (1974) Psychotherapy and obsessional disorders. In *Obsessional States* (ed. H. R. Beech). London: Methuen.

Charney, D. S., Goodman, W. K., Price, L. H., *et al* (1988) Serotonin function in obsessive–compulsive disorder. *Archives of General Psychiatry*, **45**, 177–185.

Drummond, L. M. & Gravestock, S. (1988) Delayed emergence of obsessive–compulsive neurosis following head injury: case report and review of its theoretical implications. *British Journal of Psychiatry*, **153**, 839–842.

—— & Matthews, H. P. (1988) Obsessive–compulsive disorder arising as a complication of benzodiazepine withdrawal. *Journal of Nervous and Mental Disease*, **176**, 688–691.

Dubois, F. S. (1949) Compulsion neurosis with cachexia. *American Journal of Psychiatry*, **106**, 107–115.

Emmelkamp, P. M. G. (1982) *Phobic and Obsessive–Compulsive Disorders: Theory, Research and Practice*. New York: Plenum.

—— & Kwee, K. G. (1977) Thought-stopping v. prolonged exposure in imagination for obsessional ruminations. *Behaviour Research and Therapy*, **15**, 441–444.

Foa, E. B. (1979) Failures in treating obsessive–compulsives. *Behaviour Research and Therapy*, **17**, 169–176.

—— & Goldstein, A. (1978) Continuous exposure and complete response prevention in the treatment of obsessive–compulsive neurosis. *Behavior Therapy*, **9**, 821–829.

Freud, S. (1907) Obsessions and religion. In *The Complete Psychological Works of Sigmund Freud* (ed. J. Strachey), pp. 115–127. London: Hogarth Press.

—— (1908) Character and anal eroticism. In *The Complete Psychological Works of Sigmund Freud* (ed. J. Strachey), pp.167–175. London: Hogarth Press.

—— (1926) Inhibitions, symptoms and anxieties. In *The Complete Psychological Works of Sigmund Freud* (ed. J. Strachey), pp.75–115. London: Hogarth Press.

Ghosh, A., Marks, I. M. & Carr, A. C. (1988) Therapist contact and outcome of self-exposure treatment for phobias: a controlled study. *British Journal of Psychiatry*, **152**, 234–238.

Goodman, W. K., Price, L. H., Delgado, P. L., *et al* (1990) Specificity of serotonin reuptake inhibitors in the treatment of obsessive disorder: comparison of fluvoxamine and desipramine. *Archives of General Psychiatry*, **47**, 577–585.

Gray, J. (1971) *The Psychology of Fear and Stress*. London: Weidenfeld & Nicholson.

—— (1982) *The Neuropsychology of Anxiety: An Enquiry into the Functioning of the Septohippocampal System*. Oxford: Oxford University Press.

Headland, K. & McDonald, R. (1987) Rapid audiotaped treatment of obsesssional ruminations. *Behavioural Psychotherapy*, **15**, 188–192.

Hillbom, E. (1960) After effects of brain injuries. *Acta Psychiatrica et Neurologica Scandinavica* (suppl. 142), 1–195.

Hollander, E., Fay, M., Cohen, B., *et al* (1988) Serotonergic and noradrenergic sensitivity in obsessive–compulsive disorder: behavioral findings. *American Journal of Psychiatry*, **145**, 1015–1017.

Hoover, C. F. & Insel, T. R. (1984) Families of origin in obsessive–compulsive disorder. *Journal of Nervous and Mental Disease*, **172**, 207–215.

Jenicke, M. A., Baer, L. & Greist, J. H. (1990*a*) Clomipramine versus fluoxetine in obsessive–compulsive disorder: a retrospective comparison of side-effects and efficacy. *Journal of Clinical Psychopharmacology*, **10**, 122–124.

——, ——, Summergrad, P., *et al* (1990*b*) Sertraline in obsessive–compulsive disorder: a double-blind comparison with placebo. *American Journal of Psychiatry*, **147**, 923–928.

Karno, M., Golding, J. M., Sorenson, S. B., *et al* (1988) The epidemiology of obsessive–compulsive disorder in five US communities. *Archives of General Psychiatry*, **45**, 1095–1099.

Kelly, D. H. W. (1980) *Anxiety and Emotions: Physiological Basis and Treatment*. Illinois: Thomas.

——, Richardson, A. & Mitchell-Heggs, N. (1973) Stereotactic limbic leucotomy: neurophysiological and operative technique. *British Journal of Psychiatry*, **123**, 133–140.

Kendell, R. E. & DiScipio, W. J. (1970) Obsessional symptoms and obsessional personality traits in patients with depressive illness. *Psychological Medicine*, 1, 65–72.

Kettl, P. A. & Marks, I. M. (1986) Neurological factors in obsessive–compulsive disorder: two case reports and a review of the literature. *British Journal of Psychiatry*, **149**, 315–319.

Khanna, S., Rajendra, P. N. & Channabasacvanna, S. M. (1986) Sociodemographic variables in obsessive–compulsive disorder in India. *International Journal of Social Psychiatry*, **32**, 47–54.

Klein, M. (1932) *The Psychoanalysis of Children*. London: Hogarth Press.

Lewis, A. J. (1934) Melancholia: a clinical survey of depressive states. *Journal of Mental Science*, **80**, 277–378.

—— (1935) Problems of obsessional illness. *Proceedings of the Royal Society of Medicine*, **29**, 325–336.

Lishman, W. A. (1968) Brain damage in relation to psychiatric disability after head injury. *British Journal of Psychiatry*, **144**, 373–410.

Lo, W. H. (1967) A follow-up study of obsessional neurotics in Hong Kong Chinese. *British Journal of Psychiatry*, **113**, 823–832.

Markovitz, P. J., Stagno, S. J. & Calabrese, J. R. (1990) Buspirone augmentation of fluoxetine in obsessive–compulsive disorder. *American Journal of Psychiatry*, **147**, 798–800.

Marks, I. M. (1969) *Fears and Phobias*. London: Academic Press.

—— (1981) *Cure and Care of Neurosis: Theory and Practice of Behavioural Psychotherapy*. New York: Wiley.

—— (1987) *Fears, Phobias and Rituals*. Oxford: Oxford University Press.

——, Stern, R. S., Mawson, D., *et al* (1980) Clomipramine and exposure for obsessive–compulsive rituals. *British Journal of Psychiatry*, **136**, 1–25.

——, Hodgson, R. & Rachman, S. (1975) Treatment of chronic obsessive–compulsive disorder by *in vivo* exposure. *British Journal of Psychiatry*, **12**, 349–364.

——, Lelliot, P., Basoglu, M., *et al* (1988) Clomipramine, self-exposure and therapist-aided exposure for obsessive–compulsive rituals. *British Journal of Psychiatry*, **152**, 522–534.

Mavissakalian, M., Turner, S. M., Michelson, L., *et al* (1985) Tricyclic antidepressants in obsessive–compulsive disorder: II. *American Journal of Psychiatry*, **142**, 572–576.

McDougle, C. J. & Goodman, W. K. (1990) Obsessive–compulsive disorder: recent neurobiological developments. *Current Opinion in Psychiatry*, **3**, 239–244.

——, ——, Price, L. H., *et al* (1990) Neuroleptic addition in fluvoxamine-refractory obsessive–compulsive disorder. *American Journal of Psychiatry*, **147**, 652–654.

—— & —— (1991) Obsessive–compulsive disorder: pharmacotherapy and pathophysiology. *Current Opinion in Psychiatry*, **4**, 267–272.

McGuffin, P. & Reich, T. (1984) Psychopathology and genetics. In *Comprehensive Handbook of Psychopathology* (eds H. E. Adams & P. B. Sutker), pp. 47–75. New York: Plenum.

McKeon, J. P., McGuffin, P. & Robinson, P. H. (1984a) Obsessive–compulsive neurosis following head injury: a report of four cases. *British Journal of Psychiatry*, **144**, 190–192.

——, Roa, B. & Mann, A. (1984b) Life events and personality traits in obsessive–compulsive neurosis. *British Journal of Psychiatry*, **144**, 185–189.

Mitchell-Heggs, N., Kelly, D. & Richardson, A. (1976) Stereotactic limbic leucotomy: A follow-up at 16 months. *British Journal of Psychiatry*, **128**, 226.

Monteiro, W. O., Noshirvani, H. F., Marks, I. M., *et al* (1987) Anorgasmia from clomipramine in obsessive–compulsive disorder: a controlled trial. *British Journal of Psychiatry*, **151**, 107–112.

Montgomery, M. A., Clayton, P. J. & Friedhoff, A. J. (1982) Psychiatric illness in Tourette syndrome patients and first degree relatives. In *Gilles de la Tourette Syndrome* (Advances in Neurology No. 35) (eds. A. J. Friedhoff & T. N.Chase), pp. 335–339. New York: Raven.

Myers, J. K., Weissman, M. M., Tischler, G. L., *et al* (1984) Six-month prevalence of psychiatric disorders in three communities. *Archives of General Psychiatry*, **41**, 959–967.

Nemiah, J. C. (1985) Obsessive–compulsive disorder (obsessive–compulsive neurosis). In *Comprehensive Textbook of Psychiatry* (4th edn) (eds H. I. Kaplan & B. J. Sadock), p. 906. Baltimore: Williams & Wilkins.

Noshirvani, H. F., Kasviskis, Y., Marks, I. M., *et al* (1991) Gender-divergent aetiological factors in obsessive–compulsive disorder. *British Journal of Psychiatry*, **158**, 260–263.

Palmer, H. D. & Jones, M. S. (1939) Anorexia nervosa as a manifestation of compulsion neurosis. *Archives of Neurology and Psychiatry*, **41**, 856–858.

Rachman, S. (1976) Obsessional–compulsive checking. *Behaviour Research and Therapy*, **14**, 269–277.

—— & Hodgson, R. (1980) *Obsessions and Compulsions*. New Jersey: Prentice-Hall.

Rapoport, J. L. & Wise, S. P. (1988) Obsessive–compulsive disorder: evidence for basal ganglia dysfunction. *Psychopharmacology Bulletin*, **24**, 380–384.

Rasmussen, S. A. & Tsuang, M. T. (1986) Clinical characteristics and family history in DSM–III obsessive–compulsive disorder. *American Journal of Psychiatry*, **143**, 317–322.

Salkovskis, P. M. (1983) Treatment of an obsessional patient using habituation to audiotaped ruminations. *British Journal of Clinical Psychology*, **22**, 311–313.

—— (1985) Obsessional–compulsive problems: a cognitive–behavioural analysis. *Behaviour Research and Therapy*, **25**, 571–583.

—— & Warwick, H. M. C. (1985) Cognitive therapy of obsessive–compulsive disorder: treating treatment failures. *Behavioural Psychotherapy*, **13**, 243–255.

Schilder, P. (1938) The organic background of obsessions and compulsions. *American Journal of Psychiatry*, **94**, 1397–1414.

Schneider, K. (1959) *Clinical Psychopathology* (5th edn) (trans. M. W. Hamilton). New York: Grune & Stratton.

Steinhousen, C. H. & Glanville, K. (1983) Follow-up studies of anorexia nervosa: A review of research findings. *Psychological Medicine*, **13**, 239–249.

Thoren, P., Asberg, M., Cronholm, B., *et al* (1980) Clomipramine treatment of obsessive–compulsive disorders: I. *Archives of General Psychiatry*, **37**, 1281–1285.

Toates, F. (1990) *Obsessional Thoughts and Behaviour: Help for Obsessive–Compulsive Disorder*. Wellingborough: Thorsons.

Warwick, H. M. C. & Salkovskis, P. M. (1985) Reassurance. *British Medical Journal*, **290**, 1028.

World Health Organization (1992) *The ICD–10 Classification of Mental and Behavioural Disorders*. Geneva: WHO.

Zohar, J. & Insel, T. R. (1987) Obsessive–compulsive disorder: psychobiological approaches to diagnosis, treatment and pathophysiology. *Biological Psychiatry*, **22**, 667–687.

16 Hysteria

Harold Merskey

History • Freudian concepts • Shell shock • Diagnosis and classification • Clinical presentation • Epidemic hysteria • Culturally sanctioned behaviour •Hysterical psychoses • Dissociative identity disorder • Hysterical personality disorder • Epidemiology • Aetiology • Prognosis • Treatment

---

Hysteria includes conversion and dissociative symptoms. *Conversion* is a loss or alteration of physical function, suggestive of an organic disease. *Dissociation* refers to a disturbance in the normal integrative functions of identity, memory or consciousness.

History

Traditionally the Greeks believed that the symptoms of hysteria were caused by the womb moving about the body and blocking "the channels of respiration" (Greek *hystera* = womb). If the womb was displaced upwards, there would be difficulties in swallowing and dyspnoea. This is the origin of the phrase "suffocation of the mother" in such cases. The womb could be driven down from above with the help of a pungent fumigation, or tempted back to the vaginal region by an aromatic fumigation. Hippocrates wrote that pregnancy or marriage were the best cures. Others, such as Galen, however, rejected the notion of a mobile uterus in the light of knowledge derived from dissection (Siegel, 1976).

In medieval times, and even later, hysterical illness was liable to be confused with witchcraft. In 1602, in the trial of Mary Glover, it was claimed that the 14-year-old girl had been bewitched by "an old charewoman, Elizabeth Jackson" and as a result had fallen into "fittes so fearful that all who were about her supposed she would dye and she was speechless, and blynde her neck and throat did swell depriving her of speech the lefte hand arme, and whole side were deprived of feeling and moving". Because all these symptoms commenced after a quarrel with Elizabeth Jackson and were worse in her presence, Miss Jackson was made to stand trial for witchcraft. The doctor for her defence, Edward Jorden, argued that Mary Glover's symptoms were due to natural causes rather than the result of diabolical influences and witchcraft. Regrettably he lost the case, and Elizabeth Jackson was convicted of witchcraft and imprisoned for a year.

After the rejection of his evidence, Jorden wrote his classic treatise *A Brief Discourse of a Disease called the Suffocation of the Mother* which includes an excellent clinical description of hysteria, as well as a clear statement that hysteria is mainly due to disturbances of the mind (Jorden, 1603). The historians Hunter & Macalpine (1963) commented that "Jorden's evidence was the first recorded medical defence of a woman accused of being a witch, and probably was also the first occasion when a psychiatric specialist gave evidence at a criminal trial".

The post-Renaissance view is well presented in the opening remarks of Sydenham (1697) in *Discourse on Hysteria* in which he considered the effects of mental trauma on bodily function. At that time hysteria included much that we would now regard as organic disease.

> "When the Mind is disturb'd by some grevious (sic) Accident, the animal Spirits run into disorderly motions; the Urine appears sometimes limpid, and in great quantity; the sick persons cast off all hope of recovery ... Whatsoever part of the body the Disease doth affect (and it affecteth many) immediately the symptoms that are proper to that Part appear; in the Head, the Apoplexy, which ends in a Palsy of one half of the Body, comes presently after Child-bearing; sometimes they are seiz'd with Convulsions, that very much resemble the Epilepsy, and are commonly called the Suffocation of the Womb, in which the Belly and Entrails rise upwards towards the Throat; At other times they are miserably tormented with the Hysterical Clavus (nail), in which there is a most vehement pain in the Head, which you may cover with your Thumb, the sick person in the mean time vomiting up green Matter like to that sort of Choler that has its name from Leeks."

This extract tells us that a severe stress may produce both emotional and physical changes. Some of these are observable alterations in bodily functions such as changes in the urine, apoplexy or hemiplegia, but others are changes that we would consider hysterical, such as non-epileptic fits. In the following section Sydenham included other pains, diarrhoea, dropsy, tears and laughter. Although emotional changes were recognised as part of the illness, the treatment remained physical, using venesection and medicines.

During the 19th century, knowledge of the anatomy and physiology of the spinal cord and peripheral nerves advanced, resulting in a change of emphasis. Romberg (1851) believed hysteria was "a reflex sexual neurosis", a notion which persisted in the European literature up to the end of the century. However, in France both Georget (1821) and Brachet (1847) formulated hysteria as a "neurosis", meaning that the seat of the affliction resided within the brain. Although it remained an 'organic' concept caused by a disturbance of brain function, it could still be triggered by stress, business setbacks, unhappy love affairs, and ill treatment by parents. In essence it was thought that brain function was disturbed by an unknown cause, possibly related to excessive stimulation.

Brodie (1837) appears to have been the first to make the modern distinction between effects which could be explained by structural lesions of the nervous system from those which could not, and he attributed the latter to the influence of the patient's will. Carter (1853), while discussing the role of the uterus, suggested that emotion, particularly sexual passion, played a contributory role. Sandras (1851) summarised the position as follows: "hysteria is a chronic nervous condition in which at intervals of varying length, paroxysms appear characterized by a particular sensation of choking, a severe discomfort of respiration, a pain in the head of varying severity, and clonic convulsions in all, or almost all, parts of the body".

Developing the theory that a physical symptom might result from a thought process, Reynolds (1869) wrote an article on three cases of paralysis "dependent upon idea". Charcot (1889) demonstrated that hypnosis could be used to implant an idea into the patient's thoughts and that this could later cause a symptom such as a paralysis or loss of vision. He demonstrated that when the mind caused the disorder, the symptom pattern corresponded with the patient's views, rather than conforming with anatomical and physiological knowledge. Janet (1894) suggested that conversion might take place in the patient's mind "below consciousness", an idea which was taken up and expanded by Freud. By the time Breuer and Freud came to study hysteria, it was viewed as a disorder of brain function but without specific localisation (Hirschmuller, 1989).

When Breuer & Freud (1893–5) explored their first cases with the cathartic method, they treated many symptoms, some of which we might not consider as hysterical. One of their most famous patients, Anna 0, was a wealthy 21-year-old single Viennese woman who had nursed her dying father. She presented with weakness, anorexia, a cough, great tiredness, a convergent squint, variable "contractures" of the limbs, paresis of the anterior neck muscles, alterations of consciousness and an unusual type of paraphasia in which she could speak English, but at times was quite unable to talk in German, her native tongue. Information from Ellenberger (1970) and Hirschmuller (1989) suggests that she probably had quite a severe fluctuating depressive illness, complicated by drug dependence on morphine and chloral hydrate (Merskey, 1992*b*). Later in life, the patient became a highly effective social worker, author of poems, stories and plays, the founder of a women's organisation and a social work journal, and a public figure.

The origins of the concept of the so-called hysterical personality are less ancient. At one time it was thought to be a well-defined entity, strongly associated with conversion or dissociative symptoms. Carter (1853) recognised the main characteristics such as emotional lability, intense emotion, reactive sensitivity, liveliness and vivacity, impressionability and an "affective" temperament. Kraepelin (1906) provided an impressive description of a patient with dependent traits and dramatic skill. By the 1930s the concept of hysterical personality was well established; it comprised a collection of epithets, mostly unfavourable, such as labile with shallow emotions, manipulativeness, seductiveness with frigidity, histrionic behaviour, self-centredness, vanity, exhibitionism, attention-seeking, and suggestibility. Today most of these features are included in the DSM–IV histrionic personality (American Psychiatric Association, 1994), and the ICD–10 (World Health Organization, 1992) has also adopted the term histrionic personality (see also page 787).

Freudian concepts

Freud's explanation for hysteria was both simple and mechanistic. Conflicts occurred in the unconscious and were not permitted to enter consciousness because they were too painful, but in their place hysterical symptoms appeared. For example, in the discussion of Frau Emmy Von N, Freud regarded "hysterical symptoms as the effects and residues of excitations which have acted upon the nervous system as traumas. Residues of this kind are not left behind if the original excitation has been discharged by abreaction or thought activity" (Breuer & Freud, 1893–5). Repressing the problem from consciousness protected the individual from the anxiety that was attached to the conflict. A reduction in anxiety was what Freud meant by "primary gain". The idea is often misunderstood and confused with secondary gain which refers to other benefits which may accrue additionally from an illness: for example, sympathy from relatives, or relief from normal social functions or duties.

Freud initially cast his ideas on hysteria in terms of physical changes. Hysterical symptoms were caused by a failure to discharge energy ("excitations") such as might occur in coitus interruptus. This would lead to conscious anxiety. The associated physical symptoms were known as "actual neuroses", which meant physical nervous disorders, while symptoms arising from psychological conflict were called the "psychoneuroses". Later, as the neuroses came to be regarded as purely psychological disorders, the separate concepts of actual neurosis and psychoneurosis disappeared but the word neurosis has remained. Initially, Freud and the early psychoanalysts held that sexual trauma during childhood underlay all hysterical symptoms, only later stressing the role of fantasy.

Shell shock

Conditions were so bad during the First World War, and the risk of death so great, that large numbers of men would have deserted if the punishment of death for cowardice had not been employed. Serious breakdowns in morale occurred, but there was always the possibility of an escape into illness. The military authorities could not reject this escape because many men of proven courage gave way to uncontrollable fear after protracted stress. It was not acceptable to call them cowards or to suggest their behaviour was dishonourable, much less to punish them. The British army (but not the continental armies) accepted a condition called "shell shock". The disorder was thought to be the result of changes in the nervous system caused by concussion from nearby explosions but without any evidence of external injury. The main symptoms of shell shock included tremors, blindness, deafness, a bent back, paralyses and anaesthesias, as well as virtually any other complaint. This wide variety of symptoms in the soldiers demonstrated that mental and somatic symptoms could result from severe stress, and that sexual trauma in childhood was far from essential in their production (Merskey, 1991).

Diagnosis and classification

The term hysteria has been used in many different ways. Firstly, the popular use generally denotes noisy, excited or uncontrolled behaviour. Secondly, clinicians use the term to describe a conversion or a dissociative symptom. Traditionally, those dissociative symptoms which affect the body are called conversion symptoms while the term dissociation is reserved for disturbances of mental function. Thirdly, hysteria is used to relate to a certain type of personality, the "hysterical / histrionic personality". Hysteria is classified in different ways in the DSM–IV and ICD–10 schemes. The principal difference is that ICD–10 classifies the conversion and dissociative disorders under one umbrella, the dissociative disorders, and this is viewed as the primary phenomenon. DSM–IV has a separate category for dissociation, but conversion is classified as a subtype of somatisation, and not of dissociation.

The ICD–10 scheme

According to ICD–10:

> "The common theme shared by dissociative or conversion disorders is a partial or complete loss of the normal integration between memories of the past, awareness of identity and immediate sensations, and control of bodily movements . . . In the dissociative disorders it is presumed that . . . [the] . . . ability to exercise a conscious and selective control is impaired."

ICD–10 provides brief clinical descriptions of the following traditional dissociative disorders: dissociative amnesia, fugue, stupor, trance and possession disorders, Ganser's syndrome and the alleged multiple personality disorder.

The term conversion implies that the unpleasant affect, engendered by the problems and conflicts which the patient cannot solve, is somehow transformed into the symptoms. ICD–10 describes the following types of dissociative disorders which were formerly called conversion disorders: motor disorders, convulsions, anaesthesia and sensory loss. Somatisation disorder and other somatoform disorders, including somatoform pain disorder and hypochondriasis, are presented in a section adjoining that on dissociative disorders.

The DSM–IV scheme

DSM–IV has organised the description of traditional hysterical symptoms and traits into three sections. The first covers conversion disorder, which in contrast to ICD–10 has been placed in the section on somatisation disorders. Other categories in this chapter include hypochondriasis, somatisation disorder, and somatoform pain disorder, all of which have historical links with hysteria. Next, dissociative disorders are placed in a separate group on their own. Thirdly, hysterical personality has been renamed as histrionic personality disorder, is considered an axis II disorder, and is included as one of the personality disorders. Diagnostic criteria for conversion disorder are given in Box 16.1.

In the DSM–IV scheme the essential feature of a dissociative disorder is "a disruption in the usually integrated functions of consciousness, memory, identity, or perception of the environment. The disturbance may be sudden or gradual, transient or chronic". The category of dissociative disorders includes: psychogenic amnesia, fugue, dissociative identity disorder (formerly multiple personality disorder), as well as depersonalisation disorder, and a group of disorders not otherwise specified. DSM–IV gives clear operational criteria (as well as a clinical description) for each disorder.

There appears to be at least one advantage in ICD–10 with respect to conversion symptoms. Das & Saxena (1991) found that many patients who had dissociative disorder had to be placed in the DSM–III–R category "dissociative disorder not otherwise specified" (American Psychiatric Association, 1987). With ICD–10 this group could be further classified into transient possession disorders, dissociative movement disorders, dissociative convulsions, depersonalisation states, and other dissociative and conversion disorders, so that only a small minority of cases fail to fit into any subcategory. This suggests that ICD–10 provides more detail than DSM–III–R and DSM–IV, particularly for conditions which are common in developing

Box 16.1 DSM–IV criteria for conversion disorder

A. One or more symptoms or deficits affecting voluntary motor or sensory function that suggest a neurological or other general medical condition.
B. Psychological factors are judged to be associated with the symptom or deficit because the initiation or exacerbation of the symptom or deficit is preceded by conflicts or other stressors.
C. The symptom or deficit is not intentionally produced or feigned (as in factitious disorder or malingering).
D. The symptom or deficit cannot, after appropriate investigation, be fully explained by a general medical condition, or by the direct effects of a substance, or as a culturally sanctioned behaviour or experience.
E. The symptom or deficit causes clinically significant distress or impairment in social, occupational, or other important areas of functioning or warrants medical evaluation.
F. The symptom or deficit is not limited to pain or sexual dysfunction, does not occur exclusively during the course of somatisation disorder, and is not better accounted for by another mental disorder.

Specify type of symptom or deficit:
  with motor symptom or deficit
  with sensory symptom or deficit
  with seizures or convulsions
  with mixed presentation.

Adapted with permission from DSM–IV. Copyright 1994 American Psychiatric Association.

countries. ICD–10 also identifies dissociative convulsions, a frequent phenomenon in both developed and developing countries.

Clinical presentation

Motor symptoms

One of the commonest motor presentations is loss of speech, *hysterical aphonia*. Head (1922) described how the patient may become completely mute while writing voluble accounts of his condition. The patient cannot whisper, yet can cough loudly because "from a psychological point of view, the resonant sound of a cough has nothing to do with articulated speech". In the larynx, the vocal cords remain apart on phonation, although during a cough they close normally.

Aphonia is a good example of what Head called "positive signs". He emphasised that in order to diagnose hysteria it was necessary to demonstrate two phenomena. Firstly, there should be an absence of relevant organic disease, or at least proportionate organic disease. Secondly, there should be proof of the positive signs. A third condition is also necessary for the psychiatrist: the demonstration of a psychological aetiology, often confirmed by the patient, or of psychiatric illness which is of sufficient proportion to the symptom. Stuttering is also sometimes deemed to be hysterical, but while it may occasionally have a psychological cause it rarely fulfils the criteria for conversion.

Flaccid paralysis may affect one or more limbs, or one side of the face. In a hysterical *spasm* both arm and leg are contracted on the same side of the body, the hand closed tightly, the knee flexed, and perhaps the legs and the foot drawn up. *Paralysis with contractures* is one of the most extreme examples of disability caused by hysterical illness. Spasmodic contractures due to hysteria are diagnosed much less commonly today than a century ago. Sometimes, as Head observed, spasm of the muscle at the knee or other joint actually resists the movement of the limb in the direction in which the contraction is supposed to be occurring. Traditionally these phenomena have been taken as evidence of hysteria, but a pathophysiological cause, such as a joint pain or noxious irritation in a relevant part of the body, is also possible. Paralysis of the tongue is another situation where the positive signs of hysteria may be observed.

If flaccid paralysis or spasms persist, contractures may develop. However, most contractures seen in either physical medicine or psychiatry follow from temporary failure of use of a part due to local pain, or occur after some other major illness, such as myocardial infarction. True hysterical contractures are rare. "Frozen shoulder" is a common example of these occurrences, and a partially frozen shoulder, or arm which is limited in movement, is usually related to a physical cause. The author has recently seen three patients who were said to have "psychogenic" limitation of arm movements, but on magnetic resonance imaging all had evidence of tears of one or more tendons in the rotator cuff.

Hysterical tremor is a repeated positive movement of a voluntary type, but varying in rapidity. It ceases if the patient can be persuaded unwittingly to perform some other movement with the same limb. Tremor due to simple anxiety or a physical cause should be excluded before making a diagnosis of hysterical tremor. Difficulties in walking are sometimes hysterical, as in astasia-abasia. This is a hysterical unsteadiness of gait or ataxia, characterised by incoordination which can be quite striking, as well as an inability to walk or stand still, even though all leg movements can function normally when sitting or lying down. Some patients appear to be able to perform movements which many normal individuals would find difficult to achieve even with full muscular control.

Three reported series offer different frequencies for the occurrence of motor and other symptoms, as shown in Table 16.1. Carter (1949) was treating civilians during the wartime bombardment. Hafeiz (1980) reported from the Sudan where hysterical presentations are relatively common. Ljungberg's (1957) study came from a university centre and psychiatric hospital in Stockholm. Today, in developed countries, the commonest hysterical symptoms are motor symptoms and seizures, and they most frequently present in neurological clinics.

Certain abnormal movements such as facial tics, blepharospasm, dyskinesias and the tardive dyskinesias, which were once thought to be psychological in origin, have crossed the porous boundary separating psychiatry from neurology and are now considered to be neurological in origin. The same also substantially applies to Gilles de la Tourette's syndrome (see chapter 23). The facial dyskinesias and blepharospasm also changed category after the introduction of L-dopa (Lloyd & Hornykiewicz, 1973). A small excess of L-dopa could result in a switch from a Parkinsonian state to an overt facial dyskinesia which was indistinguishable from conditions that were once diagnosed as hysterical facial abnormalities. Since then it has generally been assumed that most, if not all, of the blepharospasms and dyskinesias found in clinical practice are of neurological origin. Occasionally a blepharospasm may emerge with a depressive illness, or other emotional changes, and remit with them.

Table 16.1 Frequency (%) of occurrence of motor and other common hysterical symptoms in three series

	Carter (1949)	Ljungberg (1957)	Hafeiz (1980)
n	100	381	61
Paralysis	23	10	10
Tremor	10	10	3.3
Astasia	–	47	–
Fits	6	20	10
Aphonia	29	1.3	20
Vomiting	6	–	16
Dyspnoea	–	–	20
Blindness	3	0.8	3.3
Amnesia	23	–	3.3

Note: not all symptoms have been included, thus the columns do not add up to 100%.

As already noted, establishing the evidence for hysteria by clinical examination requires searching for discrepancies between the patient's concept of the symptom and the physician's knowledge of the relevant anatomy and physiology. For example, when a patient walks, the manner in which he moves, takes off his clothes or dresses again or gets on an examination couch may indicate a global affection that is incompatible with a specific nerve lesion or even with a hemiplegia. Hysterical paresis is marked by simultaneous contraction of agonistic and antagonistic muscles. This provides a basis for one of the favourite signs, which is to ask the patient to press one heel down on the examiner's hand on the bed while lying supine. When the patient finds that he or she cannot do it, the hand is kept under that heel and the patient is asked to lift the opposing limb, perhaps against resistance. The synergistic response of the "paralysed" leg produces pressing down of the heel while the "good" leg is lifted. "Giveway weakness" is another sign used as a diagnostic test of hysterical paralysis. The term refers to a sudden fall in resistance during the direct testing of muscle power. Although it is often held to be diagnostic of a hysterical condition, it can occur in individuals with pain who, because of the fear of the pain, do not move their limbs as requested by the examining physician.

Hysterical fits or seizures

Hysterical seizures only occur in the presence of an audience or when one is close at hand. They may be precipitated by stress, but more often they occur by virtue of the social setting. The patients tend not to fall hard or quickly to the ground, but rather more gradually. Crying may occur, but vocalisation is limited to a few words. Movements usually follow the fall, often with dramatic clutching, and sometimes there may be opisthotonos, but there is never the regular tonic–clonic sequence of epilepsy. Tongue-biting and incontinence of urine are rare in hysterical fits, while the corneal reflex is preserved and the plantar response is flexor (unless previously abnormal). Firm handling and pressure over the supra-orbital nerves (which may be painful) may arouse the patient.

By contrast, epileptic patients may have a brief aura or cry, particularly with the onset of a tonic convulsion, and are liable to hurt themselves in the fall to the floor. They generally go through regular tonic and clonic phases of muscular contraction with tongue-biting and incontinence of urine. In practice, however, the diagnosis is not so easy because anticonvulsant drugs may modify epileptic fits, and also subjects with genuine epilepsy can develop hysterical fits. In drug-treated epilepsy, the falls may be less abrupt, the characteristic pattern of tonic and clonic movements, tongue-biting and incontinence much less obvious, and sometimes, particularly with temporal lobe epilepsy, ictal behaviour is confined to a few smacking movements of the lips or face. Following an epileptic fit there may be a drug-modified automatism which can also resemble hysterical behaviour. Patients who have brief, barely noticeable partial tonic–clonic fits may afterwards have poorly-organised behaviour, appearing to be partly in touch with the environment and acting purposively (see also page 1040).

Hysterical fits are more common among epileptic patients than others, particularly if there are emotional problems or toxic levels of anticonvulsant medication. A few epileptic patients have learnt how to induce ictal discharges, and are able to induce extra fits, while others may consciously or unconsciously demonstrate an increased falling tendency. Certain tests may be of diagnostic value. The classic Hippocratic diagnostic test between epilepsy and hysteria was to pinch the skin of the abdomen, which would have no effect in the unconscious epileptic. The electroencephalogram (EEG), if available, is abnormal during an epileptic fit but normal during hysterical fits. Serum prolactin is elevated after an epileptic seizure, and this may also be a useful discriminating measure (Trimble, 1978).

Anxious patients sometimes develop phenomena which resemble fits. In the face of severe anxiety, blood pressure may fall, and this is associated with feelings of faintness, or feelings of loss of awareness of the surroundings. There is usually a brief warning before a fainting episode that allows the patient enough time to subside more gently. Fainting has numerous causes apart from anxiety, but in psychiatric practice, postural hypotension as a result of drug side-effects is the most common cause. Occasionally patients hurt themselves after a fainting episode, but the patient usually comes around quite rapidly, with the initial pallor soon returning to normal.

Anxious subjects, particularly those with phobias and panic disorders, may also *hyperventilate.* In situations such as assemblies, small spaces, and underground railway stations, these individuals feel uneasy that they cannot get their breath and as a consequence hyperventilate. Carpopedal spasms, loss of consciousness and (rarely) epileptiform convulsions may result from the fall in carbon dioxide because too much has been breathed off. Although hyperventilation has been termed hysterical, and may occur in those with hysterical personalities, the symptom is most commonly associated with phobias. It can be relieved by demonstrating to the patient how the symptom is caused (i.e. by over-breathing) and cured by re-breathing into a paper bag, or even by holding the breath.

Dizziness is also a common complaint. Such a subjective feeling of unsteadiness has often been called hysterical, but this is probably not the best label. Feelings of unsteadiness and falling are part of the syndrome of astasia-abasia mentioned above, but also occur commonly with anxiety. They should be distinguished from vertigo in which the patient feels that the environment is rotating. A further differential diagnosis of a hysterical seizure is from an automatism occurring in response to lowered blood sugar levels or other metabolic disorders; these may also mimic an epileptic automatism.

Globus hystericus

Symptoms affecting the viscera, in particular difficulty in swallowing or *globus,* have been classified as hysterical. The classical globus syndrome is defined as "median or paramedian sensation of an unidentified object or lump in the pharynx, mainly on, but also above or beneath the crico-pharyngeal level" (Lehtinen & Puhakka, 1976). The sensation may be associated with dry-swallowing or the need to dry-swallow. During eating the symptom disappears and no difficulties seem to occur in swallowing food, and nor has any weight loss been reported. Occasionally, the syndrome is experienced as a sharp sting as if by a fishbone, a soreness in the throat, or as a burning pain (Lehtinen & Puhakka, 1976). Most of the patients in that series were middle-aged women, but younger subjects and men were not exempt. Most of these patients will present to the ear, nose and throat department rather than to the psychiatric clinic. Some have a physiological anomaly, others have anxiety superimposed upon such anomalies, while a third group have a primary anxiety disorder which focuses around an excessive concern over swallowing or dryness of the mouth. A few may be suffering from depression.

Traditionally, the sensation of a ball (globus) in the throat almost always occurred in women, hence the description "suffocation of the mother". The idea of a hysterical symptom in the throat was linked with the notion that the wandering uterus blocked the channels of respiration. It is uncertain whether the early writers were describing an anxious dyspnoea or an anxious difficulty in swallowing.

Modern techniques have suggested that the majority of patients presenting with difficulty in swallowing do have some underlying physical problem. Malcolmson (1966, 1968) found that only 21% of patients with a complaint of difficulty in swallowing had a completely negative physical and radiological examination. Others found evidence of reflux oesophagitis in most patients, or elevated resting pressures in the cricopharyngeal sphincter in patients with gastric reflux. These pressures fell to normal after successful treatment. Lehtinen & Puhakka (1976) described two different types of globus pharyngis (i.e. globus hystericus), one in which the cause was mainly somatic and the other in which the cause was primarily psychological. In some centres psychological causes may predominate, but even among those it would be wrong to label all cases of "globus" as "hystericus".

Other symptoms

Vomiting and *diarrhoea* that may be psychogenic have previously been regarded as hysterical but are now rarely classified in this way. Induced vomiting such as occurs in bulimia nervosa is a deliberate disability, but there may be some overlap because hysterical symptoms are quite common in bulimia. Traumatic experiences during childhood may be a common aetiological factor for both disorders. Repeated spontaneous vomiting from intestinal obstruction is also sometimes misdiagnosed as hysterical, even to the point of a fatality. Other disorders of bowel control such as diarrhoea or constipation are sometimes caused by the misuse of laxatives, and by underlying physical disorders. Irritable bowel syndrome should not be attributed to psychological motivation (see page 729) even if psychological measures may be helpful. *Dyspnoea,* which can be psychogenic, is usually due to anxiety rather than the result of hysterical mechanisms. Retention of urine has traditionally been regarded as an hysterical symptom, but it is questionable whether retention occurs at all or to an appreciable extent for psychological reasons. Simulation of retention has also been reported.

Hysterical stupor is diagnosed on the basis of a profound diminution or absence of voluntary movement and normal responsiveness to external stimuli such as light, noise and touch. However, although there is a disturbance of consciousness, the patient is neither asleep nor unconscious. In these circumstances, and in the absence of a physical or other psychiatric disorder (particularly catatonia and severe depression), and in the presence of recent stressful events or current problems, a diagnosis of a psychogenic stupor of a hysterical type may be made. Hysterical stupor is rare and is included in ICD–10 but not in DSM–IV.

Sensory symptoms

Deafness

Hysterical deafness is quite rare in civilian clinical practice, but was common among soldiers exposed to blast injury and was then sometimes associated with hysterical paralysis and blindness. A few subjects who have had their eardrums ruptured, or suffered from industrial deafness, may also prolong or magnify an original injury particularly where compensation is an issue. Absolute hysterical deafness can be detected during sleep, because noise may waken the patient. A more subtle method of demonstrating the presence of intact hearing is to take a sleep EEG recording and then speak the patient's name during it. This may produce the characteristic K complex in the EEG that indicates a response to familiar material, although the response tends to extinguish upon repetition. Evoked potential studies can also be used to demonstrate intact auditory pathways. Incomplete hysterical deafness is rather more difficult to diagnose but may be inferred from inconsistent responses on audiological testing.

Blindness

Hysterical blindness is common in ophthalmological practice (Kathol *et al*, 1983*a,b*; Weller & Wiedemann, 1989) and is often partial rather than complete. It usually presents either as a blurring of vision or difficulty in reading in adolescents, particularly when facing examinations. Difficulty in vision is often thought to be hysterical if the patient shows tubular or spiral visual fields. The measurement of visual fields by perimetry involves moving a small spot systematically from the margin to the centre, and asking the patient to detect the spot. With normal vision the fields should be wider at a distance than close to the eye. If the size of the visual field stays the same on testing, regardless of the distance from the eye, the patient has tubular vision. A spiral change in the visual fields is obtained when the examiner, starting at one point, obtains a visual field of a given magnitude which then gradually decreases as he moves around the field in a circle. By the time the test spot has been returned to the starting point, it may only be visualised on the axis where it started in a position much closer to the centre than was originally found. In a review of the literature, Kathol *et al* (1983*a*) noted that as many as 60% of patients with functional visual loss had no evidence of psychiatric disease either at the time of testing or at follow-up. Inconsistent spiral fields, like tubular vision, may often be due to the persuasive skill of the examiner or to high suggestibility. Stress may make the patient give inconsistent replies, but these are not in themselves disabling or sufficient proof of hysteria.

Disabling blindness is a more troublesome problem. Evoked potential studies will help to demonstrate intact visual pathways. Other evidence on the processing of visual information may be obtained by using colour filters, and by finding discrepancies in reading different sizes of print at different distances. There may also be discrepancies in what the patient reports when looking at polaroid projector slides and when using polaroid goggles. A further test is to produce opto-kinetic nystagmus, which should not occur in the genuinely blind. Blepharospasm which may also be tantamount to blindness is usually due to anxiety or extrapyramidal dyskinesia, rather than hysteria.

Hallucinations that are well formed, often visual, and generally of people, are frequently hysterical. Labarre (1975) described numerous reports and instances of hallucinations associated with dissociative behaviour. Hallucinations which occur without evidence of psychological illness are not clinically important; for example, the bereaved often see or hear relatives. Profuse visual images (e.g. of trains of people passing before the eyes) were called phantasmagoria and are a normal phenomenon. Other types of hallucinations, especially at night, may result from anxiety, sensory deprivation, partly impaired consciousness before or after sleep (hypnagogic and hypnopompic hallucinations), or a combination of these causes.

Anaesthesias

A hysterical loss of sensation can involve half the entire body from top to toe, or from right to left. It may also involve the whole of a limb and characteristically has a glove or stocking distribution on the arms or legs or both. In such cases, the patient may not feel a light touch, firm pressure, pin pricks or vibration. To qualify for a diagnosis of hysteria, the distribution of the sensory loss must fail to fit in with known anatomical boundaries, but conform more with the patient's concept of physiology and anatomy. Thus, hysterical sensory loss is likely to stop sharply at the midline, but only approaches the midline if it is non-hysterical, since at this point segmental nerves overlap by one or two centimetres on each side. Similarly, vibration ought to be felt on both sides when a tuning fork is placed on the bone near the midline, because the vibration will be transmitted across the midline. Unfortunately these classical signs are often unreliable, because they sometimes occur in patients with organic disease such as acute stroke (Gould *et al*, 1986). In regional pain syndromes the existence of pain in one area of the body may elicit a regional effect that overlaps anatomical boundaries, but is still nevertheless physiological (Merskey, 1988).

Hysterical sensory loss is not very important clinically because it rarely leads to immediate complaints. In the past, pain was held to be an important hysterical symptom (Merskey & Spear, 1967), but hysterical pain is rare nowadays (Merskey, 1988); it is discussed further on page 737.

Dissociative symptoms

Hysterical amnesia is characterised by a loss of the knowledge of personal identity combined with preservation of environmental information and often complex learned information or skills. For example, a patient may claim he does not know who he is, and be oblivious to his own past, yet at the same time can play chess. Psychogenic amnesia consists of an episode of sudden inability to recall important personal information that is too extensive to be explained by ordinary forgetfulness. Hysterical amnesia most commonly presents to accident and emergency departments and then to neurologists, but is relatively rare in psychiatric clinics. The condition may be more frequent among criminals or soldiers in distress. A history of head injury or brain damage is often present in civilian cases.

Amnesic patients with an impulse to wander are said to be in a *fugue* state. The predominant disturbance is sudden unexpected travel away from home or a customary place of work. There is an inability to recall their past, and sometimes the assumption of a partial or completely new identity. Memory for recent events which may be of a traumatic or stressful nature is lost, although these aspects may emerge when other informants are available. In contrast to organic fugue states, basic self-care such as eating or washing, and simple social interactions with strangers, such as buying a ticket, asking directions or ordering a meal, are preserved. Hysterical fugue may be differentiated from post-ictal fugue because the latter usually occurs in the presence of a history of epilepsy, without stressful events or problems, and the activities and travels of the epileptic patient are less purposeful and more fragmented. ICD–10 and DSM–IV provide similar descriptions and require the exclusion of both multiple personality disorder and organic mental disorder. ICD–10 in addition requires the exclusion of excessive fatigue and intoxication.

Stengel (1941) described 25 patients with fugues, of whom 10 had epilepsy, one had schizophrenia, and several others had depression. Traumatic childhood experiences were also common in these patients. In three other series (Wilson *et al*, 1950; Barrington *et al*, 1956; Kennedy & Neville, 1957), organic brain disease, particularly head injury, was common.

Symonds (1970) observed that in his experience patients with hysterical amnesia and fugues had some awareness of counterfeiting their symptoms. Others find that it is wholly genuine, in the sense that some patients appear truly lost, and on recovery give evidence of troublesome personal problems which explain their conditions. In summary, it appears that hysterical amnesias and fugues often have an organic factor as a complication or cause, in addition to psychological contributions from depression, early childhood disturbances and current stress.

The Ganser syndrome

Ganser (1898) described three prisoner patients who showed the central feature of talking past the point.

> "The most obvious sign which they present consists of their inability to answer correctly the simplest questions which are asked of them, even though by many of their answers they indicate that they have grasped, in a large part, the sense of the question, and in their answers they betray a baffling ignorance and a surprising lack of knowledge which they most assuredly once possessed, or still possess . . . We cannot fail to recognise how in the choice of answers the patient appears to pass over deliberately the indicated correct answer and to select a false one, which any child could easily recognise as such." (Ganser, 1898)

Ganser wrote of *vorbeigehen*, meaning "passing by". The word *vorbeireden* meaning "talking past the point" has also been used. Both words essentially signify that a question is answered by deliberately neglecting the correct answer in favour of a related nonsensical response. The term "approximate answers" has also been used. Thus the colour of the sky on a fine day may be grey, a cow may have five legs, or two and two add up to five.

The Ganser symptoms reflect a specific memory defect and this should be distinguished from the complete Ganser syndrome (Scott, 1965). Ganser syndrome patients have clouding of consciousness with impairment of attention and concentration. There may also be a memory defect, anxiety, perplexity, hallucinations (often of a frightening visual type), as well as hysterical motor and sensory symptoms. Whitlock (1967*a*) found that while Ganser symptoms were common, the complete syndrome itself was rare. The syndrome has been found in individuals awaiting trial, particularly for murder charges, or for those in prison when under considerable stress. It also occurs in patients with organic brain disease such as strokes and head injury. In other cases individuals were seeking financial benefits, or had depression. Chronic schizophrenic patients may also give Ganser-like answers to questions, leading to the term the "Fatuous Syndrome" (Bleuler, 1911).

Malingering

Hysteria is distinguished from malingering on the grounds that hysterical symptoms are produced unconsciously while malingering is consciously produced. In practice the distinction can be difficult to make, and most psychiatrists try to take a patient's statements on trust. Also, both unconscious and conscious intention tend to work in the same way, resulting in the mimicry of an illness in accordance with the patient's concept of that illness. More commonly malingering is superimposed on a genuine physical or psychiatric illness.

Hurst (1940) gave two criteria for the detection of malingering: detection "in flagrante delicto" and an unforced confession. Few malingerers are so helpful as the soldier who wrote a letter on lined paper without a heading, purporting to be signed by the matron of a hospital, to the effect that "Private X is unfit to return to duty because he has a broken ankel (sic)". Some patients admit that they "bring on" their symptoms; for example, an epileptic patient who produced hysterical fits was diagnosed as attention-seeking. She later indicated that she was partly aware of what she was doing and had produced the hysterical fits in order to try to get her "proper fits" treated better. Other individuals with hysterical symptoms appear genuinely unaware of the mechanism, which is presumably unconscious. A former nurse with an hysterical gait who managed to read her own notes was horror-struck and indignant at the diagnosis. Claimants seeking large damages for personal injuries may be videotaped by insurance investigators, and some patients prove to have capacities which they solemnly swore to the doctor were lacking. In one case a patient presented with an apparent organic paralysis, but investigators succeeded in installing a camera in a hotel bedroom and filmed the paralysed individual walking around unaided. He was discovered and charged with fraud. Another patient was seen trotting vigorously in a public place, while the same man would regularly appear in the waiting room, shuffling and bent.

Flicker (1956) considered that 10% of malingerers were normal, and that as many as 5% of people malingered at the time of induction for military service. This was nearly the same proportion as occurred in the service hospitals, but only 0.03% of the latter were officially diagnosed. In his view malingering was encountered in five situations: psychosis, oligophrenia, constitutional psychopathic states, neurosis, and fear states or deficiencies of morale.

Epidemic hysteria

Hysterical symptoms communicated by social contact can affect large numbers of people. This is usually known as mass or epidemic hysteria (Sirois, 1975; Merskey, 1979). Common symptoms include convulsive jerks, headaches, sore throats, abdominal pain, belief in food-poisoning, dizziness and weakness. The syndrome is most frequent in girls' schools, but both sexes may be affected. Factory workers, nurses and other health personnel have also been involved (Kerckoff & Back, 1968; McEvedy & Beard, 1970*a,b*). Moss & McEvedy (1976) described criteria indicating that hysteria was the most likely cause for an epidemic. The epidemic disseminates most rapidly when the social group is large, and in places where social contact is maximum. During the outbreak new cases tend to start in places of high social contact, such as the school hall, the playground and the corridors, rather than the classroom. Younger girls in the 11–15 year age group are more susceptible, and the incidence of new cases tends to move to the lower end of the school as the epidemic progresses. Benaim *et al* (1973) described a possible epidemiogenic personality.

Epidemic hysteria has a long history, particularly in Europe. St John's dance appeared in Germany soon after the Black Death in 1374. Men and women formed circles and danced for hours in a wild delirium and appeared to have lost control of their senses, until at length they fell to the ground exhausted (Hecker, 1844). Another dancing plague, known as St Vitus' dance, appeared in Strasbourg in 1418, although this term was later applied to cases of chorea. Comparable outbreaks in Italy were described as 'Tarantism', being attributed to the bite of the tarantula spider which was alleged to continue its effects indefinitely. Groups of 18th century Cornish Methodists had attacks of leaping around in frenzied states and were known as the "Jumpers". An equivalent French group were known as the "convulsionnaires", while another group who took to moving on all fours and growling were known as the "Barkers". All these outbreaks probably occurred during periods of social upheaval among the affected populations, and the behaviour received popular sanction at the time.

Culturally sanctioned behaviour

Many cultures have permitted, or developed, forms of bizarre behaviour occurring in the context of extreme stress or personal difficulty. In the ICD–10 scheme, the category of dissociative disorders includes transient possession states. During these states there is a temporary loss of the sense of personal identity and awareness of the surroundings, and the individual acts as if taken over by another personality, spirit, deity or 'force'. These trance states, which are involuntary or unwanted, intrude into ordinary activities and occur outside special religious or other culturally accepted situations.

Latah (Yap, 1951, 1952) affects Malayan women who behave in a simple and compliant way, sometimes with echopraxia, echolalia, and even coprolalia. The condition usually follows a sudden fright such as seeing or stepping on a snake. Chiu *et al* (1972) found that 7 out of 50 females with latah had a definite mental illness, and another 13 had mild psychiatric disorders. They considered it to be a "socially acceptable form of attention-seeking behaviour in women". *Amok* is found in Malayan men, who after a period of brooding may suddenly seize a weapon and slay anyone within reach, until the subject himself is killed. Those who have survived are said to claim amnesia for the whole episode. Comparison can be made with the 'berserk' behaviour of Vikings (Sim, 1974). Most authors consider that amok is usually a response by a man to a desperate situation which he cannot remedy.

Piblokto or "Arctic hysteria" is described among the Inuit (Eskimos). The sufferer, usually a woman, begins to scream, and tear off and perhaps destroy her clothing, imitating the cry of an animal or a bird, before she throws herself into the snow or ice. The condition is very rare. Lehmann (1975) reported that he had seen only one case. *Wihtigo*, put forward as a psychiatric illness of the Cree, Ojibway and Salteaux Indians, involves a belief or fear that the sufferer has been transformed into a man-eating giant monster. No cases have been described in detail (Lehmann, 1975). Culturally sanctioned behaviour allows individuals to engage in wild or extreme actions, which on occasion (as in wihtigo) involve delusions or hallucinations. The connection with psychodynamic theory is not straightforward, since some of these conditions involve repression (latah, piblokto), while in others (amok, wihtigo) there is a release from repression (Merskey, 1979).

The difficult distinction between the cultural hysterical possession states and psychotic symptoms, particularly delusions of control, is considered in the Present State Examination (Wing *et al*, 1974). Possession states always occur in a state of dissociation, while delusions of control occur in clear consciousness. The cultural origins of possession states are generally obvious, as is the motivation for the symptoms, but there is no explanation for delusions of control. Cultural possession states are generally ego-enhancing in effect, since the subject becomes identified with a more powerful being. Delusions of control, on the other hand, express an experience of loss rather than acquisition of identity. Finally, delusions of control are often associated with other abnormal or psychotic experiences.

Hysterical psychoses

A small number of apparently psychotic illnesses exist that have been termed the hysterical psychoses, which differ clinically from schizophrenia and affective disorders, have different management and generally have a good prognosis. Hirsch & Hollender (1969) described a group of individuals with hysterical personality traits who became psychotic under conditions of stress. The features included delusions, hallucinations (generally visual), depersonalisation and grossly unusual behaviour, with the episodes lasting for 1–3 weeks. Mallet & Gold (1964) reported a series of 13 female patients with an illness that had at one point been diagnosed as schizophrenia, and who had made a poor response to treatment. The illness was characterised by the presence of emotional emptiness, bizarre depersonalisation phenomena, paranoid thinking, dramatic hallucinations and hysterical personality traits, and was called "hysterical psychosis". Commonly, the subject is an immigrant, with a poor command of the language of their new country, who "breaks down" under considerable stress, the illness resembling an acute schizophreniform or depressive disorder with some atypical features. Such illnesses respond more to general nursing and hospital care than to phenothiazines (Allodi, 1982). The Scandinavian notion of psychogenic psychosis (Faergeman, 1945) describes the condition well (see page 497 for further discussion). These illnesses can usually be distinguished from schizophrenia by the history of recent stress, abrupt onset, and the lack of other typical features of schizophrenia. Hallucinations, if they occur, are vivid, often visual and well formed. Today some of these patients would be diagnosed as having borderline personality disorder, which includes in its diagnostic criteria both the presence of certain personality traits previously considered to be hysterical, as well as the occurrence of brief psychotic episodes.

Dissociative identity disorder

Individuals with this diagnosis (formerly multiple personality disorder) are said to have at least two personalities, of which only one is dominant at a given time. DSM–IV mentions the occurrence of more than 100 individual identities in one person. The number of cases reported in the literature, particularly in the US, has grown enormously since the publication of the book *The Three Faces of Eve* (Thigpen & Cleckley, 1957), which received widespread publicity and was also made into a film. The book describes the transformation from "Eve White" to "Eve Black", only mentioning briefly a little later on that the new name was the patient's original one. In her autobiography (Sizemore & Pittilo, 1977), the patient describes the transition from being Chris White to Chris Costner. Costner was her maiden name and she was unhappy in her marriage. The obvious psychodynamic explanation for her second 'personality' is that she resumed her maiden name and this symbolised the denial of her marriage. DSM–IV criteria for dissociative identity disorder are:

(1) the presence of two or more distinct identities or personality states (each with its own relatively enduring pattern of perceiving, relating to, and thinking about the environment and self);

(2) at least two of these identities or personality states recurrently take full control of the person's behaviour;

(3) the inability to recall important personal information that is too extensive to be explained by ordinary forgetfulness; and

(4) the disturbance is not due to the direct physiological effects of a substance or a general medical condition.

The condition is reported most commonly in the US, but is rarely if ever seen in the UK. Those who find the condition common have noted a high frequency of extreme abuse in childhood as a common feature (Ross, 1989). Bliss (1986) suggested that multiple personality disorder is caused by autohypnosis. Much doubt has been cast on the quality of the literature describing the syndrome (Fahy, 1988), to the point where the existence of the syndrome itself has been attributed to iatrogenesis and social encouragement (Merskey, 1992*a*). Examination of the earlier literature suggests that many of the cases were misdiagnosed bipolar illness or organic disease, while other cases were induced by overt suggestion under hypnosis. No cases in the classical historical series could be seen to be 'pure', and no modern case arose spontaneously without prior knowledge of the idea. Even the case of Sybil (Schreiber, 1973) has been shown to be fallacious, appropriately enough in a television programme where Spiegel (1993) declared that the patient reported to him that the principal proponent of the diagnosis of multiple personality disorder required the patient to assume different names and identities.

Currently, multiple personality disorder or dissociative identities disorder is liable to be found with cases of the false memory syndrome, in which sometimes a psychotherapist may have pressed a patient to recollect memories of abuse. Long-forgotten memories of this type, or any type, are profoundly unreliable, and even more so when related to childhood and when they are produced for the benefit of therapists (Merskey, 1995).

Hysterical personality disorder

At one time it was thought there was a close link between hysterical personality disorder and hysterical symptoms, but this is now known to be untrue. Chodoff & Lyons (1958) showed that among 17 patients with conversion symptoms, only three had good evidence of the so-called hysterical personality. Conversion symptoms were more often a feature of immaturity and dependence rather than personality disorder, as has also been shown in the series of Ljungberg (1957) and Merskey & Trimble (1979). Hysterical personality disorder is now termed histrionic personality disorder, and is described with the other personality disorders on page 787.

Epidemiology

The incidence and prevalence of hysterical symptoms has varied across time, place and culture. For example, very high rates were observed among soldiers in the trenches during the First World War. In general psychiatric practice today the condition is rare. Two psychiatric case register studies for the period 1960–69, one from Iceland and the other from Monroe County, New York State, provide some useful data. Figures for Monroe County were 22 per 100 000 population, which was double the rate found in Iceland. In the American sample rates were higher for women, non-whites and those of low socioeconomic status (social classes 4 and 5) (Stefannson *et al*, 1976). A general population study in Sweden found the morbidity risk for hysteria to be 0.5% (Ljungberg, 1957). Higher rates of conversion symptoms are seen in psychiatric liaison practice, with figures of between 5 and 16% being given (Lazare, 1981). Pain is supposedly the most common symptom, while conversion symptoms were usually superimposed on an underlying organic disorder. When attention is focused on multiple somatic symptoms, about 10% of psychiatric in-patients are found to be affected (Bibb & Guze, 1972) and between 5–11% of psychiatric out-patients (Guze *et al*, 1971). In some underdeveloped countries rather higher rates are reported presenting to out-patient departments; for example, Hafeiz (1980) found 10% in the Sudan. There is a substantial overlap between patients who have conversion symptoms and those who have multiple somatic complaints because the latter is a common condition. Thus one out of 50 consecutive women under investigation in a university hospital medical ward had multiple somatic complaints (Woodruff, 1968). There has been a suggestion that the prevalence of hysteria has declined over the last few decades. Conversion symptoms which were once common at the turn of the century now seem to be relatively rare.

Aetiology

Genetics

Briquet (1859), who carried out one of the first family history studies in psychiatry, reported a strong familial trend for his patients with hysteria. However, this finding may be partly explained by the fact that his case material included many women with multiple somatic complaints and others with classical affective disorders. The twin study of Shields (1982) failed to demonstrate any significant genetic contribution. On the other hand, Inouye (1972) collected all the available twin studies and case reports and found 9 concordant and 33 discordant monozygotic pairs, but no concordant and 43 discordant dizygotic pairs. The lack of any dizygotic concordant pairs was a surprising finding as it appears to suggest that environmental familial effects are not important either.

Functional disorders

Major psychiatric disorder may also occasionally contribute to hysteria. In a series of 85 cases, two later developed schizophrenia and eight developed endogenous depression (Slater & Glithero, 1965). Lewis (1975) traced 98 cases from the Maudsley Hospital of whom two developed schizophrenia, and of those who had not recovered, eight had depression. Ciompi (1969) traced 38 patients surviving an average of 34 years after their first admission with hysteria, and found two with schizophrenia and two with epilepsy. In Ljungberg's (1957) series the morbidity risk was 2% for psychogenic psychosis, 3.1% for schizophrenia, and 2.4% for manic–depressive psychoses, suggesting small but definite associations.

Unipolar depression has been reported in 16–22% of cases (Merskey & Buhrich, 1975; McKegney, 1967). Also, 58% of those with hysteria had some depression (McKegney, 1967), with particularly high rates of depression being found in those with fugue states (Stengel, 1941). Recognition of depressive illness in such cases is important because it may be treatable. Bibb & Guze (1972) found depressive symptoms to be prominent in 80% of patients hospitalised with Briquet's syndrome.

Organic brain disease is another contributory factor to hysteria. In one series, around two-thirds of the cases had an accompanying cerebral disorder or preceding organic brain disease (Whitlock, 1967*b*), although in the Maudsley series only 4% had a history of organic brain disease (Lewis,

1975). An intermediate figure was given by Standage (1975) who noted that 32% of subjects with hysteria had a previous history of neurological disease, particularly epilepsy.

Pathogenic mechanisms

Consideration of the literature suggests that there are probably five ways in which physical illness relates to hysterical symptoms.

(1) An independent emotional stress may make a patient elaborate the distressing effects of an organic lesion which has already disturbed normal functioning. Thus the weak hand may become paralysed. This mechanism appeared to operate in at least 12 out of 89 cases in the author's series (Merskey & Buhrich, 1975).

(2) The occurrence of previous or intermittent physical symptoms, as in epilepsy, provides a model for the hysterical symptom. A psychological stress would then more easily produce a form of illness of which the patient had some knowledge. Past illness in a relative or a close acquaintance may also serve the same function.

(3) The unpleasant psychological implications of a physical illness, such as the discomfort and fear attached to it, may make the patient elaborate an existing symptom, or produce a fresh one.

(4) Physical illness can cause a regression in behaviour into the sick role. The advantages of the sick role range from receiving get-well cards, gifts of fruit and flowers, to relief from painful responsibilities and intrapsychic dilemmas.

(5) In an unknown way, cerebral damage may operate more specifically to produce conversion symptoms.

Concerning this last possibility, Schilder (1940) wrote that "cerebral organic syndromes may change functions of the brain in such a way as to provoke neurotic attitudes. One cannot claim similar mechanisms for traumas which afflict other parts of the body". Schilder linked this with a concept of "organic repression", according to which the organic lesion acted to produce repression in place of a psychological stress. Galin *et al* (1977) observed that hysterical conversion symptoms and psychogenic pain symptoms are more common on the left side of the body suggesting some neurological contribution, but this observation has never been properly explained. Slater & Glithero (1965) thought that organic disease might bring about a general disturbance of the personality "which results in modes of behaviour such as exaggeration, attention seeking, etc., which we naturally think of as manifestations of an hysterical personality". Whatever the underlying mechanism, physical illness, particularly organic brain disease, is an important factor contributing to the development of hysterical symptoms.

Sociological explanations

An alternative social explanation, which has not been generally accepted, was proposed by Szasz (1961). He suggested that hysterical symptoms reflect the choice of a particular social role by the patient. He argued that a person with hysterical symptoms is impersonating the physically ill in order to "achieve, maintain, or regain control over an interpersonal relationship. The patient simulates physical illness to communicate helplessness, submissiveness, weakness, dependency, etc., and this absolves him or her of any blame or responsibility." A similar, although much less harsh, sociological formulation was given by Slavney (1990). He argued that hysteria is not something which a patient has, but rather reflects something a patient *is* and something the patient *does*, and these questions can be understood by a knowledge of the patient's life story. Eisenthal & Lazare (1979) suggested that the clinician, when analysing the symptoms of any social communications, should always consider the sender, the receiver, and what the sender is symbolically saying about himself. What is the sender trying to tell the receiver? Why has this particular message been sent? What is the social setting of the communication? Finally, has the receiver understood the message? Explanations in social terms of this type are particularly helpful in understanding some hysterical states such as the Ganser syndrome.

Prognosis

The largest follow-up study (Ljungberg, 1957) found that after one year, 43% of men and 35% of women were still symptomatic. By five years these figures were 25% and 22% respectively, with little change at 10–15 years. Of those who had recovered, around 7% had relapsed by one-year follow-up. Age and intelligence had little effect, but a poor premorbid personality had an adverse effect on outcome. A more pessimistic picture was given by Slater & Glithero (1965) who conducted a nine-year follow-up study of 85 out of 112 patients who had initially been given a diagnosis of hysteria at a tertiary neuropsychiatric referral centre (The National Hospital for Nervous Diseases). Nine years later, 12 patients of the 85 traced had died, four by suicide, and the remaining 73 patients fell into three groups. At the time of the initial psychiatric referral, 19 patients had a diagnosis of hysteria or "hysterical overlay", and this was coupled with a known physical disorder. In a second group of 22 patients, an organic basis for the symptoms was eventually discovered, even though this had been missed during the index admission. In the third group the remaining 32 patients had no evidence of organic illness, but some had later developed a psychiatric disorder. Two became schizophrenic, eight had "cyclothymic depression" and one had a severe depressive illness. Seven subjects who presented initially with acute psychogenic reactions recovered well, while 14 patients developed more chronic neurotic states. This rather dismal prognosis, particularly the high mortality, has not been replicated elsewhere, possibly because the cases originated from a tertiary referral centre.

A more optimistic prognosis was given in Lewis' (1975) study in which follow-up ranged from 7 to 12 years; of the 75 subjects seven had died, of whom three had central nervous system disease and one committed suicide. Two-thirds of the survivors were sufficiently well to be working and were symptom-free. Of the remainder a few were better but still symptomatic, a few were worse and the rest unchanged. A long-term follow-up by Ciompi (1980) showed that conversion symptoms tended to disappear. Almost all those who develop hysterical symptoms in particular circumstances, such as during a war, or in epidemics of hysteria, recover completely. A good prognosis is also reported from developing countries where acute conversion symptoms are more common (Hafeiz, 1980). Overall, the outcome of conversion or dissociative symptoms is most closely related to the severity and chronicity of the disorder. Severe and dramatic illnesses may respond very well, but as with many other disorders, prolonged cases tend to persist. In all cases, the more recent the symptom the better the prognosis.

Treatment

Therapy starts during the diagnostic process. The relationship which develops between the doctor and the patient during the course of history-taking and examination is of critical importance. Occasionally an initial interview with abreactive qualities may abolish the symptoms altogether. Unfortunately, clumsy attempts are often made towards the end of the initial interview to try to persuade patients that their physical symptoms are "all in the mind" and this gives rise to misunderstandings. Patients will generally try to resist messages of this type and the psychiatrist's task is to find an effective way to circumvent this problem. Direct attempts to explain that the symptom is in the unconscious mind, or that if they were to think differently they would be cured, are ineffective. It is important in the first interview not to jump to any conclusions, and certainly not to offer them to patients without adequate supportive evidence. It is more helpful to convey an impression of uncertainty and intimate that more time is needed to form a useful opinion, rather than to create hostility by offering an unsubstantiated conclusion which fails to persuade the patient.

The management of hysterical symptoms requires patience, thoroughness and a gradual, but firm, approach. It is tempting to confront the patient: "This symptom arises from your mind, and we need to change your thoughts about it". The patient is liable to respond "Yes, I am willing to but please tell me how", and then add "I have tried very hard and nothing has happened". Other patients may simply not believe that their paralysis, which so dominates their thoughts, is otherwise non-existent. It is better to avoid attempts to explain the symptoms directly. Direct efforts at explanation very often lead to a blank wall of incomprehension, or sometimes even frank hostility.

Interviews with close relatives may yield significant information, or sometimes result in a change of attitude in the relative which may in itself be helpful. The patient may slowly begin to revise his seemingly fixed attitudes or ideas as a result of the therapist's enquiries, particularly if they broach on troublesome relationships or other sensitive areas.

Concomitant organic disease must be recognised or excluded. Approximately 60% of those presenting with classical conversion symptoms to the author's clinic were superimposed on physical disorder. The most common organic cause was toxic levels of anticonvulsant drugs and other substances, and this may present as slurred speech or altered reflexes, a cause easily remedied by a reduction in dose. Depression and occasionally schizophrenia may underlie a conversion symptom, and appropriate treatment for these disorders may also cure the hysterical symptoms.

Understanding the symptom

As already indicated, the doctor's efforts to try to understand and relieve the patient's symptoms will help to strengthen the doctor–patient relationship. Alternative suggestions as to how best to deal with the symptoms begin to appear during therapy, and relief may occur partly by a cathartic mechanism, but also because of simple practical changes that patients make in their life. Sometimes merely examining the problems at work, in the home, or in relationships may be sufficient to trigger a successful result, but in other cases more prolonged psychotherapy may be required. Attention to relationships may cause changes through a psychodynamic process.

> *Case example*
> A young woman who was engaged to be married developed pain over one eye and blurring of vision. The history indicated that she had suffered a minor blow from the buckle of the car seatbelt in her fiancé's car on a day he had taken her out. No organic basis was found for either the pain or for the blurred vision. After she had separated from her fiancé, the symptoms disappeared.

Clinicians who believe that hysterical symptoms are a message between the sender and receiver try to help the patient to become aware of both the meaning and reasons for the communication, in the hope that as more direct and appropriate behaviour is adopted, the symptoms are relinquished.

Insight psychotherapy

Prolonged psychoanalytical therapy is usually not the best treatment since the problems may either be too overwhelming, or alternatively not at all observable. However, the therapist should offer a series of 6–10 interviews with the aim of exploring emotional relationships in general, rather than simply focusing on the symptom. As in other brief psychotherapies the therapist should play a rather more active role. In these sessions, transference interpretations should be dealt with very cautiously or possibly even avoided altogether. This is because anger and hostility are often near the surface and focusing on these emotions may make the situation worse rather than better. If hostility is discussed it is better handled in terms of the patient's "emotions", "states of nervous tension" or feelings of irritability or worries concerning the situation, and their expectations from treatment, rather than by making bold interpretations about the symbolic meaning of the doctor.

Narco-analysis, as well as being diagnostic, may also be psycho-therapeutic. Narco-analysis by the injection of amylobarbitone sodium or other sedative medication was widely used in soldiers just removed from the scene of battle. Good results were obtained in this situation, but they might equally have been obtained with oral sedation and discussion. Stengel taught that narco-analysis added nothing to what could be obtained by a series of interviews, and modern evidence concurs (Piper, 1994).

Suggestion

Suggestion has been the main historical treatment and is still widely used in a variety of ways, while indirect suggestion often occurs during psychotherapy. Direct suggestion may involve retraining or behavioural techniques. Traditionally, the aphonias have often been cured by demonstrating to patients that they can still cough. This leads to the patient saying "ah", and then trying more varied syllables such as "baa, paa" until normal speech is resumed. This should always be done with a background of psychological and social support. Suggestion may also help to relieve a paralysis. In one method which is often successful, a physiotherapist offers what appears to be a series of progressively more difficult physiotherapeutic manoeuvres which are intended to improve motor function. There is then no need to challenge the patient's inner thoughts or capacity.

Hypnosis is favoured by some therapists, possibly because it is a widely accepted measure and so can provide a face-saving solution.

However, it is probably no more than an approved mode of suggestion. There is controversy over whether it is a special state, perhaps accompanied by altered consciousness, and physiologically different from normal waking or attention. State theorists believe the above, and consider that the trance condition is a special physiological alteration. This view is challenged by the absence of relevant physiological evidence which could distinguish hypnosis from other states of suggestion (Merskey, 1971). More importantly, Barber (1969) has demonstrated that task-motivating suggestions produce as much effect in hypnosis as the induction of trances. At a minimum, the procedure of offering hypnotic instructions or suggestions does frequently result in the remission of acute conversion symptoms, but rarely improves chronic ones.

Suggestion, hypnosis and psychodynamic approaches to treatment should not be advanced without giving the patient continuous implicit or explicit assurances of psychological support. This is particularly important once the material giving rise to the problem has been revealed. This is also true even when one suspects that the patient may have a degree of conscious awareness of the nature of the symptom. Symonds (1970), a neurologist, considered that all persons with hysterical amnesia that he had encountered had at least some knowledge of their complaints, but this was combined with a state of intolerable emotional turmoil, and so a consideration of the patient's self-respect required that there should always be some face-saving manoeuvre.

Social measures

Carter (1853) removed patients from environments in which they were prone to develop symptoms, and this may explain why admission to hospital is sometimes helpful. An outbreak of hysterical syndromes at a local elementary school ceased following a public announcement of the diagnosis of "mass hysteria" (Nitzkin, 1976). Sirois (1974) listed the responses to epidemics of hysteria which were effective, including isolation of affected individuals and the closing of schools. A clinician working together with a patient may find other ways to meet his needs without the patient ever becoming aware of the meaning of the symptom. Finally, the clinician can influence the patient's social milieu to respond to a patient's unstated needs, so that the symptom may no longer be necessary.

Behaviour therapy

Aversive therapy by electrical stimulation was used by Yealland (1918) with soldiers. It was much in line with the ethical position of his time, but would not be acceptable today. Lazarus (1963) reported the outcome for 27 patients with conversion or dissociative symptoms treated with behaviour therapy; a multimodal approach sometimes involving the use of hypnosis, medication or more than one therapist produced marked improvement or recovery in 19 (71%) patients after an average of 14 treatment sessions. Recovery has also been obtained with patients who had been disabled for years in spite of other approaches (Liebson, 1969; Munford *et al*, 1976). The most substantial review of the literature on this topic is by Scallet *et al* (1976) who examined 23 reports on the management of "chronic hysteria" and found that 62% of out-patients and 65% of in-patients were improved.

References

Allodi, F. (1982) Acute paranoid reaction (bouffee delirante) in Canada. *Canadian Journal of Psychiatry*, **27**, 366–373.

American Psychiatric Association (1987) *Diagnostic and Statistical Manual of Mental Disorders* (3rd edn revised) (DSM–III–R). Washington, DC: APA.

—— (1994) *Diagnostic and Statistical Manual of Mental Disorders* (4th edn) (DSM–IV). Washington, DC: APA.

Barber, T. X. (1969) *Hypnosis, a Scientific Approach*. New York: Van Nostrand.

Barrington, W. R., Liddell, D. W. & Foulds, G. A. (1956) A re-evaluation of the fugue. *Journal of Mental Science*, **102**, 280.

Benaim, S., Horder, J. & Anderson, J. (1973) Hysterical epidemic in a classroom. *Psychological Medicine*, **30**, 366–373.

Bibb, R. C. & Guze, S. (1972) Hysteria (Briquet's syndrome) in a psychiatric hospital. The significance of secondary depression. *American Journal of Psychiatry*, **129**, 224–228.

Bleuler, E. (1911) *Textbook of Psychiatry* (trans. H. A. Brill, 1951). New York: Dover Publications.

Bliss, E. L. (1986) *Multiple Personality, Allied Disorders and Hypnosis*. New York: Oxford Medical Publications.

Brachet, J. L. (1847) *Traite de l'Hysterie*. Paris: J. B. Bailliere.

Breuer, J. & Freud, S. (1893–1895) Studies on hysteria. In *Complete Psychological Works of Freud*, Vol. 2 (1955). London: Hogarth Press.

Briquet, P. (1859) *Traite Clinique et Therapeutique de l'Hysterie*. Paris: J. B. Bailliere.

Brodie, B. C. (1837) *Lectures Illustrative of Certain Nervous Affections*. London: Longman.

Carter, A. B. (1949) The prognosis of certain hysterical symptoms. *British Medical Journal*, **i**, 1076–1079.

Carter, R. B. (1853) *On the Pathology and Treatment of Hysteria*. London: Churchill.

Charcot, J. M. (1889) Lectures on the diseases of the nervous system. Delivered at La Salpetriere, 1872 (trans. T. Savill). London: The New Sydenham Society.

Chiu, T. L., Tong, J. E. & Schmidt, K. E. (1972) A clinical and survey study of Latah in Sarawak, Malaysia. *Psychological Medicine*, **2**, 155–165.

Chodoff, R. & Lyons, H. (1958) Hysteria, the hysterical personality and 'hysterical' conversion. *American Journal of Psychiatry*, **114**, 734-740.

Ciompi, L. (1969) Follow-up studies on the evolution of former neurotic and depressive states in old age. Clinical and psychodynamic aspects. *Journal of Geriatric Psychiatry*, **3**, 90–106.

—— (1980) The natural history of schizophrenia in the long term. *British Journal of Psychiatry*, **136**, 413–420.

Das, P. S. & Saxena, S. (1991) Classification of dissociative states in DSM-III–R and ICD–10 (1989 draft). A study of Indian out-patients. *British Journal of Psychiatry*, **159**, 425–427.

Eisenthal, S. & Lazare, A. (1979) The sociocultural approach. In *Outpatient Psychiatry, Diagnosis and Treatment* (ed. A. Lazare). Baltimore: Williams & Wilkins.

Ellenberger, H. F. (1970) *The Discovery of the Unconscious*. New York: Basic Books.

Faergeman, P. M. (1945) *Psychogenic Psychoses*. London: Butterworth.

Fahy, T. A. (1988) The diagnosis of multiple personality disorder. A critical review. *British Journal of Psychiatry*, **153**, 597–606.

Flicker, D. J. (1956) Malingering: a symptom. *Journal of Nervous and Mental Disorders*, **123**, 23–31.

Galin, D., Diamond, R. & Braff, D. A. (1977) Lateralization of conversion symptoms: more frequent on the left. *American Journal of Psychology*, **134**, 578–581.

Ganser, S. J. M. (1898) A peculiar hysterical state (trans. C. E. Schorer, 1965). *British Journal of Criminology*, **5**, 120–126.

Georget, M. (1821) *De la Physiologie du Systeme Nerveux*. Paris: J. B. Bailliere.

Gould, R., Miller, B. L., Goldberg, M. A., et al (1986) The validity of hysterical signs and symptoms. *Journal of Nervous and Mental Disease*, **174**, 593–598.

Guze, S. B., Woodruff, R. A. & Clayton, P. J. (1971) A study of conversion symptoms in psychiatric out-patients. American Journal of Psychiatry, 128, 643–646.

Hafeiz, H. B. (1980) Hysterical conversion: A prognostic study. *British Journal of Psychiatry*, **136**, 548–551.

Head, H. (1922) An address on the diagnosis of hysteria. *British Medical Journal*, i, 827–829.

Hecker, J. F. C. (1844) *Epidemics of the Middle Ages* (trans. B. G. Babington). London: The New Sydenham Society.

Hirsch, S. J. & Hollender, M. H. (1969) Hysterical psychoses: Clarification of the concept. *American Journal of Psychiatry*, **125**, 905–915.

Hirschmuller, A. (1989) *The Life and Work of Josef Breuer, Physiology and Psychoanalysis*. New York: New York University Press.

Hunter, R. & MacAlpine, I. (1963) Three Hundred Years of Psychiatry, 1539–1860. Oxford: Oxford University Press.

Hurst, A. F. (1940) *Medical Diseases of War*. London: Edward Arnold.

Inouye, E. (1972) Genetic aspects of neurosis. *International Journal of Mental Health*, **1**, 176–189.

Janet, P. (1894) *The Mental State of Hystericals* (trans. C. R. Corson, 1901). New York: G. P. Putnam.

Jorden, E. (1603) *A Breife Discourse of a Disease Called the Suffocation of the Mother*. Reprinted in *Witchcraft and Hysteria in Elizabethan London: Edward Jorden and the Mary Glover Case* (ed. M. MacDonald), 1991. London: Tavistock/ Routledge.

Kathol, R. G., Cox, T. A., Corbeft, J. J., *et al* (1983*a*) Functional visual loss: I. A true psychiatric disorder? *Psychological Medicine*, **13**, 307–314.

—, —, —, *et al* (1983*b*) Functional visual loss: II. Psychiatric aspects in 42 patients followed for 4 years. *Psychological Medicine*, **13**, 315–324.

Kennedy, A. & Neville, J. (1957) Sudden loss of memory. *British Medical Journal*, **11**, 428–433.

Kerckoff, A. & Back, K. W. (1968) *The June Bug: A Study of Hysterical Contagion.* New York: Appleton Century Crofts.

Kraepelin, E. (1906) Hysterical insanity. In *Lectures on Clinical Psychiatry* (trans. T. Johnstone), pp. 249–258. New York: William Wood & Co.

Labarre (1975) Anthropological perspectives on hallucinations and hallucinogens. In *Hallucinations: Experience and Theory* (eds R. K. Siegel & L. J. West). New York: Wiley.

Lazare, A. (1981) Conversion symptoms. *New England Journal of Medicine*, **305**, 745–748.

Lazarus, A. A. (1963) The results of behavior therapy in 126 cases of severe neurosis. *Behavioral Research Therapy*, **1**, 69–79.

Lehmann, F. (1975) Unusual psychiatric disorders and atypical psychoses. In *Comprehensive Textbook of Psychiatry* (2nd edn) (eds A. Freedman, H. I. Kaplan & B. J. Sadock). Baltimore: Williams & Wilkins.

Lehtinen, V. & Puhakka, H. (1976) A psychosomatic approach to the globus hystericus syndrome. *Acta Psychiatrica Neurologica Scandinavica*, **53**, 21–28.

Lewis, A. J. (1975) The survival of hysteria. *Psychological Medicine*, **5**, 9–12.

Liebson, I. (1969) Conversion reaction: a learning theory approach. *Behavioral Research Therapy*, **7**, 217–218.

Ljungberg, L. (1957) Hysteria. *Acta Psychiatrica Scandinavica* (suppl. 112).

Lloyd, K. G. & Hornykiewicz, 0. (1973) L-glutamic acid decarboxylase in Parkinson's disease: Effect of L-dopa therapy. *Nature*, **243**, 521–523.

Malcolmson, K. G. (1966) Radiological findings in globus hystericus. *British Journal of Radiology*, **39**, 583–586.

— (1968) Globus hystericus and pharyngis: A reconnaissance of proximal vagal modalities. *Journal of Laryngology and Otology*, **82**, 219–230.

Mallet, B. I. & Gold, S. (1964) A pseudoschizophrenic hysterical syndrome. *British Journal of Medical Psychology*, **37**, 59–70.

McEvedy, C. P. & Beard, A. W. (1970*a*) Royal Free epidemic of 1955: a reconsideration. *British Medical Journal*, **i**, 7-11.

— & — (1970*b*) Concept of benign myalgic encephalomyelitis. *British Medical Journal*, **i**, 1–5.

McKegney, F. P. (1967) The incidence and characteristics of patients with conversion reactions: I. A general hospital consultation service sample. *American Journal of Psychiatry*, **124**, 542–545.

Merskey, H. (1971) An appraisal of hypnosis. *Postgraduate Medical Journal*, **47**, 572–580.

— (1979) *The Analysis of Hysteria.* London: Bailliere Tindall.

— (1988) Regional pain is rarely hysterical. *Archives of Neurology*, **45**, 915–918.

— (1991) Shell shock. In *150 Years of British Psychiatry, 1841–1991* (eds G. E. Berrios & H. L. Freeman), pp. 245–267. London: Gaskell.

— (1992*a*) The creation of personalities. The production of multiple personality disorder. *British Journal of Psychiatry*, **160**, 327–340.

—— (1992*b*) Anna 0. had a severe depressive illness. *British Journal of Psychiatry*, **161**, 185–194.

—— (1995) The Analysis of Hysteria. Understanding Conversion and Dissociation. 2nd edn. London: Gaskell.

—— & Spear, F. G. (1967) *Pain: Psychological and Psychiatric Aspects*. London: Bailliere, Tindall & Cassell.

—— & Buhrich, N. (1975) Hysteria and organic brain disease. *British Journal of Medical Psychology*, **48**, 359–366.

—— & Trimble, M. (1979) Personality, sexual adjustment and brain lesions in patients with conversion symptoms. *American Journal of Psychiatry*, **136**, 179–192.

Moss, P. D. & McEvedy, C-P. (1976) An epidemic of overbreathing among schoolgirls. *British Medical Journal*, ii, 1295–1300.

Munford, P. R., Reardon, D., Liberman, R. P., *et al* (1976) Behavioral treatment of hysterical coughing and mutism: a case study. *Journal of Consulting Clinical Psychology*, **44**, 1008–1014.

Nitzkin, J. L. (1976) Epidemic transient situational disturbance in an elementary school. *Journal of Florida Medical Association*, **63**, 357–359.

Piper, A. (1994) "Truth Serum" and "Recovered Memories" of sexual abuse: a review of the evidence. *The Journal of Psychiatry and Law*, Winter (1993), 447–471.

Reynolds, J. R. (1869) Remarks on paralysis and other disorders of motion and sensation, dependent on idea. *British Medical Journal*, ii, 483–485.

Romberg, M. H. (1851) *A Manual of the Nervous Diseases of Man* (2nd edn) (trans. E. H. Sieveking). London: The New Sydenham Society.

Ross, C. A. (1989) *Multiple Personality*. New York: Wiley.

Sandras, C. M. S. (1851) *Traite Pratique des Maladies Nerveuses*. Paris: Germer, Bailliere.

Scallett, A., Cloninger, R. & Othmer, E. (1976) The management of chronic hysteria: a review and double-blind trial of electrosleep and other relaxation methods. *Disease of the Nervous System*, **37**, 347–353.

Schilder, P. (1940) Neurosis following head and brain injuries. In *Injuries of the Skull, Brain and Spinal Cord* (ed. S. Brock). Philadelphia: Williams & Wilkins.

Schreiber, F. R. (1973) *Sybil*. Chicago: Henry Regnery.

Scott, P. D. (1965) Commentary on "A Peculiar Hysterical State" by S. J. M. Ganser. *British Journal of Criminology*, **5**, 120–126.

Shields, J. (1982) Genetic studies of hysterical disorders. In *Hysteria* (ed. A. Roy), pp. 41–56. Chichester: John Wiley.

Siegel, R. E. (1976) *Galen on the Affected Parts*. Basel: S. Karger.

Sim, M. (1974) *Guide to Psychiatry* (3rd edn). Edinburgh: Churchill Livingstone.

Sirois, F. (1974) Epidemic hysteria. *Acta Psychiatrica Scandinavica* (suppl. 252).

—— (1975) *A propos* the incidence of mass hysteria. *Union Medical Canadien*, **104**, 121–123.

Sizemore, C. C. & Pittilo, E. S. (1977) *I'm Eve*. New York: Doubleday.

Slater, E. & Glithero, E. (1965) A follow-up of patients diagnosed as suffering from "hysteria". *Journal of Psychosomatic Research*, **9**, 9–13.

Slavney, P. R. (1990) *Perspectives on "Hysterics"*. Baltimore: Johns Hopkins University Press.

Spiegel, H. (1993) Comments. In *Mistaken Identities. Canadian Broadcasting Corporation, The Fifth Estate*. Ottawa: Media Tapes and Transcripts.

Standage, K. F. (1975) The etiology of hysterical seizures. *Canadian Psychiatric Association Journal*, **20**, 67–73.

Stefansson, J. G., Massina, J. A. & Meyerowitz, S. (1976) Hysterical neurosis, conversion type: clinical and epidemiological considerations. *Acta Psychiatrica Scandinavica*, **53**, 119–138.

Stengel, E. (1941) On the aetiology of fugue states. *Journal of Mental Science*, **87**, 572–599.

Sydenham, T. (1697) Discourse concerning hysterical and hypochondriacal distempers. In *Dr. Sydenham's Complete Method of Curing Almost All Diseases, and Description of Their Symptoms. To Which are Now Added Five Discourses of the Same Author Concerning Pleurisy, Gout, Hysterical Passion, Dropsy and Rheumatism* (3rd edn). London: Newman & Parker.

Symonds, C. (1970) An address given at the National Hospitals for Nervous Diseases, London, 27/02/70. In *The Analysis of Hysteria* (ed. H. Merskey), 1979. London: Balliere Tindall.

Szasz, T. (1961) *The Myth of Mental Illness*. New York: Harper & Row.

Thigpen, C. H. & Cleckley, H. M. (1957) *The Three Faces of Eve*. New York: McGraw-Hill.

Trimble, M. R. (1978) Serum prolactin in epilepsy and hysteria. *British Medical Journal*, **2**, 1682.

Weller, M. & Wiedemann, P. (1989) Hysterical symptoms in ophthalmology. *Documenta Ophthalmologica*, **73**, 1–33.

Whitlock, F. A. (1967a) The Ganser Syndrome. *British Journal of Psychiatry*, **113**, 19–30.

—— (1967b) The aetiology of hysteria. *Acta Psychiatrica Scandinavica*, **43**, 144–162.

Wilson, G., Rupp, C. & Wilson, W. W. (1950) Amnesia. *American Journal of Psychiatry*, **106**, 481–485.

Wing, J. K., Cooper, J. E. & Sartorius, N. (1974) The Description and Classification of Psychiatric Symptoms: An Instruction Manual for the PSE and CATEGO Systems. London: Cambridge University Press.

Woodruff, R. A. (1968) Hysteria: An evaluation of objective diagnostic criteria by the study of women with chronic medical illnesses. *British Journal of Psychiatry*, **114**, 1115–1119.

World Health Organization (1992) *The Tenth Revision of the International Classification of Mental and Behavioural Disorders (ICD–10)*. Geneva: WHO.

Yap, P. M. (1951) Mental disease peculiar to certain cultures: A survey of comparative psychiatry. *Journal of Mental Science*, **97**, 313–327.

—— (1952) The Latah reaction: Its pathodynamics and nosological position. *Journal of Mental Science*, **98**, 515–564.

Yealland, L. R. (1918) *Hysterical Disorders of Warfare*. London: Macmillan.

17 Hypochondriasis and other somatoform disorders

Tom Brown

Classification ● *Hypochondriasis* ● *Somatisation disorder and Briquet's syndrome* ● *Dysmorphophobia* ● *Irritable bowel syndrome* ● *Cardiac syndromes* ● *Chronic fatigue syndrome* ● *Chronic pain* ● *Münchausen's syndrome* ● *Münchausen's syndrome by proxy*

The word *hypochondriasis* literally means "below the cartilage" and was first used by Smollius in 1610 (Veith, 1965). It was applied to the various mental states that were thought to be caused by changes in the organs of the hypochondrial region, particularly the liver and spleen (Kenyon, 1976). The more recent notion that hypochondriasis is a morbid preoccupation with health only emerged in the 19th century, when Falret (1822) called abnormal beliefs about the state of one's health "hypochondria".

Previously the word had been used by Burton (1651) to describe a subdivision of melancholia, while James Boswell, who wrote in *The London Magazine* as "The Hypochondriac", also took it to mean depression. Thomas Willis (1684) is credited with being the first to make the distinction between hypochondriasis and hysteria. He regarded the latter as an organic brain disease, and so challenged the uterine view of hysteria which had prevailed for many centuries. Some hundred years later, Robert Whytt distinguished between hypochondriasis and depression and criticised those who applied the terms hypochondriasis and hysteria too loosely (Veith, 1965). Whytt's diagnostic concerns remain of interest to the present day, and argue against diagnosis by exclusion, stating that "physicians have bestowed the character of nervous on all those disorders whose nature and causes they were ignorant of". These early historical debates about hypochondriasis, its distinction from depression and the other somatoform disorders are still relevant.

Another important historical contribution was made by George Cheyne who wrote a treatise on hypochondriasis, hysteria and melancholy entitled *The English Malady* (Cheyne, 1733). Cheyne grouped psychiatric symptoms together, and under the heading of hypochondriasis he included depression, anxiety and other neurotic symptoms rather than regarding hypochondriasis as a separate syndrome. He described his own depressive and hypochondriacal symptoms, and in the preface of his book wrote that it was "intended as a legacy, and dying speech only to my fellow sufferers". Cheyne felt that the disorders were caused by the pressures of "modern living" (in the 18th century), by which he meant the influence of mechanisation, city dwelling

710

and affluence. Overeating and lack of exercise made the symptoms worse. Savill (1909) proposed that a "sedentary life" was the main cause of hypochondriasis. Whytt offered a pragmatic approach to treatment. This included the wise advice not to promise to cure the patient, plenty of exercise and a change of diet, and for severe cases, opium. A truly eclectic approach!

The famous French author Marcel Proust suffered from hypochondriasis, and an interesting account is given by Fabricant (1960). Proust suffered from asthma but this was complicated by a gross hypochondriacal preoccupation with his state of health. He spent most of the week in bed, in a specially designed room, and he communicated detailed accounts of his health to other people in his many letters. He abused a variety of drugs, indulged in many health-checking behaviours, and on the rare occasions he left home he wore numerous layers of clothing, several coats as well as padding round his neck. It is alleged that on one occasion when attending the wedding of a friend, his clothing made him so bulky that he was forced to stand in the aisle, because he could not fit in the pews!

The word 'somatisation' is derived from the Greek *soma* meaning body. It was first used early in this century by Stekel to describe neuroses that present as bodily disorders (Hinsie & Campbell, 1960). The concept has more recently been championed by Lipowski (1988), who defined it as "a tendency to experience and communicate somatic distress and symptoms which are unaccounted for by pathological findings and to attribute them to physical illness and to seek medical help for them".

The description of hypochondriasis outlined by Gillespie (1928) earlier this century paved the way for the modern concept found in DSM–IV (American Psychiatric Association, 1994) and ICD–10 (World Health Organization, 1992). Preoccupations with disease and disease conviction were at its heart, along with the notion that the symptoms persist in spite of medical reassurance. These three features form the core of the DSM–IV criteria for hypochondriasis (see Box 17.1).

Classification

ICD–9 (World Health Organization, 1978) recognised hypochondriasis as a neurotic disorder along with hysteria, anxiety states, phobias, depression and obsessive–compulsive neurosis. It provided the following definition: "a neurotic disorder in which the conspicuous features are excessive concern with one's health in general, or the integrity and function of some part of one's body, or less frequently one's mind". ICD–10 has almost abandoned the concept of neurosis altogether, but retains the word in a chapter headed "Neurotic and stress related disorders". Definitions were tightened with the advent of DSM–III (American Psychiatric Association, 1980), which split the old concepts of hysteria and hypochondriasis and proposed new concepts of the different "somatoform" disorders. The major categories of the somatoform disorders were hypochondriasis, somatisation disorder, body dysmorphic disorder, conversion disorder and somatoform pain disorder. With the possible exception of somatisation disorder, the reliability, validity and stability over time of the diagnoses have yet to be established. Recent work by Barsky (1986, 1992) has clarified understanding of the relationship between hypochondriasis and other axis I disorders, as well as providing further empirical support for the consistency of primary hypochondriasis. In practice these disorders are rarely discrete; they often overlap or even coexist with each other. Further epidemiological studies will help to clarify their relationship.

Hypochondriasis

Definition

The DSM–IV diagnostic criteria for hypochondriasis are stated in Box 17.1. Core features are the preoccupation with the fear of having or the idea

---

Box 17.1   DSM–IV diagnostic criteria for hypochondriasis

A. Preoccupation with fears of having, or the idea that one has, a serious disease based on the person's misinterpretation of bodily symptoms.

B. The preoccupation persists despite appropriate medical evaluation and reassurance.

C. The belief in Criterion A is not of delusional intensity (as in delusional disorder, somatic type) and is not restricted to a circumscribed concern about appearance (as in body dysmorphic disorder).

D. The preoccupation causes clinically significant distress or impairment in social, occupational, or other important areas of functioning.

E. The duration of the disturbance is at least six months.

F. The preoccupation is not better accounted for by generalised anxiety disorder, obsessive–compulsive disorder, panic disorder, a major depressive episode, separation anxiety, or another somatoform disorder.

Specify:

With poor insight: if, for most of the time during the current episode, the person does not recognise that the concern about having a serious illness is excessive or unreasonable.

Adapted with permission from DSM–IV. Copyright 1994 American Psychiatric Association.

---

that one has a serious disease. This is based on misinterpretation of one or more bodily signs or symptoms and is resistant to medical reassurance. Following the publication of DSM–III–R (American Psychiatric Association, 1987), it was pointed out that the definition of hypochondriasis failed to include patients whose fears of medical disorders were not accompanied by physical symptoms, for example people who fear having AIDS. Also, the distinction between the other anxiety disorders accompanied by somatic symptoms is somewhat blurred. DSM–IV did not eliminate the requirement that fears about physical health were related to misinterpretations of bodily symptoms, but gave exclusion criteria that the physical symptoms could not be better accounted for by other psychiatric disorders, particularly generalised anxiety disorder, panic disorder, obsessive–compulsive disorder, depression or other somatoform disorders.

The ICD–10 concept of hypochondriasis (called "hypochondriacal disorder") also emphasised preoccupation with the possibility of having physical disease, persistent belief in the presence of such disease and lack of response to medical reassurance. One notable difference between ICD–10 and DSM–IV is that the ICD–10 concept of hypochondriasis includes the persistent preoccupation with physical appearance, which in DSM–IV would be subsumed under the heading of body dysmorphic disorder.

Primary and secondary hypochondriasis

Kenyon (1964) took issue with Gillespie's concept of a primary discrete neurotic syndrome, claiming that hypochondriasis was "always part of another syndrome, commonly an affective one", and cast doubt on the existence of primary hypochondriasis.

Appleby (1987) and Murphy (1990) have criticised Kenyon's study, arguing that because it was conducted in a psychiatric hospital population, the sample might be biased towards a more severe group who inevitably would have a high degree of comorbidity with other syndromes. Moreover, Kenyon's definition of hypochondriasis was rather loose. It probably included a number of patients who showed little resemblance to Gillespie's earlier definition of the syndrome, which shows a better correspondence to the modern DSM–IV concept. Indeed, Appleby (1987) has reinterpreted Kenyon's data to support the notion that primary hypochondriasis does exist.

Others, such as Pilowsky (1967, 1970), have championed the concept of primary hypochondriasis, and his work has lent support to its validity. With factor analysis he showed that the triad of disease phobia, disease conviction and bodily preoccupation lay at the core of the syndrome. Barsky *et al* (1986), in a study of medical out-patients, applied the DSM–III criteria to ascertain cases of hypochondriasis, and also found that disease conviction, disease phobia and bodily preoccupation correlated significantly, indicating that the DSM–III definition was internally consistent, which is one type of reliability. However, in the same study Barsky also found that the syndrome had blurred boundaries and proposed that hypochondriasis was a dimension of abnormal illness behaviour rather than a discrete category. This complex diagnostic issue has been reviewed more comprehensively by Murphy (1990). The modern consensus is that a syndrome of primary hypochondriasis as defined by DSM–IV does exist, even though for many subjects the hypochondriacal symptoms may be secondary to depressive illness, schizophrenia or anxiety disorders.

Epidemiology

The wide variation in estimates of the prevalence of hypochondriasis probably reflects both the varying diagnostic criteria used and differences in the population being sampled. Brown (1988), in a survey of 1500 patients in general practice, found a prevalence of 0.2% for the DSM–III–R syndrome. Kenyon (1976) found that the prevalence is higher in psychiatric hospital populations (0.9% for out-patients and 1.1% for in-patients), and this study also showed that it was equally common in both sexes but more common among social class V subjects, although the latter observation remains to be confirmed.

Clinical features

Abnormal attitudes to health can take many forms, and a wide variety of bodily systems and regions may be involved in hypochondriacal syndromes. Symptoms relating to the chest, abdomen, head and neck are particularly common (Kenyon, 1964). Pain is present in more than half the patients. Headaches, chest pain, abdominal pain and lower back pain are most common. Pain syndromes are described in more detail later in this chapter, and are mentioned here only briefly as a reminder that the hypochondriacal elaboration of pain is frequent. Vague muscular pains are very common and are sometimes called "fibrositis", "fibromyalgia" or "rheumatism".

Complaints of dizziness, vertigo, hearing one's pulse beat at night, catarrh and globus sensation may present to ear, nose and throat clinics. Other patients present to general practitioners or ophthalmologists complaining of "floaters" in their eye. Sexual anxieties may sometimes assume a hypochondriacal flavour. These include concerns about sexual adequacy in general, as well as particular preoccupations concerning the size and shape of the genitalia (see section below on body dysmorphic disorder). Abdominal pain in the context of the irritable bowel syndrome, nausea and flatulence are sometimes accompanied by the complaint of having a bad taste in the mouth. Gastrointestinal symptoms may be made worse by aerophagy (swallowing air).

Doctors often agonise over whether the origin of symptoms is organic or psychological. This is probably a false dichotomy because, for many symptoms, both organic and psychological factors are aetiologically relevant. Also physical and psychiatric illness may coexist. However, it is sometimes necessary to make clinical judgements on certain symptoms. The following factors given below are said to distinguish a psychiatric diagnosis from a physical illness (McGrath & Bowker, 1987; Brown *et al*, 1990):

(1) Symptoms are ill-defined, vaguely described, or do not conform to anatomical or physiological patterns (this can be misleading – see section on Pain).
(2) Symptoms are precipitated by stressful events (but again, so can organic symptoms).
(3) Symptom severity is inconsistent with day-to-day functioning.
(4) The patient is highly suggestive.
(5) The patient has a model for the symptoms.

The concept of secondary gain, i.e. the rewards and advantages of the sick role, although relevant to the management of a many patients, is unhelpful diagnostically. Secondary gain may result from almost any illness, whether physical, psychiatric or a combination of both.

The following patient was seen by the author in the course of a study on somatoform disorders.

> *Case example*
> Mrs C. was a 66-year-old married lady. She lived with her husband who was well. For many years she had been a regular visitor to her general practitioner, and she had amassed 232 attendances with unexplained physical symptoms in the previous five years. Her repertoire of symptoms was narrow, consisting mainly of dysphagia and abdominal pain that had been present for many years. She had had a fear of cancer since adolescence, and believed her symptoms were due to malignant disease. She examined herself several times each day, feeling her neck, swallowing and looking at her throat in a mirror. She would apparently accept reassurance from her doctor during consultations, only to return to the surgery a few days later complaining of the same symptoms and the same fears. Specialist referral and numerous investigations failed to allay her fears.
> When interviewed for the study, she met DSM–III–R criteria for hypochondriasis but not for a major depressive episode. Her Beck Depression Inventory score was only 7 (low). A year after being seen in the study she was still consulting her doctor with the same frequency. On one of her visits he felt the symptom pattern had altered and sent her for a chest x-ray. In spite of a negative report, he referred her to a chest physician who performed a bronchoscopy, which revealed an inoperable squamous cell carcinoma. She died a few months later, her worst fears realised.

This patient illustrates the two common traps in managing patients with hypochondriasis. Firstly there may be an early phase of zealous over-investigation for organic disease when none is present. Secondly, almost as a reaction to this, there may follow a policy of under-investigation, even in the presence of ominous organic symptoms.

The doctor–patient relationship

Most authors on hypochondriasis comment on the strained nature of the doctor–patient relationship (Ford, 1983; Pilowsky, 1983; Stoudemire, 1988). Cohen (1966) pointed out that such patients fail to arouse any interest in their doctors.

Anger and frustration are common responses of doctors to patients with hypochondriasis. Pilowsky (1983) asserted that "medical writers appear to have been more intemperate in their description of these patients than any other". The unwillingness to accept reassurance or advice, the refusal to get better, and the criticism, implicit or explicit, of medical treatment, present doctors with a challenging test of their clinical skills and patience. This interactional problem is so common as to merit mention as one of the clinical features of the syndrome. Recognition of the distorted relationship is also of crucial importance in management.

Patients with hypochondriasis have often been described as pedantic and rather concrete thinkers. They tend to relate their medical histories in an excessively detailed and meticulous way, tolerating interruption poorly. Case records are voluminous and visits to the doctor frequent. Over-investigation by a variety of different specialists places the patient at risk of iatrogenic illness, quite apart from being an unnecessary and costly exercise.

Differential diagnosis

The differential diagnosis of hypochondriasis includes anxiety disorders, obsessive–compulsive disorders, depression, and to a lesser extent schizophrenia. A careful search for evidence of these syndromes needs to be carried out. The doctor also needs to be vigilant about the presence of organic illness. Neurological disorders, including multiple sclerosis and myasthenia gravis, are a particular pitfall, as are multi-system disorders such as systemic lupus erythematosus which sometimes causes symptoms in the absence of physical signs.

There is a very fine line between the opposite errors of compulsive over-investigation and forgetting that even those with hypochondriasis may become physically ill. It is often debated whether hypochondriasis is an obsession, an over-valued idea, a delusion, or merely an epiphenomenon of anxiety. In reality, it can be any of these things. At the mildest end of the spectrum some patients become transiently anxious about symptoms such as chest pain, palpitations or an altered bowel habit, which may occur at times of stress and usually respond to medical examination and reassurance. It is only prolonged episodes that are morbid, and for this reason DSM–IV stipulates that the condition should have lasted for more than six months.

Transient hypochondriacal symptoms occur after both stressful life events (Izdorek, 1975) and serious medical disorders (for example, cancer or ischaemic heart disease). Following such illnesses, some patients become preoccupied with any ache or pain and incorrectly misinterpret it as a sign of disease. A similar phenomenon has been reported following bereavement, when subjects adopt the symptoms of the same disorder which the deceased suffered. Appropriate medical evaluation, explanation and reassurance for patients with physical disease, or counselling for the bereaved, will usually lead to a resolution of the symptoms.

At the other end of the spectrum are hypochondriacal delusions and the so-called monodelusional hypochondriacal psychosis (see below). Depressive hypochondriacal delusions are usually mood congruent: for example, the belief that one's bowels are rotting away or one is giving off a terrible smell. In schizophrenia there is a more bizarre quality; one patient had a bewildering array of physical symptoms including chest pain, abdominal pain, urinary symptoms and swelling of the legs. He attributed his symptoms to the activity of a worm which he believed lived in his right leg.

Between these groups are patients who complain of physical symptoms, have no demonstrable physical illness, yet fail to respond to reassurance and have repeated negative physical and pathological examinations, and also lack any other primary psychiatric syndrome. For these patients, the concept of hypochondriasis as an over-valued idea is useful. Wernicke (1900) defined over-valued ideas as solitary beliefs that determine each individual's actions to a morbid degree, while at the same time being considered justified and a normal expression of their nature. Overvalued ideas and their significance in a variety of psychiatric disorders are discussed further by McKenna (1984).

Preoccupation with disease and the accompanying obsessional concern with body functioning (sometimes including checking behaviours) serve to distinguish hypochondriasis from somatisation disorder. Patients with somatisation disorder tend to be younger (at least at the onset), focus more on individual symptoms rather than on whole diseases (e.g. "I've got cancer"), as well as having a more colourful histrionic cognitive style.

Aetiology

Genetics

An adoption study of somatoform disorders divided patients into "diversiform somatisers" and "high frequency somatisers". The former group have a greater diversity of complaints, perhaps akin to somatisation disorder, while the high frequency somatisers have a narrower band of complaints. Probands with diversiform somatisation had an increased rate of male-limited alcoholism (highly heritable from father to son) (Bohman *et al*, 1984). A subsequent study (Torgersen, 1986) concluded that even if somatoform disorders were familial, the transmission may be environmental; similarity in childhood experiences seemed to influence the concordance rate for somatoform disorders.

Although evidence exists from adoption studies (Cloninger *et al*, 1984; Sigvardsson *et al*, 1986) that genetic factors may be of some relevance in patients with functional somatic symptoms, present information is insufficient to draw any conclusion on the magnitude, if any, of a genetic contribution to hypochondriasis.

Early environmental influences

Parental attitudes toward disease and early exposure to chronic disease may predispose individuals to both somatisation and hypochondriasis (Apley, 1958; Mechanic, 1964; Parker & Lipscome, 1980; Brown, 1988). Adults with somatisation disorder and hypochondriasis often had a model in childhood for their symptoms, in the form of a chronically ill parent (Brown, 1988). The pattern of parental care and protection experienced during childhood may be associated with care-eliciting behaviours in parents (e.g. seeing a doctor and complaining about physical symptoms). In a general practice population, Parker & Lipscome (1980) found that patients who scored highly for hypochondriasis rated their fathers as significantly more over-protective, and their mothers as more highly caring, than those with low ratings for hypochondriasis. High scorers described their parents as being very sympathetic and more likely to call the doctor whenever they complained about physical symptoms. Baker (1989) also provided evidence, suggesting that hypochondriasis is related to maternal over-protection. Craig *et al* (1993) reported that lack of care in childhood and early childhood illness both contribute to adult somatisation. Their hypothesis is that lack of care increases the risk of emotional disorder in the face of adversity in adult life, and early childhood illness predisposes people to interpret innocuous symptoms as being indicators of physical illness.

Sociocultural factors

Early studies which described an association with lower social class and poor education have been questioned (Lerner & Noy, 1968). Some of these studies had a sample bias towards the less educated, lower social class groups, and it is now clear that patients of all educational levels and social classes may suffer from hypochondriacal syndromes. Likewise, sweeping generalisations about the greater tendency to somatise for those in "third world" countries or broad ethnic groups may be misleading. For example, oriental Jews in Israel have a much higher rate of somatisation than European Jews but once the effects of education are taken into account this difference disappears (Lerner & Noy, 1968). The complex relationship between sociocultural factors and unexplained physical symptoms was reviewed by Katon *et al* (1982) and Kirmayer (1984). Katon *et al* (1982) suggested that culture can influence somatisation in three ways. Firstly, language may have an influence; for example, the Yoruba of Nigeria have no word in their language for depression. Secondly, there may be a cultural sanction against the open expression of emotion, so that care and rewards are only given for physical symptoms. Thirdly, culture may provide people with an idiosyncratic explanation for affective states. For example, in South America the syndrome of "susto" has most of the features of major depressive illness as well as some physical symptoms. The cultural explanation is a spiritual one, and so the cure is also a spiritual one. In Western societies, early family interactions, the systems of health care and work disability payment all tend to favour a presentation with somatic rather than psychological symptoms.

Psychoanalytic views

To Freud, the unexplained somatic symptoms were the result of repressed or undischarged libido (Freud, 1896). His successors emphasised the mechanism of displacement, in which particular parts of the body acquire a special significance and become connected with fears or phobias, instead of the fears being focused on individuals or external situations.

Alexander, one of the fathers of psychosomatic medicine, described three mechanisms in the psychogenesis of hypochondriasis. Firstly, there is a withdrawal of interest from other people into the self. Secondly, guilt feelings and an attendant need for punishment occur. Thirdly, there is displacement of anxiety. These mechanisms permit a guilt-free retreat into the sick role, which is combined with the expression of covert or even open hostility towards others, especially doctors (Alexander, 1949). Psychoanalysts have not written very much about hypochondriasis in recent years, perhaps because the sufferers are such poor candidates for psychoanalytic treatment (Pilowsky, 1983).

A sociological explanation was first proposed by Parsons (1951) who introduced the term *sick role* and highlighted the reinforcing effect of the privileges and rewards of the sick role. Mechanic (1962) used the term *illness behaviour,* by which he meant "the ways in which given symptoms may be differentially perceived, evaluated and acted (or not acted) upon by different kinds of persons". Pilowsky (1969) developed these ideas further, and his concept of *abnormal illness behaviour* has been widely used as a model for patients with unexplained physical symptoms.

Psychophysiological mechanisms

Several different mechanisms have been put forward to explain the transformation of emotion into physical symptoms. They include:

over-activity of the autonomic nervous systems with smooth muscle contraction (Sullivan *et al*, 1978); increased tension in voluntary muscles (Sainsbury & Gibson, 1954); changes in endocrine activity during arousal; and biochemical changes caused by hyperventilation (Lewis, 1959).

For poorly understood reasons, many of the patients develop an initial conviction that they have some undiagnosed disease. Anxiety becomes raised and this leads to more frequent visits to the doctor. Barsky & Klerman (1983) and Kellner (1986) suggested that this heightened anxiety leads to selective perception of sensations associated with the relevant part of the body. Patients become more aware of their own heartbeat or of normal bowel contractions. This develops into a vicious circle of increasing selective perception as well as self-examination, such as monitoring their pulse, examining faeces or urine, which raise anxiety more, and the somatic anxiety in turn leads to more physical symptoms, and so on. Hypochondriacal symptoms should be distinguished from conversion symptoms: they do not replace emotions, but rather are a consequence of emotions and reinforce the emotions (Kellner, 1986).

Measurement of hypochondriasis

The two main scales used clinically and in research to measure hypochondriasis are the Whiteley Index (Pilowsky, 1967) (see Box 17.2) and the Illness Attitude Test (Kellner, 1986), both of which have acceptable reliability and validity. The scales attempt to measure the three core elements of the DSM–IV concept of hypochondriasis (i.e. disease phobia, disease conviction and lack of response to medical reassurance). The Illness Attitude Test is a 29-item questionnaire with nine subscales including hypochondriacal beliefs, worry over illness, disease phobia and bodily preoccupation. Although the scale was not originally intended as a diagnostic scale, Kellner claims that it is a sensitive instrument for detecting hypochondriacal subjects. Kirmayer & Robbins (1991) criticised both scales, claiming that they sample only a limited range of patients' symptoms, mood and attitudes, and tell little about actual behaviour. They mainly measure "illness worry" and fail to address behavioural or communicative aspects of the patient's response to illness. One scale which attempts to do so is the Illness Behaviour Inventory (Turkat & Pettigrew, 1983).

Management

Although most of the treatment studies published so far have been uncontrolled, there is now some consensus on the best way to manage patients with hypochondriasis and the other chronic somatoform disorders. An adequate initial medical, psychiatric and social assessment is essential (Kellner, 1986; Lipowski, 1988). It is crucial at this stage that one doctor, probably the general practitioner, retains some control over the patient's

---

Box 17.2 The Whiteley Index

A. Do you often worry about the possibility that you have a serious illness?
B. Are you bothered by many pains and aches?
C. Do you find that you are often aware of various things happening in your body?
D. Do you worry a lot about your health?
E. Do you often have the symptoms of very serious illnesses?
F. If a disease is brought to your attention (through the radio, television, newspapers, or someone you know) do you worry about getting it yourself?
G. If you feel ill and someone tells you that you are looking better, do you become annoyed?
H. Do you find that you are bothered by many different symptoms?
I. Is it easy for you to forget about yourself, and think about all sorts of other things?
J. Is it hard for you to believe the doctor when he tells you there is nothing for you to worry about?
K. Do you get the feeling that people are not taking your illness seriously enough?
L. Do you think that you worry about your health more than most people?
M. Do you think there is something seriously wrong with your body?
N. Are you afraid of illness?

---

management, as these patients are often highly adept at "splitting" health professionals. In the early stages a thorough medical assessment and all appropriate investigations should be carried out. The doctor should give the patient the results of the physical examination and any special investigations in a clear, unambiguous way, possibly supplementing verbal with written information. If no disease is found, the doctor should try to shift the focus of enquiry away from medical to more psychosocial areas. It is important to introduce discussion of psychosocial issues at as early a stage as possible. To mention psychiatric disorder, or referral to a psychiatrist, after a prolonged battery of medical investigations or visits to a host of other specialists, is likely to invite the patient's wrath. It may even give some patients a feeling of being slighted, because their complaints are not being taken seriously enough.

Opinions differ on the role of reassurance at this stage in the patient's assessment. Kellner (1986) and Kirmayer & Robbins (1991) state that explanation and reassurance which is given in the context of adequate medical assessment, during an ongoing therapeutic relationship, often constitutes adequate treatment in itself. On the other hand, Warwick & Salkovskis (1985) drew attention to the dangers of providing reassurance at the wrong time as well as in the wrong kind of way. They emphasised that the reassurance should be, if possible, accompanied by an explanation, and cautioned against repeatedly trying to reassure patients by ordering yet more tests, examining them too often, or giving too many appointments. These manoeuvres may actually reinforce abnormal illness behaviours, similarly to rituals in obsessive–compulsive disorder, in that both lead to a short-term reduction of anxiety but soon the fears return accompanied by increased urges to seek further reassurance. Reassurance should be given at the right time, not prematurely before the results of independent investigations are known, or before patients have had a good opportunity to ventilate adequately all their ailments (Kessel, 1979).

Bass (1990*a*), Ford (1983), Lipowski (1988) and Pilowsky (1983) all emphasised the importance of listening carefully to all statements by patients about their symptoms and allowing adequate time for ventilation, because this is essential in the establishment of a good therapeutic alliance. It gives patients the feeling that the doctor takes them seriously and is trying to understand them. Although this is often a difficult task for the doctor, Pilowsky (1983) asserted that many patients who are given the freedom to describe their physical complaints at length will sooner or later start to talk about their psychological problems.

A useful management strategy to adopt at the outset is to explain to the patient that the aim is not the complete removal of all the physical symptoms, or a radical cure, but rather one of care. The goal is one of improved function, and exactly what this entails should be made explicit during the first few sessions. Patients also need to be told that their symptoms are not "all in your head" or "in your imagination", because they often claim that other doctors have said this to them. Although this will rarely be the case, in practice many patients will report having left a consultation with an irate feeling that their doctor has denied the reality of their symptoms or the severity of their distress. Patients find it helpful to hear the doctor accept their experience of the symptoms as well as their reported severity.

Another useful strategy is to encourage patients to view their illness as one with physical, emotional and social aspects, all of which require assessment and management. Goldberg *et al* (1989) suggested that somatising patients should be encouraged to re-attribute their bodily symptoms to psychological causes, and advocated "slowly changing the agenda" during the therapeutic interviews. Sometimes this tactic works, but with the more chronic cases it may not. Bass (1990*a*) wrote that there are dangers in moving some patients from an organic aetiology to a psychological one as they "would usually replace one distortion of reality with another". He recommended trying to get patients to see the relevance of a whole range of possible causes for their symptoms.

It is also helpful to schedule regular appointments, regular physical examinations, and also to clarify on what basis other clinical investigations will, or will not, be carried out. Regular appointments provide a certain predictability to the treatment programme, help reduce anxiety and may remove the need to increase or exaggerate the complaints to "up the stakes" in order to obtain more medical attention and further investigations. The patient's family should also be involved in ongoing management. Families (along with doctors) are sometimes potent reinforcers of abnormal illness behaviour and may also benefit from education and advice on how to handle the patient's complaints. Occasionally some family members may be so distressed by the patient's behaviour that they require treatment in their own right.

A number of psychotherapeutic approaches, including cognitive–behavioural therapy and educational work, may be helpful. Warwick & Salkovskis (1985), Salkovskis & Warwick (1986) and Salkovskis (1989) suggested that illness preoccupation, misinterpretation of bodily symptoms and anxiety are maintained by three distinct mechanisms, each accessible to treatment:

(1) increased physiological arousal
(2) selective attention in which previously unnoticed body sensations or aspects of appearance become more readily attended to (Kellner, 1986)
(3) avoidant behaviours.

Patients deal with the anxiety by indulging in obsessional checking and reassurance seeking; these maintain hypochondriacal symptoms and so are key targets in the treatment programme. This model is illustrated in Fig. 17.1.

Cognitive techniques include challenging the patient's beliefs about the nature of the symptoms and the treatment. It is useful to teach patients that autonomic arousal can heighten symptoms, and how selective attention allows them to focus on particular symptoms. Useful behavioural techniques include exposure to feared stimuli (for example, hospital visits), talking about feared illnesses, seeing films about feared illnesses; massed practice (for example, repeatedly writing illness fears down); banning reassurance seeking; and more investigations. These strategies are not always easy to implement and should only be attempted in the context of a good therapeutic relationship in suitable subjects.

Barsky *et al* (1988) described a cognitive educational treatment based on the view of hypochondriasis as a disorder of perception and cognition. Somatic sensations are experienced as abnormally intense, and are then incorrectly attributed to serious medical disorder. Therapy aims to change both the patient's sensations and the cognitive appraisal of these sensations. The treatment focuses on four factors which amplify somatic symptoms: (1) attention and expectation; (2) symptom attribution and appraisal; (3) the context used for interpreting symptoms; and (4) the role of dysphoria and dependency. The therapist educates the patient in these four areas, and discussion on these topics provides a basis for ongoing therapeutic dialogue, but it should be noted that the method has not so far been subjected to a controlled study.

Patients with hypochondriasis often take unnecessary drugs, and if possible these should be withdrawn (Bass, 1990*a*). This requires careful handling and should always be negotiated with the patient first and then carried out gradually. Drug withdrawal is more likely to be successful in the context of a good therapeutic alliance or where the patient accepts alternative ways of managing the symptoms. In the presence of a major depression, antidepressants may be helpful. Tricyclic antidepressants or mono-aminoxidase inhibitors decrease somatic symptoms in anxious subjects and also lower anxiety (Robinson *et al*, 1973; Covi *et al*, 1974). The role of the selective serotonin reuptake inhibitors has yet to be evaluated. In the absence of major depressive disorder, drugs should be used sparingly and only when the psychotherapeutic approach as described above has failed. Some patients take psychotropic drugs for hypochondriacal symptoms for many years without deriving any obvious benefit.

Somatisation disorder and Briquet's syndrome

DSM–III and DSM–IV assign a separate category to a discrete syndrome of multiple somatic complaints extending over a period of years which is termed somatisation disorder, and is also sometimes known as Briquet's

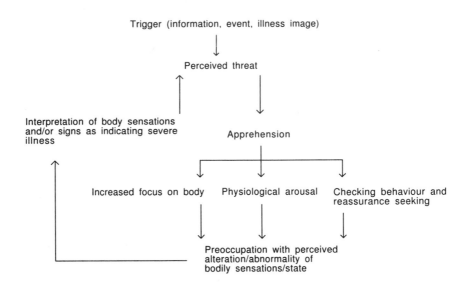

Fig. 17.1 Genesis and maintenance of hypochondriacal symptoms. Adapted from Salkovskis (1989), by permission of Oxford University Press.

syndrome. The contribution of Pierre Briquet was recently reassessed by Mai & Merskey (1980). Briquet (1869) followed up 430 of his own patients who were given a diagnosis of hysteria and described the many symptoms from which they suffered. His observations led him to reject the prevailing view that hysteria had some connection with sexual frustration, because he found the condition occurred in prostitutes, married women, virgins and widows. Indeed, he thought it less frequent in nuns than in others.

This is a chronic disorder of multiple, unexplained medical symptoms starting before the age of 30 and found primarily, but not exclusively, in women. Symptoms in almost every organ system are found, but cardiopulmonary problems, gastrointestinal complaints, and vague musculoskeletal aches and pains are particularly common. Pseudo-neurological conversion-type syndromes, such as paraesthesia, loss of vision and paralysis are not uncommon, while menstrual and sexual disorders are almost always present. The disorder results in multiple medical attendances as well as other help-seeking behaviours. Iatrogenic disease occurs as a consequence of over-investigation, polypharmacy and polysurgery. Somatisation disorder has the highest reliability, validity and stability of diagnosis of all the DSM–III somatoform disorders (Hyler & Sussmann, 1984). This is in spite of the view (which the author shares) that somatisation disorder lies at one end of a continuum of abnormal illness behaviour and is somewhat arbitrarily separated off. Studies suggest that there are many patients who have fewer symptoms than the required number for the diagnosis, but in terms of illness behaviour and day-to-day functioning they are similar to patients meeting the full criteria (Brown, 1988; Escobar *et al*, 1989).

By definition, somatisation disorder runs a chronic and often unremitting course, and it may be comorbid with depressive illness, panic disorder, drug or alcohol abuse and personality disorder (Liscow *et al*, 1986; Swartz *et al*, 1986*b*).

Reported prevalence rates vary, reflecting the different populations studied and differences in diagnostic criteria for Briquet's syndrome as defined by Guze (1967) and somatisation disorder as defined by DSM–III. Woodruff *et al* (1971) cited a prevalence rate of 1–2% in a group of hospitalised patients (drawn from the postpartum wards) but this may be an overestimate of the true prevalence. Swartz *et al* (1986*a,b*) gave a prevalence rate of 0.4% in North Carolina, while Brown (1988) found a prevalence of 0.5% in an Edinburgh general practice.

The disorder is costly, both in medical time and financially. Smith *et al* (1986) found that somatisation disorder patients accrued nine times the healthcare costs of a matched control group. In broad terms, the management approach delineated for hypochondriasis applies to somatisation disorder and to the other chronic somatoform disorders, but the structured cognitive–behavioural approach has not yet been shown to be effective for somatisation disorder.

Dysmorphophobia

According to Philippopoulos (1979): "this term comes from dysmorfia, a Greek word meaning ugliness, specifically of the face, and first appeared in the *Histories* of Herodotus referring to the myth of the 'ugliest girl in Sparta', who was taken to a shrine each day by her nurse so she might be delivered from her homeliness".

Morselli (1891) first used the term dysmorphophobia in a medical setting to refer to a subjective feeling of ugliness or of physical defect that the patient believes to be obvious to others, in spite of a normal physical appearance. Bishop (1980) pointed out the inappropriateness of the term because it is not a true phobia, but rather an obsession with bodily appearance. It was therefore renamed *body dysmorphic disorder* in DSM–III; the current DSM–IV criteria are shown in Box 17.3. As noted earlier, body dysmorphic disorder is subsumed in ICD–10 under the heading of 'hypochondriacal disorder'. The DSM–IV criteria for body dysmorphic disorder emphasise the preoccupation with an imagined defect in appearance in a person who appears to others to be normal. Where a slight anomaly is present, the person's concern is deemed grossly excessive. A typical case is described below.

Case example
James, a 31-year-old professional musician, presented to his general practitioner with a lengthy history of anxiety about what he perceived to be excessive hair loss. He also believed that his face was in some way "strange looking", and because of this he attracted the attention of others whom he believed looked at him in strange ways, particularly in public. His friends and his general practitioner reassured him that his hair loss was minimal and that his facial appearance was in no way unusual. In spite of this he spent many hours every day worrying about his appearance and checking his hair line in mirrors. He was unable to stop this, although in his better moments he could see that his concern and compulsive checking were excessive. In the past he had had analytically-based psychotherapy for similar symptoms, but on this occasion came to his general practitioner requesting either treatment with Minoxidil for his perceived hair loss or referral for cosmetic surgery. Although he was still able to work, his concerns had resulted in difficulties in interpersonal relationships and social withdrawal.

His GP persuaded him to accept psychiatric referral. A diagnosis of dysmorphophobia was made. Supportive psychotherapy and cognitive–behavioural psychotherapy (including exposure therapy and audio-visual self-confrontation) led to no improvement in his symptoms. He refused drug treatment because of his worry that it might affect his performance as a musician. After two years of psychiatric treatment there was no change in his symptomatology.

The preoccupation may be with a wide variety of perceived bodily abnormalities including facial abnormalities (such as wrinkles, spots, scars,

---

Box 17.3 DSM–IV diagnostic criteria for body dysmorphic disorder

1. Preoccupation with an imagined defect in appearance. If a slight physical anomaly is present, the person's concern is markedly excessive.
2. The preoccupation causes clinically significant distress or impairment in social, occupational, or other important areas of functioning.
3. The preoccupation is not better accounted for by another mental disorder (e.g. dissatisfaction with body shape and size in anorexia nervosa).

Adapted with permission from DSM–IV. Copyright 1994 American Psychiatric Association.

---

facial asymmetry or disproportion), hair abnormalities (including fears of baldness), preoccupations with the shape and size of the nose, eyes, ears, mouth, jaw, chin or head (Phillips, 1991). Preoccupation with the size and shape of genitalia is fairly common. In others the complaints are vague, for example, the belief that a person has a "funny face". There may also be a preoccupation with more than one body part at the same time. There is not, however, a more generalised body-image disturbance as, for example, occurs in anorexia nervosa (Thomas, 1987). Associated behaviours include checking rituals, looking in mirrors (although some patients deliberately avoid mirrors), concern that others may be looking at them or talking about them, camouflaging the perceived defect, and repeated reassurance-seeking.

The distinction from obsessive–compulsive disorder is not always easy. A patient's constant attention and concern about body parts may appear obsessional and can result in repeated repetitive checking, which may be interpreted as a compulsive behaviour. In the view of Vitiello & de Leon (1990), the distinction between the two disorders rests primarily on the nature of the thoughts and the patient's reaction to them. In obsessions the patient is bothered by intrusive thoughts or images; in dysmorphophobia (an overvalued idea) the patient's concern is with a belief in a bodily deformity. In dysmorphophobia the content of the belief always concerns somatic deformity, while in obsessive–compulsive disorder the belief may cover a variety of themes. Resistance to the thoughts is common but not always present in obsessive–compulsive disorder, while in dysmorphophobia the patient makes no attempt to resist the dysmorphophobic belief.

Dysmorphophobia is often a symptom of other underlying major psychiatric disorder, most notably schizophrenia, depressive illness or an organic brain syndrome (Andreasen & Bardach, 1977). Many authors have pointed to the association of dysmorphophobia with abnormal personality, in particular Schneider's sensitive personality disorder (Hay, 1970; Andreasen & Bardach, 1977; Thomas, 1984). Other personality types also associated with dysmorphophobia are obsessional, schizoid, narcissistic, or a mixture of these.

Little is known about the epidemiology of the disorder, although Phillips (1991) stated that it is "probably not rare". There is a slight excess among women. Onset is usually in adolescence, although there may be a mean interval of six years between onset of symptoms and presentation for treatment (Phillips, 1991); 85% of sufferers are unmarried. The natural history of the disorder has not been extensively studied, but there is some suggestion that the part of the body concerned may change with time (Marks & Mischan, 1988) and that occasionally the beliefs become delusional. In a follow-up study of patients who received cosmetic surgery as a response to their dysmorphic beliefs, a few later developed schizophrenia (Gipson & Connolly, 1975). Aetiology is unknown, and hypotheses range from psychoanalytic speculation about displacement, to biochemical theories involving serotonin dysfunction (see Phillips, 1991).

Studies of the efficacy of medication are confined to case reports because psychiatrists come across relatively few cases, but successful outcomes have been reported for both clomipramine and fluoxetine (Hollander *et al*, 1989; Tynes *et al*, 1990), which are also effective treatments for obsessive–compulsive disorder (Rapaport, 1989). No concurrent depressive illness was present in over half of these case reports, yet dysmorphic symptoms recurred if medication was decreased or discontinued. Unless the beliefs are delusional, antipsychotic medication is ineffective. Studies on psychodynamically orientated psychotherapy, behavioural therapies, exposure therapy, audio-visual confrontation and desensitisation have reported mixed results, and it is uncertain how useful these measures are.

Many patients request cosmetic surgery. In cases of a genuine minimal deformity the outcome may be good. On the other hand, when there is poor agreement on the presence of any deformity, cosmetic surgery is unlikely to be helpful. The main risks of intervening surgically with these patients derive from their unrealistic expectations of the outcome of surgery, and this will sometimes lead to an escalation of complaints and difficulties in the therapeutic relationship with surgeons, physicians and others (Fukuda, 1977). Symptom substitution may occur, with another body part becoming the focus of attention (Andreasen & Bardach, 1977). Psychiatrists, dermatologists and plastic surgeons should collaborate closely in the assessment and management of patients presenting for cosmetic surgery. Even though the consensus of opinion is that the management of body dysmorphic disorder should be psychiatric, the outcome is often poor.

Monosymptomatic hypochondriacal psychoses

The boundary between the overvalued ideas of dysmorphophobia and the delusions of monosymptomatic hypochondriacal psychosis may be blurred, and it is sometimes impossible to make the distinction (McKenna, 1984; de Leon *et al*, 1989). This difficulty has found expression in DSM–IV, which unlike its predecessors DSM–III and DSM–III–R no longer has the exclusion criterion that beliefs about abnormal appearance should "not be of delusional intensity". This means that the diagnosis of body dysmorphic disorder can now be made concurrently with a diagnosis of delusional disorder. There are claims that monosymptomatic hypochondriacal psychosis responds to the antipsychotic drug pimozide (Munro, 1978; Munro & Chmara, 1982), although the specificity of this response has been questioned (Kendell, 1983). The disorder has three main clinical presentations: dysmorphophobic delusions about particular body parts; delusional beliefs that the person is emitting an offensive odour (delusions of bromosis); and delusions of parasitosis (Ekbom's syndrome). Those who believe they have an offensive odour often bathe frequently, change their clothes, and use pungent perfumes and deodorants. This is commonest among young males (Ford, 1983) and may be associated with depression, schizophrenia and temporal lobe epilepsy (Pryse-Phillips, 1971).

Patients with delusions of infestation, usually women, often consult dermatologists. Sometimes they bring pieces of skin, hair and other particles which they show to their doctors as evidence of the infestation. The high frequency with which these syndromes present as part of a more major psychiatric disorder, particularly affective disorder, schizophrenia and organic brain syndromes (Ford, 1983), has led some to question the validity of the disorder as a separate psychiatric syndrome. DSM–IV classifies all these disorders as delusional disorder, somatic subtype, rather than as one of the somatoform disorders, and they are also discussed together with other delusional disorders on page 500.

Irritable bowel syndrome

Although this syndrome is common it should be emphasised that most patients with it do not meet diagnostic criteria for hypochondriasis. The core features of irritable bowel syndrome include: abdominal pain relieved by defaecation; a change in bowel habit; altered stool form (hard or loose watery stools); straining or urgency on defaecation with an associated feeling of incomplete evacuation; rectal bleeding; and the passage of mucus.

This is an exceedingly common disorder, and up to a third of new patients in gastroenterology clinics have functional bowel disorders (Drossman *et al*, 1988; Creed, 1990). Although there are no pathological changes in the gut, increased motor activity has been reported in some but not all studies (Creed, 1990).

The importance of psychological factors in irritable bowel syndrome has been recognised since the turn of the century (White, 1905). Anxiety or depression which meet diagnostic criteria may coincide with the onset of bowel symptoms (Craig & Brown, 1984; Creed & Guthrie, 1987; Ford *et al*, 1987). Around two-thirds of subjects with irritable bowel syndrome have experienced a threatening life-event in the 38 weeks prior to presentation

(Craig & Brown, 1984; Ford *et al*, 1987). A similar high number of life events was found among a group of patients undergoing appendicectomy who did not have an inflamed appendix (Creed, 1981). Aetiology remains uncertain, and a variety of psychological and pathophysiological mechanisms may be responsible.

Management

Patients attending gastroenterology clinics usually receive antispasmodics and bulking agents, reassurance, and education about the nature of the symptoms and their benign nature. Most will have some short-term response to this approach (Harvey *et al*, 1987). Creed (1990) highlighted the importance of the doctor–patient relationship in giving the right kind of reassurance and education. An explanation of the cause of the symptoms supplemented by written information is sometimes helpful. Possible links between the symptoms and recent life-events should be discussed, as well as any particular worries, for example, of underlying cancer.

Guthrie *et al* (1991) described a psychotherapeutic treatment which is based on establishing a sound therapeutic relationship. A daily diary of bowel symptoms and bowel habits, mood states and ongoing life-events provides material for discussion about links between physical symptoms and emotional feelings, and these are combined with relaxation techniques. Guthrie *et al* (1991) claimed that two-thirds of patients improve with this treatment. In another study using both cognitive and behavioural methods, including progressive muscular relaxation biofeedback and training in stress coping skills showed that those with low trait anxiety scores did very well with treatment (Blanchard *et al*, 1988). Antidepressants including desipramine (Greenbaum *et al*, 1987) and doxepin (Thomson *et al*, 1988) may also help. Non-directive psychotherapy combined with routine medical treatment is superior to medical treatment alone (Svedlund *et al*, 1983). In a further study, Guthrie *et al* (1993) described a randomised controlled trial of psychodynamic psychotherapy that showed that psychotherapy was superior to supportive listening, and she concluded that psychotherapy was both "feasible and effective in the majority of irritable bowel syndrome patients with chronic symptoms unresponsive to medical treatment".

Cardiac syndromes

Da Costa (1871) described 300 soldiers who became ill with cardiorespiratory symptoms and concomitant anxiety disorders during the American Civil War. He named the condition "irritable heart" and believed the aetiology was organic, but the condition is still sometimes called "Da Costa's syndrome". In practice it is difficult and possibly irrelevant to distinguish between functional cardiac and functional respiratory symptoms; they commonly coexist and for practical purposes they are best dealt with together (Bass, 1990*b*).

Epidemiology

Chest pain is a common complaint in primary care, but only a small minority of patients have any serious cardiorespiratory disease. Even among those referred to cardiac clinics around 14% have functional cardiovascular syndromes (White, 1937). Bass *et al* (1988) found that 21% of patients in a cardiac clinic had evidence of hyperventilation, while as few as 19% of the patients with chest pain had abnormal results on exercise testing. Possibly this low rate could be accounted for by a tendency to refer selectively those patients with atypical features for exercise testing.

The presenting symptoms in this group include breathlessness, palpitation, chest pain, dizziness, paraesthesiae, faints and anxiety. These symptoms may occur as a result of hyperventilation, suggesting that hyperventilation might be of aetiological relevance to these cardiorespiratory syndromes. Alternatively, hyperventilation may be an epiphenomenon which is secondary to anxiety, particularly panic disorder (Bass, 1990*b*). This distinction may be of relevance in management.

Functional breathlessness

A useful diagnostic pointer which distinguishes between patients with and without ischaemic heart disease is situational breathlessness. Breathlessness that comes on in particular situations, such as in crowds, shops, buses or other enclosed spaces, accompanied by fear and a desire to escape the situation, is more likely to be functional. The sensation of "air hunger", a feeling of smothering or suffocation, or the feeling of inability to get "enough" air into one's lungs, is also more likely to be functional except in cases of pulmonary oedema (Bass, 1984). Diagnostic difficulties include the fact that ischaemic heart disease and functional cardiorespiratory symptoms often occur together, and also that some cardiac investigations such as exercise testing are relatively non-specific.

Functional chest pain

Pain in the left inframammary or left pectoral region and pain at one site which has a sharp or stabbing quality are suggestive of functional chest pain. Pain brought on by cold or relieved by nitrates is more likely to be due to ischaemic heart disease (Bass, 1990*b*). Useful physical signs which favour a functional diagnosis include chest wall tenderness, audible gasping and sighing respiration, throat clearing, short breath-holding time, chest tightness and the inability to lie flat without bringing on breathlessness (assuming that pulmonary oedema has been excluded) (Bass, 1990*b*).

Comorbidity

Functional cardiorespiratory symptoms may occur in generalised anxiety disorder, panic disorder, major depression, other somatoform disorders, particularly somatisation disorder and hypochondriasis, as well as in the cardiac variants of Münchausen's syndrome. The somatic accompaniments of panic attacks and anxiety in these patients are sometimes attributed to physical causes, and some patients express the fear that they are having "a heart attack" during one of their panic attacks.

A subgroup of patients presenting to cardiologists with chest pain and normal coronary arteries have high rates of psychiatric morbidity and comprise around 20% of those undergoing angiography. These patients have high rates of functional disability due to symptoms of anxiety and panic, but low long-term cardiac morbidity and mortality (Bass, 1990*b*).

Aetiological factors

Bass (1990*b*) subdivides them into:

(1) *Predisposing factors* that include previous personal experience of cardiorespiratory illness, such as exposure to these illnesses in close family members or friends.
(2) *Precipitating factors*, commonly life events, particularly those threatening the individual, including witnessing the death of friends or relatives (Burns & Nicols, 1972). A recent study has shown life events to be more common than in a matched control group (Roll & Theorell, 1987).
(3) *Maintaining factors*, mostly personality traits, such as high trait levels of anxiety and hypochondriacal personality traits. More importantly perhaps, they also include iatrogenic factors such as the inappropriate prescription of cardiac medication for patients who have been reassured by their prescribing physician that they have no significant cardiac disease.

Management

As well as the history and mental state examination, a hyperventilation provocation test and measurement of end tidal pCO_2 is often useful. These will help to establish the role of hyperventilation in individual cases, and provide a useful lead into giving a patient an explanation for the symptoms as well as specific management strategies. Many patients referred to psychiatrists are taking unnecessary cardiac medication, and when indicated such medication may be withdrawn, although this should *always* be done in consultation with the cardiologist. Liaison with both the general practitioner and cardiologist is important.

Bass (1990*b*) describes the role of cognitive–behavioural therapy. The three basic processes involved in the treatment of cardiorespiratory syndromes are:

(1) attempting to replicate the symptoms. This should only be tried if organic heart disease has been excluded. Techniques include asking the patient to hyperventilate, run on the spot or to breath-hold. Such procedures may reproduce the symptoms, and will allow the patient to move on to stage 2.
(2) reattribution of somatic symptoms, and the correction of underlying assumptions about the nature of the symptoms. The patient is taught to perceive the symptoms not as a warning of impending doom, but a normal response to anxiety and hyperventilation. The therapist may give the patient written instructions about how to cope during an attack, which will also include a factual explanation of the symptoms. Instructions remind patients to slow their breathing, to remember that they have survived symptoms before, and that their symptoms do not last long.
(3) coping strategies. These include the use of positive self-statements, breathing exercises (such as slow breathing at the rate of 8–12 breaths per minute), as well as avoiding checking habits like repetitive pulse-taking, reassurance-seeking, and directly tackling ruminations about the nature of symptoms.

This cognitive–behavioural package has been demonstrated to be effective in a study by Klimes *et al* (1990). Drug treatments such as imipramine are effective among those with panic disorder or depressive illness. Other effective drugs are clomipramine, fluvoxamine and fluoxetine (Den Boer & Westernburg, 1990; Schneier *et al*, 1990) and the benzodiazepine, alprazolam (Ballinger *et al*, 1988), although benzodiazepines must be used with caution because of the risks of dependence.

The most consistent finding at follow-up is that very few of these patients have died. In Grant's (1925) follow-up study, a sixth had recovered completely, half were asymptomatic with varying degrees of disability, with the remaining third still disabled. Personality and social variables affect outcome, but there are no recent follow-up studies.

Chronic fatigue syndrome

In a now notorious study, McEvedy & Beard (1970) described the cases of some of the patients involved in the 1955 epidemic of myalgic encephalomyelitis (ME) at the Royal Free Hospital, which subsequently became known as Royal Free disease. The authors attributed the epidemic to "mass hysteria". They highlighted the high female to male sex incidence, normal investigations, and the apparent intensity of malaise and fatigue compared with the mildness of more tangible physical symptoms. They suggested that anxiety and secondary hyperventilation produced many of the observable symptoms. White (1990) criticised this study because it failed to comment on the high prevalence of lymphadenopathy and muscle pain, and also because McEvedy & Beard (1970) only reviewed the case notes of the most severely affected patients. In the last ten years the literature on chronic fatigue has proliferated, and the disorder has attracted numerous names, as shown in Box 17.4.

The debate concerning the validity, aetiology and treatment of the disorder has been acrimonious at times and even reached the floor of the House of Commons. Most psychiatrists working in this area have tried not to fall into the trap of mind/body dualism (David *et al*, 1988; White, 1989; Sharpe, 1990). Psychiatric involvement in cases of chronic fatigue syndrome may be helpful because there are often associated psychiatric disorders, and also because psychological approaches help in management (Sharpe, 1990; Butler *et al*, 1991). The precise nature of the syndrome associated with exhaustion and fatigue has proved difficult to define, and current definitions have poor reliability and validity. White (1990) provided evidence that there probably is a discrete fatigue syndrome which may follow certain infections, including glandular fever. Recent authors have pointed to the similarity between chronic fatigue syndromes and neurasthenia (Wessely, 1990). Neurasthenia was included in ICD–9 and is retained in ICD–10 (Box 17.5), but was not considered to be a sufficiently valid condition to be included in either DSM–III or DSM–IV.

ICD–10 describes two types of neurasthenia, the first characterised by increased fatigue after mental effort, with associated decline in occupational functioning, and the second with feelings of bodily or physical weakness after minimal effort, and which is accompanied by muscle aches and pains. In both types there are a variety of other physical symptoms, including dizziness, headaches and feelings of instability. ICD–10 includes the syndrome of neurasthenia in the section on somatoform disorders, but there is a separate syndrome of post-viral fatigue that includes benign encephalomyelitis; this is described in the section on neurological disorders rather than in the psychiatric section.

Epidemiology and comorbidity

Fatigue as a main symptom is common in the community, and prevalence rates of 24% (Kroenke *et al*, 1988) and 20–25% (White, 1990) are given. Norrelund & Holnagel (1979) found that 41% of women and 25% of men in a Danish population study felt "tired at present".

Fatigue is also a common presenting symptom of almost any underlying infectious disease, neurological disorder, diabetes and myxoedema (Allan, 1944). Fatigue as a symptom is included in the operational criteria for several other DSM–IV psychiatric diagnoses, including depression, dysthymia and cyclothymic personality disorder. Chronic fatigue syndrome is frequently comorbid with other psychiatric disorders. Kruesi *et al* (1989) found that 75% of patients with chronic fatigue syndrome had a history of major psychiatric illness. Concurrent major depression is most common, and figures of 36% (Manu *et al*, 1989), 46% (Kruesi *et al*, 1989) and 66% (Taerk *et al*, 1987) are given. In some cases the depression antedates the onset of the fatigue, but in others depression follows the fatigue, so it is uncertain which is the primary disorder. Somatisation disorder occurs in around 19% (Kruesi *et al*, 1989) or 15% (Manu *et al*, 1988). This is much higher than the prevalence rate in the community of 0.1–0.5% (Swartz *et al*, 1986*b*; Brown, 1988) or in hospitalised subjects (1–2%).

Aetiology

The aetiology of the disorder is probably multifactorial, with similar factors causing fibromyalgia (David *et al*, 1988; White, 1990). The muscle weakness in chronic fatigue syndrome is best explained by central rather than peripheral mechanisms (Kennedy, 1988). There is scant evidence of persistent viral infection, even in people who are severely functionally impaired (Tobi & Strauss, 1985; Buchwald *et al*, 1987). Sleep deprivation may be an additional perpetuating factor (Moldofsky *et al*, 1986).

Some have divided chronic fatigue syndrome into cases in which there is a proven infection, such as brucellosis, malaria or infective mononucleosis, and cases in which there is no proven infection. Patients with previous infections are sometimes referred to as true ME. The main differences relate to the frequency with which physical symptoms such as myalgia and dizziness are observed. Psychological symptoms, along with physical fatigue and weakness, are found equally in both syndromes. In practice the distinction is not clear-cut. Hellinger *et al* (1988) studied 60 patients with chronic fatigue, half of whom had elevated titres of antibody to the Epstein Barr virus antigen and half of whom had normal titres. There were no clinical differences between the two groups, nor was there any difference in outcome at follow-up. White (1990) has suggested that while viral illness may be a precipitant in many cases of chronic fatigue, the perpetuating

---

Box 17.4 Synonyms for chronic fatigue syndrome

Myalgic encephalomyelitis (ME)
Royal Free disease
Post-viral fatigue syndrome
Post-infectious fatigue syndrome
Neurocirculatory asthenia
Fibromyalgia

Box 17.5   ICD–10 definition of neurasthenia

Definite diagnosis requires the following:

A. Either persistent and distressing complaints of increased fatigue after mental effort, or persistent and distressing complaints of bodily weakness and exhaustion after minimal effort.

B. At least two of the following: feelings of muscular aches and pains; dizziness; tension headaches; sleep disturbance; inability to relax; irritability; dyspepsia.

C. Any autonomic or depressive symptoms present are not sufficiently persistent and severe to fulfil the criteria for any of the more specific disorders in this classification.

---

factors are usually psychological. In his follow-up study of patients with infectious mononucleosis, 60% had chronic fatigue at two months after diagnosis, but only 10% at six months, indicating that most people with the disorder recover.

The suggestion that there is an inflammation of the brain, implicit in the name "myalgic encephalitis", has never been substantiated. Summarising the evidence for an organic basis for the disorder, White (1990) states that:

> "there is intriguing evidence of abnormal immune function, persistence of viral immune response and even viral antigen persistence in the blood, muscle and faeces of highly selected patients. Unfortunately these abnormalities lack both specificity and sensitivity when applied to broader groups of patients with chronic fatigue syndrome and it is possible they may merely represent epiphenomena and be of no aetiological relevance."

Management

Treatable physical disorders should be excluded, and this may entail further history-taking, physical examination and investigations. It is unusual for the patient to reattribute physical symptoms completely to psychological symptoms and causes, given the diversity of possible aetiological factors. It is generally fruitless to argue with patients about the labelling of the disorder or its aetiology. On the other hand, it is important to try to help them to understand the relevance of psychological explanations for some of their symptoms, and this may also help them engage more easily in psychological treatment approaches.

The explanation of their illness that patients are given is crucial to successful management. White (1990) suggests the following: the doctor tells patients that their illnesses may have been precipitated by a virus, but that their continued symptoms are caused by several factors all acting together. These may include becoming unfit following the initial viral illness, muscle-weakening due to bed-rest and inactivity, and subsequent tiredness on attempting to exercise. The explanation may go on to highlight social difficulties, the role of sleep disturbance and the frustration at having been perhaps told by doctors that there was "nothing wrong". He suggests that such a complex multifactorial explanation may make it easier for the patient to accept a multifaceted treatment programme, which includes slowly increasing exercise and the gradual resumption of normal activities, treatment of concurrent depression with antidepressant drugs, and psychotherapy. The involvement of a physiotherapist and graded exercise programmes is often helpful and very acceptable to patients, particularly those who have a basically physical concept of their illness. Wessely (1990) and Sharpe (1990) proposed a cognitive–behavioural treatment which aims at tackling inactivity, because this is seen as a maladaptive strategy leading to further demoralisation, fear and depression. Treatment involves mutually agreed behavioural targets which the patient agrees to carry out, even when symptomatic. This is combined with standard cognitive techniques for treating depression and fear, with the aim of increasing the patient's self-control and mastery. Open studies suggest this programme is sometimes effective.

Chronic pain

Pain is difficult to define, possibly because of its subjective nature. Melzack & Wall (1988) wrote "pain . . . has a unique distinctly unpleasant affective quality that . . . demands immediate attention and disrupts ongoing behaviour and thought. It motivates or drives the organism into activity aimed at stopping the pain as quickly as possible." This definition contains sensory, behavioural and cognitive aspects, all of which may be relevant to its management. Similarly, Barsky (1989*b*) states "pain is a complex mental event, the product of psychological, neurochemical and neurophysiological factors. Although pain perception has a sensory component it also has affective, motivational and attitudinal components as numerous associative pathways link the sensory cerebral cortex with the limbic system." In 1979 the International Association for the Study of Pain (IASP) adopted the following definition of pain: "An unpleasant sensory and emotional experience associated with actual or potential tissue damage or described in terms of such damage". According to Barsky (1989*a*) the argument about whether pain is organic or functional is spurious as "all pain is simultaneously pathogenic and psychogenic, rather than one or the other". A comprehensive account of pain covering both organic and psychological aspects is given in Wall & Melzack (1984), and only a brief overview follows here.

Doctors frequently make value judgments about what is essentially a patient's subjective experience, and all the above definitions have a subjective component. The judgment of severity is particularly difficult in chronic pain, because the physiological accompaniments of acute pain usually attenuate with time and so are often absent among those with chronic pain.

The DSM–III and DSM–III–R criteria for somatoform pain disorder were regarded as among the least satisfactory of all somatoform disorders and have been widely criticised (Merskey, 1991; Barsky, 1989*a*). DSM–IV has made considerable changes from the DSM–III–R definition; the name has been changed to pain disorder. The definition has been broadened to include two types of pain disorder, one called "Pain disorder associated with psychological factors", and the second "Pain disorder associated with both psychological factors and a general medical condition". In addition, acute and chronic specifiers are provided for both categories. Pain resulting from general medical conditions in which psychological factors are judged to have either no role or a minimal role are not coded as mental disorders.

It is unlikely that patients with pain disorders will form a homogeneous group, and some may not even have a psychiatric disorder. Merskey (1988) has argued that hysterical mechanisms are only occasionally relevant in chronic pain syndromes. For example, in the Couvade syndrome, the husbands of pregnant women sometimes develop abdominal pain and this may be through a hysterical mechanism. Controversy still rages concerning the possible organic or psychological aetiology of syndromes such as repetitive strain injury (Littlejohn, 1986) and fibromyalgia (Moldofsky *et al*, 1975). Merskey (1990) questioned the use of clinical features like the supposed non-anatomical patterns of pain to distinguish organic from psychological syndromes. He cites the studies of Wall & Melzack (1984) who found that the receptive fields of afferent neurons in the dorsal horn of the spinal column can change and extend, suggesting that non-anatomical patterns of pain may sometimes be physiological. Various regional pain syndromes have been described. Although they are too numerous to describe in detail, some of the more common syndromes will be mentioned below.

Fibromyalgia

Fibromyalgia is a syndrome of chronic musculoskeletal aches and pains of unknown aetiology. Reliable diagnostic criteria have recently been published by the American College of Rheumatology (Wolfe *et al*, 1990). No consistent histological changes or organic pathology have been demonstrated, but there may be a reduction in the pain threshold and an increased responsiveness to noxious stimuli. Some authors such as Merskey (1991) suggest that there may be an organic basis, as yet unknown, while others point to the considerable overlap in symptomatology with chronic fatigue syndromes (Kirmayer & Robbins, 1991). White (1990) goes even further, stating that fibromyalgia and chronic fatigue syndrome "are in all probability one and the same".

Atypical facial pain

This pain may be dull or sharp and can affect almost any non-muscular part of the face, but most commonly occurs around the cheeks, eyes and jaws. It may be intermittent and is very often worse when patients feel fatigued or under a great deal of stress. Atypical facial pain should be distinguished from facial arthromyalgia, which commonly affects the temporo-mandibular joints. It is also important to distinguish it from neurological syndromes, such as trigeminal neuralgia. This is usually straightforward because atypical facial pain does not conform to the cranial nerve distribution and tends to be described in more vague terms, and does not have the intermittent shooting quality of trigeminal neuralgia. There is often a considerable time interval between the onset of symptoms and presentation, and the initial presentation is commonly to a dentist. The pain usually fails to respond to standard analgesics, but may respond to antidepressants, particularly dothiepin (Fienmann, 1985). Psychological treatment is often helpful in addition to drug treatment and consists of allaying fears concerning physical illness, educating and changing patients' beliefs concerning the nature of their symptoms. As with many other pain syndromes, treatment involves both cognitive and behavioural psychotherapy as well as straightforward explanation. In many cases the pain does not disappear or may recur.

Chronic pelvic pain

Pelvic pain is common among women attending gynaecology clinics. In recent years there has been some move away from more rigidly psychological explanations of these syndromes, towards a rather more multifactorial view of the nature of this disorder (Pearce & Beard, 1990). Although many women with pelvic pain have no discernible organic pathology, Beard *et al* (1984) has shown that 80% of women with chronic pelvic pain have pelvic venous congestion, but the identification of the congestion does not necessarily imply that it is aetiologically relevant. Psychogenic theories of pelvic pain have emphasised women's conflicts over sexuality, because it commonly occurs in association with dysmenorrhoea and dyspareunia. Treatment has included hormone therapy or cognitive psychotherapy; Farquhar *et al* (1989) showed that a combined treatment programme is superior to using either method on its own.

Low back pain

Low back pain is an extremely common presenting symptom. Nagi *et al* (1973) found that 18% of the population between the ages of 16 and 84 have persistent back pain, and rates are higher among the old, women and those with high levels of anxiety. These subjects have a generally poor view of their health and are frequent users of health services. Genuine organic diagnoses are difficult to make because there are only rarely altered reflexes or changes in neuroimaging. It is possible that an organic musculoskeletal dysfunction may underlie some of these symptoms, but the accompanying physical signs are soft and therefore difficult to diagnose reliably.

Opinions on the best treatment of chronic low back pain are varied, and are generally unsatisfactory (Yates & Currie, 1986). Treatments recommended include a rigid brace, physical rehabilitation programmes, transcutaneous electrical nerve stimulation, and psychological treatment. Baker (1989) described the core principles of psychological treatment. They are:

(1) exclusion of obvious physical disorder, particularly the exclusion of nerve-root pressure;
(2) reassurance about the absence of physical illness and the likelihood of good prognosis;
(3) discouraging the use of numerous alternative practitioners and reassuring patients they had an adequate assessment;
(4) encouraging participation in a treatment programme, which may include simple analgesics, mobilisation and a programmed increase in activity, including swimming and walking.

Differential diagnosis

Deciding whether the pain disorder or depression is primary is sometimes difficult, and when in doubt a trial of an antidepressant may be helpful. Pain may also feature in anxiety disorders, schizophrenia and dementia, but in these cases it rarely dominates the picture. It may also occur in somatisation disorder and hypochondriasis. Pain can occur as a hallucination, but this is exceedingly rare. Pain in the presence of anxiety or depression may be due to muscle contraction. Cognitive processes probably result in an exacerbation of pain in such cases.

Assessment

A variety of psychometric instruments have been developed to assess pain (for review see Pearce & Myles, 1993). Some instruments assess the sensory component of pain, for example, visual analogue scales, while others assess both sensory and affective components. Others focus on the behavioural component of pain, the impact on lifestyle, and finally on central control processes. The best-known of these is the McGill Pain Questionnaire (Melzack, 1975). This widely-used questionnaire consists of 78 adjectives arranged in 20 groups which reflect the different qualities of pain. These include words like "pricking, boring, drilling" which describe sensory experiences, and words such as "annoying, troublesome, intense, cruel" which describe emotional experiences. Subjects are asked to tick words that describe their pain and the questionnaire can be scored to arrive at an index reflecting the intensity of the words checked, as well as the number of words checked in each of the various categories. Studies of reliability have confirmed a clear distinction between the sensory and affective words.

Management

The aim of management should be to improve function and help the patient to cope better, because complete pain relief is often not possible. As with other somatoform disorders, the patient's physical state should be attended to from the outset, paying particular attention to commonly missed physical disorders such as soft tissue injury. Patients' own notions of the cause of their pain should be explored and taken seriously, but at the same time the therapist should encourage patients to see the relevance of physical, psychological and social processes as causes of the pain.

A wide variety of physical and psychological treatment methods have been applied to chronic pain. These include transcutaneous neuro-stimulation, biofeedback, hypnosis, physiotherapy, relaxation, drugs and cognitive–behavioural psychotherapy. Melzack & Wall (1988) have cited evidence that many treatments that are not helpful individually may be helpful in combination (e.g. biofeedback plus hypnosis).

Drug treatment

It appears that some tricyclic antidepressants possess analgesic properties. The best evidence is for amitriptyline, although other drugs including nortriptyline and imipramine have also been used. There is as yet no evidence that drugs acting on the serotoninergic system are more analgesic than those acting on the noradrenergic system. Sometimes the effect of a tricyclic antidepressant can be augmented by a phenothiazine. Carbamazepine may be useful for shooting pains but is unhelpful for steady, dull pains. There is some controversy about the use of opiates in chronic pain syndromes of unknown aetiology. Barsky (1989*b*) states that opiates are "generally ineffective and should be reserved for patients suffering from pain that is clearly pathogenic". It is usually unwise for psychiatrists to be drawn into prescribing opiates for non-malignant causes of pain. However, other authorities suggest that there may occasionally be a place for opiates in the management of chronic non-malignant pain, after a trial of other treatment.

Fordyce (1976) has pioneered behavioural management of pain. He places importance on *not verbally reinforcing* complaints of pain and other pain behaviours, but instead reinforcing more desirable behaviours such as exercising, talking about things other than pain, and taking part in normal social interactions. This regime is incorporated into many pain programmes, but behavioural approaches used in isolation are usually disappointing and they need to be combined with other remedies (Melzack & Wall, 1988). Cognitive therapies have attracted recent interest; they are directed at modifying pain-related cognitions and the cognitive responses to stress. Most patients completing intensive pain treatment programmes retain some symptoms but may benefit from functional improvement (Rybstein-Blinchick, 1979; Farquhar *et al*, 1989; Pearce *et al*, 1989).

Pain and litigation

In a much-quoted and influential article on compensation neurosis, Miller (1961) claimed that it was "motivated by greed, encouraged by lawyers and invariably cured by a favourable verdict", and money was thought to be the motive behind much unexplained pain. As pointed out by Merskey (1990) and by Mendelson (1982), not a single study since Miller's has supported his conclusions. On the contrary, most studies have found that many patients continue to suffer pain long after litigation has been settled. Moreover, disorders such as cervical sprain syndrome and minor head injury, which often occur in compensation claims and were previously thought to be largely psychogenic, have now been shown to have a significant organic basis (Taylor & Bell, 1966; McNab, 1973).

Münchausen's syndrome

Much of the medical literature about Münchausen's syndrome is anecdotal. This is almost inevitable bearing in mind the nature of the disorder and subsequent difficulties in studying these patients. The syndrome was given its name by Asher (1951) because sufferers, like the legendary Baron Von Münchausen, usually travel widely.

The term has now been abandoned in modern psychiatric classification; DSM–IV classifies it together with factitious disorders. Patients present with plausible physical symptoms which are factitious, and this is associated with multiple visits to hospital. Indeed, as the DSM–IV handbook points out, "the person's entire life may consist of trying to get admitted to or staying in hospital". Common symptomatic presentations include pyrexia of unknown origin, bleeding disorders, pain syndromes, haemoptysis and rashes. Requests for analgesics are particularly common and some patients are addicted to opiate drugs. They may go to extraordinary lengths to produce physical signs, such as self-instrumentation of the urethra, or even placing pieces of liver in the vagina to simulate blood clots. Lying and the use of false names are common.

It is the intentional production of symptoms and signs which helps distinguish Münchausen's syndrome from the somatoform disorders. It is usually implicit that this is a conscious process, but in practice, distinguishing what is conscious from what is unconscious is often difficult, if not impossible. One useful distinguishing clinical feature is that patients with Münchausen's syndrome very often have some physical signs, whereas in somatisation disorder these are usually absent.

The prevalence of Münchausen's syndrome is unknown. Although it has been described in both sexes, it is commoner in males and may be more frequent in the paramedical occupations (Morris, 1991). The question of motivation of these patients is a difficult one, and it is likely that a variety of factors operate. Some are seeking opiate drugs, some enjoy attention, others wish to express feelings of anger and hostility towards doctors, and a few are even trying to escape the police.

Management of Münchausen's syndrome is exceedingly difficult. In the general hospital ward there is often an angry confrontation that usually leads to the patient taking his own discharge. Once the diagnosis is suspected the patient should be approached cautiously, and preferably by a psychiatrist and physician in collaboration. If the patient can be engaged, a psychotherapeutic approach may be instituted; one study suggests that improvement may occur in some patients (Mayo & Haggerty, 1984), but in general the condition is very resistant to change.

Münchausen's syndrome by proxy

This syndrome should be seen as a form of child abuse. It has been extensively described by Meadow (1972, 1985) who drew the attention of paediatricians to this disorder. It is a form of factitious disorder in which children present with a plethora of symptoms and signs usually suggestive of a multisystem disorder, although occasionally only one system is involved. Symptoms have usually either persisted or recurred for periods of more than one year, and bleeding, neurological symptoms, rashes, glycosuria and fever are common findings. Most of the children will have seen numerous doctors; for example, one subject in Meadow's series had seen 28 different doctors. In 95% of cases the mother is the perpetrator and fabricator of both the symptoms and signs. It is unusual for the father to be involved, but occasionally other key carers, such as staff in hospitals or residential facilities, have been implicated.

The consequences of the syndrome can be extremely serious. The children have frequent admissions to hospital, are usually subjected to multiple investigations (which are often invasive), and they may suffer iatrogenic harm, as well as experiencing social harms such as missing school. In Meadow's original series, two of the 19 children had died as a result of the syndrome, while it is also possible that some of these children may grow up to become adult Münchausen's cases.

Describing the parents of children involved, Meadow (1972, 1985) points out that 50% of the mothers had had some nursing training, or were working as nurses, while around 20% had Münchausen's syndrome themselves. These mothers were noted to be overattentive in hospital, rarely leaving the ward, although seemed to show less anxiety over their child's health than would normally be expected. Sometimes they develop close relationships with the staff and may even be found engaged in fundraising activities for the hospital.

Because of the significantly raised morbidity and mortality associated with the syndrome, early diagnosis is crucial. Meadow lists a number of things which should act as warnings:

(1) children presenting with multiple, unexplained, prolonged symptoms with accompanying incongruent signs;
(2) less anxiety than would be anticipated on the part of the mother;
(3) children who appear to have multiple, often unusual, allergies;
(4) children who often have poor tolerance of offered treatments;
(5) children from large families in which other members appear to suffer from a variety of medical illnesses;
(6) families in which multiple cot deaths occur.

During investigation, careful and detailed history-taking is essential and the history should be checked from other sources, including schools, playgroups, friends and neighbours. It is also helpful to check straightforward details of the personal, social and family history as given by the mother because there are commonly fabrications in this part of the history, and discrepancies here may provide the first clue concerning the mother's dishonesty. Once the syndrome has been suspected it is important to look for a temporal association between illness events and the presence of the mother (or other key adult carers). Speaking to the family doctor and other family members will often reveal inconsistencies in the history and other diagnostic clues. The general practitioner, for example, may know that the mother has presented with a factitious disorder before, or that she has multiple unexplained symptoms herself. Sometimes it may be possible to find motives for perpetrating this type of behaviour. Some people enhance their personal status as a result of the attention they receive from having a sick child, and on occasions communities have even collected large sums of money to support the families. Not surprisingly, this can perpetuate the syndrome.

If there is suspicion in the hospital that the syndrome is present, the mother should be observed, particularly ensuring that she does not change charts or records. If new symptoms develop, samples of body fluids should be retained and checked for poisoning. In cases of bleeding it is crucial to check that the blood is that of the child. Once suspicions are strong enough, staff may need to resort to searching the mother or even excluding the parents from the ward as a diagnostic test.

If there is strong suspicion or confirmation of the diagnosis, the doctor has a statutory responsibility to inform the social services who will convene a case conference, and the child may have to be removed from the care of the mother. The perpetrator should be confronted and the diagnosis brought into the open. If possible the family should be referred to a family psychiatrist for long-term support and counselling. This is often resisted and the mother in particular will deny that she is responsible or has any need for ongoing psychotherapy.

References

Allan, F. N. (1944) The differential diagnosis of weakness and fatigue. *New England Journal of Medicine*, **231**, 414–418.

Alexander, F. (1949) *Fundamentals of Psychoanalysis*. London: Allen & Unwin.

American Psychiatric Association (1980) *Diagnostic and Statistical Manual of Mental Disorders* (3rd edn) (DSM–III). Washington, DC: APA.

—— (1987) *Diagnostic and Statistical Manual of Mental Disorders* (3rd edn, revised) (DSM–III–R). Washington, DC: APA.

—— (1994) *Diagnostic and Statistical Manual of Mental Disorders* (4th edn) (DSM–IV). Washington, DC: APA.

Andreason, N. C. & Bardach, J. (1977) Dysmorphobia: symptom or disease? *American Journal of Psychiatry*, **134**, 673–676.

Apley, T. (1958) Common demoniates in the recurrent pains of childhood. *Proceeding of the Royal Society of Medicine*, 51, 1023–1027.

Appleby, L. (1987) Hypochondriasis: an acceptable diagnosis? *British Medical Journal*, **294**, 8857.

Asher, R. (1951) Münchausen's syndrome. *Lancet*, *i*, 339–341.

Baker, G. H. B. (1989) Backache. In *Psychological Management of the Physically Ill* (eds J. H. Lacey & T. Burns), pp. 229–246. Edinburgh: Churchill Livingstone.

Ballinger, J. C., Burrows, J. D., Du Pont, R. L., *et al* (1988) Alprazolam in panic disorder and agorophobia: results from a multi-centre trial. 1. Efficacy and short term treatment. *Archives of General Psychiatry*, **45**, 413–442.

Barsky, A. J. (1989*a*) International Association for the Study of Pain (1979) Pain terms: a list with definitions and notes on usage. Recommended by an IASP sub committee on Taxonomy. *Pain*, **6**, 249–252.

—— (1989*b*) Somatization disorders. In *Comprehensive Textbook of Psychiatry* (5th edn) (eds H. I. Kaplan & B. J. Sadock). Baltimore: Williams & Wilkins.

—— & Klerman, G. L. (1983) Hypochondriasis, bodily complaints and somatic styles. *American Journal of Psychiatry*, **140**, 273–284.

——, Wyshak, G. & Klerman, G. (1986) Hypochondriasis: an evaluation of the DSM–III criteria in medical outpatients. *Archives of General Psychiatry*, **43**, 493–500.

——, Geringer, E. & Wool, C. A. (1988) A cognitive educational treatment for hypochondriasis. *General Hospital Psychiatry*, **10**, 322–327.

——, Wyshak, G. & Klerman, G. L. (1992) Psychiatric co-morbidity in DSM–III–R hypochondriasis. *Archives of General Psychiatry*, **49**, 101–108.

Bass, C. M. (1984) Unexplained chest pain: psychosocial studies in presumptive angina . MD thesis, University of London.

—— (1990*a*) Assessment and management of patients' with functional somatic symptoms. In *Somatization: Physical Symptoms and Psychological Illness* (ed. C. Bass), pp. 40–72. Oxford: Blackwell Scientific.

—— (1990*b*) Functional cardiorespiratory syndrome. In *Somatization: Physical Symptoms and Psychological Illness* (ed. C. Bass), pp. 171–206. Oxford: Blackwell Scientific.

——, Chambers, J. B., Kith, P., *et al* (1988) Panic, anxiety and hyperventilation in patients with chest pain. *Quarterly Journal of Medicine*, **69**, 949–959.

Beard, R. W., Hymen, J. W., Pearce, S., *et al* (1984) Diagnosis of pelvic varicositus in women with chronic pelvic pain. *Lancet*, **2**, 946–949.

Bishop, E. R. (1980) Monosymptomatic hypochondriasis. *Psychomatics*, **21**, 731–747.

Blanchard, A. P., Swartz, S. T., Neff, D. F., *et al* (1988) Prediction of outcome from a self regulatory treatment of irritable bowel syndrome. *Behavioural Research Therapy*, **26**, 187–190.

Bohman, M., Cloninger, C. R., Von-Knorring, A. L., *et al* (1984) Adoption study of somatoform disorder. *Archives of General Psychiatry*, **41**, 872–878.

Briquet, P. (1869) *Traite Clinique Therapeutique de l'Hysterie*. Paris: J. B. Balliere.

Brown, T. M. (1988) Somatizing disorders in an Edinburgh general practice. MPhil. thesis, University of Edinburgh.

——, Scott, A. I. F. & Pullen, I. M. (1990) *Handbook of Emergency Psychiatry*. Edinburgh: Churchill Livingstone.

Buchwald, D., Sullivan, J. L. & Komaroff, A. L. (1987) Frequency of chronic active Epstein Barr virus infection in general medical practice. *Journal of the American Medical Association*, **257**, 2303–2307.

Burns, B. H. & Nicols, M. A. (1972) Factors related to the localisation of symptoms to the chest and depression. *British Journal of Psychiatrists*, **121**, 405–409.

Burton, R. (1651) *The Anatomy of Melancholy* (eds L. Dell & P. Jordon-Smith) (1948). New York: Tudor Publishing.

Butler, S., Calder, T., Ron, M., *et al* (1991) Cognitive behaviour therapy in the chronic fatigue syndrome. *Journal of Neurology, Neurosurgery and Psychiatry*, **54**, 153–158.

Cheyne, G. (1733) *The English Malady: or, a Treatise of Nervous Diseases of all Kind; as Spleen, Vapours, Lowness of Spirit, Hypochondriacal and Hysterical Distempers* (4th edn). London: G. Strachan.

Cloninger, C. R., Sigvardsson, S., Von-Knorring, A., *et al* (1984) An adoption study of two discrete somatoform disorders. *Archives of General Psychiatry*, **41**, 863–871.

Cohen, A. (1966) The physician and the "crock". In *Practical Lectures in Psychiatry for the Medical Practitioner* (ed. G. L. Usden). Springfield, IL: Charles C. Thomas.

Covi, L., Lipman, R. S., Derogatis, L. R., *et al* (1974) Drugs and group psychotherapy in neurotic depression. *American Journal of Psychiatry*, **131**, 191–198.

Craig, T. J. K. & Brown, G. W. (1984) Goal frustration and life events in the aetiology of painful gastrointestinal disorder. *Journal of Psychosomatic Research*, **28**, 411–421.

——, Boardman, A. P., Mills, K., *et al* (1993) The South London Somatization Study and the influence of early life experiences. *British Journal of Psychiatry*, **163**, 579–588.

Creed, F. H. (1981) Life events and appendectomy. *Lancet*, **1**, 1381–1385.

—— (1990) Functional abdominal pain. In *Somatization: Physical Symptoms and Psychological Illness* (ed. C. Bass), pp. 141–170. Oxford: Blackwell Scientific.

—— & Guthrie, E. (1987) Psychological factors in irritable bowels. *Gut*, **28**, 1307–1308.

Da Costa, J. M. (1871) On irritable heart. The clinical study of a form of functional cardiac disease and its consequences. *American Journal of Medical Sciences*, **61**, 17–52.

David, A. J., Wessely, S. & Pelosi, A. J. (1988) Post viral syndrome: a time for a new approach. *British Medical Journal*, **296**, 696–699.

de Leon, J., Bott, A. & Simpson, G. M. (1989) Dysmorphobia: body dysmorphic disorder or delusional disorder somatic sub-type? *Comprehensive Psychiatry*, **30**, 457–472.

Den Boer, J. A. & Westernburg, H. G. M. (1990) Serotonin function in panic disorder: a double blind placebo controlled study with fluvoxamine and retansorine. *Psychopharmacology*, **102**, 85–94.

Drossman, D. A., McKee, D. C., Sandler, R. S., *et al* (1978) Psychosocial factors in irritable bowel syndrome. A multivariate study of patients and non-patients with IBS. *Gastroenterology*, **91**, 701–708.

Escobar, J. L., Rubiostipec, M., Canino, G., *et al* (1989) Somatic symptoms index (SSI) – a new and abridged somatization construct. Prevalence and epidemiological correlates in two large community samples. *Journal of Nervous and Mental Disorders*, **177**, 140–146.

Fabricant, N. D. (1960) *Thirteen Famous Patients*. Philadelphia: Charles E. Shulton.

Falret, J. P. (1822) *De l'Hypochondriac et du Surade*. Paris.

Farquhar, C. M., Rodgers, S., Franks, S., *et al* (1989) A randomised controlled trial of medroxyprogesterone acetate and psychotherapy for the treatment of pelvic congestion. *British Journal of Obstetrics and Gynaecology*, **6**, 1152–1162.

Feinmann, C. (1985) Pain relief by anti-depressants: possible modes of action. *Pain*, **23**, 1–8.

Ford, C. V. (1983) *The Somatising Disorders: Illness as a Way of Life*. New York: Elsevier Biomedical.

Ford, M. J., Miller, P. McC., Eastwood, J., *et al* (1987) Life events, psychiatric illness and the irritable bowel syndrome. *Gut*, **28**, 160–165.

Fordyce, W. E. (1976) Behavioral Methods for Chronic Pain and Illness. St. Louis, Mo: CV Mosby.

Freud, S. & Breuer, J. (1896) Studies on hysteria. In *Standard Edition of the Complete Psychological Works of Sigmund Freud. Vol 2.* (1955). London: Hogarth Press.

Fukuda, O. (1977) Statistical analysis of dysmorphobia in outpatient clinic. *Japanese Journal of Plastic and Reconstructive Surgery*, **20**, 569–577.

Gillespie, R. (1928) Hypochondria: its definition, nosology and psycholopathology. *Guy's Hospital Report*, **78**, 308–460.

Gipson, M. & Connolly, F. A. (1975) The incidence of schizophrenia and severe psychotic disorder in patients ten years after cosmetic rhinoplasty. *British Journal of Plastic Surgery*, **28**, 155–159.

Goldberg, D., Gask, L. & O'Dowd, T. (1989) The treatment of somatization: teaching techniques of reattributions. *Journal of Psychosomatic Research*, **33**, 689–695.

Grant, R. (1925) Observations on the after-histories of men suffering from the effort syndrome. *Heart*, **12**, 121–142.

Greenbaum, D., Mayle, G., Vanegeran, L. E., *et al* (1987) Effects of desipramine on irritable bowel syndrome compared with atropine in placebo. *Digestive Disease and Sciences*, **32**, 257–266.

Guthrie, E., Creed, F., Dawson, D., *et al* (1991) Controlled trial of psychological treatment for the irritable bowel syndrome. *Gastroenterology*, **100**, 450–457.

—, —, —, *et al* (1993) A randomised controlled trial of psychotherapy in patients with refractory irritable bowel syndrome. *British Journal of Psychiatry*, **163**, 315–321.

Guze, S. B. (1967) The diagnosis of hysteria: what are we trying to do? *American Journal of Psychiatry*, **124**, 491–498.

Harvey, R. F., Mauad, E. C. & Brown, A. M. (1987) Prognosis in the irritable bowel syndrome: a five year prospective study. *Lancet, i*, 963–965.

Hay, G. G. (1970) Dysmorphophobia. *British Journal of Psychiatry*, **116**, 399–406.

Hellinger, W. C., Smith, T. F., Van Scoire, R. E., *et al* (1988) Chronic fatigue syndrome in the diagnostic utility of antibody to Epstein Barr virus early antigen. *Journal of American Medical Association*, **260**, 971–973.

Hinsie, L. E. & Campbell, R. J. (1960) *Psychiatric Dictionary* (3rd edn). Oxford: Oxford University Press.

Hollander, E., Liebowitz, M. R., Winshel, R., *et al* (1989) Treatment of body dysmorphic disorder with serotonin reuptake blockers. *American Journal of Psychiatry*, **146**, 768–770.

Hyler, S. E. & Sussmann, N. (1984) Somatoform disorder after DSM–III. *Hospital and Community Psychiatry*, **34**, 469–478.

International Association for the Study of Pain (Sub-Committee on Taxonomy) (1979) Pain terms: A list with definitions and notes on usage. *Pain*, **6**, 249–252.

Izdorek, S. (1975) A functional classification of hypochondriasis with specific recommendations for treatment. *Southern Medical Journal*, **68**, 1326–1332.

Katon, W., Kleinman, A. & Rosen, G. (1982) Depression and somatization: I and II. *American Journal of Medicine*, **72**, 127–135, 241–247.

Kellner, R. (1986) *Somatization and Hypochondriasis*. Westport, CT: Praeger.

Kendell, R. E. (1983) Other functional psychoses. In *Companion to Psychiatric Studies* (3rd edn) (eds R. E. Kendell & E. K. Zealley), pp. 319–329. Edinburgh: Churchill Livingstone.

Kennedy, H. G. (1988) Fatigue and fatiguability. *British Journal of Psychiatry*, **153**, 1–5.

Kenyon, F. (1964) Hypochondriasis: a clinical study. *British Journal of Psychiatry*, **110**, 478–488.

— (1976) Hypochondriacal state. *British Journal of Psychiatry*, **110** , 478–488.

Kessel, N. (1979) Reassurance. *Lancet, i*, 1128–1133.

Kirmayer, L. J. (1984) Depression and somatization: I and II. *Transcultural Psychiatric Research Review*, **21**, 159–188, 237–262.

— & Robbins, J. M. (eds) (1991) *Current Concepts of Somatization: Research and Clinical Perspectives*. Washington, DC: APA.

Klimes, I., Mayou, R. & Pearce, M. J. (1990) Psychological treatment for atypical non-cardiac chest pain: a controlled evaluation. *Psychological Medicine*, **20**, 605–611.

Kroenke, K., Wood, D. R., Mangelsdorff, A. D., *et al* (1988) Chronic fatigue in primary care: prevalence of patient and outcome. *Journal of the American Medical Association*, **260**, 929–934.

Kruesi, M. J. P., Deo, J. & Strauss, S. E. (1989) Psychiatric diagnosis of patients who have chronic fatigue syndrome. *Journal of Clinical Psychiatry*, **50**, 53–56.

Lerner, J. & Noy, P. (1968) Somatic complaints in psychiatric disorder: social and cultural factors. *International Journal of Social Psychiatry*, **14**, 145–150.

Lewis, B. I. (1959) Hyperventilation syndrome: a clinical and psychological evaluation. *California Medicine*, **3**, 121–129.

Lipowski, Z. J. (1988) Somatisation: the concept and its clinical application. *American Journal of Psychiatry*, **145**, 1358–1368.

Liscow, B., Othmere, E., Penick, E. C., *et al* (1986) Is Briquet's Syndrome a heterogeneous disorder? *American Journal of Psychiatry*, **143**, 636–629.

Littlejohn, G. O. (1986) Repetitive strain syndrome: An Australian experience (Editorial). *Journal of Rheumatology*, **136**, 1004–1006.

Mai, F. M. & Merskey, H. (1980) Briquet's treatize on hysteria: a synopsis and commentary. *Archives of General Psychiatry*, **37**, 1401–1405.

Manu, P., Mathews, D. A. & Laing, T. J. (1988) The mental health of patients with a chief complaint of chronic fatigue: prospective evaluation and follow-up. *Archives of Internal Medicine*, **148**, 2213–2217.

——, Laing, T. J. & Mathews, D. A. (1989) Somatization disorder in patients with chronic fatigue. *Psychosomatics*, **30**, 388–395.

Marks, I. & Mischan, J. (1988) Dysmorphophobic avoidance with disturbed bodily perception: a pilot study of exposure therapy. *British Journal of Psychiatry*, **152**, 674–678.

Mayo, J. P. & Haggerty, J. J. (1984) Long term psychotherapy of Münchausen syndrome. *American Journal of Psychotherapy*, **38**, 571–578.

McEvedy, C. P. & Beard, W. (1970) The Royal Free epidemic of 1955: A reconsideration. *British Medical Journal*, **1**, 7–11.

McGrath, G. & Bowker, M. (1987) *Common Psychiatric Emergencies*. Bristol: Wright.

McKenna, P. J. (1984) Disorders with overvalued ideas. *British Journal of Psychiatry*, **145**, 579–585.

McNab, I. (1973) The whiplash syndrome. *Clinical Neurosurgery*, **20**, 232–241.

Meadow, R. (1972) Münchausen syndrome by proxy. *Archives of Diseases of Childhood*, **57**, 92–98.

—— (1985) Management of Münchausen syndrome by proxy. *Archives of Diseases of Childhood*, **60**, 385–393.

Mechanic, D. (1962) The concept of illness behaviour. *Journal of Chronic Diseases*, **15**, 189–194.

—— (1964) The influence of mothers on their children's health, attitudes and behaviour. *Paediatrics*, **33**, 444–453.

Melzack, R. (1975) The McGill Pain Questionnaire: Major properties and scoring methods. *Pain*, **1**, 277–299.

—— & Wall, P. D. (1988) *The Challenge of Pain*. Harmondsworth: Penguin.

Mendelson, G. (1982) Not "cured by a verdict". Effect of legal settlement on compensation claimants. *Medical Journal of Australia*, **2**, 132–134.

Merskey, H. (1988) Chronic pain syndromes and their management. In *Recent Advances in Clinical Neurology*, **5**, 87–106. Edinburgh: Churchill Livingstone.

—— (1990) Conversion symptoms revisited. *Seminars in Neurology*, **10**, 221–228.

—— (1991) The definition of pain. *European Psychiatry*, **6**, 153–159.

Miller, H. G. (1961) Accident neurosis. *British Medical Journal*, **1**, 919–925, 992–1028.

Moldofsky, H., Scarisbrick, P., England, R., *et al* (1975) Musculoskeletal symptoms and non-REM sleep disturbances in patients with fibrositis syndrome and healthy subjects. *Psychosomatic Medicine*, **37**, 341–351.

——, Lue, F. A., Ison, J., *et al* (1986) The relationship of Interleukin-1 and immune functions to sleep in humans. *Psychosomatic Medicine*, **48**, 309–318.

Morris, M. (1991) Münchausen's syndrome and factitious interests. *Current Opinion in Psychiatry*, **4**, 225–230.

Morselli, E. (1891) Sulla, dismorfofobia, e sulla, tafefobia. *Bolletinno della R. Accademia di Genova*, **6**, 110–119.

Munro, A. (1978) Monosymptomatic hypochondriacal psychoses: a diagnostic entity which may respond to pimozide. *Canadian Psychiatric Association Journal*, **23**, 497–500.

—— & Chmara, J. (1982) Monosymptomatic hypochondriacal psychosis: a diagnostic check list based on fifty cases of the disorder. *Canadian Journal of Psychiatry*, **27**, 374–376.

Murphy, M. R. (1990) Classification of the somatoform disorders. In *Somatization: Physical Symptoms and Psychological Illness* (ed. C. M. Bass), pp. 10–39. Oxford: Blackwell.

Nagi, S. Z., Riley, L. E. & Newby, L. B. (1973) A social epidemiology of back pain in a general population. *Journal of Chronic Diseases*, **26**, 769–779.

Norrelund, N. & Holnagel, H. (1979) Fatigue amongst 40 year olds. *Ugeskr Laeger*, **141**, 1425–1429.

Parker, G. & Lipscome, P. (1980) The relevance of early parental experiences to adult dependency, hypochondriasis and utilization of primary physicians. *British Journal of Medical Psychology*, **53**, 355–363.

Parsons, T. (1951) *The Social System*. New York: Free Press.

Pearce, S. & Erskine, A. (1989) Chronic pain. In *The Practice of Behavioural Medicine* (eds S. Pearce & J. Wardle), pp. 83–111. London/Oxford: The British Psychological Society and Oxford University Press.

—— & Beard, R. W. (1990) Chronic pelvic pain in women. In *Somatization: Physical Symptoms in Psychological Illness* (ed. C. Bass), pp. 206–232. Oxford: Blackwell.

—— & Myles, A. (1993) Chronic pain. In *Recent Advances in Clinical Psychiatry* (vol. 8) (ed. G. Grossman), pp. 123–142. Edinburgh: Churchill Livingstone.

Phillips, K. A. (1991) Body dysmorphic disorder: the distress of imagined ugliness. *American Journal of Psychiatry*, **148**, 1138–1149.

Phillipopoulos, G. S. (1979) The analysis of a case of dysmorphophobia. *Canadian Journal of Psychiatry*, **24**, 397–401.

Pilowsky, I. (1967) Dimensions of hypochondriasis. *British Journal of Psychiatry*, **131**, 89–93.

—— (1969) Abnormal illness behaviour. *British Journal of Medical Psychology*, **42**, 347–351.

—— (1970) Primary and secondary hypochondriasis. *Acta Psychiatrica Scandinavica*, **46**, 273–285.

—— (1983) Hypochondriasis. In *Handbook of Psychiatry 4 – the Neuroses and Personality Disorders* (eds G. Russell & L. Hersov). Cambridge: Cambridge University Press.

Pryse-Phillips, W. (1971) An olfactory reference syndrome. *Acta Psychiatrica Scandinavica*, **47**, 484–509.

Rapaport, J. L. (1989) *The Boy Who Couldn't Stop Washing: The Experience and Treatment of Obsessive Compulsive Disorder.* New York: E. P. Dutton.

Raspe, R. E. (1784) *Singular Travels, Campaigns and Adventures of Baron Münchausen.* London: Cresset Press.

Robinson, D. S., Nies, A., Ravaris, C. L., *et al* (1973) The monoaminoxidase inhibitor phenelzine in the treatment of depressive anxiety states: a controlled clinical trial. *Archives of General Psychiatry,* **28,** 407–413.

Roll, M. & Theorell, T. (1987) Acute chest pain without obvious organic cause before aged 40 – personality and recent life events. *Journal of Psychosomatic Research,* **31,** 215–221.

Rybstein-Blinchick, E. (1979) A psychiatric study of patients with supposed food allergy. *British Journal of Psychiatry,* **145,** 121–126.

Sainsbury, P. & Gibson, J. G. (1954) Symptoms of anxiety and tension and the accompanying psychological changes in the muscular system. *Journal of Neurology, Neurosurgery and Psychiatry,* **17,** 216–224.

Salkovskis, P. M. (1989) Somatic problems. In *Cognitive Behaviour Therapy for Psychiatric Problems: a Practical Guide* (eds K. Hawton, P. M. Salkovskis, J. Kirk, *et al*), pp. 235–276. Oxford: Oxford University Press.

—— & Warwick, H. M. (1986) Morbid preoccupations, health anxiety and reassurance: a cognitive behavioural approach. *Behaviour Research and Therapy,* **24,** 597–602.

Savill, T. D. (1909) *Lectures on Hysteria and Allied Vasomotor Conditions.* London: H. J. Glaisher.

Schneier, F. R., Leibowitz, M. R., Davies, S. O., *et al* (1990) Fluoxetine in panic disorder. *Journal of Clinical Psychology,* **10,** 119–121.

Sharpe, M. (1990) Chronic fatigue syndrome: can the psychiatrist help? In *Dilemmas and Difficulties in the Management of Psychiatric Patients* (eds. K. Houghton & P. Cowan). Oxford: Oxford Medical Publications.

Sigvardsson, S., Bohman, M, Von-Knorring, A. L., *et al* (1986) Genetic causes of somatization in men. *Epidemiology,* **3,** 153–185.

Smith, G. R., Monson, R. A. & Ray, D. C. (1986) Psychiatric consultation in somatization disorder. A randomised controlled study. *New England Journal of Medicine,* **314,** 1407–1413.

Stoudemire, G. A. (1988) Somatoform disorders, factitious disorders and malingering. In *Textbook of Psychiatry* (eds Talbott, Hales & Yudodsky). Washington, DC: APA.

Sullivan, M. A., Cohen, S. & Snape, W. J. (1978) Colonic myoelectrical activity in irritable bowel syndrome. *New England Journal of Medicine,* **298,** 873–883.

Svedlund, J., Sjodin, I., Olloson, J. O., *et al* (1983) Controlled study of psychotherapy in irritable bowel syndrome. *Lancet, ii,* 589–592.

Swartz, M., Blazer, D., Wodbury, M., *et al* (1986*a*) Somatization disorder in a US southern community: Use of a new procedure for analysis of medical classification. *Psychological Medicine,* **16,** 595–600.

——, ——, George, L., *et al* (1986*b*) Somatization disorder in a community population. *American Journal of Psychiatry,* **143,** 1403–1408.

Taerk, J. S., Toner, B. B. & Salit, I. E. (1987) Depression in patients with neuromyesthenia (benign myalgic encephalomyelitis). *International Journal of Psychiatry and Medicine,* **17,** 49–56.

Taylor, A. R. & Bell, T. K. (1966) Slowing of cerebral circulation after concussional head injury. *Lancet, ii,* 178–180.

Thomas, C. S. (1984) Dysmorphophobia: a question of definition. *British Journal of Psychiatry*, **144**, 513–516.

—— (1987) Anorexia nervosa and dysmorphophobia. *British Journal of Psychiatry*, **150**, 406.

Thomson, W. H. N. & St Carter, S. (1988) Intractable functional abdominal pain. *Journal of Royal Society of Medicine*, **81**, 124.

Tobi, M. & Strauss, S. C. (1985) Chronic Epstein Barr virus disease: a workshop held by the National Institute of Allergy and Infectious Disease. *Annals of Internal Medicine*, **103**, 951–953.

Torgersen, S. (1986) Genetics of somatoform disorder. *Archives of General Psychiatry*, **48**, 502–505.

Turkat, I. D. & Pettigrew, I. S. (1983) Development and validation of the illness behaviour inventory. *Journal of Behavioural Assessment*, **5**, 35–47.

Tynes, L. L., White, K. & Steketee, G. S. (1990) Towards a new nosology of obsessive compulsive disorder. *Comprehensive Psychiatry*, **31**, 465–480.

Veith, I (1965) *Hysteria: the History of a Disease*. Chicago: University of Chicago Press.

Vitiello, B. & de Loen, J. (1990) Dysmorphophobia misdiagnosed as an obsessive compulsive disorder. *Psychosomatics*, **31**, 220–222.

Wall, P. D. & Melzack, R. (eds) (1984) *Textbook of Pain*. Edinburgh: Churchill Livingstone.

Warwick, H. M. & Salkovskis, P. M. (1985) Reassurance. *British Medical Journal*, **290**, 1028.

Wernicke, C. (1900) *Grundriss der Psychiatrie*. Leipzig: Verlag von George Thieme.

Wessely, S. (1990) Old wine in new bottles: Neurasthenia and "ME". *Psychological Medicine*, **20**, 35–53.

White, H. (1905) A study of 60 cases of membranous colitis. *Lancet*, *ii*, 1229–1235.

White, P. D. (1937) *Heart Disease*. New York: Macmillan.

White, P. D. (1989) Fatigue syndrome: neurasthenia revisited. *British Medical Journal*, **298**, 199–200.

—— (1990) Chronic fatigue syndrome. In *Somatization: Physical Symptoms and Psychological Illness* (ed. C. Bass), pp. 104–140. Oxford: Blackwell Scientific.

Willis, T. (1684) *An Essay of Pathology of the Brain and Nervous Stock in which Convulsive Diseases are Treated of*. London: Dring Lee & Harper.

Wolfe, F., Smythe, H. A., Yunus, N. B., *et al* (1990) American College of Rheumatology, 1990. Criteria for the classification of fibromyalgia: Report of the multi-centre criteria committee. *Arthritis and Rheumatology*, **33**, 160–172.

Woodruff, R. A., Clayton, P. J. & Guze, S. B. (1971) Hysteria studies of diagnosis, outcome and prevalence. *Journal of the American Medical Association*, **215**, 425–428.

World Health Organization (1978) Mental Disorders: Glossary and Guide to their Classification in Accordance with the Ninth Revision of the International Classification of Diseases (ICD–9). Geneva: WHO.

—— (1992) *The ICD–10 Classification of Mental and Behavioural Disorders*. Geneva: WHO.

Yates, A. & Currie, H. L. F. (eds) (1986) *Mason and Currie's Clinical Rheumatology* (4th edn). Edinburgh: Churchill Livingstone.

Index

Compiled by Nina Boyd